Encyclopedic Reference of
Traditional Chinese Medicine

Springer
Berlin
Heidelberg
New York
Barcelona
Hong Kong
London
Milan
Paris
Tokyo

Encyclopedic Reference of
Traditional Chinese Medicine

With 85 Figures

Editor in Chief: Yang Xinrong

General Editors: Chen Anmin
                   Ma Yingfu
                   Gao Yuan
                   Gao Zhemin

Editors: Fu Bingyi
                   Sun Fang
                   Qiao Jinlin
                   Li Quan
                   Wan Shuqian
                   Hermut Werner
                   Chuang Yinfu
                   Zhu Xinsheng

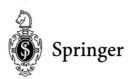

Springer

EDITOR IN CHIEF: Yang Xinrong
Center of Information for
Traditional Chinese Medicine
Marxheimer Platz 1
60326 Frankfurt
Germany

ISBN 3-540-42846-1 Springer-Verlag Berlin Heidelberg New York

Springer -Verlag Berlin Heidelberg New York
a member of BertelsmannSpringer Science+Business Media GmbH

http://www.springer.de/

© Springer -Verlag Berlin Heidelberg 2003

Printed in Germany

Typesetting: Elke Fortkamp, Heidelberg

Printed on acid-free paper   SPIN: 10780131   27/3136-5 4 3 2 1 0

Preface

The Traditional Chinese Medicine is a national treasure of China, and an important part of the treasure of the entire world as well.

The Traditional Chinese Medicine has a long history for thousands of years since the beginning of the written literature on medicine in China. Even in ancient time with very low developed culture, science, and technology, our ancestry had made a gigantic contribution to the healthy multiplying of the Chinese people of all nationalities through the application of acupuncture techniques and medicinal herbs as well as massage and Qigong.

After the People's Republic of China was founded, the administration has been standing for combining of Traditional Chinese Medicine with Western Medicine in order to use reference to each other, which has gained gratifying achievements in the treatment for a lot of ordinary illnesses and hypochondria.

With the reformation and opening of the People's Republic of China, the Traditional Chinese Medicine has been recommended to the western countries. While the voice of returning to nature is rising higher and higher, more and more friends over the world have accepted the Traditional Chinese Medicine, and many of them hope to deeply understand the Traditional Chinese Medicine, study its theory and learn how to apply medical herbs and techniques of acupuncture, massage and Qigong. In order to meet their requirements we compiled this "Encyclopedia Dictionary of Traditional Chinese Medicine", which includes about 5,000 terms with concise annotations and some color pictures. This book is compiled according to the order of the English alphabet and is convenient for reference.

Considering that the Traditional Chinese Medicine, with a long history, has wide and deep contents, this book cannot contain all the terms of it. And owing to the Traditional Chinese Medicine literatures were written in the classical literary style and the translation into English of most of their terms was not standardized and normalized, the translation of these terms remains to be discussed by specialists and linguists. So, many terms of diseases in this book have to use the terms of Western Medicine in Latin with notes for positions of diseases or their etiology and pathogenesis; at the same time, some terms have to be transliterated into English such as yin, yang, qi, zang-fu, etc.

Besides, China has a vast territory and many dialects, and the neighboring countries such as Japan, Democratic People's Republic of Korea and Republic of Korea, Viet Nam, also have their own acupuncture treatment, thus the nomenclature of acupuncture points can easily be confused. In order to avoid confusion, the terms of acupuncture in this book are taken from "Standard Acupuncture Nomenclature" WHO, 1984. The positions of the acupuncture points are shown in the General Picture of Acupuncture Points as the annex.

Acknowledgments

This book benefited from the efforts of numerous people. Foremost among them are the scholars and experts. Professor Guo Jinzhou, Hu Peixian, Gao Yongchun, Liu Guoming, Ma Changwen, Liu Yuanzhong, Jia Haijun, Zhou Zhiwen, Jiang Shengyue, Cui Tingrong, PanJindi checked and approved this book. Professor Xie Fengxun offered many elaborate color pictures of CTM herbs, and photographers Mr. Li Songlin and Mr. Bao Guotao took some fine color pictures for this dictionary.

Editor in Chief

Drugs and Treatments

A

Abalone

It is the meat of Haliotis Diversicolor Reeve or H. Gigantea Reeve (Haliotidae).
Effect. Nourishing yin and reducing fever, replenishing vital essence to improve eyesight.
Indication. Fever caused by general debility, cough, metrorrhagia, stranguria, optic atrophy, etc.

Abalone Shell

The shell of Haliotis diversicolor Reeve, H. Gigantea discus Reeve, and H. ovina Chemnitz (Haliotidae).
Effect. Removing heat from the liver, calming the liver and improving acuity of vision.
Indication. Sthenia of liver-yang or deficiency of yin leading to dizziness, blurred vision, restlessness and amnesia, conjunctival congestion, cataract, etc.

Abatement of Fever by Epistaxis

The patient suffered an epidemic febrile disease with a high fever, suddenly shows an epistaxis without inducing perspiration. After that, the fever has gone and the body becomes cool.

Abdomen (MA)

It is an auricular point.
Location. On the medial side of the lumbosacral vertebrae (MA), proximal to the border of the cavum conchae.
Indication. Abdominal pain, distention, diarrhea and acute lumbar muscle sprain.

Abdominal Distention

Symptoms. Abdominal distention, visible varicose veins, yellow skin absence of edema (or presence of slight edema) in the limbs.
Pathogenesis. Mostly caused by impairment of the liver and the spleen, qi stagnancy and blood stasis due to emotional depression, irregular diet, addiction to drink, parasitic infestation, etc.
Therapeutic Principle. Relieving the depressed liver, invigorating the spleen, regulating the circulation of qi, promoting blood circulation by removing blood stasis, and removing dampness by diuresis and destroy intestinal parasites.

Abdominal Distention due to Blood Stasis

Symptoms. Visible blood vessel In the chest and abdomen, abdominal distention like drum with excess sound by percussion, etc.
Pathogenesis. Blood stasis in abdominal superficial venules.
Therapeutic Principle. Promoting blood circulation and relieving distention.

Abdominal Distention due to Cold Deficiency

Symptoms. Abdominal distention with preference for pressing alternative onset and severe, and sometimes disappearing and mild with preference for warmth and pressing, relieved by hot diet, fatigue, anorexia, pale tongue, etc.
Pathogenesis. Mainly from spleen and stomach cold of insufficiency type.
Therapeutic Principle. Warming and invigorating the spleen and stomach.

Abdominal Distention due to Indigestion

Symptoms. Feeling of fullness of the stomach and abdomen, eructation and anorexia, or vomiting with acid regurgitation, fetid feces, etc.

Pathogenesis. Mainly caused by improper diet, retention of indigested food, dysfunction of middle-energizer in transport and disturbance of visceral function.

Therapeutic Principle. Promoting digestion to remove retention of food and regulating the stomach.

Abdominal Distention due to Internal Injury

Symptoms. Abdominal distention and uncomfortable feeling.

Pathogenesis. Qi stagnation, accumulation of indigested food, malnutrition due to parasitic infestation or deficiency of the zang-organs and fu-organs.

Abdominal Distention due to Liver-fire

Symptoms. Yellowish sclera, pain in the hypochondrium and abdominal distention, scanty dark urine and pathogeny insomnia, etc.

Pathogenesis. Spleen restricted by liver-fire.

Therapeutic Principle. Relieving the depressed liver and purging the pathogenic fire.

Abdominal Distention due to Phlegm-retention

Symptoms. Feeling of fullness in the chest and abdomen, severe palpitation, dyspnea, vomiting, abundant expectoration.

Pathogenesis. Dysfunction of the spleen and stomach in transportation leading to retention of phlegm in the abdomen.

Therapeutic Principle. Removing phlegm and fluid retention.

Abdominal Free Mass

Symptoms. Distention and fullness of the abdomen, movable sensation with pain, mass gathered intermittently with attack at no fixed time, anorexia, constipation or loose stool, etc.

Pathogenesis. Imbalance between cold and warmness, improper diet.

Therapeutic Principle. Regulating and nourishing the stomach and the spleen, promoting digestion and removing stagnacy and retention of food.

Abdominal Free Mass due to Drinking

Symptoms. Poor appetite, emaciation, vomiting and somnolence etc.

Pathogenesis. Over-drinking.

Therapeutic Principle. Relieving alcohol, resolving dampness and regulating the spleen and stomach.

Abdominal Lump due to Food

Symptoms. Difficulty in passing stools, and with movable lumps in the abdomen.

Pathogenesis. Obstruction of the intestines.

Therapeutic Principle. Regulate the function between the spleen and stomach, remove stagnancy of indigested food, clean the bowel.

Abdominal Mass due to Qi Stagnation

Symptoms. Feeling of stuffiness and tightness in the chest and stomach, abdominal and hypochondriac distention, abdominal mass that is appearing or fading at frequent intervals and mobile, etc.

Pathogenesis. Mental depression, excessive melancholy, anxiety and anger leading to disturbance functional activities of qi.

Therapeutic Principle. Disperse the depressed liver-energy and rectify it.

Abdominal Mass of Oxyuriasis

Symptoms. Large and distended abdomen, pruritus of anus and oxyurids may be visible at night, etc.

Pathogenesis. Accumulation of oxyurids due to the weakness of the spleen and stomach.

Therapeutic Principle. Nourishing the spleen and the stomach, regulating the flow of qi to dissipate blood stasis, and expelling intestinal parasites.

Abdominal Pain

Pathogenesis. Internal accumulation of pathogenic cold, retention of food, stagnation of liver-qi due to qi-stagnancy and yang deficiency of the zang-fu organs. In the clinic, it is divided into abdominal pain due to pathogenic cold, abdominal pain due to retention of food, abdominal pain due to stagnation of liver-qi and abdominal pain due to yang deficiency.

Abdominal Pain due to Blood stasis

Symptoms. Persistent abdominal fixed pain, accompanied by tenderness intolerance of pressing, more severe pain at night, etc.

Pathogenesis. Depression or traumatic injury, obstruction in meridians, or improper diet, and disorder of qi.

Therapeutic Principle. Promoting blood circulation and removing blood stasis, alleviating pain.

Abdominal Pain due to Cold Accumulation

Symptoms. Lingering abdominal pain which may be alleviated by warmth and aggravated by cold, often accompanied by diarrhea.

Pathogenesis. The deficiency of the spleen-yang injured by raw or cold food, the attack of pathogenic cold and cold accumulation.

Therapeutic Principle. Warming yang, dispelling cold and removing stagnation.

Abdominal Pain due to Deficiency of Blood

Symptoms. Lingering abdominal pain which may be more severe during hunger or overstrain, dim and black complexion, etc.

Pathogenesis. Excessive bleeding, or over-anxiety, consumption of yin blood.

Therapeutic Principle. Enriching blood and relieving middle-energizer.

Abdominal Pain due to Dry heat

Symptoms. Severe abdominal pain, stretching into hypochondriac region, thirst, obscured fever, restlessness, insomnia, dark urine without vomiting and diarrhea.

Pathogenesis. Affection by seasonal pathogenic dryness-heat, impairment of the body fluid and consumption of qi, fluid insufficiency in the stomach and intestine, and impeded circulation of qi.

Therapeutic Principle. Clear away heat and promote salivation, regulate the flow of qi to relieve pain.

Abdominal Pain due to Parasitic Infestation

Symptoms. Usually pain around the navel, which appears and disappears from time to time, or pain after meals, vomiting, ascaris, grinding teeth in sleep, etc.

Pathogenesis. Accumulation of ascaris in the intestines.

Therapeutic Principle. Expelling the parasites.

Abdominal Pain due to Qi Deficiency

Symptoms. Dull pain in abdomen which alleviated by pressing and aggravated by overstrain, lassitude and shortness of breath, etc.

Pathogenesis. Prolonged illness and qi deficiency, protracted diarrhea and qi impairment, and the impairment of middle-energizer qi because of overstrain and hunger.

Therapeutic Principle. Strengthening the middle-energizer and replenishing qi.

Abdominal Pain due to Stagnation of Liver-Qi

Symptoms. Abdominal pain without a fixed region accompanied by stuffiness in the hypochondrium, frequent eructation, fidgetiness, bitter taste, etc.

Pathogenesis. Qi-stagnation in the liver, resulting in abnormal descent or ascent of qi, usually induced by emotional upset.

Therapeutic Principle. Relieve the depressed liver and regulate the circulation of qi.

Abdominal Pain due to Summer-heat

Symptoms. Chest tightness with nausea, distention and pain in the stomach and abdomen, heavy sensation of the head and limbs, etc.

Pathogenesis. External affections of summer-heat pathogen, impairment of qi system and the stagnation of the Spleen Meridian.

Therapeutic Principle. Clearing away the summer-heat and eliminating dampness, relieving pain by regulating qi.

Abdominal Pain due to Wind-cold

Symptoms. Abdominal pain after attack by wind-cold, accompanied by chills and fever, or bombus and diarrhea.

Pathogenesis. Invasion of pathogenic wind-cold.

Therapeutic Principle. Warming the middle-energizer to dispel the wind and cold evils.

Abdominal Pain due to Yang Insufficiency

Symptoms. Occasional dull abdominal pain from time to time, which is relieved when pressed, loose stools, dim complexion, etc.

Pathogenesis. Weakened yang of the middle-energizer, internal lack of warmth and nourishment.

Therapeutic Principle. Reinforce the spleen and warm the kidney.

Abdominal Pain during Pregnancy

There are three types:

1. Cold of insufficiency type.

   Symptoms. Cold pain in the lower abdomen, which is relieved by warming.

   Pathogenesis. Deficiency of blood, stagnation of qi, disorder of nourishment of the uterine collaterals.

   Therapeutic Principle. Expel pathogenic cold from the meridian.

2. Deficiency of blood type.

   Symptoms. Dull and continuous pain in the lower abdomen, which prefers pressing, dizziness with headache.

   Therapeutic Principle. Prevent miscarriage by nourishing the blood and alleviating pain.

3. Stagnation of qi.

   Symptoms. Distending pain in the lower abdomen distention and fullness in the chest and stomach, dysphoria and irritability.

   Therapeutic Principle. Relieve the depressed liver.

Abdominal Pain with Chronic Dysentery

Symptoms. Protracted diarrhea and unrelieved pain in abdomen.

Pathogenesis. Deficiency cold of the spleen and stomach, cold qi in the body fighting against visceral-qi.

Therapeutic Principle. Warming and nourishing the spleen and stomach.

Abnormal Fetal Position

Pathogenesis. Qi stagnation or excessive fear before delivery.

Therapeutic Principle. Promoting the flow of qi to remove stagnation, or to apply moxibustion to bilateral zhiyin (BL 67) point for 15 minutes, once or twice a day until the position of the fetus is normal.

Abnormal Labor Pain

It refers to hyperactivity of the fetus in third trimester of pregnancy, slight or intermittent abdominal pain without lumbago at the time approaching to term-pregnancy. They are all signs of abnormal labor.

Abnormal Pulse

1. It indicates pathologic changes. Doctors can diagnose the disease according to the pulse. There are twenty-eight abnormal pulses.
2. It refers to the condition of the pulse of a pregnant woman during parturition.

Abortion

It refers to precocious birth after three months' pregnancy.

Pathogenesis. Excess of sexual intercourse, deficiency and impairment of qi and blood, blood heat due to kidney deficiency, etc.

Abortion by Trauma

It refers to a sensation of bearing-down pain in the waist and abdomen, vaginal bleeding in severe cases, resulting in abortion, caused by deficiency of qi, blood, and kidney, or by traumatic injuries.

Abortion within First Month of pregnancy

It refers to natural abortion within the first month of pregnancy when the embryo forms at the first stage. Usually ignorance of the pregnancy because of its similarity to menstruation.

Pathogenesis. Excess of sexual intercourse.

Therapeutic Principle. Tonifying the kidney to prevent abortion.

Abscess of Iliac Fossa with Flexed Leg

It is one kind of the disease of multiple abscesses.

Symptoms. Usually appears deep inside the iliac fossa. At the beginning the affected part can be limited on stretching and bending, with severe pain on strong stretching. Lumps can be touched in the iliac fossa, with the feeling of wave motions after the forming of pus. Aversion to cold, fever, anhidrosis, or slight sweating, reduced eating, tired, and lazy.

Therapeutic Principle. In the case of the forming of pus, cutting to open and drain is applicable.

Abscess of Internal Organs

It refers to the abscess appearing in the internal organs or in the chest and abdominal cavity. It is named differently according to the differently affected positions as lung abscess, intestinal abscess, liver abscess, gastric cavity abscess, etc.

Absence of Menstruation

It refers to amenorrhea after menarche of a puberty unmarried female without any other accompanied symptom and disorder. It is not an abnormal state.

Absent-minded and Upset

It refers to a patient's mental disturbance with incoherence and failure to control himself.

Pathogenesis. Deficiency of both the heart-yin and heart-yang. The heart cannot be warmed nourished.

Abstentions from Five Kinds of Flavors

There are two meanings.

1. A liver disease, avoiding things acrid in flavor. A heart disease, avoiding things salty in flavor. A spleen disease, abstaining from sour flavor. A kidney disease, abstaining from sweat flavor. A lung disease, avoiding things bitter in flavor.

2. One should not eat too much food of pungent flavors in qi syndrome. One should not eat too much food of salty flavor in the syndrome due to blood disorder. One should not eat too much food of bitter flavor in bone disease. One should not eat too much food of sweet flavor in fleshy disorder. One should not eat too much food of sour flavor in muscular disorder.

Acanthopanax Root-bark

It is the bark or root cortex of Acanthopanax gracilistylus W. W. Smith (Araliaceae).

Effect. Expelling wind and dampness, strengthening the tendon and bone, invigorating the liver and kidney and inducing diuresis.

Indication. Rheumatic arthralgia, spasm in the extrimities, lassitude in the waist and knees, edema and oliguria.

Accumulating Essence and Gathering Qi

It is a term in Qigong.

Essence and qi are the essential substances for training Inner Elixir Pellet. Persistent practising of Qigong can accumulate both of them to achieve the effect of dispelling diseases, keeping good health and prolonging life.

Accumulation in Viscera

There are three meanings.

1. It refers to a disease due to insufficiency of yang-qi and accumulation of yin
   Symptoms. Accumulation of pathogens in the chest and persistent diarrhea with usual diet.
   Pathogenesis. Invasion of pathogenic factor into the viscera due to deficiency of yang after exogenous febrile disease.
   Therapeutic Principle. Warming the middle-energizer to promote yang.
2. A disease marked by a lump below the costal region linking to the naval, and pain extending to the lower abdomen.

3. It refers to constipation due to uneven visceral-qi, and refusal of yin and yang to each other.

Accumulation of Cold

Symptoms. Gastric and abdominal cold pain, constipation, clear and long urine, pale complexion, aversion cold, etc.

Pathogenesis. Yang deficiency of the spleen and stomach, the attack of pathogenic cold and its stagnation in the body.

Therapeutic Principle. Warming the middle-energizer and dispelling cold and removing stagnation.

Accumulation of Damp-heat in Spleen

Symptoms. Fullness in the epigastrium and abdomen, anorexia, listlessness, loose stool, scanty, deep-colored urine and even yellow eye and skin all over the body, etc.

Pathogenesis. Accumulation and stagnation of dampness, heat transformation by damp resulting from dysfunction of the spleen in transportation and transformation.

Therapeutic Principle. Induce diuresis with bland drugs, and adjuvant aromatics to eliminate dampness.

Notice. Drugs bitter and cold in nature should not be overused.

Accumulation of Excessive Fluid

Symptoms. Cold pain in back and hypochondrium, shortness of breath, thirst and arthragra of limbs.

Pathogenesis. Yang deficiency and yin excess of the spleen, lung and kidney.

Therapeutic Principle. Reinforcing the spleen and warming the kidney, strengthening the body resistance and eliminating excessive fluid.

Accumulation of Extravasated Blood

Symptoms. Sallow complexion, spider nevus on the chest, neck and face, mass in the hypochondrium and abdomen, constipation or melena, etc.

Therapeutic Principle. Promoting blood circulation and removing blood stasis, removing stagnation and dispersing accumulation.

Accumulation of Heart-qi

Symptoms. Fullness in the chest, dysphoria with smothery sensation, heart palpitation, dryness of the throat, flushed complexion, hematemesis, swelling in the leg, etc.

Pathogenesis. Insufficiency of vital-qi, internal damage of seven emotions, diet and affection of pathogenic poison.

Therapeutic Principle. Simultaneous reinforcement and elimination, promoting the blood circulation and regulating the flow of qi.

Accumulation of Heat in Urinary Bladder

Symptoms. Distention and fullness of the lower abdomen, incontinence of urine, fever without chillness, and coma.

Pathogenesis. Stagnation of heat in the urinary bladder. The heat that combines with blood is accumulated in the bladder.

Therapeutic Principle. Clearing away heat and removing blood stasis.

Accumulation of Pathogens in Chest

Symptoms. Fullness, stuffiness and pain in the chest, epigastrium and abdomen.

Pathogenesis. Accumulation of pathogenic heat with stagnancy of fluid or phlegm in the chest.

Therapeutic Principle. Expelling the pathogenic heat, dispelling retained water, and removing accumulation.

Accumulation of Phlegm-heat in Lung

Symptoms. Fever, cough with yellowish thick sputum or blood-stained expectoration, rale, fullness in chest and diaphragm, and even heavy and short breath, chest pain, etc.

Pathogenesis. External-evil attacking the lung, leading to heat by stagnation, and phlegm blocking the collaterals of the lung.

Therapeutic Principle. Clearing away heat and expelling phlegm, and facilitating the flow of the lung-qi to relieve asthma.

Aching Pain of Limbs

Symptoms. Feeling of aching pain of the limbs, muscles and tendons.

Pathogenesis. Blockage of meridians due to attack of damp-heat and cold-dampness, deficiency of qi and blood.

Achyranthes Root   ✾ A-1

It is the root of Achyranthes bidentata Blume (Amaranthaceae).

Effect. Promoting blood circulation and removing blood stasis, reinforcing the liver and kidney, strengthening the tendons and bones, inducing diuresis for treating stranguria.

Indication. Irregular menstruation, dysmenorrhea, amenorrhea, postpartum abdominal pain due to retention of blood stasis, traumatic injuries, hematuria, dysuria, pain in the urethra, epistaxis, toothache, etc.

Acid Regurgitation

Symptoms. Sour juice rising from the stomach to the throat.

Pathogenesis. Insufficiency of qi in middle-energizer, the retention of sputum and salvia, and pathological changes of Liver Meridians.

Acne

Symptoms. Appearing on the face, chest, shoulder and the back. Follicular papula with black heads, after being pressed, white lipid comes out. In the serious case, it is red, swelling, and painful, and becomes acute folliculitis and steatadenitis.

Pathogenesis. Excess heat retention in the lung and the stomach to steam upwards the face, and the stagnation of blood-heat, or excessively eating rich, fatty diet.

Therapeutic Principle. Ventilating the lung and clearing away heat.

Aconite-cake Moxibustion

It is an indirect moxibustion method to administer moxibustion by using an aconite-cake as a interposition between the moxa cone and skin. It is applicable to patients suffering from such symptoms as impotence, seminal emission, unhealing ulcer, etc.

Acorn

It is the fruit of Quercus acutissima Carr. (Fagaceae).

Effect. Anti-diarrhea with astringents.

Indication. Prolapse of rectum due to dysentery, hemorrhoid bleeding, etc.

Acorn Shell

It is the shell of Quercus acutissima Carr. (Fagaceae).

Effect. Astringe to arrest bleeding.

Indication. Proctoptosis due to dysentery, hematochezia, metrorrhagia, leukorrhagia, etc.

Acquired Essence of Life

It is one of the essential substances derived from food and water used to maintain the vital activities and metabolism of the body and to promote the growth.

Actinolite

It is the ore of silicate mineral Actinolite, or Actinolite asbestos.

Effect. Warming the kidney and strengthening yang.

Indication. Impotence, uterine coldness, lassitude in the loins and knees, etc.

Acuminate Violet Leaf

It is the leaf of Viola acuminata Ledeb. (Violaceae).

Effect. Clearing away heat, detoxication, subduing swelling and relieving pain.

Indication. Cough with lung-heat, swelling pain due to traumatic injuries, sores, furuncle, etc.

Acupoint

It refers to a spot, where the qi of zang-fu organs and meridians and collaterals flow in and out. Generally, acupoints are divided into 3 kinds: meridian points, extra acupuncture points, and Ashi points. Acupoints on the body pertain to the meridians respectively, and the meridians are also related to certain zang and fu organs, which make the connections among acupoints, meridians and zang-fu organs inseparable.

Acupoint Block Therapy

It is a therapeutic method, referring to point-injection therapy with narcotic medicine.

Acupoint Electrometry

It has been found that the electric resistance on the skin of a point is usually lower than that of the skin areas without points. An acupuncture point surveying apparatus may determine the electrical conductivity of a point. Analysing the conductivity of representative points of each meridian helps the doctor to know the conditions of qi and blood in each meridian.

Acupoint Magnetotherapy

It refers to the treatment of diseases by means of magnetic objects acting on acupoints.

Acupuncture and Moxibustion

It is a collective term for the methods of acupuncture and moxibustion. Acupuncture is the therapy that treats diseases by puncturing acupoints and meridians with various needling tools, while moxibustion is the therapy, which treats diseases by smoking and burning points and meridians mainly with moxa. They are generally called acupuncture and moxibustion therapy.

Acupuncture and Moxibustion in the Dog Days

Acupuncture and moxibustion in hot, summer days has good preventive and curative effect on some chronic diseases which easily occur in the autumn and winter such as cough and asthma, because the weather is very hot and the yang-qi ascends.

Acupuncture Anesthesia

It refers to a method enabling the patient to accept the surgical operation in the state of mental consciousness by puncturing the points to arrest pain and regulate functions of the internal organs. This method is easy to practise and efficacious in clinical therapy.

Acupuncture Anesthesia Induction

In the course of acupuncture anesthesia, it is necessary to apply acupuncture to the patient before operation, in order to heighten the pain-endurance. It usually gives certain stimulus to the point with an electric needle. The time taken between the patient's subjective needling sensation and the start of the operation is usually 15-20 minutes.

Acupuncture Drills

Fairly thin and pliable needling instruments which are very difficult to handle skillfully without drills; one should train the strength of the fingers and master acupuncture manipulation and techniques before applying them in clinic. The commonly used drills are as follows: 1. Puncturing drills on a paper pad: Fold a piece of strawboard into a small square; tie it tightly into a pad. Insert the needle into the pad by twirling and do the same repeatedly to train the strength of fingers. 2. Puncturing drills with a cotton ball: Wrap cotton tightly with gauze and roll into a small ball, on which techniques such as inserting, lifting, thrusting, twirling, etc. should be repeatedly drilled until skillfully mastered.

Acupuncture Manipulations

It generally refers to the operating method of therapeutic acupuncture which include the needling methods of the filiform needle, the three-edged needle, the cutaneous needle, and the intradermal needle, etc.

Acupuncture Needle

Referring to sewing utensils, and later, used as medical apparatus. The needle underwent a long development process from ancient Bian Stone and bamboo needles to modern metal ones.

Acupuncture Posture

It refers to the patient's body position in the course of acupuncture therapy. The selection principle is: correct location of points, convenience for manipulation and comfortable for the patient.

Acupuncture Therapy

It has two meanings: 1. The method by which diseases are cured. 2. A general designation of all kinds of acupuncture manipulation with all kinds of needles.

Acupuncture with Filiform Needle

It refers to needling with a filiform needle alone, as opposed to electrical acupuncture, acupuncture with injection of fluids and other forms of acupuncture used in acupuncture anesthesia.

Acupuncture Zone along Meridians

It refers to the sensitive zone and area represented on the body surface due to diseases. The location of the zones and areas are in conformity with the positions of the acupoints, but a little wider.

Acupuncturist

Referring to the doctor who masters the needling methods.

Acute Angle-closure Glaucoma

Symptoms. Ocular cirrhosis, platycoria, slightly green pupil and severe hyposmia.

Pathogenesis. Stagnation of wind-fire and phlegm in the liver and irregularity of yin and yang therein, resulting in derangement of qi and blood, blocked meridians, stuffed blood and body fluid in the eyeball.

Therapeutic Principle. Removing blood stasis and eliminating stagnation. Simultaneously pay attention to making the pupil contracted, and acupuncture, moxibustion, etc. are applicable. Operative therapy is used when necessary.

Acute Appendicitis

It refers to the painful carbuncle near Tianshu (S25) point.

Symptoms. Abdominal pain and tenderness, knee flexion with difficulty to stretch, alternate attacks of chills and fever, etc.

Pathogenesis. Disorder of intestinal function, damp-heat in the interior due to improper diet, rich fatty diet, etc.

Therapeutic Principle. Clearing away heat and toxic material, eliminating heat by purgation.

Acute Conjunctivitis

Symptoms. Red eyes with swelling and pain, photophobia, epiphora and gum in the eye.

Pathogenesis. Invasion of pathogenic wind-heat into the body and upward drive of pathogenic heat to the eyes due to the wind-heat.

Therapeutic Principle. Dispelling wind, clearing away heat, and detoxicating.

Acute Convulsion

Symptoms. Back rigidity, dryness nose, lockjaw, spasm muscles or high fever, etc.

Pathogenesis. Attack of pathogenic factors when body resistance is weak.

Therapeutic Principle. Strengthening body resistance to eliminate pathogenic factors.

Acute Dacryocystitis

Symptoms. Sudden redness, swelling and burning pain in the region of the inner canthus, followed by diabrosis and suppuration in the vicinity of the inner canthus inferior to the point of Jingming (B1), obvious tenderness, or even swelling of the cheek on the same side with the affected eye.

Pathogenesis. Mostly caused by pathologic changes from dacryocystitis, or by obstruction of lacrimal cavity from heat-toxin in the heart and spleen.

Therapeutic Principle. Clearing away heat, detoxicating, subduing swelling and promoting visual acuity. If there is suppuration, it is advisable to cut it open for drainage.

Acute Eczema

Symptoms. At the beginning it is like millets, itching of the skin. When torn by scratching, yellow water flows out. It spreads fast, and soaks in stretches. In the severe case, there is even body fever.

Pathogenesis. Hyperactivity of heart-fire, stagnancy spleen-dampness, and the additional invasion of wind, stagnated in the skin and muscle.

Therapeutic Principle. Expelling wind and eliminating dampness, removing pathogenic heat from blood.

Acute Febrile Jaundice

Symptoms. A critical case of jaundice with sudden onset, rapid deterioration and poor prognosis, high fever and even coma, delirium or bloody urine, etc.

Pathogenesis. Excessive damp-heat which burns in ying and blood systems and invades the pericardium.

Therapeutic Principle. Clearing away heat, detoxicating, removing heat from the blood and inducing resuscitation.

Acute Filthy Disease

It refers to an acute exogenous febrile disease accompanied by filthy disease. There are two cases:

1. **Symptoms.** Sudden abdominal pain and unconsciousness.
   Pathogenesis. Filthy toxic factor obstructing upward due to touching and smelling filth or suffering from cold due to sleep in the open at night.
   Therapeutic Principle. Administering the drug of aromatics at once.
2. **Symptoms.** Failing to vomit and defecate.
   Pathogenesis. Dyspepsia in qi of middle-energizer.
   Therapeutic Principle. Induce vomiting right away, then regulating the flow of qi and scraping needling.

Acute Filthy Disease due to Cold

It is a type of filthy disease. There are two cases.

1. **Pathogenesis.** Excessive cold drinking, the toxin of filthy disease and pathogenic cold in the chest.
   Therapeutic Principle. Eliminating the toxin of filthy disease.
2. It refers to the filthy disease attacked by pathogenic cold.
   Therapeutic Principle. Cutaneous scraping therapy together with medicine.

Acute Infantile Convulsion

It is the infantile convulsion with sudden onset.

Symptoms. Sudden onset, coma, rolling upwards of the eyes, lockjaw, rigidity of the neck, convulsion of limbs, occasional high fever, frothy salivation, rattling sound due to phlegm in the throat, etc.

Pathogenesis. 1. Affection by seasonal expathogenic factors, 2. Stagnation of food in the stomach and intestines, 3. Sudden terror and fear.

Therapeutic Principle. According to the different pathogenes, it will be 1. Clearing heat and eliminating evils, 2. Removing heat-phlegm and calming the endopathic wind, 3. Relieving muscular spasm and tranquilizing the mind.

Acute Inflammation of Orbit with Protrusion of Eyeball

Symptoms. Acute attack, ocular pain, or even unbearable throbbing pain of eyes, sudden diminution of vision, redness and swelling of the eyelid and white, suppurative eyeball or orbit, accompanied by constitutional symptoms. In the serious case, an ulcer is formed with pus coming out, or even resulting in ocular suppuration and collapse.

Pathogenesis. Hyperactivity of fire-toxin or internal invasion thereof.

Therapeutic Principle. Clearing away heat, detoxicating, purging intense heat, removing heat from the heart and dredging the ocular orifice.

Acute Injury of Tendon and Muscle

Symptoms. Pain, swelling, hematoma and ecchymosis, dysfunction.

Cause. Injury by a sudden force, or the patient has a history of external injury.

Therapeutic Principle. It can be treated by manipulations.

Acute Laryngitis

Symptoms. General pain, headache, flushed face, red pharynx, swelling and pain of the throat, lockjaw, rale in the throat, hoarseness and dysphagia, etc.

Pathogenesis. Heat accumulation in the lung and stomach, repeated attack affection by exopathogenic wind and heat, and accumulation and obstruction of phlegm-fire and pathogenic factors in the throat.

Therapeutic Principle. Clearing away heat to relieve sore throat, and detoxicating to subdue swelling.

Acute Lymphangitis

Symptoms. Red, swelling, heat and pain in the furuncle region, followed by red streaks appearing in the medial part of the upper limbs or the lower limbs. They move towards the heart quickly. In the severe case, the patient has fever and headache, etc.

Pathogenesis. Furuncle, tinea pedis, or skin injury, infection by toxins, internal accumulation of fire-toxins.

Therapeutic Principle. Clearing away heat and removing toxic materials. Externally the therapeutic primary disease should be treated, and the red streaks should be treated with pricking therapy.

Acute Mastitis

Symptoms. Stiffness and distending thelalgia, or sore of the nipple, and fever and aversion to cold.

Pathogenesis. Absence of breast-feeding, or contradiction between the accumulated milk, and blood and qi in a healthy parturient with sufficient milk secretion.

Therapeutic Principle. Clearing away heat for detoxicating, and swelling and alleviating mental depression.

Acute Mastitis due to External Blowing

An acute and suppurative breast disease. It is caused by infection due to an injury or biting of the nipple by the baby sucking in sleep.

Acute Mastitis due to Fetus

Refers to acute mastitis, not commonly seen clinically. It is mostly due to the excessive qi of the fetus, and steaming by pathogenic heat, difficulty in healing after ulcer. Take caution in the therapeutic care of the fetus.

Acute Mastitis due to Stomach-heat

Symptoms. At its early stage, mass in the breast with distention, swelling and painful sensation, difficulty in lactation, general discomfort, alternative attacks of chill and fever.

Pathogenesis. Improper diet, accumulation of heat in the stomach meridian, broken nipple, difficulty in lactation due to exogenous fire-toxin invasion leading to obstruction in the meridians and collateral.

Therapeutic Principle. Clearing away heat and dispelling masses.

Acute Necrosis of Scrotum

Symptoms. At the beginning, red swelling of the scrotum. Then the scrotum soon becomes dark purple and begins to ulcerate, with peculiar odor, accompanied by aversion to cold, and fever. The skin of the scrotum may even become necrotic with perforation in a large area, with the testicle exposed.

Pathogenesis. Local dirt, usual lying on the damp ground or the impaired liver-kidney essence, and the attacking of exopathogen.

Therapeutic Principle. Removing heat from the liver, removing dampness by diuresis, and detoxicating.

Acute Non-suppurative Infection of Testicle

Symptoms. Swelling and painful testicle, but without suppuration after contracting mumps.

Pathogenesis. Spreading of wind-heat to the Liver Meridian after contracting mumps.

Therapeutic Principle. Clearing away heat and detoxicating.

Acute Otitis Media in Infant

Symptoms. Swelling pain in the ear of the infant, fever, aversion to cold and crying with fear during sleeping.

Pathogenesis. Ulceration due to water soaked in the external acoustic meatus.

Therapeutic Principle. Removing heat from the liver.

Acute Pharyngitis

Symptoms. Swelling and pain of the throat, sufficiency of phlegm and saliva, tachypnea, headache, reddish complexion, or even lockjaw, and dysphagia.

Pathogenesis. Mostly caused by heat accumulation in the lung and stomach, inward invasion of pathogenic toxin, which results in upward flow of wind-phlegm.

Therapeutic Principle. Dispelling wind evil, clearing away heat, resolving phlegm and detoxicating.

Acute Postauricular Abscess

It refers to a disease, similar to retroauricular subperiosteal abscess.

Symptoms. Pressing pain in the region of the mastoid process, or even perforation of ulcer.

Therapeutic Principle. Clearing away heat and toxic material, and removing blood stasis to promote pus discharge. If there is an abscess, an operation is required.

Acute Pyogenic Infection of Finger Tip

Symptoms. Abscess under the finger tip, rather difficult to subdue and dispell.

Pathogenesis. Traumatic infection and the accumulation of fire-toxin in the finger and the toe.

Therapeutic Principle. Clipping the finger tip to drain the pus, clearing away heat and detoxicating.

Acute Pyogenic Infection of Right Buttock

It refers carbuncle of the buttock appearing in the crease under the right buttock.

Acute Scleritis

Symptoms. Diminution of vision, dryness and discomfort of the eyes pancorneal opacity, and in severe cases ulceration with yellow watery discharge.

Pathogenesis. Caused by infantile malnutrition due to failure of the spleen yang to ascend and excess of the heat in the liver.

Therapeutic Principle. Strengthening the spleen and promoting digestion, and preventing secondary infection.

Acute Throat Trouble

It is a general designation of multi-acute diseases in relation to the throat. It is divided into acute laryngeal trouble, chronic laryngeal trouble, laryngeal erosion, laryngeal trouble with lockjaw, retropharyngeal trouble, etc. The therapeutic principle is clearing away heat, detoxicating, resolving sputum, and removing stagnation.

Acute Throat Trouble with Whitish Surface

Symptoms. Discomfort in the throat and tonsils, or ulceration with purplish-red macules.

Pathogenesis. Caused by invasion of exterior pathogenic cold and interior fire-accumulation.

Therapeutic Principle. Clearing away heat, expelling cold, nourishing yin and tonifying the kidney.

Acute Thyroiditis

Symptoms. Acute or subacute, with mass formation on either side of the neck, unchanged color, slight burning heat, pain spreading to the occiput or the back of the ear, usually accompanied by fever, headache, seldom by suppuration.

Pathogenesis. Attacking of wind-warm pathogen and wind-fire in the lung and the stomach, with the internal stagnation of the liver-qi and stomach-heat to cause the upward rising of the accumulated heat with phlegm.

Therapeutic Principle. Relieving the depressed the liver and removing heat, dispelling phlegm and subduing swelling.

Acute Tonsillitis

Symptoms. Red swelling and pain of tonsils with white and yellow purulent spots on the surface, dysphagia, halitosis and constipation, alternate attacks of chills and fever.

Pathogenesis. Caused by obstruction of the lung and stomach, fumigation and steaming of fire-toxin, or by qi stagnation and blood stasis, coagulation of phlegm-fire, or by yin insufficiency of the liver and kidney, and flaring up of deficiency fire.

Therapeutic Principle. Dispelling wind, removing heat from the lung, dispelling phlegm.

Acute Tuberculosis

Symptoms. Cough, fever, night sweat, vexation, dry mouth, hemoptysis, emaciation, etc.

Pathogenesis. Debilitated body constitution accompanied by infection of tuberculin.

Therapeutic Principle. Nourishing yin, invigorating qi and removing hectic fever.

Acute Ulcerative Angina

It refers to a severely infectious disease.

Symptoms. Redness, swelling and pain in the throat with rapid erosion, short breath and rale, hoarseness, alternate attacks of chills and fever.

Pathogenesis. Mostly caused by flaring up of pathogenic toxin to the pharynx due to affection by epidemic toxic factors.

Therapeutic Principle. Clearing away heat and removing toxic material, relieving sore throat and eliminating ulcer.

Acute Warming

It refers to a method of immediate oral use of the drug of warming interior to rescue the patient form the serious condition of deficiency of yang and excess of yin.

Acutifoliatepodocarpium Herb

It is the whole herb of Desmodium racemosum (Thunb.) DC. (Leguminosae).

Effect. Eliminating pathogenic wind and dampness, dissipating blood stasis and promoting the subsidence swelling.

Indication. Dyspnea, arthralgia due to wind-dampness, metrorrhagia and metrostaxis, acute mastitis, traumatic injuries, etc.

Adder's Tongue Herb

It is the whole herb of Ophioglossum pedunculosum Desv. Or Ophioglossum thermale Kom. (Ophioglossaceae).

Effect. Clearing away heat, detoxicating, nourishing the lung to arrest cough, promoting blood circulation and dissipating blood stasis.

Indication. Acute mastitis, bronchitis, chronic pharyngitis furuncle, scabies, traumatic injuries, swelling pain due to blood stasis, etc.

Addiction to One of Five Flavors

Five flavors refer to pungent, sweet, sour, bitter, and salty taste. The habitual preference for one of the five flavors may give rise to diseases, e.g. preference for pungent food may bring about constipation, aphtha or hemorrhoids and overeating sweet food may cause abdominal distention and acid regurgitation.

Adding Sweet Drug for Restoring Body Fluid

It is a therapy, referring to adding sweet drug in the drugs to promote the production of body fluid and moisturizing the viscera.

Adhesive Plaster

It refers to the herbal plaster sticking to the skin on external application.

Function. It can subdue swelling and stop pain, drain the pus and get rid of putrefaction, promote tissue regeneration and astriction, expel wind and eliminate dampness, regulate qi and promote blood circulation.

Adhesive Plaster for Post-moxibustion Sore

Referring to the adhesive plaster for moxibustion with suppuration. After direct moxibustion, the plaster is put on the region in order to induce the formation of the post-moxibustion sore and protect its surface.

Adhesive Plaster Substitute for Moxibustion

Referring to the adhesive plaster, applying to the umbilical region and keeping it there until a heat sensation appears in the region.

Indication. Cold due to insufficiency in the lower-energizer, weakness of genuine-qi, diarrhea with abdominal pain, shortness of breath, etc.

Adjuvant drugs

It has three implications. 1. It refers to drugs which assist the principal and assistant drugs to increase their therapeutic effect or treat less important symptoms by itself. 2. It refers to drugs that eliminate the principal and assistant drugs' negative action. 3. It refers to drugs which are aimed at dealing with possible vomiting in serious cases after taking the drugs, also with side effect. The drugs possess the properties opposite to those of the principal drugs in compatibility, but produce supplementing effect in the therapy of diseases.

Adrenal (MA)

It is an auricular point.

Location. At the tip of the lower protuberance on the border of the tragus.

Function. Clear heat and alleviate pain, expel endogenous wind and relieve convulsion.

Indication. Rheumatic arthritis, mumps, mandibular lymphnoditis, malaria tertian, dizziness, pruritus, pain and hypoacusis resulting from streptomycin poisoning.

Advanced Menstruation

Symptoms. Menstruation coming one week or more ahead of due time.

Pathogenesis. Mostly caused by qi deficiency or blood heat.

Therapeutic Principle. In the case of qi deficiency, invigorating qi as commander in charge of blood circulation to regulate menstruation; in the case of excess heat, clearing away heat from blood to regulate menstruation; in the case of heat deficiency type, nourishing yin and clearing away heat to regulate menstruation.

Affection by Dampness

It refers to disease due to invasion of pathogenic dampness into the skin and muscula stria. It can be divided into the exterior affection by dampness and the interior affection by dampness.

Affection by Exogenous Pathogenic Factors

It refers to any of the six external etiological factors (wind, cold, heat, dampness, dryness, and fire) or other noxious factors, which invade the skin, hair, and muscle, or enter the body from the mouth and nose. At the beginning, patients have occurrences such as cold and heat or the upper respiratory tract infection.

Affection of Facial Orifices by Pathogen

It refers to the pathologic change caused by the attack of pathogen-qi into the ear, eye, nose, mouth, etc.

Affection of Kidney by Cold-dampness

Symptoms. Chiefly by pain, feeling of coldness and heaviness on the waist region, difficulty in turning the back and the symptoms are exacerbated upon cold, etc.

Pathogenesis. Mostly caused by asthenia kidney and invasion of cold and damp.

Therapeutic Principle. Warming the spleen and the kidney, removing dampness and promoting diuresis.

Affine Cudweed

It is the whole herb of Gnaphalium affine D. Don (Compositae).

Effect. Eliminating phlegm, relieving cough and expelling wind-dampness.

Indication. Profuse cough, asthma, common cold due to wind-cold, favism, rheumatic arthralgia, leukorrhea, sores and furuncles, etc.

Afternoon Fever

It refers to fever occurring from about 3 to 5 o'clock in the afternoon. It is mainly caused by deficiency of yin.

Agalactosis

It refers to lack of lactation or ischogalactia after childbirth.
There are two cases:

1. **Symptoms.** Pale complexion and lips, and poor appetite and tiredness without distention and fullness sensation in the breast.
   Pathogenesis. Insufficiency and deficiency of qi and blood, a poor source from which milk is produced.
   Therapeutic Principle. Invigorating qi and nourishing blood, and promoting lactation as an auxiliary measure.
2. **Symptoms.** Distending pain in the breast, oppressed feeling in the chest and general fever.
   Pathogenesis. Stagnation of liver-qi, and obstruction of milk.
   Therapeutic Principle. Relieving depressed liver, dispelling accumulation and promote lactation.

Age Moxa Cones

Referring to the method of deciding the number of moxa cones applied to the patient, namely, the number of moxa cones equal to the age of the patient.

Agkistrodon Acutus

It is the dried corpus of Agkistrodon acutus (Crotalidae) with viscera extracted.
Effect. Dispelling pathogenic wind, dredging the meridian and relieving muscular spasm, alleviating itching.
Indication. Rheumatic arthralgia with spasm of muscles, facial hemiparalysis, numbness of the extremities, hemiplegia due to apoplexy, leprosy, tetanus and acute and chronic infantile convulsion.

Ailanthus Bark

It is the root bark or trunk bark of ailanthus altissima (Mill) Swingle (Simarubaceae).
Effect. Clearing away heat, eliminating dampness, astringing the intestines, stopping bleeding, arresting leukorrhea and destroying parasites.
Indication. Chronic diarrhea, chronic dysentery, abnormal uterine bleeding, metrorrhagia, metrostaxis, leukorrhea, scabies, tinea and ascariasis.

Air Potato Yam

It is the rhizome of Dioscorea bulbifera L. (Dioscoreaceae).
Effect. Dissolving lumps and treating goiter, clearing away heat and removing toxic substances, dispelling heat from the blood and arresting bleeding.
Indication. Goiter in the neck, sores, carbuncles and other suppurative skin infections, snake bite, hematemesis, epistaxis, etc.

Alangium Root

It is fibrous root or the bark of the root of Alangium chinense (Lour.) Harms or A. platanifolium Harms (Alanginaceae).
Effect. Expelling pathogenic wind, removing the obstruction in the meridians and collaterals, dispersing blood stasis and relieving pain.
Indication. Rheumatic arthralgia, numbness of the extremities, lumbago due to overstrain and traumatic injuries bleeding wounds and snake bite.

Alcoholic Consumption

It refers to the impairment of the intestine and stomach caused by prolonged habitual misuse of alcohol.

Alcoholic Jaundice

Symptoms. Jaundice, vexation, dryness of nasal cavity, abdominal fullness, anorexia and frequent inclination to vomiting, etc.

Pathogenesis. Excessive intense damp-heat due to indulgence in alcohol and the cholorrhea due to gallbladder heat.

Therapeutic Principle. Clearing away heat and eliminating dampness, removing alcoholic poison.

Alcoholic Phlegm

There are two meanings.

1. **Symptoms.** Indigestion of drinking, loss of appetite and vomiting with acid regurgitation, etc.

   Pathogenesis. Phlegm due to the accumulation of alcoholic dampness.

   Therapeutic Principle. Alleviate alcoholism and removing dampness.

2. **Symptoms.** Asthma, cough with phlegm.

   Pathogenesis. Invasion of original phlegm by drinking and fatty food.

   Therapeutic Principle. Relieving asthma, removing dampness by diuresis, resolving phlegm and ventilating the lung.

Alcoholic Stagnancy

Symptoms. Yellowish sclera and dry mouth, abdominal distention and anorexia, etc.

Pathogenesis. Alcoholic stagnancy due to indulgence in alcohol.

Therapeutic Principle. Removing stagnancy and relieving alcohol.

Algid Malaria

Symptoms. Light fever and great chills, absence of thirst, stuffiness in the chest and epigastrium, lassitude and fatigue.

Pathogenesis. Mostly caused by pathogenic cold accumulating in the interior, and the invasion of malarial evils in cold autumn.

Therapeutic Principle. Harmonize and regulate the exterior and interior; warm yang to dispel pathogenic factors.

Alienation due to Lochioschesis

Symptoms. Puerperal delirium, singing, dancing, incessant talking, laughing, curs-

ing in rage, feeling of restlessness, even climbing up and over the wall, biting and fisting others, etc.

Pathogenesis. Retention of lochia and blood stasis that goes reversely upward and attacks the heart.

Therapeutic Principle. Sending down abnormally ascending qi and removing blood stasis, tranquilizing the mind.

All Diseases Resulting from Qi Disorder

Various diseases are all caused by the functional disturbance of the activities of qi. For instance, when one is attacked by the external evils, the qi stagnation in the body will turn to heat.

Alleviating Water Retention

It refers to a therapy of clearing and regulating water passage and removing dampness and promoting diuresis.

Indication. Edema all over the body, dysuria, bodily indolence, anorexia, fullness in the stomach, loose stools, etc.

All the Pulses from Same Origin

It refers to the meridians all over the body of the same origin. Although there are so many meridians in the whole body, they are all governed by the heart and the lung.

Aloe

It is the concentrated substances drained from the liquid of Aloe vera L. and A. ferox Mill (Liliaceae).

Effect. Removing heat from the liver, relieving constipation and destroying parasites.

Indication. Constipation due to accumulation of heat, infantile dyspepsia and malnutrition of child, tinea and scabies.

Aloe Flower

It is the flower of Aloe vera L. Var. chinensis (Haw.) Berger.

Indication. Cough, hematemesis and gonorrhea.

Alopecia Areata

Symptoms. Sudden occurrence of loss of hair in a circular or irregular form, resulting in smooth and bright skin. It is divided into the syndrome of wind-dryness due to deficiency of blood, the syndrome of blood stasis due to stagnation of qi, the syndrome of deficiency of liver-kidney essence.

Pathogenesis. Deficiency of blood, attacking of pathogenic wind, excessive wind and blood dryness, or by stagnation of liver-qi, over-exertion or blood stasis due to stagnation of qi.

Therapeutic Principle. Nourishing the blood to expel wind, or regulating the flow of qi and promoting blood circulation to remove stasis, or tonifying the liver and kidney. The therapy may also be given by rubbing the affected area with fresh ginger or a tap with plum-blossom needle locally, or fumigate the affected parts with a moxa-stick until the skin turns reddish.

Alternate Attacks of Chills and Fever

It refers to alternate attacks of chills and fever, which can be found in half exterior and half interior syndrome, such as malaria, etc.

Alum

It is the extracted crystalline mineral salt from alunite.

Effect. Detoxicating, destroying parasites, expelling dampness, relieving pruritus, arresting bleeding and diarrhea, clearing away heat and eliminating sputum.

Indication. Externally as an antiparasitic and antipruritic agent for sores, ulcers, scabies, tinea, eczema; internally as an astringent for hematemesis, epistaxis, hemafecia, chronic dysentery, epilepsy and mania.

Amber

It is the yellowish or brownish fossil resin, formed by changing under the earth for many years.

Effect. Relieving convulsion and allaying excitement, activating blood circulation and removing blood stasis, inducing diuresis and treating stranguria.

Indication. Palpitation, insomnia, dreaminess, infantile convulsion, epilepsy, urodynia and hematuria due to acute urinary infection and urinary calculus.

Ambergris

The dried substance formed in the intestines of sperm Physeter catodon L. (Physeter catodon).

Effect. Promoting the circulation of blood and qi, resolving masses, expelling wind and relieving pain, inducing diuresis and curing stranguria.

Indication. Cough and dyspnea due to reversed flow of qi, masses in the abdomen, pain in the chest and abdomen and stranguria.

Amenorrhea

It refers to absent menstruation in a female over 18 years old, or suppression of menstruation for more than three months. It is divided into amenorrhea due to blood insufficiency, amenorrhea due to blood depletion, amenorrhea due to kidney deficiency, amenorrhea due to qi stagnation and blood stasis, etc.

Amenorrhea due to Blood Depletion

It refers to amenorrhea caused by severe anemia.

Pathogenesis. Mostly caused by exhaustion of essence and blood due to early marriage, multireproduction, excessive sexual intercourse, prolonged breast feeding, persistent illness and internal injury due to overstrain.

Therapeutic Principle. Nourishing yin and blood to promote menstruation.

Amenorrhea due to Deficiency of the Liver and Kidney

Symptoms. Delayed menarche, or delayed menstrual cycle and gradually diminished discharge of menstruation, or amenorrhea, dizziness, tinnitus, soreness and weakness of the lumbus and knees, dry mouth and throat, dysphoria with tidal fever and sweating etc.

Pathogenesis. Asthenia constitution, premature marriage or multiple childbirth.

Therapeutic Principle. Nourishing the liver and kidney.

Amenorrhea due to Parasitic Infestation

It refers to amenorrhea caused by parasitic infestation.

Therapeutic Principle. Killing the parasites and nourishing blood to restore normal menstruation.

Amenorrhea due to Stagnation of Blood

Pathogenesis. Emotional frustration, accumulation of qi and blood, or external pathogenic cold in delivery or internal cold.

Therapeutic Principle. Removing stasis and promoting blood circulation to induce menstrual flow. If it is caused by cold, it should warm the meridian.

Amenorrhea due to Stagnation of Phlegm-dampness

Symptoms. A small amount of menstrual blood that is pale and thin, fullness and tightness in the chest and hypochondrium, physical lassitude, profuse leukorrhea.

Pathogenesis. Dysfunction of the spleen in transportation, excessive phlegm-dampness inside the body.

Therapeutic Principle. Strengthen the spleen and reduce phlegm.

Amenorrhea due to Stagnation of Qi

Symptoms. Amenorrhea, mental depression, dysphoria, irritability, distention in the hypochondrium and lower abdomen.

Pathogenesis. Stagnation of the liver-qi and impeded circulation of qi due to depression and anger.

Therapeutic Principle. Promoting the circulation of qi to relieve stagnation and regulate menstruation.

Amenorrhea due to Weakness of the Spleen and Stomach

Symptoms. Absence of menses past the age of menarche, amenorrhea, severe palpitations, shortness of breath and listlessness, fatigue, anorexia, stuffiness in the abdomen and watery stools, etc.

Pathogenesis. Constitutional weakness of the spleen and stomach, or improper diet and overworking.

Therapeutic Principle. Invigorate the spleen and tonify the stomach.

Amenorrhea in Virgins

It refers to amenorrhea of the unmarried.

Pathogenesis. Weak constitution, disorder of the liver and spleen, leading to blood deficiency of Front and Back Meridians.

Therapeutic Principle. Enriching qi and nourishing blood to regulate menstruation; but, in the case accompanied by mental depression leading to stagnation of qi and blood, it is necessary to relieve the depressed liver to regulate the circulation of qi, and promote blood circulation to remove blood stasis.

Amenorrhea with Edema

Symptoms. Edema of the body and limbs after amenorrhea.

Pathogenesis. Pathogenic cold-dampness injuring the Front and Back Middle Meridians and Uterine Collaterals.

Therapeutic Principle. Promote the circulation of qi and blood.

American Ginseng   ✿ A-2

It is the root of Panax quinquefolium L. (Araliaceae).

Effect. Invigorating qi and nourishing yin, removing internal heat and promoting the secretion of body fluid.

Indication. Asthma and cough with blood-tinged sputum, listlessness of the limbs, thirst, deficiency of the body fluid, dryness in the mouth and tongue, etc.

Amnesia

A symptom marked by declination of memory and easy forgetfulness.

Pathogenesis. Mostly caused by over anxiety, breakdown of the coordination between the heart and the kidney.

Ampelopsis Root

The rhizome of Ampelopsis japonica (Thunb.) Makino (Vitaceae).

Effect. Clearing away heat and detoxicating, relieving swelling and pain, promoting wound healing and regeneration of the tissue.

Indication. Subcutaneous swelling, burns and scalds, scrofula, hemorrhoids, dysentery with bloody stool, etc.

Amur Adonis

The whole herb of Adonis amurensis Reg. et Radde (Ranunculaceae) with root.

Effect. Exerting a tonic effect on the heart to induce diuresis.

Indication. Palpitation, edema, epilepsy, etc.

Anal Fissure

Symptoms. Constipation, periodic anal pains in defecation with little flow of blood.

Pathogenesis. Injury and toxic infection of anal skin due to blood-heat, dryness in the intestines, constipation, excessive force in dejection.

Therapeutic Principle. Clearing away heat, moistening intestines and loosing the bowel to relieve constipation.

Anal Fistula

Symptoms. Sore with fistula, flow of pus, pain and scratching itch.

Pathogenesis. Mainly caused by diabrosis of carbuncle, cellulitis or sore around anus, which is refused to heal.

Therapeutic Principle. Surgical operation or taking orally antipyretic and antidote.

Analogical Febrile Disease

It is a general term for febrile disease similar to exogenous febrile disease. This kind of disease looks similar to febrile disease, but different in nature from each other.

Analogical Heatstroke

It refers to fever by deficiency of blood due to overwork, which is similar to sunstroke.

Symptoms. Hot skin and flushed face, polydipsia and susceptibility to drinking, etc.

Therapeutic Principle. Replenishing qi, nourishing yin and blood.

Anal Pruritus in Children

Symptoms. The infant feels anus pruritus, serious at night, with crying and sleeplessness.

Therapeutic Principle. Clearing away heat, drying damp, and killing the pinworms to relieve the pruritus.

Pathogenesis. Prolonged excessive eating of sweet and fatty foods, leading to damp-heat stasis in the large intestine, and the presence of pinworms in the anus.

Anal Sinusitis

Symptoms. Feeling of anal malaise, occasional stabbing pain, occasional slight blood in constipation.

Pathogenesis. Improper diet, or disturbance of parasitic infestation, growing of damp-heat in the interior, which flows down to the anus. It may also be caused by injury and infection of toxins due to dryness of intestines and constipation .

Therapeutic Principle. Clearing away heat and promoting diuresis or treatment by operation.

Anasarca

Symptoms. Sluggishness of heavy limbs and impeded movement, edema, in some cases accompanied by cough and dyspnea.
Pathogenesis. Stagnation of fluid due to deficiency of the spleen, retention of excessive fluid in the superficial tissues.
Therapeutic Principle. Warming the lung to reduce waterly phlegm.

Anasarca with Dyspnea

Symptoms. Edema all over the body, fullness in the abdomen, dyspnea.
Pathogenesis. Mostly caused by deficiency of the spleen and kidney, fluid retaining inside and going up to the lung.
Therapeutic Principle. Strengthening the spleen, nourishing the kidney and warming yang to promote diuresis.

Anatomical Landmarks on Body Surface

Referring to the prominences and depressions of bones, the outline of muscles and the wrinkles of the skin, etc. This can be observed and touched on the surface of a living body. They are divided into fixed anatomical signs and moving landmarks.

Anemia

It refers to insufficiency of blood and body fluid.
Symptoms. Dizziness and blurred vision, pale complexion, fatigue and weakness, etc.
Pathogenesis. Mostly caused by serious disease and prolonged illness, insufficiency of blood and qi in the body at ordinary time, weakness of middle-energizer, spleen and stomach, or improper diet.
Therapeutic Principle. Invigorating qi and enriching blood.

Anger

Symptoms. Unbearable anger, ascending heat attacking the heart, shortness of breath.
Therapeutic Principle. Disperse and rectify the depressed liver-energy.

Angina Pectoris

It is a dangerous disease with precordial pain.
Symptoms. Continuous violent pain in the heart and chest, which may spread to the shoulders and back, left upper arm, throat, gastric cavity and abdomen, etc. It is accompanied by shortness and rapidness of breath, dyspnea, palpitation, cold limbs, etc.
Pathogenesis. Mainly caused by deficiency of yin, yang, qi and blood in the heart, accumulation of cold and heat, stagnation of phlegm, stagnation of qi, and blood stasis, etc.
Therapeutic Principle. Revive the yang by resuscitation and promoting blood circulation to remove blood stasis.

Angioma

Symptoms. It is similar to hemangioma, dark red, purple blue colors in the skin of the angioma body, softness and hardness in part.
Pathogenesis. Stagnation of qi, blood stasis, the blockage of meridians and collaterals, and together with affection of exopathogens.
Therapeutic Principle. Eliminating pathogenic heat from the blood, dissipating blood stasis and promoting the subduing of swelling or an operation is advisable.

Angle of Cymba Conchae (MA)

An auricular point, also called Prostate (MA).
Location. At the medial superior angle of cymba conchae.
Indication. Prostatitis, urethritis.

Angle of Needle Insertion

Referring to the angle formed by the body of needle and the skin surface of the acupoint. Clinically, according to the anatomic characteristic of the acupoint and the demand of the needling method, different insertion angles are adopted. The insertion angles are commonly divided into three types: perpendicular insertion (approx. 90 degrees), oblique insertion (30-60 degrees) and transverse (horizontal) insertion (10-20 degrees).

Anhidrosis

It refers to the disease of no sweating when there should be sweating.

Pathogenesis. Blocking of striae of skin, muscle, due to summer-heat and dampness or wind and cold.

Ankle (MA-AH 2)

It is an auricular point.

Location. At the middle point between Heel (MA-AH 1)and Knee (MA-AH 3).

Indication. Ankle diseases, sprain of ankle.

Ankyloglossia

Refers to the tip of tongue cannot stretch out or draw back or turn freely, due to shortened sublingual vessels and ligament. It hinders the infant from drinking milk and speaking clearly.

Anmian (Ex)

One of the extraordinary points, there are two such points:

Location. Anmian 1, midway between Yifeng (TE17) and Yiming (Ex); Anmian 2, midway between Fengchi (G20) and Yiming.

Indication. Insomnia, dizziness, headache, palpitation, epilepsy, hysteria, etc.

Manipulation. Puncture perpendicularly 0.8-1.2 cun.

Anorectal Carcinoma

It is the advanced stage of rectal cancer of anal canal.

Therapeutic Principle. Removing blood stasis, clearing away heat and toxic material. In the early stage, an operation is the main method.

Anorexia

It refers to poor appetite.

Pathogenesis. Deficiency of qi in the middle-energizer, or the dysfunction of the spleen due to food retention.

Antelope's Horn

The horn of Saiga tatarica L. (Bovidae).

Effect. Purging intense heat from the liver to improve acuity of vision and clearing away heat and detoxicating expelling wind and relieving spasm.

Indication. Infantile convulsion, apoplexy, epilepsy, spasm, headache, dizziness and bloodshot eyes due to liver-fire and skin eruptions etc.

Anterior Ear Lobe (MA)

An ear point, also named neurasthenia point.

Location. In the 4th area of the ear.

Indication. Neurasthenia and toothache.

Anterior-posterior Midline

One of the mark lines of head acupuncture, from the center between the eyebrows to the inferior border of the external occipital protuberance.

Anterior-posterior Point Association

It refers to a method of the combination of points. Selecting and combining simultaneously the involved acupuncture points on the thoracic-abdominal region with those on the lumbodorsal region to use coordinately. For example, to cure cough with dyspnea, select Shanzhong (CV 17) and Tiantu (CV 22) on the chest, and Dingchun (Ex-B) and Feishu (B 13) on the back.

Anthelmintic

A general name for drugs with a major effect on expelling or poisoning parasites. Mainly used for ascariasis, enterobiasis, ancylostomiasis, etc., but also for treating the syndromes caused by parasites.

Antitragic Apex (MA)

It is an ear point.

Location. On the tip of antitragus.
Function. Ventilating the lung and relieving asthma, clearing away heat and detoxifying, and dispersing pathogenic wind.
Indication. Asthma, trachitis, parotitis, cutaneous pruritus and epididymitis.

Antler

It refers to the horn of Cervus nippon Temminck (Cervidae) and various growing ossified horn of male deer.
Effect. Reinforcing the kidney and supporting yang, promoting blood circulation and subduing swelling, strengthening the tendons and bones.
Indication. Infections on the body surface, acute mastitis, pain due to the retention of blood, etc.

Antler Glue

It is the colloid substance concentrated by decocting the antler.
Effect. Tonifying the liver and kidney, replenishing vital essence and blood, and arresting bleeding.
Indication. Insufficiency of the kidney-yang, deficiency of the essence and blood, emaciation due to consumption and stopping bleeding.

Anuresis

It refers to retention of urine.
Pathogenesis. Usually caused by stagnation of lung-qi and heat in the lung, the accumulation of damp-heat in the bladder.
Therapeutic Principle. Clearing away heat, relieving the depressed liver, promoting diuresis.

Anus Hemorrhoid

The pile growing close to the region of anus.
Therapeutic Principle. In the internal therapy, removing pathogenic heat and cool the blood, dispelling wing and removing dampness by diuresis. In the external therapy, it is advisable to follow the method of ligation, drying the hemorrhoid, operations, etc.

Anus-lifting Respiration

A form of breath-regulating method in Qigong.
Method. Drawing up the anus and the perineum with slight mind-will while inhaling and relaxing them while exhaling.
Indication. Gastroptosis, proctoptosis or hysteroptosis.

Anus (MA-H 5)

An auricular point, also called Hemorrhoid Nucleus Point.
Location. On the helix, on the level of the lower border of the superior antihelix crus, i.e. between the lower rectal portion point and the urethra point.
Indication. Internal and external hemorrhoids.

Anus Swelling

It refers to the burning, reddened swelling and prolapsed anus.
Pathogenesis. Mostly caused by descending of accumulated heat into the anus of children, or difficulty in defecation with an excessive effort.
Therapeutic Principle. Clearing away heat and loosing the bowels.

Anxiety Impairs Spleen

It means that the excessive worry and over-anxiety may suppress the splenic functions.
Symptoms. Poor appetite, abdominal distention, loose stools, tiredness, etc.
Therapeutic Principle. Strengthening the spleen and replenishing qi.

Apes and Monkeys Pinching Fruits

One of massage manipulations for children.
Operation. Pinch the skin of the snail bone with two hands, pulling and releasing, and repeat the movements for many times.
Function. Dispersing phlegm and premoting qi circulation and strengthening spleen and stomach.

Indication. Food stagnancy, phlegm syndrome caused by cold wetness evil, and malaria.

Aphasia and Paralysis

One type of disease with loss of voice when speaking.

Symptoms. Flaccid tongue with inability to speak.

Pathogenesis. Mainly caused by internal exhaustion, impairment and upward reversed flow of kidney-qi.

Therapeutic Principle. Replenishing and restoring the kidney-qi.

Aphasia due to Acute Throat Trouble

Symptoms. Sudden swelling and pain of the throat with lockjaw, cyanosis of face and lips, loss of speech, and watery nasal discharge.

Therapeutic Principle. Dispel pathogenic wind and eliminate phlegm.

Aphonia

Symptoms. Hoarseness of voice or articulation

Pathogenesis. It can be divided into deficiency syndrome caused by the yin and qi deficiency of both the lung and kidney; Excess syndrome due to the invasion of external pathogen into the lung.

Therapeutic Principle. Nourishing the lung and kidney.

Aphonia due to Cough

Symptoms. Cough, hoarseness of voice, painful in the throat, or cough of long duration, fever with aversion to cold, etc.

Pathogenesis. Mostly caused by long duration cough due to heat.

Therapeutic Principle. Moistening the lung, clearing the pharynx and dispersing pathogenic factors.

Aphonia during Pregnancy

Symptoms. Hoarse voice or even aphonia during the later period of pregnancy.

Pathogenesis. Mostly caused by failure of the kidney-yin to nourish the tongue due to obstruction of uterine collaterals by the growing fetus.

Therapeutic Principle. Nourish yin and supplement the kidney.

Aphtha

Usually occurring in malnourished children.

Pathogenesis. Dampness and heat in the interior and deficiency of stomach-yin.

Therapeutic Principle. Clearing away heat and promoting diaphoresis.

Aphthous Stomatitis

Symptoms. White erosive spots, or even erosion in the mouth cavity.

Pathogenesis. Long accumulation of damp-heat in the Spleen Meridian which is transmitted into toxic heat, and damp-heat steaming in the mouth.

Therapeutic Principle. Clearing away heat and removing dampness.

Apoplectic Stroke

This term has two meanings: 1. It refers to apoplexy due to endogenous wind. 2. It refers to clinic manifestations, similar to those of apoplexy, but in fact they are not genuine apoplexy.

Apoplexy

Symptoms. Sudden collapse, coma, deviation of the mouth and eyes, hemiplegia and dysphasia.

Pathogenesis. Mostly caused by qi-deficiency, overstrain and the rising of liver-yang caused by insufficiency of kidney-yin, leading to imbalance of yin and yang and derangement of qi and blood. Worry, anger and over-drinking are common predisposing causes of the disease. Clinically divided into apoplexy involving zang and fu, and apoplexy involving the meridians and collaterals.

Apoplexy due to Fright
Symptoms. Sudden unconsciousness from fright but without facial paralysis and hemiplegia.
Therapeutic Principle. Tranquilizing the mind, calming the fright, and inducing resuscitation.

Apoplexy due to Prostration
It refers to apoplexy with syncope of the visceral relationship, such as mouth opened, enuresis, hand flaccidity, closed eye, and snore.
Therapeutic Principle. Warming yang and promoting the flow of qi to restore the vital function from collapse.

Apoplexy due to Reversed Flow of Qi
A type of apoplexy due to exogenous wind evil.
Symptoms. Sudden fainting, unconsciousness, lockjaw, convulsion of the hands and feet, cold feeling throughout the body, absence or less saliva in the mouth etc.
Pathogenesis. Stagnation of the seven emotions (joy, anger, melancholy, anxiety, sorrow, fear and fright), and up-rising qi.
Therapeutic Principle. Regulating qi and dispersing the stagnation, and lowering the adverse rising qi.

Apoplexy in Pregnancy
1. **Symptoms.** Apoplexy involving the meridians and collaterals: numbness of limbs, facial hemiparalysis, even hemiplegia.
   Pathogenesis. Mostly caused by blood deficiency in pregnancy, lack of nourishment of the meridians and zang-fu organs, and invasion of pathogenic wind leading to imbalance of yin and yang.
   Therapeutic Principle. Nourish the blood, prevent miscarriage and calm the endopathic wind.

2. Apoplexy involving zang-fu organs: sudden coma, accumulation of excessive phlegm and saliva in the throat, unconsciousness.
   Therapeutic Principle. Expel wind to remove phlegm for resuscitation.

Apoplexy Involving Collaterals
A kind of syndrome of apoplexy referring to pathogenic factor in the collaterals.
Symptoms. It is a mild apoplexy, facial palsy and numbness of the skin, etc.
Therapeutic Principle. Promote blood circulation, clearing and activating the meridians and collaterals.

Apoplexy Involving Meridians and Collaterals
A type of relatively milder apoplexy than the one involving zang-fu, deviation of eyes and mouth, muscular and skin numbness, hemiplegia, dysphasia, etc.

Apoplexy Involving Zang and Fu
Symptoms. A type of relatively serious apoplexy, paralysis of limbs, coma and aphasia, etc.
Pathogenesis. Sudden upward movement wind-yang and phlegm-fire stirring each other up, leading to upward qi and blood, and mental confusion.

Apoplexy of Deficiency Type
Symptoms. Sudden unconsciousness, stiff tongue and retardation in speech, facial hemiparalysis, with lassitude and disability of limbs, and spontaneous sweating, etc.
Pathogenesis. Due to overstrain, weakness of the spleen and stomach, exhaustion of the primordial qi.
Therapeutic Principle. Strengthening the spleen and replenishing qi, clearing and activating the meridians and collaterals.

Apoplexy of Excess Type
Symptoms. A sudden coma, lockjaw, clenched fists, stiffness and spasm of limbs.
Pathogenesis. Obstruction of qi and phlegm.
Therapeutic Principle. Restoring consciousness and removing phlegm for resuscitation.

Apoplexy of Yang Syndrome
Symptoms. Red face and lips, lockjaw, eyes looking upward, stiffness of nape, trembling and dizziness and vexation and thirst, etc.
Pathogenesis. The occlusion due to phlegm-heat, the stagnancy of cold and heat, the obstruction of phlegm and qi.
Therapeutic Principle. Eliminating phlegm for resuscitation.

Appendix (MA)
One of the auriculo-acupuncture points.
Location. Between Large Intestine (MA-SC 4) and Small Intestine (MA-SC 2).
Indication. Simple appendicitis and diarrhea.

Appliance for Needle-Insertion
An auxiliary tool used in acupuncture, which can relieve pain because the needle is inserted quickly into the skin by means of a spring apparatus. It is made of metal or plastic. Apply acupuncture manipulations after the needle is inserted into the skin.

Application of Hemorrhoid Complicated by Anal Fistula
The therapy of using medicine for external application on the hemorrhoid. The method is divided into application of medicine and inserting medicine. It is suitable for the initial internal hemorrhoids, or hemorrhoids complicated by anal fistula.

Apricotleaf Ladybell Root
The root of Adenophora trachelioides Maxim. (Campanulaceae).
Effect. Clearing away heat, detoxicating and resolving phlegm.
Indication. Pulmonary infection with dry cough, sore throat, diabetes, and boils, furuncles, etc.

Apricot Kernel ⊛ A-3
The ripe seed of Prunus mandshurica (Maxim) Koehne, of Prunus sibirica L. or Prunus armeniaca L. (Rosaceae).
Effect. Relieving cough and asthma and moistening the intestines to relax the bowels.
Indication. Cough with asthma, constipation due to dryness.

Apricot Plum Root and Leaf
The root or leaf of Prunus simonii Carr. (Rosaceae).
Effect. Promoting flow of qi and blood circulation, alleviating pain.
Indication. Traumatic injury, pain due to blood stasis, hematemesis and gonorrhea.

Arctium Fruit ⊛ A-4
The ripe seed of Arctium lappa L. (Compositae).
Effect. Dispelling wind and heat, detoxicating, promoting skin eruption and alleviating itching, easing the throat and subduing swelling.
Indication. Cough due to affection by exopathogenic wind-heat, swollen and sore throat, early stage of measles, skin infection subcutaneous swelling, mumps, etc.

Areca Flower
The male flowerbud of Areca catechu L. (Palmae).
Effect. Strengthening the stomach, quenching thirst and relieving cough.
Indication. Epigastric and abdominal distention, loss of appetite, vomiting due to dampness blockage of middle-energizer,

excessive thirst due to summer-heat, cough, etc.

Areca Peel

It is the peel of Areca catechu L. (palmaceae).

Effect. Activating qi circulation, relieving the stagnation of intestine, promoting diuresis and alleviating edema.

Indication. Stuffiness and distention in the epigastrium and abdomen, dyschezia, beriberi and edema, etc.

Areca Seed

The ripe seed of Areca catechu L. (Palmae).

Effect. Anthelmintic for taeniasis, ascariasis, removing stagnation, promoting flow of qi and inducing diuresis.

Indication. Parasitosis in the intestinal tract, food retention and stagnation of qi, abdominal distention, constipation or diarrhea, edema, etc.

Argyi Fruit

The fruit of Artemisia argyi Levl. et Vant. (Compositae).

Effect. Improving eyesight and strengthening yang.

Indication. Blurred vision due to deficiency of liver-yin and kidney-yin, pain in the waist and knees and infertility due to cold in the womb.

Argyi Leaf   ✿ A-5

The leaf of a perennial shrub Artemisia argyi Levl. Vant. (Compositae).

Effect. Stop bleeding by warming the meridians, expel cold and relieve pain.

Indication. Bleeding of deficiency cold, cold of insufficiency type in lower-energizer, cold pain in the abdomen, irregular menstruation, dysmenorrhea, leukorrhagia, cough and asthma, eczema and dermatitis etc.

Arisaema Cum Bile

It is the processed product of arisaema with the mixture of ox bile.

Effect. Drying dampness to eliminate-phlegm and relieving convulsion and spasm.

Indication. Convulsion, apoplexy due to heat-phlegm, epilepsy, mania, etc.

Aristolochia

It is the dried ripe fruit of Aristolochia contorta Bge., or Aristolochia debilis Sieb. et Zucc. (Aristolochiaceae).

Effect. Clearing away heat from the lung, eliminating phlegm, relieving cough and asthma, and lower blood pressure.

Indication. Cough due to the lung-heat, chronic cough with the bloody phlegm due to the lung deficiency, hemorrhoid bleeding due to intestine heat and swelling and painful hemorrhoids, hypertension with heat syndrome.

Ark Shell

It is the shell of Arca granoca L. and A. Subcrenata Lischkel, or A. inflata Reeve (Arcidae).

Effect. Eliminating phlegm and removing blood stasis, softening hard lumps and dissolving nodes.

Indication. Scrofula, masses in the abdomen, hyperacidity and nodular swelling.

Arm Numbness

Symptoms. Pain in the joints and muscles linking up the arm and shoulder girdle with difficulty in lifting, supporting, and doing activities of flexion and extention.

Pathogenesis. Invaded by wind-cold and damp pathogen due to blood deficiency, resulting in unsmooth passages of meridians and vessels.

Therapeutic Principle. Nourishing blood and expelling wind, dispelling cold, removing dampness, and removing the obstruction in the meridians and collaterals.

Aromatic Drugs for Resolving Dampness

Effect. Promoting the elimination of pathogenic dampness, invigorating the spleen and strengthening the stomach.

Indication. Epigastric dullness, abdominal distention, nausea and acid regurgitation, loose stool, anorexia, lassitude etc.

Arrhythmic Pulse

It refers to uneven pulse, which is slow and has three beats or five beats per respiration, belonging to knotted pulse.

Arrival of Qi at the Affected Area

A term in acupuncture. It refers to a needling sensation to reach the affected area by means of manipulations. As a result, a better curative effect can be achieved.

Arsenolite

It is the material processed from the ore of Arsenolite or Arsenopyrite.

Effect. Externally treating wound and internally eliminating phlegm and relieving asthma.

Indication. Tinea, sores, scabies scrofula, hemorrhoids, asthma due to cold-sputum, and malaria.

Arteries of the Twelve Meridians

The arteries along the courses of the twelve meridians, of which the pulse can be easily felt. The undulatory points of the meridians are as follows: The Lung Meridian: Zhongfu (L 1), Yunmen (L 2), Tianfu (L 3), Xiabai (L 4), Chize (L 5), Jingqu (L 8); The Heart Meridian: Jiquan (H 1), Shaohai (H 3); The Pericardium Meridian: Laogong (P 8); The Large Intestine Meridian: Hegu (LI 4), Yangxi (LI 5), Shouwuli (LI 13); The Small Intestine Meridian Tianchuang: (SI 16); The Triple Energizer Meridian Erheliao: (TE 22); The Stomach Meridian: Daying (S 5), Xiaguan (S 7), Renying (S 9), Qichong (S 30), Chongyang (S 42); The Bladder Meridian: Weizhong (B 40); The Gallbladder Meridian: Tinghui (G 2), Shangguan (G 3); The Spleen Meridian: Jimen (Sp 11), Chongmen (Sp12); The Kidney Meridian: Taixi (K3), Yingu (K 10), and The Liver Meridian: Taichong (Liv 3), Xingjian (Liv 2), Zuwuli (Liv 10), Yinlian (Liv11).

Artery in Front of Ear

It belongs to Triple-energizer Meridian, located in the sunken place in front of tragus. From here, the prosperity and decline of the ear-qi can be detected.

Arthralgia

Symptoms. Pain in limb joints.

Pathogenesis. Invasion of pathogenic wind, cold and dampness, stagnation of phlegm and blood stasis which leads to obstruction of meridians and collaterals, or failure in nourishing muscles due to deficiency of blood.

Arthralgia due to Cold

Symptoms. Cold and pain of limbs and inability of joints to flex and stretch, aversion to cold and preference for warming, etc.

Pathogenesis. Attack of pathogenic cold into the joints and collaterals resulting in qi and blood stagnancy.

Therapeutic Principle. Warming yang and dispelling cold and activating collaterals to relieve pain.

Arthralgia due to Dampness

There are two meanings:

1. It refers to arthralgia syndrome caused by excessive dampness.

   Symptoms. Swelling with heaviness sensation in joints, paralysis in one part of the body, inability to turn one side of the body, etc.

   Therapeutic Principle. Eliminating dampness, dredging the meridians and expelling wind.

2. It is a kind of beriberi.

Arthralgia due to Phlegm Stagnation

Symptoms. Protracted arthralgia with swelling and distortion, or subcutaneous nodule and lump, etc.

Pathogenesis. Stagnation of phlegm in meridians and collaterals.

Therapeutic Principle. Eliminating phlegm and promoting blood circulation.

Arthralgia due to Summer-dampness

Symptoms. Aching pain and heaviness of limbs, flushed face and oliguria with dark urine, etc.

Pathogenesis. Attack into muscles and skin, and collaterals by pathogenic summer-dampness in summer and autumn.

Therapeutic Principle. Dispelling dampness and relieving stagnation.

Arthralgia during Pregnancy

Symptoms. Fever, excessive pain of joints, heaviness sensation of the limbs, stuffy nose, etc.

Pathogenesis. Impairment of muscular striae due to affection of pathogenic dampness.

Therapeutic Principle. Eliminating dampness to prevent abortion.

Arthralgia of Heat Type

Symptoms. Pain and swelling of limb joints, listlessness, sore throat, fever, scanty and dark urine, etc.

Pathogenesis. Heat transmitted from pathogenic wind-dampness, accumulation of pathogenic heat in meridians and collaterals and joints, stagnation of qi and blood.

Therapeutic Principle. Eliminate dampness, clear heat, and invigorate collaterals to relieve pain.

Arthralgia with Irritability

Symptoms. Arthralgia accompanied by vexation and restlessness.

Pathogenesis. Conjoint invasion by wind and dampness or impairment qi and blood, the nutrient and superficial defensive system or invasion of the kidney by pathogenic heat.

Arthroncus of Knee

Symptoms. At the beginning, the knee mostly shows slight swelling, then pain, local red swelling or white swelling, then the thigh becoming thin.

Pathogenesis. Mostly caused by the deficiency of three yang meridians, the external attacking of pathogenic wind, and the concretion of severe pathogenic cold.

Therapeutic Principle. Warming yang and dispelling dampness, reinforce the body resistance to eliminate pathogens.

Arthropathy due to Deficiency of Blood

Symptoms. Numbness of the skin, frequent soreness and pain in joints, pale or sallow complexion, etc.

Pathogenesis. Usually caused by deficiency of qi and blood, or blockage of qi, blood and meridians due to sweating by strain, or sleeping in wind with the invasion by pathogenic factors.

Therapeutic Principle. Nourishing blood, invigorating qi, together with expelling wind, cold, dampness pathogen.

Asafoetida

It is the gum-resin of Ferula fukanensis K. M. Shen F. Sinkiangensis K. M. Shen (Umbelliferae).

Effect. Promoting digestion and destroying parasites.

Indication. Masses in the abdomen, abdominal pain due to parasitic infestation, meat stagnancy, malaria and dysentery.

Ascariasis of Biliary Tract

Symptoms. Sudden onset of colic in the upper abdomen (below the xiphoid process), in crying with trembling, sweating over the entire body, vomiting, shivers and fever, etc.

Pathogenesis. Upward movement of the intestinal ascarids into the biliary tract. It is induced by diarrhea, constipation, fever, pregnancy, incorrect application of ascaridole, stimulation due to cold, etc.

Therapeutic Principle. Disperse the depressed gallbladder qi, relieve epigastric distention and regulate the stomach.

Ascites due to Parasitic Infestation

It refers to ascites caused by schistosomiasis.

Symptoms. Abdominal distention and fullness like a drum, slight edema of limbs, reddish spots and stripes on the face, etc.

Therapeutic Principle. Killing parasites and detoxicating.

Ash Bark

The bark of a deciduous arbor Fraxinus rhynchophylla Hance, or F. Bungeana DC. (Oleaceae).

Effect. Clearing away heat drying dampness and detoxicating, removing intensive acuity of sight.

Indication. Diarrhea due to pathogenic heat, acute dysentery with purulent and bloody stool, leukorrhegia, bloodshot, swollen and painful eyes, etc.

Ashi Point

A category of acupoints which have no fixed location, but are selected as acupoints according to tenderness or pain at the site of sensitivity.

Asian Butterflybush Root or Stem

The root and stem of Buddleia asiatica Lour (Loganiaceae).

Effect. Dispelling wind, eliminating dampness, removing the obstruction in the meridians and destroying parasites.

Indication. Fever due to wind-cold, headache, joints with difficulty in flexion and extension, abdominal distention due to the spleen dampness, dysentery, erysipelas, traumatic injuries, etc.

Asiatic Toddalia Root

It is the root or bark of Toddalia asiatica Lam (Rutaceae).

Effect. Expelling the wind, alleviating pain, dissipating blood stasis and arresting bleeding.

Indication. Rheumatic arthralgia, traumatic injuries, hematemesis, epistaxis, amenorrhea, dysmenorrhea, etc.

Asparagus Root

It is the root tuber of Asparagus cochinchinensis (Lour.) Merr. (Liliaceae).

Effect. Removing dryness, heat from the lung, purging fire, tonifying yin.

Indication. Dry cough with sticky sputum, phthisical cough with hemoptysis, impairment of yin by febrile diseases with manifestations of dry mouth, thirsty feeling, diabetes, constipation due to dryness of the intestines, etc.

Asphyxia at Birth

It refers to fetal asphyxia after delivery. Clearing away amniotic fluid from mouth as soon as possible and light patting on the back will rescue the life of the newly born baby.

Aspongopus

It is the body of Aspongopus chinensis Dallas (Pentatomidae).

Effect. Promoting the qi circulation, relieving pain, warming the kidney and reinforcing yang.

Indication. Pain in the hypochondrium, epigastric distention and pain, lumbago due to deficiency of kidney-yang and impotence.

Assembled Meridians

It generally refers to the site where two or more of the meridians come together. For example, the ear is the mustering site of the assembled meridians, and genuine qi of many meridians flows up to the ear. As a result, there are corresponding points of the five zang and six fu organs and all parts of the body on the ear. Therefore, pricking relevant points on the ear can treat diseases of all parts of the body.

Assembling Puncture

A needling method, also named triple puncture, to puncture the center of the affected area, one needle on both sides with two needles. It is used for treating deep-rooted arthralgia in small areas.

Assisting Manipulation

Referring to nipping, pressing, snatching, and pinching the region with fingernails where the meridians distribute in order to insert the needle easily.

Asthenia-cold of Large Intestine

Symptoms. Loose stool, indigestion anorexia, cold limbs, waist soreness, dull pain and cold feeling in the abdomen, etc.
Pathogenesis. Asthenia-cold of the spleen and the kidney.

Asthenic Foot

Symptoms. Weakness of feet, difficulty in walking.
Pathogenesis. Deficiency of the spleen and kidney qi and insufficiency of essence and blood.

Asthenopia

Symptoms. Blurred vision.
Pathogenesis. Emaciation due to persistent illness and lack of qi and blood, insufficiency of the liver kidney, spleen and stomach or trauma of the head, etc. This results in the eye's failure to get nutrition of essence-qi from the five zang and six fu organs.
Therapeutic Principle. Diagnosis and therapeutic based on overall analysis of the patients symptoms and signs.

Asthma

A disease with a combination of wheezing syndrome and dyspnea syndrome. This disease is clinically divided into asthma due to cold fluid retention, asthma due to phlegm-heat, asthma due to deficiency of the spleen, asthma due to deficiency of the lung, and asthma due to deficiency of the kidney.
Pathogenesis. Retention of phlegm and fluid in the body.

Asthma due to Consumptive Injury of Genuine Qi

Symptoms. Gasping and shortness of breath, sweating with worse asthma on slight exertion, emaciation and nervous fatigue, even cyanosis of lips and nails, palpitation, edema of limbs.
Pathogenesis. Protracted asthma and cough, the injury of genuine qi after a severe disease, the deficiency of kidney-yang, and the failure of the kidney to receive qi.
Therapeutic Principle. Warming yang and reinforcing the spleen, tonifying the kidney to receive qi.

Asthma due to Deficiency of Lung-qi

Symptoms. Asthma with shortness of breath and low rale, listlessness etc.
Pathogenesis. Lack of primordial qi, or yin deficiency of the lung due to the weakness of the body or protracted cough.
Therapeutic Principle. Restoring the lung-qi and clearing the lung. If it is ascribable to the lung deficiency and the lack of the body fluid, nourishing the lung and promoting the production of the body fluid.

Asthma due to Fire Wrapped by Cold

Symptoms. Aversion to cold and anhidrosis, cough and rapid breath, dysphoria and fullness in the chest, etc.
Pathogenesis. Accumulated phlegm-heat, attack of cold on the exterior portion of the body, and the obstruction of the lung-qi.
Therapeutic Principle. Dispelling the cold in the exterior and clearing away the heat in the interior.

Asthma due to Improper Diet

Symptoms. Short and urgent respiration with sound of wheezing in the larynx, distensile pain in the stomach, vomiting in the serious case.

Pathogenesis. Overeating and improper diet.

Therapeutic Principle. Relieving asthma by lowering the adverse flow of lung qi, and regulating the stomach and strengthening the spleen.

Asthma due to Kidney Deficiency

Symptoms. Tidal fever in the afternoon, red face and headache, restlessness, tinnitus, soreness of the loin, cold lower limbs, etc.

Pathogenesis. Deficiency of the kidney and impairment of the lung by excessive fire.

Therapeutic Principle. Tonifying the kidney to stop fire and clearing away heat from the lungs to moisturize dryness.

Asthma due to Phlegm-heat

Symptoms. Cough with gasping, loud rale in the throat, flushed complexion, fever with sweating, thick yellow sputum which is difficult to discharge, thirst, dysphoria, cough inducing pain of chest.

Pathogenesis. Accumulation of wind heat and phlegm and impairment of the lung in purifying and descending.

Therapeutic Principle. Clear heat, disperse phlegm and relieve asthma.

Asthma due to Qi Deficiency

Symptoms. Spontaneous perspiration, shortness of breath, fatigue and listlessness etc.

Pathogenesis. Lack of genuine qi, or qi deficiency of the spleen and lung.

Therapeutic Principle. Replenishing and restoring primordial qi.

Asthma due to Retention of Cold Fluid

Symptoms. Dyspnea respiration, rale in the throat, cough with thin or frothy sputum, aversion to cold, anhidrosis, headache, mostly occurring in winter or when attacked by pathogenic cold.

Pathogenesis. Phlegm and pathogenic wind-cold blocking the respiratory tract.

Therapeutic Principle. Dispel cold and facilitate the flow of the lung-qi to relieve asthma.

Asthma due to Reversed Flowing of Stomach-qi

Symptoms. Asthma with extreme thirst or wheezing sound in the throat.

Pathogenesis. Adverse rising of stomach-fire, or the obstruction of phlegm and food.

Therapeutic Principle. Lowering the adverse flow of stomach-qi and regulating the stomach, removing phlegm and relieving asthma.

Asthma due to Spleen Deficiency

Symptoms. Asthma with weak speech, pale complexion, anorexia, gastric mass, excessive sputum, lassitude, abdominal distention and loose stool, etc.

Pathogenesis. Dysfunction of the spleen in transportation leading to retention of water-dampness and the formation of phlegm and turbidness.

Therapeutic Principle. Strengthen the spleen and replenish qi, remove phlegm to stop asthma.

Asthma due to Stagnation of Profuse Phlegm

Symptoms. Cough, stuffiness of the chest, rapidly breathing with phlegmatic sound.

Pathogenesis. Phlegm accumulation.

Therapeutic Principle. Dispersing phlegm and relieving asthma.

Asthma of Febrile Disease

It refers to two diseases:

1. The symptoms of dyspneic respiration and restlessness occurring in febrile disease.

   Symptoms. Fever with aversion to cold, restlessness, fullness and oppression in the abdomen, etc.

   Therapeutic Principle. Eliminating the pathogenic factor and relieving asthma.

2. The syndrome of asthma caused by affection by exopathogen, stagnating in the lung, and the lung qi failing to disperse.

   Symptoms. Asthma, rapid breathing, distention and oppression in the chest, thin and whitish phlegm, accompanied by headache with aversion to cold.

   Therapeutic Principle. Promoting the dispersing function of the lung, relieving asthma, and relieving exterior syndrome.

Asthma with Phlegm

A kind of phlegm syndrome, usually seen in dyspnea of deficiency type and excess type.

Therapeutic Principle. Dispelling sputum and relieving asthma.

Asthma with Wheezing

Symptoms. Shortness of breath, wheezing in the throat, choking in the chest, cough with phlegm.

Pathogenesis. Retention of phlegm in the lung with the affection by exopathogen, the impairment by diet, emotion and overstrain.

Therapeutic Principle. Expelling pathogen, ventilating the lung qi, removing phlegm, reinforcing the spleen and kidney.

Asthma with Wheezing due to Deficiency of the Lung

Symptoms. Short breath, week speech, pale complexion, spontaneous sweating and aversion to wind, stuffy nose, sneezing, fatigue, etc.

Pathogenesis. Insufficiency of lung-qi resulting from a protracted illness, and fail-ure of qi to transport body fluid, leading to stagnation of phlegm in the lung.

Therapeutic Principle. Enrich lung-qi, resolve sputum and relieve asthma.

Astragalus Root   ⊛ A-6

The root of Astragalus membranaceus (Fisch.) Bge., and A. Mongholicus Bge. (Leguminosae).

Effect. Tonifying qi, lifting the sunken yang, reinforcing the spleen and stomach, consolidating superficial resistance, relieving infection, promoting pus discharge and tissue regeneration and inducing diuresis to cure edema.

Indication. Deficiency of the spleen-qi and lung-qi, listlessness, anorexia, proctoptosis due to chronic diarrhea, spontaneous sweating, edema, scanty urine, numb extremities, arthralgia sores, hemiplegia, etc.

Atractylodes Rhizome   ⊛ A-7

The rhizome of Atractylodes Lancea (Thunb.) DC. or A. Chinensis (DC.) Koidez (Compositae).

Effect. Depriving dampness, activating the spleen, dispelling wind and removing dampness, removing nebula to improve the visual acuity.

Indication. Dyspepsia due to the accmulation of dampness, wind-cold, dampness arthralgia syndrome, swelling pain in the loins and legs, and night blindness.

Atrophic Debility of Bones

Symptoms. Lassitude in the waist and knees, inability to stretch the knee straight, atrophic and flaccid muscles of the lower limbs, difficult in movement, etc.

Pathogenesis. Mainly from heat of Kidney-qi or impairment of the kidney by pathogenic heat, exhaustion of genital essence and insufficiency of marrow due to withered bone.

Therapeutic Principle. Tonifying the kidney and supplementing essence, nourishing yin to eliminate heat, etc.

Atrophic Rhinitis

Symptoms. Constant dripping of stinking and bloody discharge from the nose, headache and dizziness, often seen in nasal sinusitis.

Pathogenesis. Mostly caused by prolonged past-recovery rhinorrhea.

Attack by Pestilent Factors

Symptoms. A kind of apoplectic stroke, deadly cold hands and feet, sudden mental confusion, incoherent speech, coma, trismus.

Pathogenesis. Attack of filthiness or evil-qi.

Therapeutic Principle. Awake the patient from unconsciousness with fragrant drugs.

Attack by Pestilent Factors during Pregnancy

It refers to the pregnant woman is attacked by sudden and severe pain in the heart and abdomen.

Pathogenesis. Exposure to pathogenic factors.

Therapeutic Principle. Strengthening the body resistance and preventing abortion.

Attacking Pathogens before Tonifying

It refers to a therapeutic method, e.g. a therapy to attack the pathogenic factors first and then giving tonic for recuperation.

Attack of Pestilent Factors

Symptoms. Sudden loss of consciousness with cold limbs.

Pathogenesis. Affection by noxious factors or pathogenic factors.

Attack of Water and Cold on the Lung

Symptoms. Cough with asthma, thin and whitish sputum, dyspnea, accompanied by fever and aversion to cold.

Pathogenesis. The lung is attacked by pathogenic cold and dampness, which make excessive fluid flowing upward, leading to obstruction of the lung-qi.

Attack of Water Pathogen

Symptoms. Borborygmus and diarrhea, palpitation and short breath, inability to lie on one's back and cyanosed lips, etc.

Pathogenesis. Water pathogen running down into the stomach and intestines and invading upward the heart and lung.

Therapeutic Principle. Clearing the lung and inducing diuresis.

Attack on Heart by Retained Fluid

Symptoms. Palpitation and dyspnea, general edema, usually seen in heart failure.

Pathogenesis. Retained fluid in the body which flows upward and leads to the disorder of the heart due to yang insufficiency of both the spleen and the kidney.

Attack on Taiyang Meridians by Wind

One of the two types of Taiyang Meridians syndromes. Taiyang Meridians refer to small Intestine Meridian, and Bladder Meridian.

Symptoms. Fever and sweating, aversion to wind and slow pulse.

Therapeutic Principle. Regulating the nutrient and superficial defensive system, dispelling wind and relieving the muscles.

Attribute of Five Flavors

A drug has five flavors that enter five zang organs. The sour, bitter, sweet, pungent, and salty are accessible to the liver, heart, spleen, lung, and kidney respectively. According to drug attributes diseases can be treated.

Aucklandia Root

It is the root of Aucklandia lappa Decne (Compositae).

Effect. Promoting flow of qi circulation, regulating the spleen and stomach and alleviating pain.

Indication. Abdominal distention and pain due to stagnation of qi in the spleen and stomach, belching, nausea, vomiting, anorexia, borborygmus, diarrhea, cholecystalgia, jaundice, etc.

Auditory Hallucination

Mostly found in patients with alienated disease.

Pathogenesis. Depression of qi generating the fire and phlegm forming due to the scorching of body fluid, leading to the phlegm-fire disturbing mental activity.

Aural Distention

Symptoms. Intra-aural distention and subjective sensation of obstruction, heaviness sensation in head, conjunctive congestion, etc.

Pathogenesis. Invasion of pathogenic wind-cold and obstruction of meridian-qi.

Therapeutic Principle. Dispelling wind to clear away heat and dispersing pathogenic factors to clear the aural passage and orifice.

Aural Itching

Symptoms. Itching in the ear, or even unbearable tickling in the serious case.

Pathogenesis. Mostly caused by invasion of wind with damp-heat and pathogenic toxin interspersed on the aural skin and muscle.

Therapeutic Principle. Dispelling Pathogenic wind to relieve itching.

Aurale Sore

Symptoms. Reddish swelling in the external auditory canal.

Pathogenesis. Upward flowing and steaming of damp-heat from the liver and gallbladder.

Therapeutic Principle. Clearing away heat from the liver and gallbladder, eliminating dampness and subduing swelling.

Auricle Erosion

Symptoms. The auricle ulcer with reddish erosion.

Pathogenesis. Damp-heat in the Liver Meridian.

Therapeutic Principle. Removing damp-heat from the liver and gallbladder.

Auricular Fistula

It refers to a fistula in the postauricular region, often with discharge of clear and thin pus; as a result, the opening of a fistulous orifice stays unhealed for a long time.

Therapeutic Principle. Consists mainly in operating on the local part.

Auscultation and Olfaction

One of the four examination methods, consisting of listening and smelling. The doctor can diagnose the clinical status by listening to abnormal voices and sounds from the patients and by smelling odour of the diseased body.

Autumn-dryness Disease

Symptoms. Cough and less phlegm, dry mouth and throat, dryness of skin.

Pathogenesis. Pathogenic dryness in autumn that can be divided into warm-dryness syndrome and cool-dryness syndrome.

Therapeutic Principle. Wetting dryness, therapy according to the different symptoms.

Autumn Elaeagnus Fruit

The root, leaf, and fruit of Elaeagnus pungens Thunb. (Elaegnaceae).

Effect. Clearing away heat, promoting diuresis and arresting bleeding.

Indication. Cough, diarrhea, dysentery, stranguria, metrorrhagia and metrostaxis, leukorrhagia, etc.

Auxiliary Manipulations

It refers to some cooperative manipulations applied in the needling process to determine certain points, help insertion and withdrawal of the needle, and regulate the needling sensation.

Aversion of Five-Zang Organs

It refers to that the five-zang organs are apt to be impaired by pathogenic factors, e.g. the heart, lung, liver, spleen, and kidney, averse to heat, cold, wind, dampness and dryness respectively.

Aversion of Liver to Wind

According to TCM the liver is called the organ of wind and wood. The function of the liver is ascending qi and its qi is related to wind. Some syndromes, such as wind stroke syndrome in old people, infantile convulsion rheumatism, numbness, itching, spasm, and epilepsy are usually seen in diseases of the liver.

Aversion of Lung to Cold

The lung is most vulnerable to direct attack of cold, easily impair yang-qi as external defence and is stagnated in the lung, thus resulting in all kinds of syndromes.

Aversion to Cold

A symptom referring to fear of cold.
Pathogenesis. Stagnation of pathogenic factors in the exterior of the body, or weakness of defensive energy.

Aversion to Cold due to Phlegm Retention

Symptoms. Fear of cold all over the body or only in the back, poor appetite, heavy limbs, etc.
Pathogenesis. Phlegm in the thoracic diaphragm preventing yang-qi from passing.
Therapeutic Principle. Activating yang and resolving phlegm.

Aversion to Food

Referring to anorexia.

Pathogenesis. Impairment of the spleen and stomach due to improper diet.

Aversion to Heat

A syndrome referring to fear heat.
Pathogenesis. Exopathogen, or hyperactivity of fire due to yin deficiency, and stomach-heat, etc.

Aversion to Wind

Referring to fear of wind.
Pathogenesis. Exogenous pathogenic factors which attack defensive system.
Therapeutic Principle. Expelling wind and relieving exterior syndrome.

Avoidance of Eating Cereals

A term in Qigong. Some practitioners practise Qigong to such an extent that they are able to avoid eating cereals for some time, only drinking a little water to maintain life activity.

Avoidance of Looking and Listening

A term in Qigong. In Qigong practice, it is necessary to droop the eyelids and concentrate the mind on the lower abdomen by "inward vision" at Dantian to achieve the aim of concentrating mind-will to practise without any disturbance from external things and sound.

Avoiding Invigorator in Treating Excess Syndrome

It refers a principle of administering drugs.
The invigorator is not allowed treating an excess syndrome, lest invigorator should make the syndrome more excessive.

Avoiding Purgation in Treating Deficient Syndrome

It refers a principle of administering drugs.
The purgation is not allowed treating a deficient syndrome, lest purgation should impair primordial qi badly and make the syndrome more deficient.

Axillary Balm Herb

It is the whole herb of Melissa axillaris (Benth) Bakh. f. (Labiatae).

Effect. Clearing away heat and removing toxic substances.

Indication. Numbness due to wind-dampness, hemoptysis, epistaxis, cutaneous pruritus, sores, rashes, metrostaxis, leukorrhea, etc.

Axillary Choerospondias Fruit

It is the dried fruit of Choerospondias axillaris (Roxb.) Burtt et Hill (Anacardiaceae).

Effect. Promoting flow of qi and blood circulation, nourishing the heart and tranquilizing the mind.

Indication. Stagnancy of qi and blood stasis, obstruction of qi in the chest, palpitation with shortness of breath, irritability, etc.

Aztec Marigold Flower

It is the capitulum of Tagetes erecta L. (Compositae).

Effect. Calming the liver to stop endogenous wind, clearing away heat and removing phlegm.

Indication. Dizziness, giddiness, acute conjunctivitis, infantile convulsion, common cold with cough, acute mastitis, etc.

B

Babylon Weeping Willow Flower

It is the flower of Salix babylonica L. (Salicaceae).

Effect. Removing pathogenic wind, inducing diuresis, ceasing bleeding and dissipating blood stasis.

Indication. Wind edema, jaundice, hemoptysis, hematemesis, hemafecia, stranguria complicated by hematuria and amenorrhea in women.

Babylon Weeping Willow Leaf

It is the leaf of Salix babylonica L. (Salicaceae).

Effect. Removing toxic materials, clearing away heat, enhancing skin eruption, inducing diuresis.

Indication. Small pox and rash without adequate eruption, cloudy urine, boils, furuncles and swellings and toothache.

Babylon Weeping Willow Root

It is the root or fibrous root of Salix babylonica L. (Salicaceae).

Effect. Enhancing diuresis, treating stranguria, releasing wind and dampness.

Indication. Stranguria, gonorrhea, edema, jaundice, pain caused by pathogenic wind-dampness and impetigo.

Babylon Weeping Willow Twig

It is the branch of Salix babylonica L. (Salicaceae).

Effect. Removing pathogenic wind, enhancing diuresis, relieving pain and expelling swelling.

Indication. Pain caused by pathogenic wind-dampness, stranguria, gonorrhea, dysuria, furuncles and gum swelling.

Back Marasmus

Referring to a syndrome of emaciation and prominent backbone. The diagnosis and treatment of the syndrome should be in accordance with the principle of the therapy of the main disease.

Back Middle Meridian

Referring to one of the eight extra meridians. Starting at the perineum, running upward along the midline of the spinal column to the back of the neck, turning anteriorly over the top of the head and ending at the middle of the upper gum on the face. The Back Middle Meridian governs the yang meridians of the body.

Back Rigidity

Symptoms. Failure to bow forward of the body.

Pathogenesis. Attack of wind pathogen, stagnation of dampness or insufficiency of the kidney-qi, leading to spasm of muscles of vertebrae.

Back-shu Meridian

Referring to the back meridian, linking yang-shu organs. The Bladder Meridian is called Back-shu Meridian also because it is in charge of the Back-shu points of the zang-fu organs.

Back-shu Points

1. Referring to a name of a group of classified meridian acupuncture points, the points into which the meridian qi of zang and fu organs infuse at the back. All of them are located at the first sideline of the Bladder Meridian in the dorsolumbar region. Diseases related to zang or fu organs frequently lead to ab-

normal reactions such as tenderness or sensitivity at those points. These points therefore help in diagnosis and treatment.

2. Referring to a general term for all the meridian acupuncture points on the back.

Bafeng (Ex-LE 10)

It is a set of extra acupuncture points.

Location. At the junction of the red and white skin proximal to the margin of the webs between each two neighboring toes, on both left and right sides, eight points in all.

Indication. Headache, toothache, snake-bite, redness and swelling at the dorsum of foot, numbness of toes, etc.

Method. Puncture 0.3 cun obliquely up-wards or prick, till bleeding, moxibustion is applicable.

Bahua (Ex-B)

It is a set of extra acupuncture points.

Location. On the body back, take 1/4 of the distance between the two nipples as the side of an equilateral triangle, place the vertex angle on Dazhui (GV 14) point, and the base side is horizontal. The two points are at the tips of the two basal angles. Move the triangle down and place the vertex angle on the midpoint between the above two points, another two points at the basal angles of this triangle. Move the triangle downward another two times, and you will get four more points. All eight points are called Bahua, the upper six called Liuhua (Ex-B).

Indication. General weakness, emaciation, painful joints, night sweating, cough, etc.

Method. Perform moxibustion 3-7 moxa cones or 5-15 minutes with warming moxibustion.

Baichongwo (Ex-LE 3)

Referring to an extra acupuncture point.

Location. 3 cun above the medial superior corner of the patella of the thigh while the knee flexed, i.e. 1 cun above Xuehai (Sp 10).

Indication. Rubella, eczema, cutaneous pruritus, sores on the lower body.

Method. Puncture perpendicularly 1-1.5 cun. Perform moxibustion 3-7 moxa cones or 5-15 minutes with warming moxibustion.

Baihuanshu (B 30)

A meridian acupuncture point.

Location. On the sacrum, at the level of the 4th posterior sacral foramen, 1.5 cun lateral to the median sacral crest.

Indication. Leucorrhea, hernia, emission, irregular menstruation, lumbocrural pain.

Method. Puncture perpendicularly 1-1.5 cun. Perform moxibustion 3-7 moxa cones or 5-15 minutes with warming moxibustion.

Baihui (GV 20)

A meridian acupuncture point.

Location. On the head, 7 cun directly above the midpoint of the posterior hair-line, or at the midpoint of the line connecting the apexes of both ears.

Indication. Headache, dizziness, palpitation due to fright, amnesia, epilepsy, hysteria, tinnitus, stuffy nose, proctoptosis, hemorrhoid, diarrhea.

Method. Puncture 0.5-0.8 cun horizontally. Perform moxibustion 4-5 moxa cones or 5-10 minutes with warming moxibustion.

Baikal Skullcap Root   ✿ B-1

It is the root of Scutellaria baicalensis Georgi (Labiatae).

Effect. Removing heat and dampness, purging fire, eliminating toxic substances, ceasing bleeding and preventing abortion, lower the blood pressure.

Indication. Damp-heat dysentery, jaundice, heat stranguria, suppurative infections on the skin, cough due to heat in the lung; epidemic febrile diseases with high fever, dire thirst; excessive fetal movement due to the attack of pathogenic heat; hematemesis, hemafecia, metrorrhagia, metrostaxis, etc.

Bailao

An extra acupuncture point.
Location. 2 cun above Dazhui (GV 14) and 1 cun lateral to the posterior midline.
Indication. Scrofula.
Method. Perform moxibustion.

Baked Ginger

It is the baked ginger till it gets slight dark on the surface and brown inside.
Effect. Warming the meridians and ceasing bleeding.
Indication. Bleeding due to cold of deficiency type, such as hematemesis, hemafecia, metrorrhagia, metrostaxis, etc.

Baldness

Symptoms. Complete loss of hair.
Pathogenesis. Poor nourishing of the hair resulting from malnutrition after disease and delivery, or excessive worry and anxiety, yin deficiency and insufficiency of blood.
Therapeutic Principle. Nourishing the kidney, yin and the blood.

Balsam Pear Moxibustion

Referring to one type of indirect moxibustion.
Method. Putting a slice of a raw balsam pear on the sore and a burning moxa cone on the balsam pear.
Indication. Carbuncle.

Bamboo Juice

It is the juice obtained from the baked bamboo stem of Bambusa tuldoides Munro, and Phyllostachys nigra (Lodd.) Munro var. henonis (Mitf.) stapt ex Rendle (Gramineae).
Effect. Removing pathogenic heat and phlegm.
Indication. Accumulation and obstruction of phlegm resulting from the lung-heat,

heat cough with thick phlegm, apoplexy, epilepsy, etc.

Bamboo Leaf

It is the leaf of Phyllostachys nigra (Lodd.) Munro var. henonis (Mitf) Stapt ex Rendle (Gramineae).
Effect. Relieving heat, restlessness, enhancing the production of body fluid and diuresis.
Indication. Restlessness and thirst resulting from febrile disease, infantile convulsion, excessive heart-fire, canker sores in the mouth, scanty dark urine, heat stranguria, etc.

Bamboo Needle

Referring to puncturing with a bamboo chopstick to cause bleeding, or to use as a fire needle. In recent years, seven sewing needles are horizontally put at the end of a bamboo chopstick to percuss the skin as a cutaneous needle.

Bamboo Shavings

It is the intermediate part of the bamboo stem of Bambusa tuldoides Munro, and Phyllostachys nigra (Lodd.) Munro var. henonis (Mitf) stapf ex Rendle (Gramineae).
Effect. Removing heat-phlegm, restlessness and vomiting.
Indication. Cough because of the lung-heat, cough with yellow and thick sputum, vexation, restlessness and vomiting resulting from stomach-heat.

Bamboo Shoots

It is the young plant of Phyllostachys nigra (Lodd). Murro var. henonis (Mitt.) Stapf ex Rendle (Gramineae).
Effect. Ceasing phlegm.
Indication. High fever, headache, dizziness during pregnancy, palpitation resulting from fright, infantile convulsion, etc.

Baohuang (B 53)

A meridian acupuncture point.

Location. On the buttocks, the level of the 2nd posterior sacral foramen, 3 cun lateral to the median sacral crest.

Indication. Borborygmus, abdominal distention, pain along spinal column, dysuria and constipation, pudendal swelling.

Method. Puncture 0.8-1 cun perpendicularly. Perform moxibustion 3-7 moxa cones or 5-15 minutes with warming moxibustion.

Baomen and Zihu (Ex-CA)

Two extra acupuncture points.

Location. 2 cun to the left and right of Guanyuan (CV 4).

Indication. Female sterility, vaginal bleeding during pregnancy, abdominal pain, dystocia, leukorrhea, etc.

Method. Puncture perpendicularly 1-1.5 cun. Perform moxibustion 3-5 moxa cones or 5-15 minutes warming moxibustion. Contraindicated in pregnancy.

Basis of Acquired Constitution

Referring to the spleen and the stomach. Both provide the body with the substance and energy to keep the vital activities by the digestion, absorption, and transportation of food.

Basket Fern

It is the thick stem of Dryopteris crassirhizoma Nakai (Aspidiaceae), the rhizome and leafstalk of Lunathyrium acrostichoides (Sw.) Ching (Athyriaceae), Woodwardia unigemmata (Makino) Nakai, Osmunda japonica Thunb. (Blechnaceae).

Effect. Killing parasites, removing heat and toxic materials, and ceasing bleeding.

Indication. Various kinds of parasites in the intestines, common cold caused by wind-heat, maculae, eruptions, mumps, epistaxis, hematemesis, hemafecia, metrorrhagia, metrostaxis, etc.

Bathing Face with Foulaged Hands

Referring to one of self-manipulation.

Operation. Warm up both hands through rubbing, keep the palms close to the forehead immediately and scrub down to the chin with force for about 10 times.

Function. Calming the mind and reinforcing fitness and health.

Indication. Insomnia and dreamful sleep.

Batryticated Silkworm

It is the rigidified larval worm of Bombyx mori L. (Bombycidae), which died due to the infection of batryticated bacterium before spitting silk.

Effect. Removing calm the endopathic wind to arrest convulsion alleviating pain, removing phlegm and resolving masses.

Indication. Spasm and clonic convulsion, such as infantile convulsion, epilepsy, etc.; headache caused by wind-heat, bloodshot, swollen and painful eyes, sore throat, scrofula, etc.

Baxie (Ex-UE 9)

It refers to a set of extra acupuncture points.

Location. Four points on the dorsum of each hand, at the junction of the red and white skin behind the margin of the webs between fingers when a loose fist is made, both left and right sides, eight in all.

Indication. Numbness and pain of fingers, headache, stiff neck, sore throat, toothache, eye diseases, malaria, snakebite, etc.

Method. Puncture obliquely 0.3-0.5 cun or prick to cause little bleeding. Moxibustion is applicable.

Bazhuixia (Ex-B)

Referring to an extra acupuncture point.

Location. On the posterior midline, in the depression below the spinous process of the 8th thoracic vertebra.

Indication. Malaria.

Method. Puncture obliquely 0.5-1 cun. Perform moxibustion 3-5 moxa cones or 5-10 minutes with warming moxibustion.

Bean Curd

It is the processed product obtained from the seed of Glycine max (L.) Merr. (Leguminosae).

Effect. Adjusting yin, the stomach, enhancing the production of the body fluid, moistening, removing heat, detoxicating.

Indication. Bloodshot eyes, diabetes, chronic dysentery with frequent relapse.

Beat the Heavenly Drum

Referring to a massage manipulation.

Operation. Rub helixes with hands for several times, and then tight-press the two ears with the centers of palms and flick the occiput with the index, middle and ring fingers closed together for 30-40 times.

Function. Nourishing the kidney and removing heat.

Indication. Preventing tinnitus and deafness.

Bee Sting

Referring to an injury caused by a bee's sting.

Symptoms. In the slight case, localized red, swelling, heat and pain, but no body symptoms. In the severe case, localized flare, swelling, severe pain, or sore caused by infection, with dizziness, nausea, vomiting, etc.

Therapeutic Principle. For the slight case, no need to treat; for the severe case, externally and heat-clearing and detoxifying drugs used internally.

Beeswax

It is the wax secreted from Apis cerana Fabricius or Apis mellifera Linnaeus (Apidae).

Effect. Ceasing secretion, enhancing wound healing and regeneration of the tissue and removing pain.

Indication. Ulcer hard to healing, erosion of ecthyma, injury, burns and scalds, etc.

Behcet's Syndrome

Symptoms. Bloodshot eyes, blue canthus and ulceration of the oral cavity, throat, and anus and genitalia, accompanied by mental trance, sleepiness, restlessness all the time, poor appetite, etc.

Pathogenesis. Prolonged damp-heat and pathogenic germs.

Therapeutic Principle. Removing heat and drying damp, detoxicating and sterilizing.

Beijiazhongjian (Ex-B)

An extra acupuncture point.

Location. In the infraspinous fossa of the scapula bone, at the central point of a triangle formed by connecting the lateral, superior and inferior points of the scapula.

Indication. Manic-depressive psychosis.

Method. Perform moxibustion 3-5 moxa cones or 5-10 minutes with warming moxibustion.

Belamcanda Rhizome

It is the rhizome of Belamcanda chinensis (L.) DC. (Iridaceae).

Effect. Removing heat, detoxicating, relieving phlegm and sore-throat.

Indication. Swollen and sore throat, abundant accumulation of phlegm and fluid, cough caused by the lung-heat, dyspnea, scrofula, etc.

Below Belt

Generally referring to gynecological diseases, such as menstruation, leukorrhea, pregancy, and delivery since these diseases occur at the body parts below the belt.

Belpharospasm

Symptoms. Uncontrollable tic of the eyelid, the disease worsens when the patient either overworks, or overuses his eyes, or suffers from insomnia. However, it remits after he has a good rest.

Pathogenesis. Blood deficiency of the heart and spleen, or stirring up of endopathic wind of deficiency type.

Therapeutic Principle. Nourishing the heart, spleen, and blood to cease wind.

Belt Meridian

It is one of the Eight Extra Meridians. It starts below the hypochondrium and runs transversely round the waist and abdomen.

Beltleaf Primrose Flower

It is the flower of Primula vittata Bur. et Franch (Primulaceae).

Effect. Removing heat, relieving dampness, purging the liver fire and ceasing bleeding.

Indication. Infantile convulsion due to acute febrile disease, acute gastroenteritis and dysentery.

Bend Needling

Referring to an abnormal condition of the needle that was bent caused by some reasons during acupuncture. Rapid and forceful withdrawal may cause more pain of the patient, even break needles. For slightly bending needle, withdraw it slowly; for severely case, shake it gently and withdraw it carefully by following the course of bend.

Benshen (G 13)

A meridian acupuncture point.

Location. On the head, 3 cun lateral to Shenting (GV 24), 0.5 cun in the hairline of the midline of forehead.

Indication. Headache, vertigo, epilepsy, infantile convulsion, stiffness and pain of the neck and nape, pain in the chest and hypochondrium, apoplexy and unconsciousness.

Method. Puncture horizontally 0.5-0.8 cun. Perform moxibustion 1-3 moxa cones or 3-5 minutes with warming moxibustion.

Benzoin

It is the dried resin of Styrax tonkinensis (Pierre) Craib ex Hart. (Styracaceae).

Effect. Wake patient from consciousness and eliminate phlegm, enhancing circulation of qi, reinforcing blood circulation and removing pain.

Indication. Phlegm syncope, apoplexy, stagnation of qi, sudden syncope, coma, pain in the chest and abdomen, postpartum bruise and infantile convulsion.

Berberis Root

It is the root and branch of Berberis amurensis Rupr.; Berberis poiretii Schneid. or Berberis thunbergii DC. (Berberidaceae).

Effect. Removing heat, relieving dampness, purging sthenic fire and detoxicating, lower blood pressure.

Indication. Acute enteritis, dysentery, jaundice, scrofula, pneumonia, conjunctivitis, boils, metrorrhagia, metrostaxis, hypertension, leukopenia etc.

Beriberi

Symptoms. Myosthenia of lower limbs, difficulty in walking.

Pathogenesis. Invasion of wind-wet, or impairment caused by a rich, fatty diet, leading to an accumulation of dampness and producing heat, the damp-heat flowing downward to the lower limbs.

Beriberi Damp-heat

Symptoms. Pain all over the body, swelling and pain in the lower part of the legs and feet, reddish and swollen feet and knees with pyogenic infection and ulcerous disease of skin, endless pus leading to pain or itches, etc.

Pathogenesis. Due to the damp and heat.

Therapeutic Principle. Removing damp-heat and detoxifying.

Betel Pepper Fruit-spike

It is the fruit-spike of Piper betle L. (Piperaceae).

Effect. Warming the middle-warmer to ease upset of the stomach and spleen, removing masses and eliminating phlegm.

Indication. Cold pain in the chest and abdomen, vomiting, diarrhea, abdominal pain due to parasite, cough with dyspnea, etc.

Biandu (Ex-UE)

An extra acupuncture point.

Location. On the flexor aspect of the forearm, between the tendons of the long palmar muscle and radial flexor muscle of the wrist, approximately 4 cun above the crease of the wrist.

Indication. Enlargement of the inguinal lymph nodes.

Method. Puncture 0.8-1.5 cun perpendicularly. Perform moxibustion 3-5 moxa cones or 5-10 minutes with warming moxibustion.

Bigflower Ladyslipper Rhizome

It is the root, rhizome, and flower of Cypripedium macranthum Sw. (Orchidaceae).

Effect. Being good for enhancing diuresis, eliminating swelling, enhancing blood circulation, dissipating blood stasis, removing wind-dampness and pain.

Indication. Common edema, leukorrhea, stranguria, pain resulting from pathogenic wind-dampness, traumatic injuries, etc.

Bighead Atractylodes Rhizome   ⊛ B-2

It is the rhizome of Atractylodes macrocephala Koidz. (Compositae).

Effect. Tonifying qi and enhancing the spleen, removing dampness and enhancing diuresis, ceasing sweating and preventing abortion.

Indication. Poor appetite, loose stool resulting from deficiency of the spleen, epigastric and abdominal distention, phlegm retention, edema, incessant sweating caused by debility, threatened abortion, etc.

Bignay Chinalaurel Root

It is the root, leaf, and fruit of Antidesma bunius (L.) Spr. (Euphorbiaceae).

Effect. Increasing the production of body fluid to quench thirst, reinforcing blood circulation and detoxicating.

Indication. Thirst because of cough, traumatic injuries, and suppurative infections on the body surface.

Biguan (S 31)

A meridian acupuncture point.

Location. At the front side of the thigh and on the line linking the anteriosuperior iliac spine and the superiolateral corner of the patella, at the level of the perineum when the thigh is flexed, in the depression lateral to the sartorius muscle.

Indication. Paralysis of lower extremities, numbness of foot, pain in the lumbar muscles, muscular contraction leading to the failure of the muscle to flex and extend.

Method. Puncture perpendicularly 0.6-1.2 cun. Perform moxibustion 3-5 moxa cones or 5-10 minutes with warming moxibustion.

Bihuan (Ex-HN)

An extra acupuncture point.

Location. At the face, on the border between the highest point of the outward protruding spot of nasal ala and face.

Indication. Furuncle, brandy nose, etc.

Method. Puncture subcutaneously 0.3-0.5 cun or prick till bleeding.

Bijian (Ex-UE)

An extra acupuncture point.

Location. At the palmar side of the forearm, 5 transverse finger-widths above the middle point of the crease of wrist, and between the long palmar muscle and radial carpal flexor muscle.

Indication. Furuncle and sores.

Method. Puncture perpendicularly 0.5-1 cun. Perform moxibustion 3-5 moxa cones or 5-10 minutes with warming moxibustion.

Bijiaoezhong (Ex-HN)

An extra acupuncture point,

Location. In the depression slightly above the highest part of the nasal bone.

Indication. Epilepsy opisthotonus, apoplexy, dreaminess, somnolence, jaundice.
Method. Puncture subcutaneously 0.3-0.5 cun. Moxibustion if needed.

Biliu (Ex-HN)
An extra acupuncture point.
Location. Above Heliao (LI 19) at the midpoint of the right nostril.
Indication. Apoplexy, facial paralysis, stuffy nose, nasal discharge, rhinitis, prosopalgia, spasm, etc.
Method. Puncture obliquely 0.3-0.5 cun.

Binao (LI 14)
A meridian acupuncture point.
Location. At the lateral side of the arm, on the line linking Quchi (LI 11) and Jianyu (LI 15), 7 cun above Quchi.
Indication. Scrofula, spasmodic rigidity of the neck, pain in the shoulder and arm and eye diseases.
Method. Puncture perpendicularly 0.5-1 cun, or puncture obliquely upwards 0.8-1.2 cun. Perform moxibustion 3-5 moxa cones or 5-10 minutes with warming moxibustion.

Bingfeng (SI 12)
A meridian acupuncture point.
Location. At the center of the suprascapular fossa of the spine of scapula, directly above Tianzong (SI 11), in the depression when the arm is lifted.
Indication. Pain in scapular region, soreness and numbness of the upper limb.
Method. Puncture perpendicularly or obliquely 0.5-1 cun. Perform moxibustion 3-5 moxa cones or 5-10 minutes with warming moxibustion.
Notice. Do not puncture the needle towards the region above the supraclavicular fossa to avoid hurting the lung.

Birchleaf Pear Fruit
It is the fruit of Pyrus betulaefolia Bge. (Rosaceae).

Effect. Astringing the lung and anti-dysentery with astringents.
Indication. Cough and diarrhea.

Bird-Pecking Moxibustion
Referring to a type of moxa-stick moxibustion.
Method. With the burning end of a moxa stick over an acupuncture point, move it up and down in a way similar to the bird pecking to give the part for moxibustion a stronger but intermittent hot stimulation, no fixed distance between the moxa stick and the part to be performed moxibustion.

Bird-Pecking Needling
It is a needling method referring to the manipulation of needling by vertical pricking with a shallow depth but high frequency, similar to the pounding method but with a lighter force.

Bishizitou (Ex-UE)
An extra acupuncture point.
Location. In the palmar aspect, on the radial border of the forearm, 3 cun above the level with Taiyuan (L 9).
Indication. Jaundice.
Method. Perform moxibustion 5-7 moxa cones.

Bistort Rhizome   ❀ B-3
It is the rhizome of Polygonum bistorta L. (Polygonaceae).
Effect. Removing heat and detoxicating, releasing dampness, enhancing the subsidence of swelling.
Indication. Dysentery resulting from damp-heat pathogenic, diarrhea with purulent and bloody stool, tenesmus, skin and external diseases resulting from noxious heat, canker sores, edema, etc.

Bite by Rabid Dog
Symptoms. Headache and weakness, vomiting with less eating, and feeling tight in the throat, followed by mania, fear, difficulty in swallowing and breathing, and

hydrophobia. A few days later, paraplegia and platycoria, etc. might appear.

Pathogenesis. The bite by a rabid dog and the attacks of its toxin into the body.

Therapeutic Principle. Clearing away blood stasis with potent drugs to detoxicate, making timely complete debridement and injection of fabies vaccine.

Bitter Orange Flower

It is the flower-bud of Citrus aurantium L. var. amara Engl. (Rutaceae).

Effect. Smoothing the liver, adjusting the stomach and flow of qi.

Indication. Stuffiness and fullness in the chest, distending pain in the abdomen, vomiting and poor appetite.

Bitter Orange Immature

It is nearly ripe fruit of Citrus aurantium L. or Citrus wilsonii Tanaka and Poncirus trifoliata (L.) Raf (Rutaceae).

Effect. Reinforcing circulation of qi to alleviate stagnation in the middle-energizer and eliminating food stagnancy.

Indication. Abdominal distention and pain caused by stagnation of the spleen-qi and sinking of qi in the middle-energizer.

Black Carp

It is the meat of Mylopharyngodon piceus (Richardson) (Cyprinidae).

Effect. Nourishing qi and releasing dampness.

Indication. Beriberi with damp arthralgia syndrome.

Black Edema

Referring to a disease.

Symptoms. Serious swelling of the feet with the sunken trace while pressed, heavy and sore feelings in the waist, cold arms and legs.

Pathogenesis. The dysfunction of the kidney.

Therapeutic Principle. Promoting diuresis by warming yang.

Blacken Saussurea Herb

It is the whole herb of Saussurea nigrescens Maxim. (Compositae).

Effect. Reinforcing blood circulation, restoring menstrual flow, removing wind, dampness, and heat and enhancing eyesight.

Indication. Irregular menstruation, hectic fever because of the consumptive disease, eye diseases, etc.

Blackish Jaundice

Symptoms. Yellowish body without moisture, blue eyelids, blackish face, irritability, blackish faeces, contracture of the urinary bladder, etc.

Pathogenesis. Mostly owing to alcoholic jaundice and prolonged jaundice caused by sexual intemperance, deficiency and failure of the liver and kidney, and internal obstruction and stagnancy.

Therapeutic Principle. Reinforcing the body resistance, nourishing the liver and kidney.

Blackish Menstruation

Symptoms. Liquid with the color of black soybean coming from the vagina of a woman, ropy, dilute and often stinks, or continuous black bloody vaginal discharge or leukorrhea.

Pathogenesis. Mostly caused by weakness and blood exhaustion.

Therapeutic Principle. Regulating menstruation, nourishing blood and qi strengthening the spleen.

Black Measles

Symptoms. Purple-black dense rashes, high fever with spasm, unconsciousness, delirium, etc.

Pathogenesis. Repeated affection of pathogenic factors, deficiency of the body resistance, excessive measles toxin entering the nourishing system and pericardium, then impairing the liver.

Therapeutic Principle. Clearing heat from the ying system cooling the blood, calming the endopathic wind and inducing resuscitation.

Black Nightshade Herb

It is the whole herb of Solanum nigrum L. (Solanaceae).

Effect. Removing swelling heat, detoxicating and enhancing blood circulation.

Indication. Furuncle, subcutaneous swelling, erysipelas, traumatic injuries, edema and dysuria.

Black Sesame

It is the ripe seed of Sesamum indicum L. (Pedaliacene).

Effect. Nourishing the vital essence and blood, moistening and promoting laxation of the bowels.

Indication. Dizziness and dim eyesight resulting from the deficiency of the vital essence and blood, constipation resulting from deficiency of blood, insufficiency of body fluid and dryness of the intestines, etc.

Black Soybean

It is the seed of Glycine max (L.) Merr. (Leguminosae).

Effect. Strengthening blood circulation, inducing diuresis, releasing and toxication.

Indication. Edema with ascites, beriberi caused by noxious wind, jaundice, general edema, disease after childbirth due to affection of wind, trismus, suppurative infections on the skin.

Black Soybean Skin

It is the black seed skin of Glycine max (L.) Merr. (Leguminosae).

Effect. Nourishing blood and removing wind.

Indication. Dysphoria with smothery sensation caused by yin deficiency, night sweat, vertigo, headache, etc.

Bladder (MA)

An ear point.

Location. At the anterior and inferior border of the inferior antihelix crus.

Indication. Lumbago, sciatica, cystitis, enuresis, uroschesis and occipital headache.

Bladder being Responsible for Storage of Fluid

The bladder possesses the function of storing urine transformed by the body fluid. The body fluid stored in the bladder is transformed by the qi activities of the kidney-yang into two parts, the small part is transformed into qi to moisten zang-fu organs, and the large part is transformed into urine to be discharged from the body.

Bladder Distention

Symptoms. Fullness feeling in the lower abdomen, dysuria, etc.

Pathogenesis. Cold accumulation in the bladder.

Therapeutic Principle. Warming yang, transmitting qi and enhancing the circulation of water within the body.

Bladder Dysfunction

Symptoms. Frequent urination, urgent urination and pain in micturition or dysuria or retention of urine, or enuresis and even incontinence of urine.

Pathogenesis. Due to the dysfunction of the kidney.

Bleeding before Cupping

Referring to one of the cupping methods.

Manipulation. Blood-letting with a three-edged or cutaneous needle, followed by cupping, so as to withdraw a small amount of blood.

Indication. Soft tissue injury, sprain, pain of the shoulder and back, or lumbago resulting from pathogenic wind-dampness, etc.

Notice. Not to apply the method to patients with anemia or those susceptible to bleeding, or the positions where big blood vessels lie.

Bleeding Caused by Excessive Heat

Referring to a kind of blood trouble.

Symptoms. High fever, excessive thirst, dry stools, yellow urine, foul breath, bitter taste, etc.

Pathogenesis. Heat sufficiency in the lung and stomach.

Therapeutic Principle. Relieving heat from the lung and stomach, and cooling down the blood to cease bleeding.

Bleeding Caused by Impairment of Liver Meridian

Symptoms. Bleeding in bright red or dark black color, asthma with restlessness, flushed complexion, or fullness and pain in the hypochondrium, dysphoria with smothery sensation, etc.

Pathogenesis. Impairment of the liver by anger, the reversed liver-qi leading to blood disorder.

Therapeutic Principle. Adjusting qi and blood.

Bleeding from Distant Part

Symptoms. Bleeding after defecating, indicating the bleeding position being far from the anus. The disease should be carefully examined and treated differently from the common syndrome.

Bleeding from Gum

Pathogenesis. 1. Gingivitis due to excessive heat in the stomach. 2. Due to deficiency of the kidney-yin and burning in the interior of deficiency of fire, mostly without pain and swell.

Therapeutic Principle. For the former, removing heat and fire; for the latter, nourishing yin to reduce fire.

Bleeding from Infantile Navel

Symptoms. The navel bleeding after cutting off the umbilical cord for a long time.

Pathogenesis. Due to improper flow of the blood resulting from the excessive heat in the interior.

Therapeutic Principle. Cooling the blood and ceasing bleeding.

Bleeding from Nine Orifices

Symptoms. The bleeding from the mouth, nose, ears, eyes, urethra (including the vagina) and the anus.

Pathogenesis. Due to the affection of pathogen of epidemic disease, or poisoning, sudden fright, etc.

Therapeutic Principle. According to the disease, tonifying method for deficiency type and the method of purgation and reduction for excess syndromes.

Bleeding from Upper Orifices

Symptoms. Bleeding from nose, tooth, eyes, ears, single orifice bleeding in light case and orifices in severe case, etc.

Pathogenesis. The failure of qi to manage the blood circulation or bleeding resulting from pathogenic heat.

Therapeutic Principle. Regulating qi, and relieving heat from blood to cease bleeding.

Bleeding Resulting from Exhaustion of Qi

Referring to a morbid state of bleeding.

Symptoms. Menorrhagia, metrorrhagia and metrostaxis, hemafacia, fatigue, pale complexion, pale tongue, little fur.

Pathogenesis. Deficiency and sinking of qi, e.g. the deficiency of the spleen qi sinking, resulting from qi deficiency and inability to keep blood flowing within the blood vessels.

Blepharitis Ulcerosa

Symptoms. Ulcer growing on the eyelid, slight itching and swelling at the early stage, gradually leading to red ulceration, pus forming, or chill and fever alternatively.

Pathogenesis. Stagnancy of fire-toxin and upward attack of pathogenic heat.

Therapeutic Principle. Removing heat, swelling, and intense heat and detoxicating.

Blepharoptosis

Symptoms. Ptosis of the upper eyelid covering the pupil, difficulty in looking up, poor movement of the eyeball and double vision in serious cases.

Pathogenesis. Mostly caused by congenital defect, deficiency of kidney qi, accompanied by insufficiency of the spleen, affection by exopathogenic wind or due to trauma.

Therapeutic Principle. Reinforcing the spleen, replenishing qi, dispelling the wind and regulate the meridian.

Blin Conyza Herb

It is the whole herb of Conyza blinii Levl. (Compositae).

Effect. Removing inflammation, heat and detoxicating.

Indication. Otitis media, acute conjunctivitis, toothache resulting from pathogenic wind-fire, stomatitis, laryngopharyngitis, etc.

Blood Ague

Symptoms. Bleeding or hemafecia or start of menstruation from attack of ague.

Pathogenesis. The attack of ague.

Therapeutic Principle. Preventing the attack of ague, reinforcing blood circulation and ceasing bleeding.

Blood Arthralgia

Symptoms. Numbness of extremities, joint pain, etc.

Pathogenesis. Deficiency of qi and blood, or sleeping in the wind, or the invasion of wind-pathogens in perspiration result from labor, occlusion of blood and qi.

Therapeutic Principle. Adjusting qi and the nutrients and activating yang to remove arthralgia.

Blood as Mother of Qi

The blood is the material base of qi, which depends on it. Pathologically, when blood is deficient and hemorrhagic, qi is deficient, and exhaust, blood stasis leading to qi stagnation. Clinically, the method of invigorating qi is always used with adjuvant method of enriching blood. The method of promoting qi circulation is used with adjuvant one of promoting blood circulation to eliminate blood stasis.

Blood-cold

Symptoms. Lower abdominal pain or the mass in the abdomen, cold limbs, irregularity of menstrual cycle, cold pain in the lower abdomen, dark purple menstruation with blood clot.

Pathogenesis. Attack of pathogenic cold into the interior, or excess of yin-cold in the interior.

Therapeutic Principle. Warming the meridians, removing cold, and regulating blood circulation, and releasing blood stasis.

Blood Constipation

Symptoms. Often seen in the aged, parturients, protracted illness and trauma, etc.

Pathogenesis. Blood deficiency and loss of body fluid and the dysfunction of intestine, or blood stasis resulting from trauma and stagnation of qi.

Therapeutic Principle. Tonifying blood and loosing the bowel to remove constipation.

Blood Deficiency in Heart and Liver

It is a pathogenesis, referring to pathological status of blood deficiency as well as the deficiency of the heart and the liver.

Symptoms. Palpitation, amnesia, insomnia, dreamful sleep, dizziness, tinnitus, dull and pale complexion, dry eyes and hypopsia, numbness of the extremities scanty menstruation,

Pathogenesis. Both blood deficiency in the heart and the liver.

Therapeutic Principle. Tonifying the blood to nourish yin and invigorating the heart and liver.

Blood Depletion

It is a disease.

Symptoms. Amenorrhea.

Pathogenesis. Resulting from the depletion of reservoir of blood.

Therapeutic Principle. Nourishing blood and adjusting menstruation.

Blood Exhaustion

Symptoms. Pale face, losing hair, irritability, palpitation and shortness of breath, dysphasia, etc.

Pathogenesis. The insufficient congenital essence, over-strain, or severe chronic disease leading to impairment of the spleen and stomach, severe deficiency of qi and blood, impairment of zang-fu.

Therapeutic Principle. Nourishing qi, yin, blood, and the body.

Blood Fetus

It is a one of the symptom complex of false pregnancy.

Symptoms. Amenorrhea with a pregnancy-like abdomen.

Pathogenesis. Blood stasis.

Therapeutic Principle. Reinforcing blood circulation, removing stasis and adjusting menstruation.

Blood-heat

Symptoms. Hemoptysis, hematemesis, hematuria, hematochezia, etc.

Pathogenesis. Sudden excess of yang-qi, transformed into fire and attacking the blood system, resulting from dysphoria, overwork, anger, intemperance in sexual life.

Therapeutic Principle. Removing pathogenic heat from blood.

Blood-heat Amenorrhea due to Emaciation

Symptoms. Amenorrhea, flushed face with tidal fever, red tongue with little fur.

Pathogenesis. The emaciated figure, yin and blood deficiency and internal weakness and heat.

Therapeutic Principle. Nourishing blood, qi, and reinforcing yin and removing heat.

Blood-letting Puncturing and Cupping

Referring to a treatment method.

Indication. Neurosism, gastrointestinal neurosis, erysipelas, neurodermatitis, and acute or chronic soft tissue injury.

Method. Prick to bleeding with a three-edged needle or a thick needle, and then leading to the enhancement of the therapeutic efficacy of blood pricking technique.

Blood-letting Therapy

It is a therapeutic technique.

Indication. Tonsillitis, neurodermatitis, allergic dermatitis, acute sprain, heat-stroke, etc.

Method. Prick the superficial blood vessels till a small amount of blood comes out with a three-edged needle, a small eyebrow-like knife or a cutaneous needle.

Notice. Do not use the method in patients with a tendency to bleed or patients with angioma.

Blood Moving

Symptoms. Various kinds of bleeding, such as epistaxis, hemoptysis, hematemesis, hemafecia, hematuria, etc.

Pathogenesis. Pathogenic heat damaging collaterals to force blood reverse.

Blood Phase

1. Referring to the blood range. If a disease occurs in blood phase, mainly to treat blood, in the patient with deficiency of blood, to enrich and nourish the blood; in the blood-heat patient, to remove heat and cool the blood; in the patient with blood stasis, to promote blood circulation by removing blood stasis, etc.

2. Referring to the disease that woman suffer from amenorrhea followed by edema, to reinforce blood circulation and adjust menstrual flow.

Blood Pimple

Symptoms. Sudden flesh pimples with itching and pain all over and loss of appetite.

Pathogenesis. The disturbance of the blood system caused by internal excessive wind-heat.

Therapeutic Principle. Relieving heat from blood and ceasing the endogenous wind.

Blood Prostration

Referring to the pathological changes of collapse due to profuse hemorrhage.

Symptoms. Pale complexion, emaciation, dizziness, dim eyesight, cold limbs etc.

Pathogenesis. The congenital malnutrition, or anxiety and worry overstrain, intemperance in sexual life or deficiency of blood sea result from chronic bleeding.

Therapeutic Principle. Enriching blood and qi and ceasing bleeding.

Blood, Qi, Essence and Vitality

Referring to the human life origins from vital essence keeping qi and blood functioning and whose presentation is vitality. Vitality depends on qi, blood, and essence, which are the material bases, and is produced on the basis of the functional activities of zang-fu organs, which in turn, are affected by vitality. So, blood, qi, essence and vitality are indispensable in the human life activities.

Blood-red Euonymus Herb

It is the whole herb of Bulbophyllum radiatum Lindl. (Orchidaceae).

Effect. Removing wind, dampness, swelling, pain, pathogenic heat from blood and reinforcing blood circulation.

Indication. Epilepsy induced by terror caused by high fever, rheumatic arthralgia, numbness of the tetraplegia, painful swelling in the joints, subcutaneous swelling, sore throat and traumatic injuries.

Blood-red Iris Root and Rhizome

It is the rhizome and root of Iris sanguinea Donn. (Iridaceae).

Effect. Eliminating food stagnancy and enhancing diuresis.

Indication. Stomachache and abdominal pain.

Blood Retention

Symptoms. Delirium, fullness, distention and pain in the lower abdomen.

Pathogenesis. Stagnated blood with pathogenic heat accumulated in the lower-energizer.

Therapeutic Principle. Removing the pathogenic heat to eliminate stagnation.

Blood Retention caused by Phlegm Stagnation

It is divided into two kinds.

1. **Symptoms.** Fullness in the chest, alternatively fever and cold, fixed pain in affected part.
   Pathogenesis. Stagnated phlegm and blood stagnation, and the conflict of phlegm and blood.
   Therapeutic Principle. Eliminating phlegm after removing blood stasis or both methods together.
2. **Symptoms.** Fixed pain in affected area while pressing, haematemesis, epistaxis, black stool.
   Pathogenesis. The stagnation of qi resulting from the loss of blood, and production of phlegm after a long period, conflicting with blood.
   Therapeutic Principle. Removing phlegm and blood stasis.

Blood Retention due to Internal Injury

Symptoms. Spastic pain in the chest and hypochondrium or the lower abdomen.

Pathogenesis. Internal injury.

Therapeutic Principle. Warming and nourishing qi and blood, relieving stasis and enhancing blood circulation.

Blood-spitting

Symptoms. Spitting of saliva with blood.

Pathogenesis. Deficiency of the spleen, and failure of the liver to store blood, or insufficiency of the kidney fluid.

Blood Stasis

Referring to blood stasis in the body.

Symptoms. 1. Local stabbing pain at certain region and aggravated by pressing on at night; 2. pelidnoma and swelling on injured skin, with hard and fixed mass; 3. bleeding of caked and dark purple blood; 4. darkish complexion, squamous and dry skin, cyanotic lips and nails, dark purple tongue or with ecchymoses and petechiac and varicose veins under the tongue.

Pathogenesis. Unsmooth circulation or stagnation of blood and retention of blood in meridians or zang-fu organs, resulting from qi deficiency, qi stagnation, blood-cold, blood-heat and trauma.

Blood Stasis Amenorrhea due to Emaciation

Symptoms. Less amount of menstrual blood with deep-purple color, clotting, and gradually disappearing, emaciation and flushed face, dark-blue tongue with ecchymoses.

Pathogenesis. The emaciated figure, yin deficiency and blood stasis.

Therapeutic Principle. Nourishing blood, removing heat, regulating the flow of qi and resolving phlegm.

Blood Stasis due to Injury

Symptoms. For retention of blood in muscle and skin, swelling pain and cyanosis; for that in ying and defense, blood stagnation and fever; for that in chest and hypochondrium, fullness sensation and choking feeling; and for that in zang and fu, extravasated blood and blood lump.

Cause. Resulting from the escape and overflow of blood from meridians and retention of blood in body tissues caused by trauma, bearing or other external injury.

Therapeutic Principle. Reinforcing blood circulation, releasing blood stasis.

Blood Stasis due to Qi Stagnancy

Symptoms. Distention and pain, ecchymosis, and abdominal mass.

Pathogenesis. Owing to qi disorder, leading to the blockage of the blood flow, even the blood stasis.

Therapeutic Principle. Supplementing qi, reinforcing blood circulation and removing blood stasis.

Blood Stasis Inside

Symptoms. Local redness, swelling, pain, cyanosis, ecchymosis, dark purplish tongue, etc.

Cause. Owing to external injury, leading to bleeding from vessels and meridians, retention of extravasated blood within the body, abnormal flow of blood and qi, and accumulation of blood stasis, also leading to edema.

Therapeutic Principle. Reinforcing blood circulation, removing blood stasis.

Blood Stasis in the Chest

1. Referring to the yang syndrome of febrile disease marked by endless hematemesis and epistaxis, stashing in the upper-energizer.

   Symptoms. Distention, fullness, pain in chest and stomach, body fever, manic state, amnesia, dark stool and normal amount of urine.

   Pathogenesis. yang syndrome of febrile disease.

   Therapeutic Principle. Removing heat, cooling blood and eliminating stasis.

2. Referring to woman cases.

   Symptoms. Blood stasis and pain in the chest, involving rigidity in the chest and back, or prickly pain.

   Pathogenesis. Invasion of heat lasting for a long time without being cured.

   Therapeutic Principle. Adjusting blood circulation and removing blood stasis.

Blood Stranguria

Referring to the stranguria of hematuria, which includes two types.

1. **Symptoms.** For the excess type, difficulty and stabbing pain of micturition, dark red urine, sometimes with blood clot, dysphoria, yellow tongue fur, etc.

   Therapeutic Principle. Removing heat, treating stranguria, ceasing bleeding.

2. **Symptoms.** For the deficiency type, light red urine, slight pain and difficulty of micturition, lassitude in loin and legs, fatigue, pale tongue, etc.

   Therapeutic Principle. Nourishing yin, removing heat, regulating qi and ceasing blood.

Blood Vessel

Referring to the meridian through which the qi and blood circulate. It originates in the heart and depends on it.

Bloody and Purulent Stool

Symptoms. Passing stool with blood and pus.

Pathogenesis. Invasion of the stomach and the intestines by epidemic pathogenic summer-heat, damp-heat, or improper diet, obstruction of fu-qi, stagnation of blood and qi.

Bloody Cough Caused by Blood Stasis

Symptoms. Cough often with the smell of fish in the throat, coughing up purplish and blackish blood, lying only on one side; otherwise more severe cough and breathing shortly and sluggish complexion, blackish rim of the eyes, etc.

Pathogenesis. Blood stasis stagnating the lung collateral.

Therapeutic Principle. Reinforcing the blood circulation, eliminating blood stasis and ceasing coughing.

Bloody Goiter

Referring to one of the goiters.

Symptoms. Goiter with purplish red skin color with red veins and thread-like things on it.

Therapeutic Principle. Releasing heat, nourishing yin, softening hard masses and removing blood stasis.

Bloody Mass

Referring to one of the eight types of mass.

Symptoms. Lumbago preventing the patient from leaning backward and forward, and contracture and pain in the lower abdomen resulting from accumulation of qi. If accompanied by accumulation of pathogenic wind and cold in the vagina with an open cervical orifice of the uterus, and irregular menstruation, it will affect childbearing.

Pathogenesis. Unstrained diet, at the advanced stage of menstruation, damaging the zang-fu organs (viscera) and making the menstrual blood, instead of going downward, flow and remain in between the stomach and intestines to gang up with cold and heat, leading to formation of mass.

Therapeutic Principle. Regulating qi circulation and dissipating stasis.

Bloody Stool in Menstruation

Symptoms. Bloody bowel movements during menstruation.

Pathogenesis. Prefer to pungent diet, prolonged accumulation of stagnated heat and disturbance of vital meridian to force blood to flow freely.

Therapeutic Principle. Clearing away heat, detoxicating, and adjusting qi and blood.

Blue-black Stripe

Symptoms. Blue and purple-black collateral branches of the infantile index finger.

Pathogenesis. The serious pathogens accumulated in the blood vessels, symbolizing a dangerous syndrome.

Blue Plantainlily Flower

It is the flower of Hosta ventricosa (Salisb.) Stearn. (Liliaceae).

Effect. Reinforcing flow of qi and blood circulation and invigorating qi.
Indication. Female asthenia, metrorrhagia and leukorrhagia.

Blue Vitriol

It is the hydrous cupric sulfate formed from the oxided cupric sulfide mineral by decomposition, or the artificial hydrous cupric sulfate. ($CuSO_4 \cdot 5H_2O$).
Effect. For oral administration vomiting endopathic wind-phlegm and toxication; detoxicating, astringing dampness, curing carbuncle and relieving the necrotic tissue for external use.
Indication. Accumulation of wind-phlegm, sore throat, epilepsy, accidental poisoning, aphthae, etc.

Bluish Cataract

Symptoms. At the beginning, unremarkable discomfort, gradual cirrhosis of the eyeball, slight bluish pupil and contraction of visual field, eventually leading to blindness.
Pathogenesis. Yin deficiency of the liver and kidney.
Therapeutic Principle. Calming the liver to cease wind. External treatment is recommended.

Bluish Lips

Symptoms. Blue color of mouth and lips.
Pathogenesis. Less blood and spleen-cold syndrome or rage.

Bluish White

Symptoms. Distending pain of the eyeball, photophobia and lacrimation, the purplish-red swelling projection in the white near the margin of the black. Repeated attack, in serious case, results in blindness.
Pathogenesis. Mostly caused by fire stagnation and blood stasis that close in and fumigate the white.
Therapeutic Principle. Relieving pathogenic fire to regulate the circulation of qi or reinforcing the body resistance.

Blunt Needle

Referring to a needling tool, one of the Nine Needles of the ancient times. Clinically used to compress the meridians and points instead of entering the skin for dredging the collaterals and meridians, particularly suitable for those who are afraid of needling.

Blurred Head and Eye

Symptoms. Head dizziness and heaviness with blurred vision.
Pathogenesis. Retention of wind, dampness, heat and phlegm in the house of intelligence, and also due to the hyperactivity of liver-yang.

Blurring of Vision

Symptoms. Hypopiesia and blurred vision with no extraocular abnormality of the eyes.
Pathogenesis. Damp-heat and turbid phlegm upward and disturbing the facial orifice, or qi stagnation and blood stasis, or insufficiency of qi, blood and body fluid, leading to visual lustrelessness.
Therapeutic Principle. Eliminating phlegm, dredging the orifice and reinforcing blood circulation to eliminate blood stasis for the excess type. Reinforcing flow of qi and nourishing blood for the deficiency type.

Blurring of Vision Accompanied by Restlessness

Symptoms. Fullness in the chest and restlessness and blurred vision.
Pathogenesis. Disturbance of mental activity by pathogenic heat.

Boat-fruited Sterculia Seed
✿ B-4

It is the ripe seed of Sterculia scaphigera Wall. (Sterculiaceae)
Effect. Facilitating flow of the lung-qi, clearing the bowels and removing constipation.
Indication. Inflammation of throat and hoarseness in phonation, headache and conjunctival congestion due to the consti-

pation resulting from accumulation of heat, etc.

Body Acupuncture

It refers to the method of puncturing the meridian or extra acupuncture points at each part of the body for treating the diseases. It is versus auricular and scalp acupuncture, etc.

Body Fluid

1. Referring to the components of body fluid from water and food, and flowing to the skin and muscles with the qi of three-energizer, nourishing muscles and skin. Both sweat and urine are from the body fluid.
2. Referring to saliva.

Body Fluid and Blood from the Same Source

Referring to the close relationship between blood and body fluid both in the source and function. They both are gained from water and food, belonging to yin-liquid, and nourishing and moisturizing all parts of the body.

Bog Marshcress Herb

It is the whole herb of Rorippa islandica (Oed.) Borb. (Cruciferae).

Effect. Removing pathogenic heat and dampness, detoxication, enhancing diuresis, and subduing swelling.

Indication. Jaundice, edema, stranguria, sore throat, subcutaneous swelling scalds, burns, etc.

Boil

Symptoms. Local skin redness and swelling, burning pain, itching, pus and blood in rupture, etc.

Pathogenesis. The invasion of noxious pathogenic factor, and the transmission of the stagnated pathogenic factor into heat impairing the skin, muscle, qi and blood.

Therapeutic Principle. Eliminating pus, heat and detoxicating.

Boil of Meatus Acusticus Externus

Symptoms. Suppurative carbuncle on external auditory meatus, red swelling and pain.

Pathogenesis. Heat accumulation in the liver and stomach, flaring up of pathogenic fire, or affection of external wind heat and pathogenic toxin fumigating the ear.

Therapeutic Principle. Removing heat, pathogenic fire and toxin.

Boil of Tongue

Symptoms. Furuncle on the tongue with swelling and cracks and bleeding, ozostomia, constipation, etc.

Pathogenesis. Excessive heat in the heart and stomach or deficiency of qi.

Therapeutic Principle. Purging pathogenic fire and detoxicating. For deficiency of qi case, tonifying the kidney and clearing away fire.

Bone Exhaustion

Symptoms. Haggard face, tinnitus, pain with inability to raise limbs, severe toothache, difficulty in urination or rachiagia, darkish complexion and edema of face, etc.

Pathogenesis. Impairment of the kidney and insufficiency of marrow caused by withered bone.

Therapeutic Principle. Nourishing for therapy.

Bone-knitting with Poplar

Referring to one of bone-setting operations in ancient time. It is suitable for comminuted fracture and inability of connection resulting from defect fractured end. Poplar is used and embedded between both fractured ends as a bridge, for rejoining, regenerating, and reuniting of bones.

Bone Proportional Measurement

It refers to the method for locating the meridian acupuncture point, in which the proportional cun of width and length of any parts of the body are measured in accordance with the main superficial marks of the bones.

Bone-separating Pad

It is a pad made of paper or cotton, folded into a strip-shaped fixation pad, used to separate the ulna from the radius after reduction.

Bone Separation with Clipping Method

Referring to a therapeutic manipulation. It can be used for a reduction manipulation for double fracture of diaphysis, such as fracture of ulna and radius, tibia and fibula, and metacarpal and metatarsal bones, etc.

Method. The mantipulator clips the two bones oppositely from both sides with his fingers, in order to separate both fractured sections, then, directs them to each other in a way like a single fracture.

Bone-setting by Massage

Referring to a treatment of orthopedic and traumatological diseases by manipulation of massage, including eight manipulations of bonesetting that is touching, reuniting, holding, lifting, pressing, rubbing, pushing, and kneading.

Boor's Mustard Seed

It is the seed of Thlaspi arvense L. (Cruciferae).

Effect. Enhancing acuity of vision.

Indication. Conjunctive congestion with swelling, pain, and shed tears.

Borax

It is the crystal powder extracted from Borax.

Effect. Removing heat, detoxicating for external use and internally removing heat from the lung, eliminating phlegm.

Indication. Aphthae boil of the mouth and the tongue, pharyngitis, conjunctivitis, phlegm-fire, thick and yellow sputum, etc.

Borborygmus

It is divided into two types: deficiency and cold in bowels.

Symptoms. For the deficiency type, fullness in the abdomen; for patients with cold in the bowels, lienteric diarrhea.

Therapeutic Principle. For the former, reinforcing the spleen and replenishing qi. For the latter, warming the middle-energizer to remove cold.

Borneol

It is the crystalline compound derived by distilling the tree trunk of Dryobalanops aromatica Gaertn. f. (Dipterocarpaceae) and then cooling the distillate, or obtained from the processed sublimate of the leaf of Blumea balsamifera DC. (Compositae); or the synthetic borneol made from turpetine oil or camphor.

Effect. Waking the patient from unconsciousness, removing heat and pain, removing nebula to improve visual acuity.

Indication. Coma and excess syndrome of stroke caused by high fever and apoplexy; ulcers, sore throat, canker sores, eye diseases, etc.

Bottle Gourd Peel

It is the dried peel of lagenaria siceraria (Molina) Standl. var. depressa Ser. (Cucurbitaceae).

Effect. Enhancing diuresis and ceasing swelling.

Indication. Severe edema and ascites.

Bow-shaped Mass and Hypochondriac Mass

Symptoms. Strips of muscular mass projecting on each side of the navel, the mass is sometimes painful and sometimes not, is called bow-shaped mass. The mass in the hypochondria, not obvious but painful if touched, called the hypochondriac mass.

Pathogenesis. By improper diet, injury to the spleen and stomach, accumulation of cold and phlegm, and stagnation of qi and blood.

Therapeutic Principle. Adjusting qi flow, releasing stagnancy and the mass, reinforcing blood circulation.

Boxleaf Syzygium Root

It is the root or root bark of Syzygium buxifolium Hook et. Arn. (Myrtaceae).

Effect. Reinforcing the spleen, enhancing diuresis, removing asthma and blood stasis.

Indication. Common edema, traumatic injuries, scalds and asthma in children.

Boyangchi

Referring to a massage point.

Location. Equivalent to the Zhigou (TE 6) acupoint.

Operation. Kneading manipulation is often used.

Function. Being good at relaxing bowels, enhancing urination and removing headache.

Indication. Constipation, dysuresia and headache.

Branches of Twelve Regular Meridians

Twelve branches from the regular meridians, entering the chest and abdomen and passing up to the head.

Breakdown of Normal Physiological Coordination between Heart and Kidney

Symptoms. Dysphoria, insomnia, palpitation, spermatorrhea and lassitude in waist and knees.

Pathogenesis. Imbalance between the kidney-yin and the heart-yang due either to deficiency of the former or to excess of the latter.

Breaking of Muscle and Tendon

Symptoms. Local pain, ecchymoma and dysfunction.

Cause. Due to the external force and incised wounds causing broken muscles and tendons.

Therapeutic Principle. Local fixation or surgical operation.

Breaking of the Inserted Needle

Referring to accidental breaking of a needle in the body during acupuncture.

Cause. Due to the needle itself being impaired, too heavy manipulation while needling, or a sudden change of the patient's position.

Notice. Before needling, examine the needles carefully; during needling, avoid sudden and heavy manipulation; and advise the patient not to change his position.

Therapeutic Principle. If the broken part sticks out of the skin, remove it with fingers or forceps; if the broken part is completely under the skin, a surgical operation is necessary.

Breast Cellulitis

Referring to the pyogenic infective disease in the deep part of the breast.

Symptoms. The mass of the breast, hard and slightly painful, unchanged skin color, gradual enlarging, cold physique with feverish body.

Pathogenesis. The stagnation of liver-qi, the steaming of accumulated stomach-heat.

Therapeutic Principle. Relieving the depressed liver, removing the stomach-heat, toxins, hard masses, cutting open and draining for pus if necessary.

Breast Nodules Caused by Phlegm Turbidity

Symptoms. Besides the common symptoms of breast-nodules usually accompanied by vertigo, nausea, oppressive feeling in the chest and fullness in the gastric region, poor appetite and diarrhea, cough with sputum and salivation.

Pathogenesis. Mainly owing to melancholy and anxiety impairing the spleen and leading to the stagnation of phlegm in the collaterals of the breast.

Therapeutic Principle. Removing phlegm and the obstruction in the collaterals.

Breast Nodules caused by Yin Deficiency

Symptoms. Besides the common symptoms of breast nodules also tidal fever flush of zygomatic region, dizziness, tinnitus, pain in the back and waist, tiredness, etc.

Pathogenesis. Mostly due to yin deficiency of the liver and kidney, leading to failure to nourish the meridians.

Therapeutic Principle. Nourishing the liver and kidney.

Breast Swelling during Pregnancy

Symptoms. Distending pain in the woman's breast between the 7th and 8th month pregnancy.

Pathogenesis. Due to the liver-qi stagnation, blood stasis caused by qi stagnancy, impeded meridians and collaterals, and blocking of the mammary tube.

Therapeutic Principle. Smoothing the liver, adjusting the circulation of qi and removing heat.

Bright Complexion

It refers to the bright and shiny face. It can be seen in the edema patients. Due to retention of water within the muscles and skin.

Bright Red Tongue with Little Fur

It can be seen in the patient with yin deficiency syndrome.

Symptoms. Flushing of zygomatic region, dry throat, tidal fever, night sweat, insomnia and dreamful sleep.

Pathogenesis. Excessive fire due to deficiency of yin, and failure of insufficiency of both the stomach-qi and stomach-yin to produce fur.

Bright Red Tongue with Yellow and Thick Fur

It can be seen in the patient with interior heat syndrome.

Symptoms. High fever, flushed face, thirst, restlessness, hyperhidrosis, etc.

Pathogenesis. Excessive interior heat, full qi and blood in vessels of tongue body, exhaustion of body fluid.

Bristles

It is the hair of Sus scrofa domestica Brisson (Surdae).

Indication. Metrorrhagia and metrostaxis and scalds.

Broad Bean

It is the seed of Vicia faba L. (Leguminosae).

Effect. Nourishing the spleen and removing dampness.

Indication. Watery distention and food obstruction in diaphragm.

Broad Bean Flower

It is the flower of Vicia faba L. (Leguminosae)

Effect. Relieving heat from the blood and stopping bleeding.

Indication. Hemoptysis, hypertension, dysentery with blood stool, leukorrhea.

Broad Bean Shell

It is the seed coat of Vicia faba L. (Leguminosae).

Effect. Good urination and relieving dampness.

Indication. Edema, dysuria and inpetigo.

Broadleaf Common Valeriana Rhizome

It is the rhizome of Valeriana jatamansii Jones, and Valeriana officinalis L. var. latifolia Miq. (Valerianaceae).

Effect. Enhancing blood circulation flow of qi, removing cold and adjusting menstruation.

Indication. Gastric and abdominal pain resulting from attack of measles, vomiting, diarrhea, edema of the lung-qi, common cold resulting from wind-heat, irregular menstruation, cough resulting from internal injury caused by overstrain, etc.

Broadleaf Cudweed Herb

It is the whole herb of Gnaphalium adnatum (Wall ex. DC.) Kitam. (Compositae).

Effect. Removing heat and detoxicating.

Indication. Dysentery, infantile convulsion, aphthous ulcer, noxious carbuncles and traumatic bleeding.

Broadleaf Vetch Herb

It is the tender stem and leaf of Vicia amoena Fisch (Leguminosae).

Effect. Removing pain, wind, and dampness, enhancing blood circulation and relaxing muscles.

Indication. Pathogenic wind-dampness pain, traumatic injuries, infantile eczema of scrotum, etc.

Bromhidrosis

Symptoms. Particular odor of the sub-axillary sweat.

Pathogenesis. Mostly due to the stagnation of damp-heat in the interior, or by heredity.

Therapeutic Principle. Powders of tangerine and alum are used in the external treatment, removing heat and dampness.

Bronchial Wheezing

Symptoms. Rapid breathing with wheezy sound.

Pathogenesis. Owing to the damage of the lung-qi due to the latent summer-heat and impairment of the purifying and descending function of the lung.

Bronchial Wheezing Caused by Wind-phlegm

Symptoms. Laryngeal rale, tachypnea, dyspnea or even inability to lie on the back, etc.

Pathogenesis. Invasion of pathogenic wind into the lung, and phlegm, blocking the air passage, leading to adverse flow of the lung-qi.

Therapeutic Principle. Enhancing the dispersing function of the lung, removing wind phlegm and the adverse flow of qi.

Bronchial Wheezing of Cold Type

Symptoms. Shortness of breath, rale in the throat, stuffiness in the chest, cough with thin and sticky sputum, etc.

Pathogenesis. Attack of the lung by wind cold, cold fluid in the interior, obstruction of the phlegm in the respiratory tract.

Therapeutic Principle. Warming the lung, removing cold, phlegm and asthma.

Broomcorn Millet

It is the seed of Panicum miliaceum L. (Gramineae).

Effect. Tonifying qi and reinforcing the middle-energizer.

Indication. Diarrhea, morbid thirst, vomiting, hiccups, cough, stomachache, infantile thrush, scalds, etc.

Broom Cypress Fruit ⊛ B-5

It is the ripe fruit of Kochia scoparia (L.) Schrad. (Chenopodiaceae).

Effect. Removing heat, itching and enhancing diuresis.

Indication. Dysuria, dribbling and painful micturition; skin exudative dermatitis and pruritus.

Broomrape Herb

It is the whole herb of Orobanche caerulescens Steph. or Orobanche pycnostachya Hance (Orobanchaceae).

Effect. Nourishing the kidney and reinforcing the muscles and tendons.

Indication. Chills and pain in the waist and knees, impotence and seminal emission, etc.

Brown Sugar

It is the processed brown crystal produced from the stem liquid of Saccharum sinensis Roxb. (Gramineae).

Effect. Reinforcing the middle-energizer, calming the liver, enhancing blood circulation and removing blood stasis.

Indication. Lochiorrhea, dry mouth with vomiting, dysentery with bloody stool.

Brucea Fruit

It is the ripe seed of Brucea javanica (L.) Merr. (Simarubaceae).

Effect. Removing vegetation, heat, keeping from attack of malaria, curing dysentery and externally cauterizing, and detoxicating.

Indication. Ague, dysentery with bloody stool due to noxious heat, chronic diarrhea, furunculosis, verruca, clavus, etc.

Brygmus

Symptoms. Grinding of teeth during sleeping.

Pathogenesis. Due to pathogenic fire of the stomach and the heart, or parasites in children's abdomen.

Therapeutic Principle. Removing the stomach-heat, relieving intense fire and killing intestinal parasites.

Buckeye Fruit

It is the fruit of Aesculus chinensis Bge. or A. wilsonii Rehd. (Hippocastanaceae).

Effect. Smoothing the depressed liver and adjusting flow of qi, and enhancing the activities of the stomach.

Indication. Oppressed feeling and distending pain in the chest resulting from stagnation of the liver-qi and stomach-qi, abdominal distention and distending pain in the breasts, etc.

Buck Wheat

It is the seed of Fagopyrum esculentum Moench. (Polygonaceae).

Effect. Being good at the functional activity of the stomach, keeping the adverse qi flowing downward and eliminating food stagnancy.

Indication. Acute abdominal pain accompanied by vomiting and diarrhea, retention of food in the stomach.

Buerger Lespedeza Root

It is the root of Lespedeza buergeri Miq. (Leguminosae).

Effect. Removing exterior syndromes, phlegm, enhancing diuresis and blood circulation.

Indication. Exterior syndromes resulting from affection by wind-heat exo-pathogens, such as headache, cough, stranguria with turbid urine, metrorrhagia, metrostaxis and female abdominal pain resulting from blood stasis.

Bulang (K 22)

A meridian acupuncture point.

Location. On the chest, in the 5th intercostal space, 2 cun lateral to the anterior midline.

Indication. Chest pain, cough, asthma, vomiting, anorexia, acute mastitis.

Method. Puncture obliquely or along the skin 0.5-0.8 cun. Perform moxibustion 3-5 moxa cones or 5-10 minutes with warming moxibustion.

Notice. Deep insertion should be avoided for preventing the internal organs from injuring.

Bulging of Fontanel in Infant

Symptoms. For an infant, swelling fontanel like pile.

Pathogenesis. Eating milk improperly, sometimes hungry, sometimes full, or hot or cold, damaging the spleen and stomach and leading to incoordinated viscera and qi upward.

Therapeutic Principle. For soft and red due to heat, removing heat; for firm and hard due to cold, dispersing cold.

Bunge Hackberry Bark

It is the bark, trunk, or branch of Celtis bungeana B1. (Ulmaceae).
Effect. Removing cough and dispelling phlegm.
Indication. Chronic bronchitis.

Bur Beggarticks Herb

It is the whole plant of Bidens tripartita L. (Compositae).
Indication. Tracheal catarrh, laryngopharyngitis and dysentery.

Burmacoast Padauk Wood

It is the heartwood of Pterocarpus indicus Willd. (Leguminosae).
Effect. Eliminating swelling and removing pain.
Indication. Pyogenic infections and traumatic bleeding.

Burmann Cinnamon Bark

It is the bark of Cinnamomum burmannii (Ness) B1. (Lauraceae).
Effect. Warming the middle-energizer, removing cold and dispelling wind-dampness.
Indication. Abdominal distention, gastric and abdominal pain, rheumatic arthralgia, swelling carbuncles and traumatic injuries.

Burmann Sundew Herb

It is the whole herb of Drosera burmanni Vahl. (Droseraceae).
Effect. Detoxicating, removing infantile malnutrition, eliminating inflammation, the necrotic tissue and heat.
Indication. Dysentery, cough because of the lung-heat, sore throat, infantile dyspepsia and otopyosis.

Burning Moxibustion

Referring to a type of moxibustion.

Method. Scorching the skin at the acupoint directly, causing blister and suppuration.

Burns and Scalds

Symptoms. In the light case and superficial symptoms as local red swelling, heat, pain, blisters, anaphylactic feeling or putrefaction appear in part. In the severe case, the injury is big and deep, the pain vanishes and the skin is like leather, even fever, coma, dissociation of yin and yang.
Cause. Due to boiling water, flame, electricity, radioactive rays or chemical substances, etc.
Therapeutic Principle. In the slight case, burn adhesive plaster can be used for the external treatment. Replenishing the vital essence and removing heat, reinforcing yang-qi and rescuing emergent collapse, clearing up the ying system, removing heat from the blood and toxic substances for the severe case. For the deficient syndrome invigorating qi and enriching the blood.

Burnt Needle

It is a treatment method.
Method. Burn needle red, then puncture into points, suitable for interior cold syndrome of deficiency type, and for exerting pus in carbuncles.

Burong (S 19)

A meridian acupuncture point.
Location. On the upper abdomen, 6 cun above the center of the umbilicus and 2 cun lateral to the anterior midline.
Indication. Abdominal distention, vomiting, stomachache, poor appetite, cough, asthma, hematemesis, precordial pain, chest, back and hypochondriac pains.
Method. Puncture perpendiculary 0.5-0.8 cun. Perform moxibustion 3-5 moxa cones or 5-10 minutes with warming moxibustion.

Burreed Tuber

It is the tuber of Sparganium stoloniferum Buch-Ham. (Sparganiaceae).

Effect. Reinforcing blood circulation to eliminate blood stasis and adjusting flow of qi to remove pain.

Indication. Abdominal pain result from amenorrhea due to the stagnation of qi and blood stasis, masses in the abdomen, stagnation of qi result from retention of food.

Bush-cherry Seed

A name of herb medicine. It is the ripe seed of Prunus humilis Bge. or P. joponica Thunb. (Rosaceae).

Effect. Moistening the bowels, removing edema and constipation, and enhancing diuresis.

Indication. Constipation and edema.

Bush Cinquefoil Leaf   ⊛ B-6

It is the leaf of Potentilla fruticosa (L.) Rydb. (Rosaceae).

Effect. Removing summer-heat and the heart-fire, adjusting menstruation and reinforcing the stomach.

Indication. Dizziness caused by summer-heat, blurred vision, disorder of the stomach-qi and irregular menstruation.

Butterfly-bush Flower

It is the flower-bud of Buddleia officinalis Maxim. (Loganiaceae).

Effect. Removing heat from the liver, enhancing acuity of vision and eliminating nebula.

Indication. Bloodshot, swollen and painful eyes caused by the heat in the liver, photophobia, delacrimation, oculopathy, marginal blepharitis, etc.

Buttock (MA-AH)

It is an auricular point.

Location. At the lateral 1/3 of the inferior antihelix crus.

Indication. Pain of the buttock, lumbosacral pain, sciatica.

C

Cairo Morning-glory Herb
It is the root or stem leaf of Lporuoea cairica (L.) Sweet (Convolvulaceae).
Effect. Removing heat, detoxicating, relieving swelling and pain, inducing diuresis.
Indication. Cough caused by lung heat, sore throat, dysuria, hematuria, boils and pyogenic infections, etc.

Cake-separated Moxibustion
Referring to a kind of the separated moxibustion.
Method. Moxibustion of the medicated cake on the selected point or the affected part.
Indication. Stomachache caused by cold of deficiency type, vomiting, diarrhea, apoplexy, impotence and premature ejaculation.

Calamine
It is a natural ore Smithsonite (zinc carbonate) ($ZnCO_3$).
Effect. Enhancing acuity of vision and releasing nebula, dampness, and promoting tissue regeneration.
Indication. Redness of eyes, ulcerative marginal blepharitis, ulcer resistant to healing skin and exudative skin infections.

Callosity
Referring to the result of thickened, painful skin on the sole of the foot.
Symptoms. Thickened skin on the sole, pain when walking, and even difficult to walk.
Pathogenesis. Owing to the unfitness of shoes and socks, long time friction, leading to the stagnation of qi and blood, and loss of nourishment of the skin and muscle.
Therapeutic Principle. Soaking the foot with warm water and then apply a paste called Wumei Gao, foot repairing if needed.

Calomel
It is the mercurous chloride (Hg_2Cl_2) made by the method of sublimation with mercury, alum and salt, etc.
Effect. Externally, use for detoxicating and killing parasites; internally, enhancing diuresis and relaxing the bowels.
Indication. Scabies, tinea, syphilis, non-union of ulcers, watery distention, difficulty in urination and defecation.

Camereed Spiralflag Rhizome
It is the rhizome of Costus speciosus (Koen.) Smith (Zingiberaceae).
Effect. Enhancing diuresis and releasing edema.
Indication. Edematous swelling, gonorrhea, carbuncle swelling, malignant boil, etc.

Camphor
It is the branch, stem, root and leaf of Cinnamomum camphora (L.) Presl (Lauraceae), from which the camphor is extracted.
Effect. Releasing pain and dampness, killing parasites, and inducing resuscitation.
Indication. Scabies, tinea, toothache, traumatic injuries, loss of consciousness, etc.

Camphor-tree Fruit
It is the fruit of Cinnamomum camphora (L.) Presl (Lauraceae).

Effect. Removing pain, cold and dampness, enhancing circulation flow of qi.

Indication. Vomiting, diarrhea, abdominal pain resulting from cold in the stomach, poisoning swellings, etc.

Camphor-tree Leaf

It is the leaf of Cinnamomum camphora (L.) Presl (Lauraceae).

Effect. Removing pain, wind and dampness, and killing parasites.

Indication. Arthralgia due to pathogenic wind-dampness, traumatic injuries, scabies and tinea, etc.

Camphor-wood

It is the wood of Cinnamomum camphora (L.) Presl (Lauraceae).

Effect. Removing cold and dampness, enhancing blood and qi circulation.

Indication. Distending pain in the chest and abdomen, migratory arthralgia, scabies, tinea, traumatic injuries, beriberi, etc.

Canker Sore

Symptoms. Infantile perleche with white erosion, pain with a little swelling.

Pathogenesis. Mostly owing to the damp-heat going up from the spleen and stomach to the mouth and lips or by congenital toxin.

Therapeutic Principle. Detoxifying, removing damp and heat.

Canton Ampelopsis Root

It is the root or whole herb of Ampelopsis cantoniensis (Hook. et Arn) Planch. (Vitaceae).

Effect. Removing heat and detoxicating, dispersing wind and expelling exogenous pathogen.

Indication. Prevention of common cold osteomyelitis, acute lymphadenitis, acute mastitis, pemphigus, eczema, erysipelas, abscess, etc.

Canton Fairybells Root and Rhizome

It is the root and rhizome of Guangdong Disporum cantoniense (Lour.) Merr. (Liliaceae).

Effect. Removing heat, detoxicating, relaxing muscles and tendons, and activating the flow of qi and blood in the collaterals.

Indication. High fever, hectic or tidal fever resulting from consumption, rheumatic arthralgia, dysmenorrhea, carbuncles, cellulitis, sores, furuncles, traumatic injuries, etc.

Canton Salomonia Herb

It is the whole herb of Salomonia cantoniensis Lour. (Polygaleae).

Effect. Detoxicating, releasing pain.

Indication. Innominate swelling and pain, toothache and nebula.

Cape-gooseberry Herb

It is the whole herb of Physalis peruviana L. (Solanaceae).

Effect. Removing swelling, pain and heat, enhancing flow of qi.

Indication. Swollen and sore throat, cough, abdominal distention, hernia, etc.

Cape Jasmine Flower

It is the flower of Garaenia jasminoides Ellis. (Rubiaceae).

Effect. Removing heat from the lung and the heat from the blood.

Indication. Cough owing to the lung-heat and epistaxis.

Cape Jasmine Fruit

It is the ripe fruit of Garaenia jasminoides Ellis. (Rubiaceae).

Effect. Removing the pathogenic fire, relieving restlessness, inducing diuresis, removing heat from the blood and detoxicating.

Indication. Vexation and insomnia caused by febrile disease, oppressed feeling in the chest, coma, delirium, jaundice, heat stranguria.

Carambola Fruit

Iti s the fruit of Averrhoa carambola L. (Oxalidaceae).

Effect. Removing heat, enhancing the production of body fluid, inducing diuresis and detoxicating.

Indication. Cough owing to wind-heat, excessive thirst, erosion of the mouth, toothache and stranguria owing to the passage of urinary stone.

Carambola Leaf

It is the leaf of Averrhoa carambola L. (Oxalidaceae).

Effect. Enhancing diuresis and detoxicating.

Indication. Dysuria, pruritus owing to blood heat, subcutaneous swelling, scabies and tinea.

Carbuncle Complicated by Septicaemia

Symptoms. Dark and sunken heads of furuncle, stretching swelling, headache with chills and fever, chest tightness and dysphoria, nausea and vomiting.

Pathogenesis. Weakened body resistance and failure in removing pathogenic factors.

Therapeutic Principle. Removing heat and toxic material.

Carbuncle of Eyebrows

Symptoms. Black, hard, and painful swelling around the eyebrows and forehead, becoming carbuncle after ulceration.

Pathogenesis. Due to the noxious heat attacking the two meridians of the heart and the liver.

Therapeutic Principle. Removing intense heat and detoxicating.

Carbuncle of Leg

Symptoms. Large Carbuncle on the leg, unbearable pain.

Pathogenesis. Owing to sitting on damp ground in childhood, and the penetration of wind and cold dampness into the bone marrow.

Therapeutic Principle. Bundle it immediately with bundling drugs at the beginning, and Wutong Wan, Xingxiao Wan for oral administration.

Carbuncle on Coccygeal Region

Symptoms. Deep abscess appears at the tip of coccyx. At the beginning, it is like an air bladder of a fish, later the carbuncle becoming red, hard and painful. For the excess syndrome it has the flow of cheesy pus or fresh blood, for the deficiency syndrome it has the flow of diluted pus, both easily develop into fistula.

Pathogenesis. Owing to the deficiency of three yin and the multiple abscess resulting from phlegm-dampness of turbid qi in Back Middle Meridian.

Carbuncle on Dorsum of Foot

Symptoms. At the start, swelling and pain on the dorsum of foot, later becoming pustule and ulcerating.

Pathogenesis. Owing to downward flow of damp-heat, or long-standing blood stasis.

Therapeutic Principle. Reinforcing blood flow and removing blood stasis, heat and toxic material.

Carbuncle on Dorsum of Hand

Symptoms. Like prickles at the beginning, later painful, red, swelling and ulceration quickly.

Pathogenesis. Owing to the stagnancy of wind, fire and dampness in the three yang meridians.

Therapeutic Principle. Removing superficies syndrome through diaphoresis, and detoxicating.

Carbuncle on Palate

Symptoms. Difficulty in opening and closing the mouth, difficulty in stretching and protruding the tongue, red nose with nasal discharge, fever with chills.

Pathogenesis. Caused by the accumulation of heat pathogen in the tri-energizer.

Therapeutic Principle. Removing heat, detoxicating, evacuate pus with knife or needle if the pus is ripe.

Carbuncle on Shoulder

Symptoms. Serious, red swelling at the beginning, small carbuncles like apricots, while the large ones are like peaches.

Pathogenesis. Mostly due to the attack by pathogenic wind into the suture of bones and its retention with dampness to transform heat.

Therapeutic Principle. The treatment of external carbuncle is recommended.

Carbuncle on Sole

Symptoms. The pain of the Yongquan (K1) point along the kidney meridian in the center of the sole.

Pathogenesis. Owing to the deficiency and the affection of dampness of the kidney, and the stagnancy of damp-heat.

Therapeutic Principle. In the case of pain in the sole and the ankle, nourishing the kidney and removing dampness by diuresis; and sole pain of a fat person, removing heat, dampness and phlegm.

Carbuncle with Heads

The acute suppurative disease.

Symptoms. In the early phase, swelling blocks in the affected part, millet-like pus heads, red color, pain with fever. During ulceration, putrefaction on the surface of the carbuncle, like a honeycomb, fever. At the healing stage new muscle grows.

Pathogenesis. Mostly owing to the disharmony between nutrient system and defence system, the stagnation of qi and blood, the external affection of the six climatic conditions, the improper diet, the sexual strain, etc.

Therapeutic Principle. For the early phase and during ulceration, removing toxin heat, and enhancing diuresis, adjusting the nutrient. For the pus, cutting and draining the pus.

Carcinoma of Breast

Symptoms. Mammary masses, hardness without pain, no appreciable boundary, after ulceration, like a cauliflower with blood.

Pathogenesis. Caused by anger and anxiety, invasion of the hyperactive qi of the liver and the spleen.

Therapeutic Principle. Relieving the depressed liver resolving masses, tonifying qi and blood.

Cardiac Beriberi

One of critical cases in beriberi.

Symptoms. Beriberi with palpitation, dyspnea and vomiting, etc.

Pathogenesis. Mainly due to the pathogenic dampness, accumulation of excessive heat, invasion of the heart by pathogenic factors.

Therapeutic Principle. Warming yang, removing heat from blood, dampness and toxic material.

Cardiac Orifice (MA-IC 7)

An ear point.

Location. At the lateral 1/3 of the inferior aspect of the helix crus.

Indication. Cardiac spasm, neurogenic vomiting.

Carp

It is the meat or whole body of Cyprinus carpio L. (Cyprinidae).

Effect. Good at enhancing diuresis, removing swelling, keeping the adverse qi flowing downward and enhancing lactation.

Indication. Edema, beriberi, jaundice, cough with dyspnea, galactostasis, etc.

Carp Gallbladder

The gallbladder of Cyprinus carpio L. (Cyprinidae).

Effect. Removing heat, nebula and swelling, enhancing eyesight.

Indication. Bloodshot, swollen and painful eyes, optic atrophy, cataract, sore throat, etc.

Carp Scale

It is the scale of Cyprinus carpio L. (Cyprinidae).

Effect. Releasing blood stasis, pain and ceasing bleeding.

Indication. Hematemesis, hemoptysis, metrorrhagia and metrostaxis, leukorrhagia, abdominal pain caused by blood stasis.

Carrot Fruit

It is the root of Daucus carota L. var. sativa DC. (Umbelliferae).

Effect. Strengthening the spleen and relieving food stagnancy.

Indication. Indigestion, chronic dysentery and cough.

Cassiabark-tree Immature Fruit

It is the tender fruit of Cinnamomum cassia Presl. (Lauraceae).

Effect. Warming the middle-energizer invigorating yang removing cold and relieving pain.

Indication. Cold pain in the gastric cavity, vomiting.

Cassia Seed

It is the ripe seed of Cassia tora or C. obtusifolia L. (Leguminosae).

Effect. Relieving heat from the liver, constipation, enhancing eyesight, moistening the bowels.

Indication. Bloodshot, swollen and painful eyes, photophobia, cataract, poor and blurred vision, constipation, etc.

Castor bean Seed

It is the seed of Ricinus communis L. (Euphorbiaceae).

Effect. Removing swelling, constipation and stagnancy, and detoxicating.

Indication. Boils and pyogenic infections, scrofula, inflammation of the throat, scabies, leprosy, tinea, sores, edema, constipation, etc.

Castor Root

It is the root of Ricinus communis L. (Euphorbiaceae).

Effect. Removing convulsion, muscle spasm, wind and blood stasis.

Indication. Tetanus, epilepsy, rheumatalgia, pain owing to blood stasis in traumatic injuries, scrofula, etc.

Cataractopiesis with Gold Needle

Referring to a technique to pluck the cataract with a needle.

Method. Insert a specially made cataract needle into the incision (2.5 mm long and at the place 4 mm away from the subtemporal corneal margin) to pluck the cataract away from the pupil, and make the cataract sink to the lower place of the eye.

Indication. The weak and aged patients suffering from cataract and senile cataract.

Catechu

Obtained by evaporating the liquid of the branch and heartwood of Acacia catechu (L.) Willd (Leguminosae); another kind of catechu, or by evaporating the liquid of the tender branch with leaf of Uncaria gambier Roxb. (Rubiaceae).

Effect. Ceasing dampness, astringing ulcers and promoting tissue regeneration and ceasing bleeding.

Indication. Eczema, ulcer, ulcerative gingivitis, canker sores and traumatic bleeding, etc.

Catgut Embedding

Method. Embed a piece of catgut subcutaneously or inside the muscle at acupoint for continuous stimulation. Generally, the acupoints are selected on the abdomen, back and the four limbs where the muscles are well developed. 1 or 2 points will be embedded each time.

Indication. Chronic gastritis, chronic bronchitis, asthma, psychoneurosis and sequela of infantile paralysis, etc.

Cat-tail Pollen

It is the pollen of Typha angustifolia L. (Typhaceae), or other plants of the same genus.

Effect. Ceasing bleeding, enhancing blood circulation to dissipate blood stasis.

Indication. Bleeding, for examples, hemoptysis, epistaxis, hematuria, hamatochezia, metrorrhagia, metrostaxis, traumatic bleeding, as well as cardiac or abdominal pains, postpartum abdominal pain, dysmenorrhea, etc.

Cat-tail Rhizome

It is the rhizome of Tupha angustata Bory. et Chaub. (Thyrhaceae) with some tender stem, or many other species of the same genus.

Effect. Removing swelling and heat from the blood, enhancing diuresis.

Indication. Consumptive fever in pregnancy, threatened abortion with vaginal bleeding, diabetes, aphtha of the mouth and tongue, dysentery of heat type, stranguria, leukorrhea, edema, etc.

Caustic Nose

Symptoms. Itching eruption on the nose.

Pathogenesis. Due to the perspiration, affected by pathogenic wind and combination of pathogenic wind and dampness.

Therapeutic Principle. Releasing wind and ceasing itching.

Cauterization

It refers to one kind of ocular therapy.

Method. By using a specially made cautery or a pyropuncture needle to cauterize the affected part, with the purpose of hemostasis and precaution against repeated attack of pathologic changes. The method is good at curing some external oculopathy while drugs are not helpful.

Cauterization with Folium Cannabis

It refers to a form of moxibustion.

Method. Collecting the fresh leaves and flowers of cannabis, pound to make cones, applying the cones on the diseased area for moxibustion.

Indication. Scrofula.

Cavalerie Clearweed Herb

It is the whole plant of Pilea cavaleriei Levl. (Urticaceae).

Effect. Removing heat, cough and phlegm, detoxicating.

Indication. Cough resulting from tuberculosis and malignant boil resulting from toxic heat.

Cayenne Pepper   ◈ C-1

It is the fruit of Capsicum frutescens L. (Solanaceae).

Effect. Warming the middle-energizer, removing cold, inducing appetite and digestion.

Indication. Abdominal pain owing to accumulation of cold, vomiting, diarrhea, frostbite, scabies, tinea, etc.

Cayenne Pepper Stem

It is the stem of Capsicum frutescens L. (Solanaceae).

Effect. Removing cold, dampness and blood stasis.

Indication. Cold and pain resulting from the wind-dampness, frostbite, etc.

Centipede   ◈ C-2

It is the whole body of Scolopendra subspinipes mutilans L. Koch. (Scolopendridae).

Effect. Removing muscle spasm, toxic substances, masses and obstruction in the meridians to alleviate pain.

Indication. Spasm and convulsion, for examples, acute and chronic infantile convulsion, tetanus, apoplexy; skin and external diseases.

Centipeda Herb

It is the whole herb of Centipeda minime (L.) A. Br. et Aschers. (Compositae) with flower.

Effect. Releasing wind, cold, dampness, nebula and clearing the nasal passage.

Indication. Common cold, pertussis, abdominal pain caused by eruptive disease, amebic dysentery, malaria, traumatic injuries, snake bite, etc.

Central Rim (MA)

An auricular point.
Location. Between the tip of antitragus and helix notch.
Function. Good in taking care of the brain and calming the mind.
Indication. Intellectual undergrowth, enuresis, and vertigo.

Central-square Needling

Referring to one of the 12 needling methods.
Method. Superficially puncture with one needle at the center of the affected area and another four around it.
Indication. Cases of relatively widespread and superficial cold arthralgia.

Cervical Vertebrae (MA-AH 8)

An auricular point.
Location. On the antihelix, a curved line from the helix-tragic notch to the bifurcation of the superior and inferior antihelix crus can be divided into five equal parts. The lower 1/5 of it is cervical vertebrae.
Function. Reinforcing the spine and nourishing the marrow.
Indication. Stiff neck, cervical spondylopathy syndrome.

Chahua (Ex-HN)

An extra point.
Location. On the head, 1.5 cun directly above Touwei (S 8).
Indication. Furuncle on head and face, migraine, etc.
Method. Puncture along the skin 0.3-0.5 cun. Apply moxibustion 1-3 moxa cones or 3-5 minutes with warming moxibustion.

Chalazion

Symptoms. At the beginning, it refers to a pit-like nodule in the eyelid, but not red and painful, then affected eyelid feels heavy and pendent, purplish red on the medial side of the eyelid.
Pathogenesis. Owing to mixture of heat in the stomach and intestine with qi, blood and phlegm dampness in the eyelid.
Therapeutic Principle. Removing heat, resolving phlegm and promoting the circulation of blood to resolve the nodule. Operation is preferable if needed.

Chancre

Belonging to syphilis.
Symptoms. For males, the chancre, on the penis, balanus, prepuce; for females, on the labia major pudendum, labia minor pudendum, vagina, etc.
Therapeutic Principle. Releasing heat and toxic materials from blood.

Changqiang (GV 1)

A meridian point.
Location. 0.5 cun below the tip of the coccyx, no the midpoint between the tip of the coccyx and the anus.
Indication. Diarrhea, dysentery, constipation, bloody stool, hemorrhoids, epilepsy, pain in the lumbar, itch in the pubic region, back rigidity, etc.
Method. Puncture obliquely 0.5-1.0 cun upward in front of the coccyx.
Notice. Do not puncture through the rectal tube in case of infection. Apply moxibustion 3-7 moxa cones or 5-15 minutes with warming moxibustion.

Changgu (Ex-CA)

An extra point.
Location. 2.5 cun lateral to Shenque (CV 8).
Indication. Diarrhea and dysentery, poor appetite and indigestion.
Method. Puncture perpendicularly 1.0-1.5 cun. Apply moxibustion 5-7 moxa cones or 10-15 minutes with warming moxibustion.

Changrao (Ex-CA)

An extra point.

Location. 2 cun lateral to Zhongji (CV 3), in the same position as of Guilai (S 29).
Indication. Constipation.
Method. Apply moxibustion with the moxa cone, which number is the same as that of the patient's age.

Changyi (Ex-CA)
An extra point.
Location. In the lower abdomen, 2.5 cun lateral to Zhongji (CV 3).
Indication. Constipation.
Method. Apply moxibustion with the moxa cone, which number is the same as that of patient's age.

Chapped Lips
A symptom.
1. **Symptoms.** Dry and cracked lips, and red and dry tongue.
   Pathogenesis. Due to the excessive heat in the spleen, the insufficiency of yin-fluid and malnutrition of lips.
2. Referring to harelip or cracked lips due to traumatic injury.

Chastetree Fruit
It is the fruit of Vitex rotundifolia L. and V. trifolia L. (Verbenaceae).
Effect. Removing wind and heat from the body, and improving acuity of vision.
Indication. Swollen and painful eyes, toothache, intractable migraine, headache, etc.

Chaulmoogra Seed
It is the ripe seed of Hydnocarpus anthelmintica Pier. (Flacourtiaceae).
Effect. Removing wind and dampness, detoxicating and killing parasites.
Indication. Leprosy, syphilis, scabies and tinea, etc.

Chengfu (B 36)
A meridian point.
Location. On the posterior side of the thigh, at the midpoint of the inferior gluteal crease.

Indication. Hemorrhoids, stiffness and pain in the lumber, sacral, gluteal and femoral regions.
Method. Puncture perpendicularly 1-2 cun. Apply moxibustion 3-5 moxa cones or 5-10 minutes with warming moxibustion.

Chengguang (B 6)
A meridian point.
Location. On the head, 2.5 cun directly above the midpoint of the anterior hairline and 1.5 cun lateral to it or 1.5 cun posterior to wuchu (B 5).
Indication. Headache, dizzines, blurred vision, vomiting, stuffy nose with nasal discharge, febrile disease etc.
Method. Puncture subcutaneously 0.3-0.5 cun. Apply moxibustion 1-3 moxa cones or 3-5 minutes with warming moxibustion.

Chengjiang (CV 24)
A meridian point.
Location. On the face, in the depression at the midpoint of the mentolabial groove.
Indication. Deviation of the eye and mouth, tight lip, swelling of face, sudden loss of voice, toothache, bleeding from the gum, epilepsy, incontinence of urine, etc.
Method. Puncture obliquely 0.3-0.5 cun. Apply moxibustion 5-10 minutes with warming moxibustion.

Chengjin (B 56)
A meridian point.
Location. On the back, below the spinous process of the 2nd thoracic vertebra, 3 cun lateral to Chengshan (B 57), at the center of the calf muscle belly, 5 cun below Weizhong (B 40).
Indication. Pain in the leg, soreness and heavy sensation in the knee, contraction of the waist area and back, hemorrhoids.
Method. Puncture perpendicularly 1.0-1.5 cun. Apply moxibustion 3-5 moxa cones or 5-10 minutes with warming moxibustion.

Chengling (G 18)

A meridian point.

Location. On the head, 4 cun above the anterior hairline and 2.25 cun lateral to the midline of the head, 1.5 cun behind Zhongying (G 17).

Indication. Headache, dizziness, pain in the eye, rhinorrhea, epistaxis, stuffy nose with plenty of nasal discharge.

Method. Puncture subcutaneously 0.3-0.5 cun. Apply moxibustion if needed.

Chengman (S 20)

A meridian point.

Location. In the upper abdomen, 5 cun above the center of the umbilicus and 2 cun lateral to the anterior midline.

Indication. Stomachache, vomiting, abdominal distention, borborygmus, anorexia, dyspnea, hemoptysis, pain in the hypochondrium.

Method. Puncture perpendicularly 0.5-1.0 cun. Apply moxibustion 3-5 moxa cones or 5-10 minutes with warming moxibustion.

Chengming (Ex-LE)

An extra point.

Location. On the medial side of the leg, 3 cun straight above Taixi (K 3).

Indication. Epilepsy and edema of the lower extremities.

Method. Puncture perpendicularly 0.5-1.0 cun. Apply moxibustion 3-7 moxa cones or 5-15 minutes with warming moxibustion.

Chengqi (S 1)

A meridian point.

Location. On the face, with the eyes looking straight forward, directly below the pupil, in the depression of the infraorbital ridge.

Indication. Red, swelling and pain of the eye, night blindness, deviation of the eye and mouth, epiphora, headace, dizziness.

Method. Puncture perpendicularly 0.3-0.7 cun along the infraorbital ridge slowly, and step by step.

Notice. Do not prick deep and cause hematoma. Moxibustion is forbidden.

Chengshan (B 57)

A meridian point.

Location. On the posterior midline of the leg, between Weizhong (B 40) and Kunlun (B 60) about 8 cun below Weizhong.

Indication. Pain in the waist area and the back, spasm with pain in the leg, hemorrhoids, constipation, beriberi, epistaxis, epilepsy, etc.

Method. Puncture perpendicularly 0.5-1.0 cun. Apply moxibustion 3-4 moxa cones or 5-10 minutes with warming moxibustion.

Chengu (Ex-LE)

An extra point.

Location. On the fibula side of the knee joint, the highest point of the external epicondyle of femur.

Indication. Lumbago, carbuncle on the coccygeal region, carbuncle adjacent to the anus, etc.

Method. Puncture shallowly to bleeding.

Chenjue (Ex-B)

An extra point.

Location. On the back, at the margin of the superior-medial angle of the scapula, at the place touched by the extremity of the middle finger when the arms are cross each other.

Indication. Walking in madness, abnormal emotions of joy, anger, sorrow and weeping, pain in the scapula, etc.

Method. Puncture 0.5-0.8 cun obliquely. Apply moxibustion 3-5 moxa cones or 5-10 minutes with warming moxibustion.

Cherokee Rose Fruit

It is the ripe pseudofruit or the ripe receptacle without thin hip (the flesh of cherokee rose-hip) of Rosa laevigata Michx. (Rosaceae).

Effect. Ceasing spontaneous emission, inducing diuresis, astringing the bowels and ceasing diarrhea.

Indication. Emission, spermatorrhea, enuresis, leukorrhagia owing to deficiency of the kidney, chronic diarrhea and dysentery, as well as proctoptosis, hysteroptosis, metrorrhagia and metrostaxis, etc.

Cherry Fruit

It is the fruit of Prunus pseudocerasus Lindl. (Rosaceae).
Effect. Nourishing qi and removing the wind and dampness.
Indication. Paralysis, hypoesthesia of limbs, lumbago owing to pathogenic wind-dampness, frostbite, etc.

Cherry Leaf

It is the leaf of Prunus pseudocerasus Lindl. (Rosaceae).
Effect. Reinforcing the spleen, ceasing bleeding and detoxicating, warming the stomach.
Indication. Indigestion owing to cold in the stomach, diarrhea, hematemesis, suppurative skin diseases, etc.

Cherry Nut

It is the nut of Prunus pseudocerasus Lindl. (Rosaceae).
Effect. Enhancing eruption and detoxicating.
Indication. Measles with insufficient eruption, cellulitis, scar, etc.

Chervil Larkspur Herb

It is the whole herb of Delphinium anthriscifolium Hance (Ranunculaceae).
Effect. Releasing pain, wind, dampness, detoxicating.
Indication. Rheumatalgia, hemiparalysis, carbuncle, furuncle, tinea and leprosy.

Chest (MA)

An auricular point.
Location. On the border of the cavity of the ear and on the medial side of Thoracic Vertebra (MA).
Indication. Oppressive feeling and pain in the chest, mastitis, and insufficient lactation.

Chest Lump

Referring to the lump.
Symptoms. Depressed fullness in the chest, the obstruction of the diaphragm and anorexia, etc.
Pathogenesis. Owing to the overeating of raw, cold and greasy food.
Therapeutic Principle. Releasing distention, fullness and the obstruction.

Chestnut ⊛ C-3

It is the shelled seed of Castanea mollissima Bl. (Fagaceae).
Effect. Tonifying the stomach, the spleen, and the kidney, reinforcing the bones and muscles, enhancing blood flow and ceasing bleeding.
Indication. Regurgitation of food from the stomach, diarrhea, paralysis of the loins and legs, hematemesis and bloody stool.

Chestnut-like Sore

Symptoms. Soft, yellowish and chestnut-like granules on the medial side of the eyelid, and often with trachoma. The granules of similar size and clear periphery in the lower eyelid, and with photophobia, lacrimation, itching, astringency, and pain.
Pathogenesis. Mostly owing to obstruction of pathogenic wind, dampness and heat in the eyelid.
Therapeutic Principle. Removing wind and heat, and promoting diuresis.

Chest Pain

Symptoms. Chest pain, oppression with nervousness, shortness of breath, cough and dyspnea, etc.
Pathogenesis. Usually owing to the stagnation of the liver-qi, the obstruction of blood stasis, the attack of yang-qi in the chest by pathogenic cold, inert yang-qi in the chest.
Therapeutic Principle. Smoothing the liver, enhancing the blood circulation, removing phlegm and cold, and warming yang, etc.

Chest Pain due to Emotional Factors

Symptoms. For the excess type, stuffiness of qi in the chest, pain caused by distention with no fixed locations. For the deficiency type, dull pain in the chest, pain relieved in pressing.

Pathogenesis. Disorder of seven emotions leading to the stagnation of qi.

Therapeutic Principle. For the excess type, adjusting the flow of qi and educing the upflow of qi. For the deficiency type, tonifying the stomach and warming the spleen.

Chest Pain due to Fluid Retention

Symptoms. Chest stuffiness with mild epigastric pain, cough with phlegm, etc.

Pathogenesis. Due to retention of excessive fluid in the chest.

Therapeutic Principle. Warming the lung to eliminate sputum.

Chest Pain Radiating to Back

It is usually found in the syndromes of obstruction of qi in the chest, epigastric ache, etc.

Chicken Blood

It is the blood of Gallus gallus domesticus Brisson (Phasianidae).

Effect. Removing wind and obstruction in the meridians, enhancing blood flow.

Indication. Infantile convulsion, facial palsy, flaccidity, fracture conjunctival congestion and lacrimation, carbuncle, cellulitis, tinea, and skin external disease.

Chicken-bone Herb

It is the whole herb of Abrus fruticulosus Wall. ex Wight et Arn. (Leguminosae).

Effect. Removing blood stasis and heat, detoxicating and smoothing the liver.

Indication. Hepatitis with jaundice, gastralgia, acute mastitis, scrofula and traumatic injuries.

Chicken Breast

Symptoms. Protruding sternum, just like the chicken's sternum.

Pathogenesis. 1. Due to rickets. 2. For the infant, long-term cough and swelling lungs with excessive sputum, maybe leading to high breast and shortness of breath, but different from the chicken breast of the rickets.

Chicken Gallbladder

It is the gallbladder of Gallus gallus domesticus Brisson (Phasianidae).

Effect. Detoxicating, releasing cough and phlegm, and enhancing eyesight.

Indication. Pertussis, chronic bronchitis, infantile (bacillary) dysentery, etc.

Chicken Liver

It is the liver of Gallus gallus domesticuse Brisson (Phasianidae).

Effect. Nourishing the liver and kidney.

Indication. Blurred vision owing to deficiency of the liver-qi, infantile malnutrition and vaginal bleeding during pregnancy.

Chicken Meat

It is the meat of Gallus gallus domesticus Brisson (Phasianidae).

Effect. Warming the middle-energizer, nourishing qi, vital essence and marrow.

Indication. Emaciation owing to consumptive disease, deficiency in middle-energizer with anorexia, diarrhea, diabetes, edema, frequency of micturition, metrostaxis, leukorrhea, postpartum hypogalactia, etc.

Chickenpox

An acute infantile infectious disease.

Symptoms. Fever, muscular eruption, papular eruption, herpes and crust on the skin and mucosa step by step.

Pathogenesis. Mostly owing to pathogenic factors in the exterior affections and the interior stagnant damp-heat.

Therapeutic Principle. Removing wind, heat, toxic substance and dampness. Warming and drying should be avoided.

Chicken's Gizzard Membrane

It is the lining membrane of the gizzard of Gallus gallus domesticus Brisson (Phasianidae).

Effect. Strengthen the stomach and improve digestion, relieve nocturnal emission and inducing decomposition of calculi.

Indication. Dyspepsia, infantile indigestion, enuresis, emission, stone of urinary system and gallstones.

Chilblains

Symptoms. Mostly occurring on the exposed positions, the hand and the foot, the auricle, and the face, etc; first pale, gradually purple, red spots, with naturally burning pain, itching or numbness, even ulcer to form boils.

Cause. Resulting from attacks of cold to the body.

Therapeutic Principle. Warming yang for removing cold, and adjusting nutrient and defence system.

Childhood Malnutrition with Kidney Syndrome

Symptoms. Thin and weak physique, gum bleeding or ulceration, hyperhidrosis, myasthenia of limbs.

Pathogenesis. Owing to malnutrition and the latent heat stagnated in the interior, or the inadequate kidney-qi.

Therapeutic Principle. Tonifying the kidney and the spleen.

Childhood Malnutrition due to Improper Diet

Referring to a morbid state, a child eating much food but thin body.

Symptoms. High fever, dry mouth, night sweat, dry skin, dried and withered hair, abdominal distention.

Pathogenesis. Mostly owing to the deficiency of the spleen and stomach.

Therapeutic Principle. Treatment should be based on the disease involving heart, liver, kidney, lung and spleen respectively.

Chimai (TE 18)

A meridian pain.

Location. On the head, at the center of the mastoid process, at the junction of the upper 2/3 and lower 1/3 of the line along the helix linking Yifeng (TE 17) and Jiaosun (TE 20).

Indication. Headache, deafness, tinnitus, blurred vision, infantile convulsion, vomiting, diarrhea and dysentery.

Method. Puncture subcutaneously 0.3-0.5 cun or prick to bleeding. Apply moxibustion with 1-3 moxa cones or 3-5 minutes with warming moxibustion.

Chinaberry Tree Bark

It is the root bark or trunk bark of Melia azedarach L. and M. toosendan S. et Z. (Meliaceae).

Effect. Killing parasites and curing tinea.

Indication. Ascariasis, ancylostomiasis, enterobiasis, porrigo and scabies.

Chinao (Ex-UE)

An extra point.

Location. On the midline of the back side of the forearm, 6 cun above the midpoint of the dorsal transverse crease of the wrist.

Indication. Mental disorder, numbness of the upper limbs or paralysis, etc.

Method. Puncture perpendicularly 1.0-1.5 cun or throught to the subcutaneous region of the opposite side.

Chinarood Greenbrier Rhizome

It is the rhizome of Smilax china L. (Liliaceae).

Effect. Enhancing diuresis, releasing pyogenic infections, wind and dampness.

Indication. Arthralgia, numbness of the muscles, diarrhea, dysentery, edema, stranguria, furuncle, pyogenic infections, scrofula and hemorrhoid.

Chinese Aloes Leaf

It is the leaf of Aloe vera L. var. Chinensis (Haw.) Berger or Aloe vera L. (Liliaceae).

Effect. Removing intense heat, recovering menstrual flow, killing parasites and detoxicating.

Indication. Gonorrhea, hematuria, amenorrhea, infantile convulsion, scald, hemorrhoids, scabies and subcutaneous swelling, etc.

Chinese Angelica Root

It is the root of Angelica sinensis (Oliv.) Piels. (Umbelliferae).

Effect. Nourishing blood, enhancing blood circulation, removing pain and moistening the bowels.

Indication. Irregular menstruation, amenorrhea, menorrhagia, abdominal pain owing to cold deficiency, pain resulting from blood stasis, sores, carbuncles and other pyogenic skin infections, traumatic injuries, etc.

Chinese Arborvitae leaf and Twig

It is the twig and leaf of Biota orientalis (L.) Endl. (Cupressaseae).

Effect. Releasing heat from the blood, phlegm and cough, and ceasing bleeding.

Indication. Various bleeding, for examples, hematemesis, epistaxis, hematuria, metrorrhagia, metrostaxis, and traumatic bleeding.

Chinese Arborvitae Seed

It is the seed of Biota orientalis (L.) Endl. (Cupressaceae).

Effect. Tonifying the heart, calming the mind, moistening the bowel and removing constipation.

Indication. Palpitation, severe palpitation, insomnia, dreaminess, constipation resulting from deficiency of yin and insufficiency of blood and dryness of the intestines.

Chinese Astilbe Herb

It is the whole herb of Astilbe Chinensis (Maxim) Franch. et Sav. (Saxifragaceae).

Effect. Removing wind, heat and cough.

Indication. Common cold owing to wind-heat, cough, headache and pantalgia.

Chinese Asystasiella Rhizome or Herb

It is the rhizome or whole herb of Asystasiella neesiana (Wall.) Lindau (Acanthaceae).

Effect. Ceasing bleeding, removing blood stasis, clearing away heat and detoxicating.

Indication. Hemoptysis, hemafecia, traumatic bleeding, sprain, abscess and swollen, and sore throat.

Chinese Bayberry Fruit

It is the fruit of Myrica rubra Sieb. et Zucc. (Myricaceae).

Effect. Enhancing the production of the body fluid, adjusting the stomach, and releasing stagnancy.

Indication. Extreme thirst, vomiting, diarrhea, dysentery, etc.

Chinese Bayberry Root

It is the root of Myrica rubra Sieb. et Zucc. (Myricaceae).

Effect. Adjusting flow of qi, ceasing bleeding and removing blood stasis.

Indication. Stomachache, vomiting, hernia, hematemesis, metrorrhagia, hemorrhoidal bleeding. etc.

Chinese Berberry Root

It is the root or the stem bark of Berberis sargentiana Schneid, Berberis barchypoda Maxim, Berberis, dictyophylla Franch. Var. epruinosa Schneid (Berberidaceae).

Effect. Enhancing diuresis and removing heat and blood stasis.

Indication. Dysentery with blood stool jaundice, sore throat, bloodshot eyes and traumatic injuries.

Chinese Blistering Beetle

It is the insect of Mylabris phalerata Pall. or M. cichorii L. (Meloidae)

Effect. Eliminating toxic material, promoting pus drainage, removing blood stasis and lumps.

Indication. Carbuncles, neurodermatitis, scrofula, bite by rabid dog; amenorrhea and abdominal masses also for cancer of liver, esophagus, and stomach.

Chinese Buttercup Herb

It is the whole herb of Ranunculus chinensis Bge. (Ranunculaceae).

Effect. Detoxicating, removing swelling, preventing malaria and killing parasites.

Indication. Hepato-splenomegaly, ascites, malaria, carbuncles, furuncles and neurodermatitis.

Chinese Cassia Tree-bark

It is the trunk bark or thick branch bark of Cinnamomum cassia Presl (Lauraceae).

Effect. Removing cold and relieving pain, warming the middle-warmer and invigorating yang.

Indication. Aches in the loins and knees, impotence, frequent urination; gastric and abdominal pain, poor appetite and loose stool, etc.

Chinese Chive Leaf

It is the leaf of Allium tuberosum Rottler (Liliaceae).

Effect. Warming the spleen and stomach, promoting qi circulation, releasing blood stasis and removing toxic substances.

Indication. Stuffiness in the chest, regurgitation, hematemesis, hematuria, dysentery, proctoptosis and traumatic injuries.

Chinese Chive Root

It is the root and bulb of Allium tuberosum Rottler (Liliaceae).

Effect. Warming the middle-energizer, promoting qi circulation and removing blood stasis.

Indication. Stuffiness in the chest, abdominal distention owing to dyspepsia, leukorrhea with reddish discharge, tinea, sores and traumatic injuries.

Chinese Chive Seed

It is the seed of Allium tuberosum Rottler (Liliaceae).

Effect. Tonifying the liver and kidney, warming the loins and knees, reinforcing yang, and stopping emission.

Indication. Impotence, weakness and cold pain in the loins and knees owing to deficiency cold of the kidney-yang, emission, nocturia, leukorrhagia owing to unconsolidation of the kidney-qi, etc.

Chinese Chive-separated Moxibustion

Referring to a type of indirect moxibustion with Chinese chive.

Method. Pound the washed and cleaned chive with roots into jelly and make coin-like cakes, then put a cake on the surface of the sore with a moxa cone upon it, and with the moxa cone for moxibustion.

Indication. Skin and external diseases, etc.

Chinese Clinopodium Herb

It is the whole herb of Clinopodium chinensis (Benth.) O. Kuntze. (Labiatae).

Effect. Expelling wind and heat, detumescence by detoxification.

Indication. Common cold, heatstroke, acute cholecystitis, enteritis, dysentery, parotitis, mastadenitis, boils, furuncles and other pyogenic infections on the skin, etc.

Chinese Clovershrub Root

It is the root of Campylotropis macrocarpa (Bge) Rehd. (Leguminosae).

Effect. Tendon relaxation and activation of blood circulation.

Indication. Numbness of limbs and hemiplegia.

Chinese Crossostephium Leaf

It is the leaf of Crossostephium chinense (L.) Mak. (Compostiae).

Effect. Expelling pathogenic wind, eliminating dampness, subsidence of swilling and detoxicating pyogenic infections.
Indication. Carbuncles and innominate toxic swelling.

Chinese-date

It is the ripe fruit of Ziziphus jujuba Mill. (Rhamnaceae).
Effect. Nourishing the spleen, qi, blood, calming the mind and moderating the properties of other drugs.
Indication. Deficiency of qi in the middle-energizer, weakness of the spleen and stomach, poor appetite, loose stool, and female hysteria, etc.

Chinese Edelweiss Root

It is the root of Leontopodium sinense Hemsl. (Compositae).
Effect. Detoxicating, releasing heat, inflammation and pain.
Indication. Tonsillitis, laryngopharyngitis, etc.

Chinese Elder Herb

It is the whole herb or root of Sambucus chinensis Lindl. (Caprifoliaceae).
Effect. Removing blood stasis, wind, dampness, enhancing blood circulation.
Indication. Rheumatalgia, nephritic edema, beriberi, general edema, dysentery, jaundice, chronic trachitis, carbuncles, swellings, fracture, etc.

Chinese Fevervine Herb ⊛ C-4

It is the whole herb and root of Paederia scandens (Lour.) Merr. (Rubiaceae).
Effect. Strengthen the stomach, promote digestion and clear away summer heat, eliminate phlegm and relieve cough dampness, and detoxicating.
Indication. Pain owing to pathogenic wind-dampness, diarrhea, dysentery, abdominal pain, general edema owing to deficiency of qi, dizziness, inappetence, hepatosplenomegaly, scrofula and acute appendicitis.

Chinese Fir Bark

It is the bark of Cunninghamia lanceolata (Lamb.) Hook. (Taxodiaceae).
Effect. Eliminating retention of fluid and removing edema, clearing away heat and toxic material.
Indication. Edema, beriberi and burns.

Chinese Fir Leaf

It is the leaf of Cunninghamia lanceolata (Lamb.) Hook. (Taxodiaceae).
Effect. Dispelling wind and dampness, relieving pain.
Indication. Chronic bronchitis, toothache, pemphigus and burns.

Chinese Fir Wood or Twig

It is the heart-wood and branch of Cunninghamia lanceolata (Lamb.) Hook (Taxodiaceae).
Effect. Releasing the pathogens of fetid odour, pain, noxious dampness and keeping the adverse qi flowing downward.
Indication. Fulminant carbuncle caused by wind-dampness, beriberi, and distending pain in the chest and abdomen.

Chinese Gall

It is the insect on the leaf of Rhus chinensis Mill or R. Potaninii Maxim (Anacardiaceae).
Effect. Reduce the fire, dissolve phlegm, astringe the lung and the intestine, relieve diarrhea, arrest perspiration and relieve nocturnal emission, stop bleeding.
Indication. Chronic cough owing to deficiency of the lung, protracted diarrhea, emission, spontaneous perspiration, metrorrhagia and metrostaxis, etc.

Chinese Gentian Root

It is the root of Gentiana scabra Bunge or G. triflora Pall. or G. manshurica Kitag. (Gentianaceae).
Effect. Removing heat, dampness and fire from the liver and gallbladder.
Indication. Jaundice caused by damp-heat, perineal swelling, pruritus leukorrhagia, eczema, fire of excess type

in the liver and gallbladder, headache, bitter taste in the mouth, dry throat, bloodshot eyes; excessive heat of the liver meridian, high fever, epilepsy induced by terror, convulsions of the extremities, etc.

Chinese Hibiscus Flower ⊛ C-5

It is the flower of Hibiscus rosa-sinensis L. (Malvaceae).

Effect. Removing heat from the lung and blood, sputum, and detoxicating.

Indication. Cough owing to phlegm-fire, epistaxis, dysentery, reddish and whitish turbid urine, subcutaneous swelling and fulminant carbuncle.

Chinese Hibiscus Leaf

It is the leaf of Hibiscus rosa-sinensis L. (Malvaceae).

Effect. Removing heat from blood and detoxicating.

Indication. Subcutaneous swelling, fulminant carbuncle and epistaxis.

Chinese Holly Fruit

It is the fruit of Ilex cornuta Lindl (Aquifoliaceae).

Effect. Tonifying yin, invigorating vital essence and reinforcing collateral flow.

Indication. Fever owing to yin-deficiency, stranguria with turbid urine, metrorrhagia, leukorrhagia, muscular pain.

Chinese Holly Root

It is the root of Ilex cornuta Lindl (Aquifoliaceae).

Effect. Nourishing the liver and kidney and removing pathogenic wind-heat.

Indication. Lassitude loin and knees, arthralgia, headache and toothache due to pathogenic wind.

Chinese Honeyiocust Fruit

It is the fruit of Gleditsia sinensis Lam. (Leguminosae).

Effect. Removing phlegm and causing resuscitation, promoting lactogenesis and relaxing bowels (external use) etc.

Indication. Stagnation of stubborn phlegm, cough and dyspnea with chest tightness, unsmooth expectoration.

Chinese Honeyiocust Spine

It is the spine of Gleditsia sinensis Lam. (Leguminosae).

Effect. Removing pus and toxin, enhancing blood circulation and treating boils.

Indication. Suppurative infections on the skin at the early stage, for examples, sores, carbuncles, furuncles and boils, and non-rupture of carbuncles.

Chinese Ligusticus Rhizome

It is the rhizome of Ligusticum sinensis Oliv. or L. jeholense Nakai et Kitag. (Umbelliferae).

Effect. Expelling the exogenous evils from the body surface, removing cold, wind, dampness and pain.

Indication. Parietal headache, migraine owing to affection by exopathogenic wind-cold and arthralgia owing to wind-cold-dampness.

Chinese Lizard-tail

It is the whole plant of Saururus chinensis (Lour.) Baill. (Saururaceae).

Effect. Removing swelling and heat, inducing diuresis, and detoxicating.

Indication. Nephritis edema, mast-adenitis, jaundice, beriberi, stranguria with turbid urine, leukorrhea and suppurative infections on the skin.

Chinese Lobelia

It is the whole plant of Lobelia chinensis Lour. (Companulaceae).

Effect. Removing swelling and heat, inducing diuresis, detoxicating.

Indication. Ascites and edema, snake bite, bee or scorpion injuries, boils, furuncles and other pyogenic infections on the skin, jaundice, diarrhea, dysentery, eczema, etc.

Chinese Mahonia Leaf

It is the leaf of Mahonia bealei (Fort.) Carr,
Mahonia fortunei (Lindl.) Fedde or
Mahonia japonica (Thunb.) DC.
(Berberidaceae).

Effect. Recovering qi, removing heat,
cough and sputum, detoxifying and promoting the subsidence of swelling.

Indication. Hemoptysis owing to tuberculosis, hectic or tidal fever with night sweat,
dizziness and tinnitus, vexation and
bloodshot eyes, etc.

Chinese Milkwort Herb

It is the whole herb with root or root of
Polygala chinensis L. (Polygalaceae).

Effect. Clearing   away   heat,   and
detoxication removing blood stasis,
enhancing blood circulation, stagnancy of
indigested food.

Indication. Productive cough, dysentery,
infantile malnutrition, scrofula, traumatic
injuries and snake bite.

Chinese Olive

It is the fruit of Canarium album (Lour.)
Raeusch. (Burseraceae).

Effect. Relieving heat from the lung, eliminating sore throat, enhancing the production of body fluid and detoxicating.

Indication. Swollen and sore throat, excessive thirst, hematemesis, owing to cough,
bacillary dysentery, epilepsy, puffer
poisoning.

Chinese Pennisetum Herb

It is the whole herb of Pennisetum
alopecuroides (L.) Spr. (Gramineae).

Effect. Enhancing acuity of vision and
removing blood stasis.

Indication. Bloodshot and painful eyes.

Chinese Pholidota Pseudobulb

It is the pseudobulb or whole herb of
Pholidota chinensis Lindl. (Orchidaceae).

Effect. Tonifying yin, removing heat from
the lung and damp elimination.

Indication. Dizziness, headache, cough,
hematemesis, nocturnal emission, dysentery, leukorrhea and infantile malnutrition.

Chinese Photinia Leaf

It is the dried leaf of Photinia serrulata
Lindl. (Rosaceae).

Effect. Releasing pathogenic wind, dispelling obstruction in the meridians and
nourishing the kidney, strengthening the
tendons and bones, relieving pain.

Indication. Arthritis of wind type, aching
pain in the back and loins, flaccidity of the
lower limbs owing to the kidney deficiency, migraine and rubella.

Chinese Pink Herb

It is the whole herb of Dianthus superbus
L. and D. chinensis L. (Caryophyllaceae)
with flower.

Effect. Clearing away heat enhancing
blood circulation, inducing menstruation
and diuresis and treating stranguria.

Indication. Scanty dark urine, pain in
micturition and suppression of menses
owing to blood stasis.

Chinese Redbud Bark

It is the bark of Cercis chinensis Bge.
(Leguminosae).

Effect. Enhancing   blood   circulation,
recovering menstrual flow, releasing
swelling and toxic substances.

Indication. Wind-cold-wetness type of
arthralgia, amenorrhea, inflammation of
the throat, stranguria, subcutaneous
swelling, etc.

Chinese Rose   ⊛ C-6

It is the flower bud or budding flower of
Rosa chinensis Jacq. (Rosaceae).

Effect. Enhancing blood circulation, regulating menstruation and removing
swelling.

Indication. Stagnation menstruation, distending pain in the chest and abdomen
and amenorrhea.

Chinese Sage

It is the whole herb of Salvia chinensis Benth. (Labiatae).

Effect. Checking upward adverse flow of qi, detoxicating, removing masses and ceasing leukorrhagia.

Indication. Dysphagia, dyspnea resulting from retention of phlegm, suppurative infections on the skin, scrofula and leukorrhea.

Chinese Skink

It is the whole body of Eumeces chinensis (Gray) (Scincidae).

Effect. Enhancing diuresis, smoothing and resolving hard masses.

Indication. Dysuria, stranguria due to the passage of urinary stone, malignant boil, etc.

Chinese Small Iris Flower

It is the flower of Iris pallasii Fisch. var. chinensis Fisch. (Iridaceae).

Effect. Removing heat, detoxicating, ceasing bleeding and enhancing diuresis.

Indication. Inflammation of the throat, hematemesis, difficulty of urination, stranguria, hernia, carbuncles, etc.

Chinese Small Iris Seed

It is the seed of Iris pallasii Fisch. var. chinensis Fisch. (Iriaceae).

Effect. Detoxicating, releasing heat, dampness by diuresis, and ceasing bleeding.

Indication. Jaundice, dysentery, hematemesis, leukorrhea, inflammation of the throat, carbuncles, sores.

Chinese Soapberry Seed

It is the seed of Sapindus mukorossi Gaertn (Sapindaceae).

Effect. Relieving heat, phlegm, removing food stagnancy and killing parasites.

Indication. Swelling pain resulting from inflammation of the throat, cough with asthma, dyspepsia, leukorrhea, malnutrition, carbuncles, tinea, pyogenic infections, etc.

Chinese Starjasmine Stem

It is the stem and leaf of a vine herb Trachelospermum jasminoides (Lindl.) Lem. (Apocynaceae).

Effect. Expelling wind-dampness and dredging, obstruction in the meridian and heat from the blood.

Indication. Rheumatic arthralgia, spasm of muscles, inflammation of the throat and subcutaneous swelling.

Chinese Sumac Leaf

It is the leaf of Rhus chinensis Mill. (Anacardiaceae).

Effect. Removing sputum, cough and detoxicating.

Indication. Cough, hemafecia, dysentery with bloody stool, night sweat, skin and external diseases.

Chinese Sumac Fruit

It is the fruit of Rhus chinensis Mill (Anacardiaceae).

Effect. Enhancing the production of body fluid, nourishing the lung, releasing fire in the lung, resolving phlegm, ceasing sweating and dysentery.

Indication. Phlegm-dyspnea, inflammation of the throat, jaundice, night sweat, dysentery, carbuncle and seborrheic dermatitis.

Chinese Sumac Root

It is the root of Rhus chinensis Mill. (Anacardiaceae).

Effect. Relieving wind, dampness and swelling, and softening hard masses.

Indication. Fever caused by cold, cough, diarrhea, watery distention, rheumatalgia, etc.

Chinese Trumpete-creeper Flower ⊛ C-7

It is the flower of Campsis grandiflora (Thunb) K. Schum (Bignoniaceae).

Effect. Enhancing blood circulation, relieving wind, blood stasis and pathogenic heat from blood subduing swelling and detoxicating.

Indication. Amenorrhea caused by stagnation of blood, masses in the abdomen, and itching all over the body, traumatic injury, poisonous snake bites.

Chinese Waxgourd   ⊛ C-8

It is the fruit of Benincasa hispida (Thunb.) Cogn. (Cucurbitaceae).

Effect. Detoxicating, releasing heat and phlegm, inducing diuresis.

Indication. Edema, beriberi, stranguria, cough with dyspnea, vexation caused by summer-heat, diabetes, diarrhea, dysentery, subcutaneous swelling, fish poisoning, etc.

Chinese Waxgourd Seed ⊛ C-9

It is the seed of Benincasa hispida (Thunb.) Cogn. (Cucurbitaceae).

Effect. Removing heat from the lung, resolving phlegm and enhancing the discharge of pus.

Indication. Cough caused by the lung-heat, pulmonary abscess and acute appendicitis.

Chinese Waxmyrtle Bark

It is the bark of Myrica rubra Sieb. et Zucc. (Myricaeae).

Effect. Enhancing blood circulation, ceasing diarrhea, detoxicating and relieving nebula and pain.

Indication. Dysentery, nebula, toothache, traumatic injuries, scald, burn, malignant boil and scabies, etc.

Chinese Weeping Cupress Resin

It is the resin seeped from the trunk of Cupressus funebris Endl. (Cupressaceae).

Effect. Releasing pathogenic wind, detoxicating and enhancing the tissue regeneration.

Indication. Headache caused by wind-heat, leukorrhea and stranguria with turbid urine.

Chinese Weeping Cupress Twig

It is the branch and leaf of Cupressus funebris Endl (Cupressaceae).

Effect. Ceasing bleeding and releasing heat from blood.

Indication. Hematemesis, dysentery with bloody stool and scalds.

Chinese Wingleaf Prickhyash Fruit

It is the fruit of Zanthoxylum planispinum Sieb. et Zucc. (Rutaceae).

Effect. Removing cold, pain and intestinal roundworms.

Indication. Cold in the stomach, abdominal pain owing to ascariasis, toothache and moist sores.

Chinese Wolfberry Bark

It is the bark of Lycium chinensis Mill. (Solanaceae).

Effect. Releasing heat from blood and from lung, bringing down hectic fever, lower blood pressure.

Indication. Blood-heat caused by yin-deficiency, hectic fever with night sweat caused by consumption, cough with dyspnea, hematemesis, diabetes, toothache caused by fire of deficiency type, hypertension, insect bite, etc.

Chinese Yam Rhizome

It is the rhizome of Dioscorea opposita Thunb. (Dioscoreaceae).

Effect. Enriching qi and yin, reinforcing the spleen, lung and kidney.

Indication. Diarrhea owing to hypofunction of the spleen, poor appetite, loose stool, chronic cough and dyspnea owing to lung deficiency, emission owing to the kidney deficiency, profuse leukorrhea and diabetes, etc.

Chinese Yangtao   ⊛ C-10

It is the fruit of Actinidia Chinensis Planch. (Actinidiaceae).

Effect. Removing heat, relieving thirst and treating stranguria.

Indication. Excessive thirst, diabetes, jaundice, stranguria due to the blockage of urinary stone and hemorrhoid.

Chirp-like Tinnitus

Symptoms. Anxiety and irritability, insomnia and dreamy, tinnitus as insects chirping.
Pathogenesis. Usually caused by the obstruction of wind-phlegm in the collaterals or internal blood stasis.

Chize (L 5)

An acupoint.
Location. On the cubital crease, in the excavation of the radial border of the biceps muscle of the arm.
Indication. Cough, asthmatic breath, tidal fever, distention and fullness of chest and hypochondrium, vomiting, pain in the elbow and arm, etc.
Method. Puncture perpendicularly 0.5-1.0 cun or prick with three-edged needle to cause little bleeding, and perform warm moxibustion to the point for 5-10 minutes.

Chloasma

Symptoms. Yellowish-brown or black spots appearing on the face, mostly of the female, in different size and shape, but not protruded out of the skin.
Pathogenesis. Owing to the deficiency of kidney or stagnation of the liver qi.
Therapeutic Principle. Tonifying the kidney and enriching the blood.

Chlorite-schist

Referring to two kinds of chlorite-schists, i.e. black and gold, the black is chlorite-schist, and the gold is mica-schist.
Effect. Keeping the adverse qi flowing downward, checking hyperfunction of the liver and removing convulsion and phlegm.
Indication. Excess syndrome of dyspnea and cough owing to reversed flow of qi and epilepsy owing to accumulation of phlegm.

Cholera Morbus due to Cold

Symptoms. Vomiting or diarrhea, or continuous vomiting and diarrhea, colic pain in abdomen, cold limbs, purplish lips and spasm of legs if serious.
Pathogenesis. Owing to constitutional yang deficiency, internal damage by cold and raw food, and invasion of exogenous cold-dampness.
Therapeutic Principle. Adjusting the middle-energizer, warming the stomach and removing cold.

Cholera Morbus due to Heat

Symptoms. Abdominal colic, vomiting and diarrhea, oppressed feeling in chest, fever, thirst, and dark urine.
Pathogenesis. Owing to improper diet or exposure to summer-heat or damp-heat, filthiness in the middle-energizer.
Therapeutic Principle. Removing heat and dampness, filth and turbidity.

Cholla Root and Stem

It is the root and stem of Opuntia dillenii Haw (Cactaceae).
Effect. Enhancing blood circulation and flow of qi, removing heat and detoxicating, subduing swelling.
Indication. Pain caused by disorder of qi in the chest and stomach, mass in the abdomen, dysentery, hemorrhoidal bleeding, cough, sore throat, and ambustion, snake bite, etc.

Chonggu (Ex-HN)

An extra point.
Location. On the posterior midline of the nape, at the inferior edge of the spinous process of the 6th cervical vertebra.
Indication. Common cold, cough, malaria, rigidity of the neck, bronchitis, epilepsy, etc.
Method. Puncture perpendicularly 0.5-1.0 cun. Apply moxibustion 5-7 moxa cones or 10-15 minutes with warming moxibustion.

Chongmen (Sp 12)

An acupoint.

Location. 3.5 cun lateral to the midpoint of the upper margin of the pubic symphysis.

Indication. Abdominal pain, diarrhea, hernia, pain of the hemorrhoid, metrorrhagia and metrostaxis, leukorrhagia, dribbling of urine, etc.

Method. Puncture perpendicularly 0.5-1.0 cun (avoid puncturing blood vessel) and perform moxibustion to the point for 5-15 minutes or 3-5 units of moxa cones.

Chong-qi Invading Kidney

Symptoms. Vertigo, aversion for cold, nausea, vomiting, epigastric fullness, abdominal distention, etc.

Pathogenesis. Owing to the wrong treatment of the vital vessel disease with the diaphoretic and purgative methods, leading to the reversed flow of qi, thus, in turn, affecting the kidney.

Therapeutic Principle. Adjusting the flow of qi and the stomach, lowering the adverse flow of qi and removing the cold, smoothing the flow of yang-qi.

Chong-qi Invading Liver

Symptoms. Contracture in the abdomen, exacerbation of pain after meal, fever, somnolence, etc.

Pathogenesis. Owing to the wrong treatment of the vital vessel disease with the diaphoretic and purgative methods, leading to the reversed flow of qi, thus, in turn, affecting the liver.

Therapeutic Principle. Removing heat, soothing the liver, invigorating qi and nourishing the blood.

Chong-qi Invading Lung

Symptoms. Dry throat and mouth, dizziness and palpitation, etc.

Pathogenesis. Owing to wrong treatment of the vital vessel disease with the diaphoretic and purgative methods, leading to the reversed flow of qi, thus, in turn, affecting the lung.

Therapeutic Principle. Nourishing qi and yin, enhancing production of the body fluid.

Chongyang (S 42)

An acupoint.

Location. At the tip of the dorsum of foot, 5 cun above Neiting (S 44).

Indication. Abdominal distention, heaviness sensation in the limbs, toothache, indigestion, edema of the face, facial paralysis, flaccidity of the foot, madness, swelling and pain of the instep, pain and paralysis of the lower extremities, etc.

Method. Puncture 0.3-0.5 cun (avoid puncturing blood vessel), and perform moxibustion to the point for 3-5 minutes.

Christina Loosestrife Herb

It is the whole herb of Lysimachia christinae Hance (Primulaceae).

Effect. Promoting diuresis, relieving stranguria, removing dampness, jaundice, toxins and swelling.

Indication. Cholelithiasis and infectious hepatitis, stranguria of heat type, urinary stone, edema, and skin infection.

Chronic Asthma

Symptoms. Rale in the pharynx, fear of cold, cough, fever and sweat respectively according to whether asthma is resulting from heat or from cold.

Pathogenesis. Due to accumulation of retained phlegm in the lung.

Therapeutic Principle. Reinforcing the flow of the lung-qi, removing phlegm during the attack stage, and enriching the lung and nourishing kidney at the remission stage.

Chronic Cough

Symptoms. Long time cough.

Pathogenesis. Usually owing to accumulation of exopathogen in the body, internal injury of zang organs and fu organs, deficiency of qi and blood, deficiency of both the lung and the spleen.

Therapeutic Principle. Treating in accordance with the syndromes, reinforcing the spleen, the kidney and the lung.

Chronic Deafness

It is a deficiency syndrome.
Symptoms. The protracted deafness.
Pathogenesis. Owing to the deficiency of qi, blood, liver-yin and kidney-yin.

Chronic Diarrhea

Symptoms. Prolonged incurable diarrhea with prolapse of rectum.
Pathogenesis. Usually owing to qi collapse.
Therapeutic Principle. Recovering qi and inducing astringency.

Chronic Dysentery

Symptoms. Intermittent diarrhea, difficult recovery tenesmus.
Pathogenesis. Owing to weakened body, accumulation of damp-heat, stirring-up of fire caused by stagnation of qi, or by deficiency of the spleen and kidney.
Therapeutic Principle. Nourishing the kidney and the spleen, and removing dampness and heat.

Chronic Eczema

Symptoms. Thick, dry and lacerated skin, sensation of itching with white broken scurf when the diseased areas is scratched.
Pathogenesis. Owing to the stagnation pathogenic wind in the muscles and skin.
Therapeutic Principle. Removing wind, moistening, and killing parasites.

Chronic Infantile Convulsions due to Dysfunction of Spleen

Symptoms. Convulsions, after vomiting and serious diseases, cyanotic complexion with pale lips, sweat on the forehead, and cold limbs.
Pathogenesis. Deficiency of the stomach and spleen, and exhaustion of the spleen-yang.
Therapeutic Principle. Warming the middle-energizer and strengthening the spleen and vital energy and restoring yang.

Chronic Suppurative Otitis Media

Symptoms. Black pus shedding from inside the ear.
Pathogenesis. Osteoporosis of the ear caused by deficiency of the kidney.
Therapeutic Principle. Tonifying the kidney, enhancing the circulation of primordial qi, removing dampness and turbid fluid.

Chronic Ulcer Dripping with Exudation

Symptoms. Broken skin and ulcerated muscle in the affected parts, black and sunken, hard to heal.
Pathogenesis. Owing to the deficiency and weakness of the body or spleen deficiency caused by chronic disease, and the invasion of dampness.
Therapeutic Principle. Mainly nourishing the spleen and removing dampness.

Chronic Ulcer of Shank

It is a chronic ulcer on the lower limbs.
Symptoms. In the early phase, itching and then painful, with red swelling. Later, ulcerate, with stink and dirty water, pus and blood flowing out.
Pathogenesis. Due to downward flow of damp-heat and the stagnation of qi and blood.
Therapeutic Principle. Enhancing blood circulation, releasing obstruction in the meridians.

Chrysanthemum Flower

⊛ **C-11**

It is the anthodium of Chrysanthemum morifolium Ramat. (Compositae).
Effect. Removing wind, heat and toxic substances, enhancing eyesight.
Indication. For the type of wind-heat and epidemic febrile diseases at the early stage, fever, dizziness and headache; conjunctival congestion with swelling

pain owing to wind-heat in the liver or owing to the flaming-up of excessive liver-fire; headache, dizziness owing to up-stirring of endogenous, etc.

Chuanshijiu (Ex-LE)

An extra point.
Location. On the anterior side of the leg, lateral to the spine of the tibia, 3 cun above the midpoint of the line connecting the medial and external malleolus.
Indication. Pulmonary tuberculosis.
Method. Moxibustion.

Chuanxiong Rhizome

It is the rhizome of Ligusticum chuanxiong Hort. (Umbelliferae).
Effect. Enhancing blood circulation and flow of qi, removing pathogenic wind and pain.
Indication. Irregular menstruation, dysmenorrhea, amenorrhea, pain in the hypochondrium, numbness of the limbs, traumatic injuries, etc.

Chunli (Ex-HN)

An extra point.
Location. In the mouth, at the midpoint of the mucoid membrane of the lower lip, opposite to Chengjiang (CV 24).
Indication. Jaundice, foul breath, edema of face, gingivitis, stomatitis, etc.
Method. Prick to cause little bleeding.

Cicada Slough

It is the slough shed by the numph of cicada Cryptotympana atrata Fabr. (Cicadidae).
Effect. Removing convulsion, spasm, pathogenic wind-heat, sore-throat, nebula, enhancing eruption, improving eyesight.
Indication. Fever, headache, cough, sore throat owing to affection of exopathogenic wind-heat, slow eruption of measles in children, bloodshot eyes, oculopathy, nocturnal fretfulness in infants, tetanus, etc.

Cigong (Ex)

An extra point.
Location. 2.5 cun lateral to the midpoint of the symphysis pubis.
Indication. Diarrhea, dysentery, irregular menstruation.
Method. Puncture perpendicularly 0.5-1.0 cun. Apply moxibustion 5-7 moxa cones or 10-15 minutes with warming moxibustion.

Ciliao (B 32)

An acupoint.
Location. In the sacral region, opposite to the second posterior sacral foramen, interior and inferior to the posterior superior iliac spine.
Indication. Lumbosacral pain, leukorrhea with reddish discharge, irregular menstruation, dysmenorrhea, sterility, nocturnal emission, dysuria, diarrhea, constipation, hemorrhoid and hernia.
Method. Puncture perpendicularly 1.0-1.5 cun and perform moxibustion to the point with 3-7 units of moxa cones or for 5-15 minutes.

Ciliate Bugle Herb

It is the whole herb of Ajuga ciliata Bge. (Labiatae).
Effect. Releasing swelling and heat from the blood, and reducing fever.
Indication. Hemoptysis resulting from the lung-heat, tonsillitis, pharyngitis, laryngitis, traumatic injuries, sprain, etc.

Cinnabar

It is the mineral ore of Cinnabaris (hexagonal system) hydragyrum sulfide.
Effect. Calming the mind and removing heat and toxins.
Indication. Irritability, severe palpitation, insomnia, infantile convulsion and epilepsy, carbuncles, furuncles, sore throat, canker sores.

Cinnamon Oil

It is the volatile oil of Cinnamomum cassia Presl (Lauraceae), distilled from the dried branch and leaf with vapour.

Effect. Reinforcing the stomach and removing pathogenic wind.

Indication. Syndrome of weakness of the spleen and the stomach; syndrome of wind-dampness and cutaneous pruritus for external use.

Cinnamon Twig

It is the twig of Cinnamomum cassia Presl. (Lauraceae).

Effect. Induce sweating to expel the pathogenic factors from the body surface, warming the meridians and reinforcing yang.

Indication. Common cold of wind-cold type obstruction of qi in the chest, chest pain, palpitation, phlegm retention owing to deficiency of the heart and spleen, and also amenorrhea, dysmenorrhea, abdominal masses owing to pathogenic cold in the blood, etc.

Circling

It refers to a needling manipulation. After inserting the needle superficially into the subcutaneous region, slope the body of the needle and make the handle of the needle circle around. Mainly used on the abdomen. The left spiraling with the needle pressed is reinforcing manipulation while the right spiraling with the needle lifted is reducing manipulation.

Citron Fruit

It is the fruit of Citrus medica L. Citrus wilsonii Tanaka (Rutaceae).

Effect. Smoothing the liver, adjusting flow of qi, reinforcing the spleen and removing phlegm.

Indication. Pain in the hypochondrium and chest owing to the stagnation of the liver-qi; gastric and abdominal distention and pain, belching, anorexia, vomiting, cough with profuse phlegm, etc.

Citrusleaf Glye Rootosmis

It is the root and leaf of Glycosmis citrifolia (Willd.) Lindl. (Rutaceae).

Effect. Removing pathogenic wind, phlegm, food stagnancy and blood stasis.

Indication. Cough owing to common cold, abdominal pain owing to retention of food, traumatic injuries and frostbite.

Clam Shell

It is the shell of Meretrix meretrix L. and Cyclina sinensis Gmelin (Veneridae).

Effect. Removing hard masses, phlegm and heat from the lung.

Indication. Phlegm dyspnea caused by the lung heat, cough, goiter, etc.

Clavicle (MA-SF 5)

An auricular point.

Location. Divide the scapha area into 6 equal parts, of which, from up to bottom, the 6th part is the clavicle.

Indication. Periarthritis of the shoulder.

Clavus

It is a disease, mostly on the foot which sinks deeply in the flesh, like a chicken eye.

Symptoms. Cuticle peg, like a pea, in grey and yellow color, hard, seriously painful when pressed.

Pathogenesis. Owing to long time pressing or friction on the sole of foot or between toes.

Therapeutic Principle. External treatment mainly.

Clear Complexion

Referring to one of ten methods by observing the complexion of a patient. Clear, bright, and moist complexion referring to yang syndrome, indicating without exhaustion of the vital-qi, strong resistance and favourable prognosis.

Clearing away Heat and Causing Resuscitation

It means using drugs, with inducing resuscitation and removing heat simultaneously for the heat syndromes, for example, coma with high fever, raving, restlessness, dry lips and teeth, limb convulsion and infantile convulsion.

Clearing away Heat and Producing Salivation

It means using drugs with cold in nature and producing salivation and ceasing thirst, for treating the diseases with exhaustion of heat and body fluid.

Clearing Away Heat and Promoting Diuresis

It means using the drugs to treat syndromes resulting from dampness and heat. The indications are such as chest tightness and abdominal distention, poor appetite, bitter taste or sore throat, yellow dark urine, etc.

Clearing away Heat in Qi System

It means using drugs with pungent flavor and cool property or these of bitter flavor and cold property, for treating heat syndromes in qi system, such as high fever, aversion to heat, profuse perspiration, thirst preferring to cold drink. yellow and dry fur, slippery rapid or slippery full pulse.

Clearing away Heat to Stop Bleeding

It means using the drugs with clearing away heat, cooling blood and ceasing bleeding in nature, for ceasing bleeding due to blood heat.

Clearing Summer-heat and Reinforcing Qi

It refers to a therapeutic method for removing summer-heat, enhancing qi circulation and production of the body fluid. This method is good at treating the syndromes due to impairing and exhausting body fluid and qi by summer-heat pathogens.

Clearing away Summer-heat and Removing Dampness by Diuresis

This treating method is good at treating the syndromes due to summer-heat and dampness, such as fever, dysphoria, thirst, and urinary incontinence.

Clear Thick Water

1. Referring to sour thick water. Put cooked millet into cold water for 5-6 days, and let it sour with white foam on the surface.
2. Referring to storing the water, rice washed but without rice, till sour. Clear thick water is cold and sweet and sour to the taste in nature. The drugs decocted with it can adjust the middle-energizer to ventilate qi, restoring consciousness, inducing appetite and digestion, removing thirst.

Clear Wine

Recently called rice wine.

Effect. Enhancing menstrual flow, removing cold, and adjusting qi and blood.

Cleft Points

It refers to the clefts where the meridian qi meeting together and converges. There are 16 such points altogether. They are usually used in treating acute diseases or persistent ailments of zang and fu organs belonging to their own meridians.

Clematis Florida Thunb

It is the root or the whole herb of Clematis florida Thunb. (Ranunculaceac).

Effect. Removing wind and dampness, and restoring menstrual flow.

Indication. Migratory arthralgia and apoplexy.

Climacterium

It refers to some symptoms that women commonly appear before or after the period of menopause, such as irregular menstruation, dizziness, palpitation, irritability, sweating, abnormal emotional changes, etc.

Climbing Fig Stem

It is the stem and leaf of Ficus pumila L. (Moraceae).

Effect. Removing wind, dampness, enhancing blood circulation and detoxicating.

Indication. Rheumatic arthralgia injuries, carbuncle, deep-rooted carbuncle, furuncle, boil, etc.

Climbing Groundsel Herb

It is the whole herb of Senecio scandens Buch.-Ham. (Compositae).

Effect. Removing heat, detoxicating, poisoning, killing parasites, enhancing acuity of vision.

Indication. Various acute inflammation, bloodshot eyes owing to pathogenic wind-fire, conjunctivitis, febrile disease, lobar pneumonia, tonsillitis, jaundice, toxemia, septicemia, suppurative infections on the body surface, eczema, trichomonal vaginitis, etc.

Clonic Convulsion

Symptoms. Stretching out and drawing back the limbs with palms opening and closing.

Pathogenesis. Owing to the extreme heat, the deficiency of yin-fluid and the excess of yang, up-stirring of the liver, the attack of pathogenic wind in the meridians and collaterals.

Therapeutic Principle. Calming the liver, ceasing the wind, removing endogenous wind and convulsion.

Clonic Convulsion during Pregnancy

Symptoms. Spontaneous spasm of the pregnant woman's extremities with alternate contracting and relaxing of the muscles.

Pathogenesis. Mostly due to original blood deficiency and blood collection to nourish the fetus after pregnancy leading to yin and blood insufficiency of the liver and kidney, failure of nourishing the tendon.

Therapeutic Principle. Calming the liver, nourishing blood.

Closed Injury of Muscle and Tendon

Symptoms. Injury of muscles and tendons of body, pain, ecchymoma and dysfunction.

Cause. Owing to the action of external force.

Therapeutic Principle. Manipulations, acupuncture and moxibustion.

Clotting Menstrual Blood

It is a disease and a syndrome, including two types:

1. **Symptoms.** Clotting with unbearable pain in the lower abdomen and aversion to touch.

   Pathogenesis. Mostly due to blood stasis resulting from the qi stagnation leading to clotting in menstrual blood.

   Therapeutic Principle. Removing stasis to adjust menstruation.

2. **Symptoms.** Clotting with whitish or dark menstrual blood, distending pain in the lower abdomen, and numb lips.

   Pathogenesis. Caused by coagulation due to blood cold leading to clotting in menstrual blood.

   Therapeutic Principle. Removing pathogenic cold from the meridian.

Cloudy Complexion

It is a diagnostic method, one of ten methods of observation of complexion. Cloudy and dim complexion indicates decline of the vital-qi, lower resistance and unfavourable prognosis.

Cloudy Internal Oculopathy

Symptoms. Glaucoma, with the pupil, with vague expression like dense smog in the rain at dusk, and constant headache without dizziness.

Pathogenesis. Usually due to yin deficiency and fire hyperactivity with internal wind-phlegm.

Therapeutic Principle. Releasing wind and phlegm, calming the liver and nourishing yin.

Clove

It is the flower-bud of Eugenia caryophyllata Thunb. (Myrtaceae).

Effect. Warming the middle-energizer, the kidney, sending down the upward adverse flow of qi and strengthening yang.

Indication. Vomiting owing to cold syndrome of the stomach, hiccups, poor appetite, diarrhea, deficiency of the kidney-yang, impotence and flaccidity of lower limbs.

Club-moss

It is the whole herb of Lycopodium clavatum L. (Lycopodiaceae) with root.

Effect. Removing pathogenic wind, cold, dampness, swelling, relaxing muscles and tendons and enhancing blood circulation.

Indication. Arthralgia with stiffness, skin numbness, flaccidity of limbs, edema and traumatic injuries.

Clump Hair

It refers to the hair on the skin of the dorsal aspect of the proximal phalange of the big toe, where the Dadun (Liv 1) of Foot-jueyin Meridian is.

Clumpy Pricking

It is a type of needling manipulations, referring to shallow and scattered pricking around the acupoints, mostly with three-edged needles.

Cluster Mallow Seed

It is the ripe seed of Malva verticillata L. (Malvaceae).

Effect. Promoting diuresis, relieving stranguria, stimulating milk secretion and inducing abortion, lubricating the intestines and releasing constipation.

Indication. Edema, dysuria, dribbling and painful micturition.

Coarse Dyspnea

Symptoms. Dyspnea with a coarse voice in febrile diseases and edema with abdominal distention.

Pathogenesis. Mostly owing to external invastion by six evils, internal injury due to improper diet, emotional frustration, weakness due to long illness, etc.

Cochinchina Momordica Seed

It is the ripe seed of Momordica cochinchinensis (Lour.) (Cucurbitaceae).

Effect. Removing swelling, lumps and toxic substances.

Indication. Suppurative infections on the body surface, for examples, sore, carbuncles, furuncles and boils, scrofula, hemorrhoid, innominate inflammatory swelling, tinea and sore.

Cockscomb Flower ⊛ C-12

It is the flower of Celosia cristata L. (Amaranthaceae).

Effect. Releasing heat from the blood and ceasing bleeding.

Indication. Hemorrhoid bleeding, dysentery, hematemesis, hemoptysis, metrorrhagia in women, leukorrhea with reddish discharge.

Coconut Root-bark

It is the root-bark of Cocos nucifera L. (Palmae).

Effect. Ceasing bleeding and removing pain.

Indication. Epistaxis, stomachache, vomiting, diarrhea, etc.

Coix Seed

It is the ripe seed of Coix lachryma-jobi L. var. mayuen (Roman.) Stapf (Gramineae).

Effect. Excreting dampness, reinforcing the spleen, removing dampness, numbness, heat and pus, inducing diuresis.

Indication. Dysuria, edema, diarrhea owing to hypofunction of the spleen, rheumatic arthralgia, spasm of muscles, pulmonary abscess and intestinal abscess.

Cold Abscess

Acute inflammatory abscess without such syndromes as red, swelling, heat and pain, often seen in the diseases of tuberculosis of bone and joint, and scrofula.

Cold Accumulation

Symptoms. Abdominal pain, relieved by pressing hard with hand or object, vomiting of watery fluid.

Pathogenesis. Mostly due to the invasion of pathogenic cold, leading to the accumulation.

Therapeutic Principle. Warming the middle-energizer and removing cold.

Cold Accumulation in Large Intestine

Symptoms. Anorexia abdominal dull pain, constipation, tastelessness.

Pathogenesis. Pathologic changes of constipation due to the accumulation and retention of pathogenic cold-qi in the large intestine, commonly occurring in the senile decay patients.

Therapeutic Principle. Relaxing the bowls with drugs of warm nature.

Cold Ache

Symptoms. Cold leading to pain, especially in upper-energizer and middle-energizer.

Therapeutic Principle. Warming yang, removing cold and pain.

Cold against Cold

It is a treatment principle. Referring to the fact that during the cool and cold seasons the principal drugs with cold and cool properties are forbidden to be used, except for excess heat syndrome, for protecting the yang-qi.

Cold and Pain below Umbilicus during Pregnancy

Symptoms. Abdominal distention, cold and pain below the umbilicus, frequent clear urine, loose stool, etc.

Pathogenesis. Owing to original weakness of the spleen and stomach, and overeating of raw and cold food during pregnancy.

Therapeutic Principle. Warming and nourishing the spleen, and the middle-energizer, and prevent abortion.

Cold-apoplexy

A type of apoplectic stroke.

Symptoms. Stiffness of the body, lockjaw, shaking of the limbs, sudden dizziness and anhidrosis.

Pathogenesis. Owing to the sudden attack of pathogenic cold.

Therapeutic Principle. Warming the interior and removing cold.

Cold-application at Acupoints

It refers to a therapeutic method. Applying cold stimulation on the acupoints for the treatment of diseases, for example, filling the umbilicus with alum and dropping some water on it to treat difficult urination and defecation. In modern times, spreading a proper amount of some cryogens, such as ethylene chloride and carbon dioxide, etc. on the points, instead of water.

Cold Compress

It refers to a treatment.

Method. Putting cold water or pieces of ice on some areas of the body.

Function. Reducing fever and ceasing bleeding.

Cold-dampness

1. It is a cause of disease. Cold-damp pathogen blocking the circulation of yang-qi, leading to impeded blood flow, painful skin and muscle, arthritis with muscle contracture, etc.
2. Referring to a syndrome.

Symptoms. Intolerance of cold and cold limbs, abdominal distention, diarrhea or edema, etc.

Pathogenesis. Owing to stagnant dampness in the spleen or owing to hypofunction of the spleen and kidney, resulting in stagnation of dampness.

Therapeutic Principle. Warming yang and inducing dampness.

Cold Diarrhea in Child

Symptoms. Pale stool, abdominal pain and borborygmus.

Pathogenesis. Owing to wind and cold entering the organs due to cutting umbilical cord without careful nursing.

Therapeutic Principle. Adjusting and nourishing the spleen and stomach, removing cold by warming up.

Cold due to Fire

Symptoms. Dry cough without sputum, feverish sensation, dry mouth, pharyngeal pain, etc.

Pathogenesis. Owing to affection of wind-heat, and pathogenic dryness-fire.

Therapeutic Principle. Removing wind, heat, and moistening dryness.

Cold due to Heart Deficiency

Symptoms. Cardiac and abdominal pain, susceptibility to sorrow, cold sweat, etc.

Pathogenesis. Owing to the insufficiency of the heart-qi, deficiency and exhaustion of the heart-yang.

Therapeutic Principle. Tonifying blood, heart, qi, and calming the mind.

Cold during Menstruation

Symptoms. The repeated attack of stuffy nose and rhinorrhea, headache, numbness and pain in the joints of the limbs, gradual recovery after menstruation.

Therapeutic Principle. Nourishing the liver, adjusting menstruation, removing heat and inducing diaphoresis.

Cold Edema

Symptoms. Abdominal distention and fullness, vomiting and diarrhea and cold limbs, etc.

Pathogenesis. Owing to the invasion of pathogenic cold.

Therapeutic Principle. Warming yang, reinforcing the spleen and inducing diuresis.

Cold Excess Syndrome

Symptoms. Distention and fullness in the chest and abdomen, cold limbs, or abdominal pain, constipation, etc.

Pathogenesis. Usually owing to invasion of pathogenic cold into visceral organs, or by stagnation of cold phlegm and turbid dampness.

Therapeutic Principle. Warming the middle-energizer to disperse cold.

Cold Feeling of Whole Body

Symptoms. Cold feeling of the whole body, foul breath, constipation, etc.

Pathogenesis. Owing to the invasion of the pathogenic heat and yang excess, separating yin outside.

Therapeutic Principle. Removing and inducing the stagnation.

Cold Feet or Cold Tips of Fingers

Symptoms. Cold feet or only cold tips of fingers.

Pathogenesis. Mostly due to deficiency and cold of the spleen and stomach.

Therapeutic Principle. Warming the middle-energizer, removing cold.

Cold Grapple

Referring to grapple of upper heat with lower cold, its clinical syndrome is vomiting mainly.

Cold Hiccups

Symptoms. Successive hiccups, slight at dawn but serious at dusk, chilly hands and feet, etc.

Pathogenesis. Due to attack of cold and wind or injury by cold drinking.

Therapeutic Principle. Warming the middle-energizer, removing cold. For the deficiency-cold of the kidney, warming and nourishing the spleen and kidney.

Cold in Both Exterior and Interior

Referring to the coexistence of exterior and interior syndrome of cold.

Symptoms. Headache, general pain, chills, anhidrosis, abdominal pain, diarrhea, cold limbs.

Pathogenesis. Owing to the affection of exopathogenic cold, the impairment of the interior by raw and cold food, or the syndrome of internal cold with the affection of exopathogenic cold.

Therapeutic Principle. Removing the exterior syndromes and warming interior.

Cold in Four Seasons

Symptoms. Stuffy, running nose, sneezing, cough, headache, aversion to cold, fever and discomfort of whole body.

Pathogenesis. Owing to the attack of wind-cold in four seasons.

Therapeutic Principle. Removing exterior syndrome and the pathogenic factor.

Cold Injuring Physique

Referring to the cold pathogenic factor injuring configuration and constitution of a human body, and leading to aversion to cold, headache, pains in the body, and anhidrosis.

Cold Limb

1. It is a symptom referring to cold hands and feet.
2. It is a symptom and disease.
   Symptoms. Severe pain in the chest and abdomen, cold hands and feet, restlessness and inappetence, etc.
   Pathogenesis. Owing to excessive yin cold, qi stagnation and blood stasis.

Therapeutic Principle. Warming the middle-energizer, removing pain, cold, adjusting qi.

3. It refers to a type of prolonged headache.
   Symptoms. Headache and toothache for a long time.
   Pathogenesis. Severe cold attacking to brain and spinal cord.
   Therapeutic Principle. Removing pain, cold, calming the adverse rising qi.

Cold Limb due to Ascaris

Symptoms. Sudden severe pain in the stomach, even cold limbs, restlessness, nausea, vomiting, spitting roundworm sometimes, but normal after pain.

Pathogenesis. Owing to dysfunction of the spleen and stomach, the disturbance by ascaris in the biliary tract, the qi obstruction of the liver and gall bladder.

Therapeutic Principle. Removing pain and killing ascaris.

Cold Limbs due to Excessive Heat

1. Referring to cold limbs, even coma.
   Symptoms. Fever and headache first, then coma, cold limbs, or restlessness, insomnia, burning heat in the chest and abdomen, constipation, dark urine, etc.
   Pathogenesis. Owing to excessive pathogenic heat.
   Therapeutic Principle. Removing accumulated heat.
2. Referring to the feverish sensation in the palms and soles owing to the deficiency of yin and excess of yang.

Cold Limbs in Children due to Excess of Heat

Symptoms. Deadly cold limbs with high fever and a feeling of burning in the chest and abdomen, dryness of the tongue, thirst, irritability, dark urine or constipation.

Pathogenesis. Usually owing to excess pathogenic heat and stagnation of yang-qi.

Therapeutic Principle. Calming mind, adjusting qi, removing heat and inducing mental resuscitation.

Cold Limbs in Children due to Pathogenic Cold

Symptoms. Deadly cold extremities and body, cyanotic, white urine.

Pathogenesis. Mostly caused by exhaustion of yang at the lower-energizer and excess of yin-cold.

Therapeutic Principle. Recuperate the depleted yang and rescue the patient from danger.

Cold Malignant Malaria

It is a type of malignant malaria.

Symptoms. Feeling cold but little heat, vomiting, diarrhea, or even coma and speechlessness.

Pathogenesis. Owing to constitutional yang deficiency.

Therapeutic Principle. Removing dampness, turbid qi, and heat from the heart to restore to consciousness.

Cold Moxibustion

It is a type of moxibustion.

Method. Putting the medicine on certain acupoints only, without any heat resources, also named moxibustion without heat, opposed to heat moxibustion.

Cold Needling

It refers to the pure needling, different from warm needling.

Coldness due to Heaven-penetrating

It is a needling technique, opposite to heat-producing needling, a comprehensive utilization of reducing needling technique.

Method. First insert the needle to the deep part, lift it quickly and thrust it slowly, and withdraw the needle to the medium part, then to the shallow part in the same way.

Indication. The technique is good at treating the heat syndrome.

Coldness due to Qi Deficiency

Symptoms. Cold limbs, sallow complexion, fatigue, etc.

Pathogenesis. Owing to the internal impairment due to overstrain, the deficiency both qi and blood.

Therapeutic Principle. Reinforcing the middle-energizer and tonifying qi.

Coldness of Genitals

Symptoms. For women, subjective cold sensation in the vagina, and even cold pain in the lower abdomen, affecting child bearing.

Pathogenesis. Owing to internal coldness due to deficiency of kidney-yang.

Therapeutic Principle. Nourishing the kidney, reinforcing yang, and removing cold from meridians.

Coldness with Flaccidity

Symptoms. Flaccidity and coldness of hands and feet.

Pathogenesis. Owing to long time disease of flaccidity, disorder of the qi circulation, abnormal rising and falling of flow of qi and imbalance between yin-qi and yang-qi.

Cold of Deficiency Type

Symptoms. Sallow and dim complexion, inappetence, profuse watery salivation, distending pain in the abdomen, feeling comfortable in warmth, lucid and thin leukorrhea for women, lassitude in loin and back, copious clear urine, loose stool.

Pathogenesis. Owing to insufficiency of genuine qi with cold.

Therapeutic Principle. Warming and tonification.

Cold of Liver Meridians

Symptoms. Pain in the chest, difficult to raise arms and to turn round, vomiting, etc.

Pathogenesis. Owing to invasion of pathogenic cold into the liver.

Therapeutic Principle. Smoothing the depressed liver and removing cold.

Cold of Lung Meridians

Symptoms. Cough, vomiting of the turbid spittle, shortness of breath.

Pathogenesis. Owing to the invasion of the pathogenic cold into the lung.

Therapeutic Principle. Warming the lung, removing cold.

Cold Pain

Symptoms. There are two cases: for cold pathogen attacking the stomach, pain in gastric cavity, preferring warmth and pressing; for cold pathogen attacking joints, cold pain, and limitation of joint movement.

Cold Penetration into Uterus

Symptoms. Sudden stop of menstruation with unbearable pain in the abdomen and hypochondrium, and loss of appetite.

Pathogenesis. Owing to invasion of pathogenic cold into vital meridian through the opening orifice of the uterus during menstruation.

Therapeutic Principle. Enhancing blood circulation, adjusting menstruation, removing cold and warming yang.

Cold Phlegm

Including three meanings:

1. Phlegm syndrome owing to cold.
2. Phlegm syndrome owing to the attack of the lung by wind-cold, and excess cold in the spleen.
   Symptoms. Aversion to cold, headache and cough with clear, thin and white sputum, etc.
   Therapeutic Principle. Warming the lung and removing phlegm.
3. Phlegm accumulation in the chest owing to dysfunction of the spleen, stomach, and deficiency of yang-qi.
   Symptoms. Anorexia, stuffiness in the chest and thin and weak physique.
   Therapeutic Principle. Warming the spleen and removing phlegm.

Cold Stagnancy

It is a syndrome.

Symptoms. Watery vomiting, sometimes accompanied by abdominal mass or hernia, copious clear urine, etc.

Pathogenesis. Owing to the cold stagnancy in the interior.

Therapeutic Principle. Warming the middle-energizer, removing cold.

Cold Stranguria

Including three meanings:

1. **Symptoms.** Chills first, and then frequent urination with pain.
   Pathogenesis. Owing to deficiency of the kidney-qi, cold qi in the lower-energizer.
   Therapeutic Principle. Warming the kidney and removing cold, enhancing diuresis.
2. **Symptoms.** The stranguria with cloudy urine like rice water.
   Pathogenesis. Owing to the insufficiency of the kidney yang and excess of cold, the mixture of clearness and turbidity.
   Therapeutic Principle. Removing turbidity from clearness.
3. **Symptoms.** Stranguria with blood.
   Pathogenesis. Owing to deficiency cold of the lower-energizer, cramping sensation in the lower abdomen, hematuria with pain or frequent urination, etc.
   Therapeutic Principle. Warming the kidney and ceasing bleeding.

Cold Stroke

Symptoms. Aversion to cold, body pain, anhidrosis and fever, for exterior cold type; abdominal pain and diarrhea, for the interior cold type.

Pathogenesis. Owing to the disease due to pathogenic cold.

Therapeutic Principle. Warming and removing pathogenic cold.

Cold-stroke Syndrome of Taiyang Meridian

Symptoms. Aversion to wind-cold, headache, arthralgia, general pain, anhidrosis, vomiting, dyspnea, cough, etc.

Pathogenesis. Owing to wind-cold pathogen tightening the exterior, closed defense system and depressed nutrient system, and obstruction of the lung-qi.

Therapeutic Principle. Inducing diaphoresis, reinforcing the flow of the lung-qi, and removing asthma.

Cold Stroke with Yin Syndrome

It refers to the direct attack of pathogenic agent on the three yin meridians. Including three types:

1. **Symptoms.** In the case of attack of cold on taiyin, chills and trembles, vomiting and diarrhea without thirst, etc.
   Therapeutic Principle. Warming the middle-energizer, removing cold.
2. **Symptoms.** In the attack of cold on shaoyin, chills and cold limbs, diarrhea with cold and clear water in stool.
   Therapeutic Principle. Warming and recuperating the kidney yang.
3. **Symptoms.** In the case of attack of cold on jueyin, chills and trembles, diarrhea with clear water in stool.
   Therapeutic Principle. Recuperating depleted yang and rescuing the patient from collapse.

Cold Sweat

Symptoms. Sweating with chills.

Pathogenesis. Mostly owing to the deficiency of yang-qi and difficult to cease sweating.

Therapeutic Principle. Warming yang and tonifying qi.

Cold Syndrome in Heart

Symptoms. Oppressed feeling in chest and vexation, like pungent sensation after eating ginger and garlic, and even pain due to contraction between the heart and back.

Pathogenesis. Owing to the invasion of the heart meridians by pathogenic cold and yang-qi closure.

Therapeutic Principle. Removing cold from the skin and enhancing the flow of yang-qi.

Cold Syndrome of Deficiency Type

Symptoms. Dull and pale complexion, anorexia, distention and pain in the epigastrium and abdomen, chills, lassitude, loose stool, copious clear urine, etc.

Pathogenesis. Owing to the deficiency of yang-qi.

Therapeutic Principle. Warming and invigorating yang-qi.

Cold Syndrome of Middle-Energizer

There are two meanings:

1. **Symptoms.** Sudden vertigo, unconsciousness, cold extremities, stiffness of the body, lockjaw, etc.
   Pathogenesis. Sudden invasion of cold pathogen.
   Therapeutic Principle. Dispersing cold pathogen.
2. **Symptoms.** Abdominal pain, relieved by pressing, cold extremities, anorexia and loose stool, etc.
   Pathogenesis. Cold deficiency in the middle-energizer, yang in sufficiency and dysfunction of the spleen and stomach.
   Therapeutic Principle. Warming and nourishing the spleen and stomach.

Cold Syndrome of Stomach

Symptoms. Gastralgia relieved by warmth but more serious by cold, watery vomiting.

Pathogenesis. Attacks of cold pathogen on stomach or impairment of stomach-yang due to excess of cold raw food.

Therapeutic Principle. Warming the stomach and removing cold.

Cold Syndrome Manifested as Colic

1. **Symptoms.** Spasm in the abdomen, pain around umbilicus, cold sweat, chill and cold extremities.
   Pathogenesis. Owing to yang deficiency of the spleen and the stomach, and stagnation of yin cold in the abdomen.

Therapeutic Principle. Removing dampness, cold, pain, and enhancing the circulation of qi.

2. **Symptoms.** Cold and pain of the scrotum.

   Pathogenesis. Owing to invasion of the liver meridians by the pathogenic cold-damp.

   Therapeutic Principle. Warming the liver, removing cold.

Cold Syndrome of Deficiency Type in Tri-energizer

Symptoms. Cold in tri-energizer of deficiency type simultaneously appearing in the three portions of tri-energizer: In the upper-energizer, deficiency of the heart and the lungs, listlessness, shortness of breath and weakness of voice; in the middle-energizer, deficiency of the spleen and the stomach, abdominal pain, increased borborygmus and chronic diarrhea; in the lower-energizer, deficiency of the liver and the kidney, polyuria or enuresis, chronic diarrhea, abdominal distention and heaviness sensation in the limbs.

Cold Type and Heat Type Malnutrition

1. **Symptoms.** For the heat type of malnutrition, short course, redness and ulceration of nose, hectic fever, and dysphoria, heat sensation in the abdomen and cold feet, etc.

   Therapeutic Principle. Removing heat, enhancing production of body fluid and invigorating the spleen.

2. **Symptoms.** For the cold type malnutrition, long course, darkish complexion, and swelling of the eyelids, weakness, poor appetite and diarrhea with blue-white foam.

   Therapeutic Principle. Warming the middle-energizer and reinforcing the spleen and stomach.

Cold Type Consumption

1. **Symptoms.** Sallow complexion, emaciation and lassitude, stuffiness and fullness in the epigastrium, abdominal pain with dysentery and cold limbs, etc.

   Pathogenesis. Mostly owing to the deficiency of qi and blood, imbalance of yin and yang, exhaustion of vital essence.

   Therapeutic Principle. Warming yang and recovering qi.

Cold Type Dyspnea

There are two meanings:

1. It refers to dyspnea due to deficiency of yang and too much cold.

   Therapeutic Principle. Warming yang to lower qi.

2. It refers to dyspnea due to wind-cold.

   Therapeutic Principle. Smoothing lung qi, removing cold.

Cold Upper Extremities

Symptoms. Cold arms and hands with spasm, difficulty in flexion and extention, sometimes thorax fullness and distress, cough and cardialgia.

Pathogenesis. Due to qi-retrogression and disturbance of the Lung Meridian of Hand Taiyin and the Heart Meridian of Hand-Shaoyin of the arms, often seen in blood deficiency.

Therapeutic Principle. Nourishing yin and blood, and clearing and activating the meridians.

Cold Vomiting

Symptoms. Pale complexion and cold limbs, fullness in the epigastrium and nausea, vomiting with water and phlegm.

Pathogenesis. Mostly owing to yang deficiency of the spleen and stomach, retention of phlegm and fluid in the epigastrium and the failure of descending of the stomach-qi.

Therapeutic Principle. Removing phlegm retention with warm drugs in nature.

Colic due to Ascaris

Symptoms. Abdominal angina and cold limbs, with vomiting and defecation of ascaris, etc.

Pathogenesis. Due to disturbance of ascaris in the abdomen.

Therapeutic Principle. Releasing colic by removing the ascaris and warming the stomach.

Collapse due to Massive Hemorrhage

Symptoms. Huge amount of hemorrhage, with pale complexion, cold limbs, sweating and asthma

Therapeutic Principle. Invigorating qi and curing collapse to cease blood immediately, and nourishing yin and supplementing blood for deficiency of yin and blood.

Collapse during Coitus

Symptoms. Sudden collapse of male or female during sexual intercourse.

Pathogenesis. Mostly owing to deficiency of kidney, over exciting during sexual intercourse.

Therapeutic Principle. Emergency treatment for collapse, nourishing yang.

Collapse-syndrome of Apoplexy Involving Zang and Fu

Symptoms. Deep coma, closing of eyes, opening of mouth, relaxed hand, incontinence of urine, nasal snore, little respiratory, cold limbs.

Pathogenesis. Owing to the deficiency of genuine qi and the sudden collapse of the primary-yang.

Therapeutic Principle. Recovering collapse, supplementing qi and restoring yang.

Collateral branch of the Large Meridian

It is the name for meridians and collaterals, referring to the branches derived from the meridians and netted throughout the human body. The collateral branch of the Large Meridian including the Fifteen Collaterals as the main, also including the minute collaterals, superficial venules and superficial collaterals.

Function. Linking meridians, transporting qi and blood, being response to and treating diseases.

Collateral of Foot-jueyin

It is one of the Fifteen Collaterals. Its name is Ligou (Liv 5). The collateral branching from Ligou, 5 cun above the medial malleolus, and running to the Foot-Shaoyang Meridian, its branch passing along the tibia, ascending to the testes, and linking at the penis.

Collateral of Foot-shaoyang

It is one of the Fifteen Collaterals. The collateral branching from Guangming (G 37), 5 cun above the external malleolus, and going to the Foot-jueyin Meridian, running downwards and linking the dorsum of the foot.

Collateral of Foot-shaoyin

It is one of the Fifteen Collaterals. The collateral branching from Dazhong (K 4) at the heel posterior to the medial malleolus, and running to join the meridian of Foot-taiyang, the branch going upwards parallel to its own meridian to the region below the pericardium, and running outwards through the part of the loin and spine.

Collateral of Foot-taiyang

It is one of the Fifteen Collaterals, the collateral of Foot-taiyang branching from Feiyang (B 58), 7 cun above the lateral ankle, running towards the Meridian of Foot-shaoyin.

Collateral of Foot-taiyin

It is one of the Fifteen Collaterals. The collateral of Foot-taiyin branching from Gongsun (Sp 4), 1 cun posterior to the 1st segment of the great toe, and running towards the Stomach Meridian of Foot-yangming, one branch getting into the abdomen, and linking with the intestines and stomach.

Collateral of Hand-jueyin

Referring to one of the Fifteen Collaterals, branching from Neiguan (P 6) on the collateral, coming out between the tendons at 2 cun from the wrist, and going up along its regular meridian, crossing the pericardium and joining the heart network.

Collateral of Hand-Shaoyang

Referring to one of the Fifteen Collaterals. The said collateral derived from Waiguan (TE 5) point, going round along the lateral arm from 2 cun posterior to the wrist, getting into the chest, and emerging with the Meridian of Hand-jueyin.

Collateral of Hand-Shaoyin

Referring to one of the Fifteen Collaterals. The said collateral branching from Tongli (H 5) and going toward the Meridian of Hand-taiyang at 1 cun from the wrist. Its branch coming out at 1.5 cun from the wrist, up to the heart along the Meridian of Hand-taiyang, linking with the root of the tongue, and then gathering the eye network.

Collateral of Hand-taiyang

Referring to one of the Fifteen Collaterals. The said collateral is branched from Zhizheng (SI 7) point, goes inward into the Meridian of Hand-shaoyin from 0.5 cun posterior to the wrist, its branch going up through the elbow, and spreading at shoulder joint.

Collateral of Hand-taiyin

Referring to one of the Fifteen Collaterals. The said collateral derived from supraclavicular fossa, and going toward the Meridian of Hand-yangming from 0.5 cun posterior to the wrist. Its branch emerging with the Meridian of Hand-taiyin, straight to the palm, and spreading at thenar eminence.

Collateral of Hand-yangming

Referring to one of the Fifteen Collaterals. The said collateral branching from Pianli (LI 6) and going to the meridian of Hand-taiyin, at 3 cun from the wrist. One branch going through Jianyu (LI 15) up to the angle of the mandible, spreading to the teeth, the other branch getting into the ear through the angle of the mandible, joining the main meridians, linking at the ear.

Collateral of the Front Middle Meridian

Referring to one of the Fifteen Collaterals, also named Jiuwei (CV 15), for it spreads down to the abdomen from Jiuwei.

Collateral of the Same Yin

Referring to the branch collateral of Foot-taiyang meridian at the leg, running from the point 5 cun above the external malleolus, to the Meridian of Foot-jueyin, then going along the meridian to spread over the dorsum; therefore, so named the collateral of the same yin.

Collateral Pricking

It is a needling method.

Method. Pricking and clumpy pricking on the superficial collateral with a three-edged needle or cutaneous needle to cause proper bleeding.

Indication. Acute tonsillitis, acute conjunctivitis, acute sprain, heat stroke, apoplexy coma, acute gastroenteritis, headache, hypertension, pulmonary edema, etc.

Notice. Avoid injury to arteries. The method is forbidden for patients with weak constitution, hypoglycemia, hypotension and pregnant women.

Collaterals

Generally referring to all kinds of collaterals running everywhere like a network from large to small, including large collaterals, superficial collaterals, superficial venules minute collaterals, and thready collaterals.

Function. Reinforcing the relationship between the interior meridian and exterior meridian, and running to the organs and tissues which the meridians fail to pass through.

Collateral Shu

Referring to the acupoints of floating collateral meridian.

Collaterals Located at the Thenar Eminence

Referring to the collaterals at the internal posterior aspect of thenar eminence. Based on the changes of color and lustre of collaterals located at the thenar eminence, some enterogastric diseases can be diagnosed clinically, for example, blue color indicating cold syndrome of the stomach, red indicating heat syndrome of the stomach and intestine, etc.

Colophony

It is the residue left after the distillation of the turpentine oil from the crude oleoresin of Pinus massoniana Lamb. (Pinaceae).
Effect. Killing parasites, releasing dampness, toxic substances and enhancing tissue regeneration.
Indication. Scabies, tinea, protracted sores and ulcer; subcutaneous swelling and chronic cough with dyspnea.

Color Blindness

Symptoms. Failure to distinguish the color, loss of red distinguish, called red blindness. Loss of green distinguish, called green blindness, loss of both red and green distinguish, called complete color blindness.
Pathogenesis. Mostly caused by congenital defect, deficiency of the liver and kidney, derangement of qi and blood of the eye's collaterals.
Therapeutic Principle. Nourishing the liver and kidney and regulating the function of the brain.

Coltsfoot Flower   ✤ C-13

It is the flower-bud of Tussilago farfara L. (Compositae).
Effect. Nourishing the lung and adjusting the adverse flow of qi, removing cough and phlegm.
Indication. Cough resulting from many diseases.

Comain Children

Symptoms. Coma in children, loss of consciousness, flushed face and gasping for breath, wheezing sound in the throat.
Pathogenesis. Owing to internal stagnation of phlegm, heat.
Therapeutic Principle. Removing pathogenic heat, phlegm and induce resuscitation.

Combination of Back-shu with Front-mu Points

Referring to one type of point prescription. It refers to the combination of the back-shu points with the front-mu points relating to the zang-fu organs affected by diseases. For example, selecting Weishu (B 21) and Zhongwan (CV 12) for the treatment of the gastrosis symptom, while Pangguangshu (B 28) and Zhongji (CV 3) for the treatment of the bladder disease.

Combination of Distal-proximal Points

Referring to the compatible method for selecting points in acupuncture, that is, the selection of both the distal and proximal points related to the disease in acupuncture. One example for stomach diseases, the distal points selected are Neiguan (P 6) and Zusanli (S 36), while the proximal one is Zhongwan (CV 12).

Combination of Points on Meridians with the Same Name

Referring to the cooperative selection of points on meridians with the same name on the hand and foot, e.g. both Hand- and Foot-taiyin or Hand- and Foot-yangming etc., linking with each other, these meridians have a cooperative function in treating diseases. It means that points of the meridians with the same name on the upper or lower part of the body can cooperatively be selected.

Combination of Primary Collateral Points

Referring to one type of point prescription. With the method, taking the primary point of the diseased meridian as the main, combining with the collateral point on the meridian with exterior-interior relation with the diseased meridian as the auxiliary.

Combination of the Anterior-posterior Points

It is a type of point prescription, anterior referring to the face, head, chest and abdomen; posterior referring to occipital and lumbodorsal regions. Coordinately using the points in the anterior and posterior to treat diseases of the five sense organs and internal organs. For example, Jingming (B 1) and Fengchi (G 20) for ophthalmopathy; Lianquan (CV 23) and Yamen (GV 15) for inability to speak due to stiff tongue; Zhongwan (CV 12) and Weishu (B 21) for stomachache, etc.

Combination of the Superior-inferior Points

Referring to selecting acupoints both above and below the lumbar region for treating some diseases. For example, select Neiguan (P 6) on the upper extremity and Zusanli (S 36) on the lower for treating stomachache; Hegu (LI 4) on the upper extremity and Neiting (S 44) on the lower for treating sore throat, etc.

Combined Pathogens

Referring to two or more kinds of pathogen-qi joining together and invading the human body.

Combined Spicebush Root

It is the root of Lindera strychnifolia (Sieb. et Zucc.) Villar (Lauraceae).

Effect. Removing cold, alleviating pain, enhancing qi circulation, and warming the kidney.

Indication. Fullness in the chest owing to accumulation of cold with stagnation of qi; pain in the hypochondrium, epigastric and abdominal distention and pain, dysmenorrhea, nocturia, enuresis, etc.

Combined Syndrome of Taiyang and Shaoyang Meridians

It refers to simultaneous occurrence of the syndrome of the Taiyang Meridian and the syndrome of the Shaoyang Meridian.

Symptoms. Diarrhea, vomiting, fever and aversion to cold.

Therapeutic Principle. For the case of more severe pathogenic factors of Shaoyang than those of Taiyang, removing heat to stop diarrhea.

Combined Syndrome of Taiyang and Yangming

Referring to simultaneous occurrence of the syndrome of the Taiyang Meridian and that of the Yangming Meridian.

Symptoms. Fever, fear of cold, headache, rigidity of the neck, no sweating, dyspnea, fullness in the chest, dysphoria, delirium, abdominal pain and tenderness, and failure in defecation. There are different conditions due to different pathogenic affection.

Therapeutic Principle. Removing exterior syndrome at first, for those with more severe Taiyang disease; for those with more severe yangming disease, mainly removing interior syndrome; for those with the same degree of exterior and interior syndrome, treating both the exterior and interior syndromes.

Combing Manipulation

Referring to massage manipulation.

Operation. Glide-comb on the affected part gently with the whorled surface of the fingers in one direction, with five fingers slightly flexed and parted naturally.
Function. Releasing stagnancy.
Indication. Stasis of liver-qi, breast carbuncle, etc.

Commencement of Static Qigong

A term in Qigong, referring to beginning to practise sitting meditation, during the practice, removing all distracting thoughts, calming down mind, and concentrating mindwill to enter a natural and comfortable state of Qigong.

Common Aeschynomene Herb

It is the whole herb of Aeschynomene indica L. (Leguminosae).
Effect. Removing heat, wind, diuresis, swelling and detoxicating.
Indication. Common cold owing to windheat, jaundice, dysentery, abdominal distention, stranguria, subcutaneous swelling, etc.

Common Andrographis Herb

It is the whole plant of Andrographis paniculata (Brum. f.) Nees (Acanthaceae).
Effect. Releasing heat, toxic materials and dampness, antineoplastic.
Indication. Epidemic diseases, headache, asthma and cough owing to the lung-heat, pulmonary abscess, swollen and sore throat, carbuncles, furuncles, subcutaneous swelling, snake bite, eczema, malignant mole chorionic epithelioma.

Common Argyreia Stem and Leaf

It is the stem leaf of Argyreia acuta Lour (Convolvulaceae).
Effect. Removing pain, wind, phlegm, cough, ceasing bleeding.
Indication. Heat cough, phlegm dyspnea, hematemesis, metrorrhagia, metrostaxis, traumatic injuries, rheumatalgia and noxious carbuncles.

Common Aspidistra Rhizome

It is the rhizome of Aspidistra elatior Bl. (Liliaceae).
Effect. Enhancing blood circulation, releasing obstruction in the meridians, and the pathogenic heat to induce diuresis.
Indication. Traumatic injuries, lumbago, abdominal pain owing to amenorrhea, headache, toothache, diarrhea, stranguria from urolithiasis, etc.

Common Bombax Bark ⊗ C-14

It is the bark of Gossampinus malabarica (DC.) Merr. (Bombacaceae).
Effect. Enhancing diuresis, blood circulation, removing heat, swelling.
Indication. Chronic gastritis, gastric ulcer, diarrhea, dysentery, aches in the loins and knees, swelling resulting from sores, traumatic injuries, etc.

Common Bombax Flower

It is the flower of Gossampinus malabarica (DC.) Merr. (Bombacaceae).
Effect. Enhancing diuresis, removing heat, swelling and ceasing bleeding.
Indication. Diarrhea, dysentery, metrorrhagia, suppurative infections on the skin, bleeding.

Common Canscora Herb

It is the whole herb of Canscora lucidissima (Levl. et Vant.) Hand. -Mazz. (Gentianaceae).
Effect. Enhancing blood circulation, removing heat, pain, detoxicating.
Indication. Cough owing to the lung-heat, hepatitis, jaundice, stomachache, snake bite and traumatic injuries.

Common Carpesium Fruit

It is the dried mature fruit of Carpesium abrotanoides L. or Daucus carota L. (Compositae).
Effect. Killing parasites in the intestines.
Indication. Disease owing to parasites in the intestines.

Common Cissampelos Herb

It is the whole herb of Cissampelos pareira L. (Menispermaceae).

Effect. Removing pain, ceasing bleeding and enhancing tissue regeneration.

Indication. Traumatic injuries, crush injury, traumatic bleeding, etc.

Common Cnidium Fruit

It is the fruit of Cnidium monnieri (L.) Cusson (Umbelliferae).

Effect. Nourishing the kidney, reinforcing yang, depriving dampness and relieving itching.

Indication. Impotence, sterility owing to uterine coldness; leukorrhea owing to cold-dampness, lumbago owing to damp arthralgia, pudendal damp itching, enuresis and frequent micturition, eczema, scabies and tinea.

Common Cold

Referring to the exterior syndrome.

Symptoms. Fever, chills, stuffy and running nose, sneezing, cough, etc.

Pathogenesis. Mostly owing to attack of pathogenic wind together with epidemic pathogen on the defensive exterior of the body.

Therapeutic Principle. Removing the exterior syndrome and the pathogen.

Common Cold Complicated by Spasm

Symptoms. Often seen in infants: fever, headache, sweating, ringing in the nose, retching, spasm of extremities, and eyes looking upward.

Pathogenesis. Caused by common cold and wind evil.

Therapeutic Principle. Removing wind, releasing the muscular spasm.

Common Cold due to Summer-heat and Dampness

Referring to a type of common cold.

Symptoms. Aversion to cold with mild sweating, heavy sensation of the head, soreness and heavy pain of joints of the body, fullness of the epigastrium, vomiting, nausea, loose stool, scanty yellow urine.

Pathogenesis. Owing to pathogenic wind with pathogenic summer-heat and dampness attacking the lung and superficial defence.

Therapeutic Principle. Removing summer-heat and dampness, expelling the evil factors from the body surface, and regulating the inner body.

Common Cold due to Wind-cold Pathogen

Referring to a type of common cold.

Symptoms. Severe chills, mild fever, anhidrosis, stuffy nose, sneezing, cough, aching feeling of the body, headache.

Pathogenesis. Owing to wind-cold pathogen.

Therapeutic Principle. Removing wind and cold pathogens, enhancing the dispersing function of the lung.

Common Cold due to Wind-heat Pathogen

Referring to one type of common cold.

Symptoms. Slight chills but severe fever, sweating, stuffy and dry nose, sore throat, thirst, cough with yellow thick sputum.

Pathogenesis. Owing to attack of wind-heat.

Therapeutic Principle. Removing wind, heat and nourishing lung-qi.

Common Cold with Convulsion

Referring to the disease and syndrome of the infant.

Symptoms. Bad sleep with crying, fright, even high-fever and convulsion.

Pathogenesis. Owing to the infant unable to bear the cold and heat, easy to be frightened and apt to be affected by the exterior pathogens.

Therapeutic Principle. Removing heat and pathogens.

Common Cold with Fever

It is a disease and syndrome for the infant.

Symptoms. Aversion to cold, fever, stuffy and running nose, flushed face, parched lips, thirst, dysphoria, etc.

Pathogenesis. Caused by the infant's weak digestion, easily to be attacked by the external pathogens. Once the infant is affected by the external pathogens, the stagnation of heat can be found by combining interior and exterior pathogens.

Therapeutic Principle. Removing exterior syndrome for releasing the interior heat.

Common Curculigo Rhizome

It is the rhizome of Curculigo orchioides Gaerth. (Amaryllidaceae).

Effect. Warming the kidney, reinforcing yang, releasing cold and dampness, strengthening the tendons and bones.

Indication. Impotence, cold sperm, incontinence of urination, cold pain in the chest and abdomen.

Common Ducksmeat Herb

It is the whole herb of Spirodela polyrrhiza (L.) Schleid (Lemnaceae).

Effect. Induce sweating to expel the exogenous evils from the body surface and enhancing skin eruption, removing swelling, pathogenic wind, itching, inducing diuresis.

Indication. Macula without adequate eruption, urticaria due to pathogenic wind-heat, cutaneous pruritus, edema.

Common Evolulus Herb

It is the whole plant of Evoloulus alsinoides L. (Convolvulaceae).

Effect. Invigorating the function of the spleen and dispersing dampness, tonifying kidney to stop emission.

Indication. Jaundice, dysentery, stranguria with turbid urine, seminal emission, enuresis, leukorrhagia, nail-like boil swelling and scabies.

Common Fennel Fruit ⊛ C-15

It is the dried ripe fruit of Foeniculum Vulgare Mill. (Umbelliferae).

Effect. Removing cold, pain, adjusting flow of qi and the stomach.

Indication. Abdominal pain owing to invasion of cold, vomiting owing to cold in the stomach, poor appetite, abdominal distention and pain, etc.

Common Flowering Quince Fruit

It is the ripe fruit of Chaenomeles speciosa (Sweet) Nakni. (Rosaceae).

Effect. Relaxation of the body, enhancing the flow of qi and blood in the meridians and collaterals, releasing dampness and recovering normal functioning of the stomach.

Indication. Arthralgia owing to wind dampness, spasm of muscles, swelling pain owing to beriberi, vomiting, diarrhea, etc.

Common Heron's Bill Herb

It is the aerial herb of Erodium stephanianum Willd, or Geranium wilfordii Maxim. (Geraniaceae).

Effect. Releasing heat, wind-dampness, obstruction in the meridians and collaterals, ceasing dysentery and diarrhea, and detoxicating.

Indication. Rheumatic arthralgia, numbness and spasm, aching pain of muscles and bones, diarrhea, dysentery, subcutaneous swelling.

Common Hogfennel Root

It is the root of Peucedanum praeruptorum Dunn and P. decursivum Maxim. (Umbelliferae).

Effect. Directing qi downwards, removing phlegm, and dispelling wind-heat.

Indication. Obstruction of the lung-qi, asthma, cough, thick sputum.

Common Jasmin Orange Leaf

It is the branch and leaf of Murraya paniculata (L.) Jack. (Rutaceae).

Effect. Enhancing the flow of qi and blood circulation, releasing the wind, dampness and pain.
Indication. Gastric abscess, rheumatalgia, orchitis, poisoning swelling, scabies, skin pruritus, swelling and pain owing to trauma.

Common Kontweed Herb

It is the dried aerial parts of Polygonum aviculare L. (Polygonaceae).
Effect. Inducing diuresis and treating stranguria, killing parasites and removing itching.
Indication. Scanty dark urine, dribbling and painful micturition, skin eczema and pudendal pruritus.

Common Lantana Leaf

It is the leaf or the twig with flower of Lantana Camara L. (Verbenaceae).
Effect. Detoxicating, removing swelling, wind and ceasing itching.
Indication. Subcutaneous swelling, noxious dampness, scabies, fulminant sores, etc.

Common Lophatherum Leaf

It is the leaf of Lophatherum gracile Brongn. (Graminaceae).
Effect. Removing heat, restlessness, quenching thirst and inducing diuresis.
Indication. Canker sores in the mouth, dysuria, heat stranguria, vexation, etc.

Common Mappianthus Stem

It is the whole plant or stem of Mappianthus iodoides Hant-Mazz. (Icacinaceae).
Effect. Adjusting menstruation, enhancing blood circulation, releasing wind and dampness.
Indication. Irregular menstruation, dysmenorrhea, amenorrhea and rheumatic arthralgia.

Common Melastoma Herb

It is the whole herb of Melastoma candidum D. Don (Melastomataceae).

Effect. Removing swelling, heat and toxic substances, enhancing blood circulation.
Indication. Traumatic injuries, suppurative infections on the skin and galactostasis.

Common Monkshood Mother Root

It is the tuber of Aconitum carmichaeli Debx. (Ranunculaceae).
Effect. Removing wind, dampness, pathogenic cold from the body to stop pain.
Indication. Arthritis of cold-dampness with pain, chest and abdominal cold pain, migraine, and pain owing to traumatic injuries.

Common Pulse

Referring to a pulse condition, the normal pulse, 4 beats per respiration, not floating, not deep, even and gently, moderate force and regular rhythm, representing the stomach-qi, vigour and force.

Common Rockvine Herb or Root

It is the whole herb or root of Tetrastigma obtectum (Wall.) Planch. (Vitaceae).
Effect. Removing wind, dampness, enhancing blood circulation and detoxicating.
Indication. Headache, rheumatic arthritis, multiple abscess and suppurative skin diseases.

Common Sage Herb

It is the whole plant of Salvia plebeia R. Br. (Labiatae.)
Effect. Enhancing diuresis, releasing heat from blood, detoxicating and killing parasites.
Indication. Hemoptysis, hematemesis, hematuria, metrorrhagia, metrostaxis, gonorrhea, swollen and sore throat.

Common Scopolia Root

It is the root of Anisodus luridus Link et Otto. (Solanaceae).
Effect. Removing spasm and pain.

Indication. Stomachache, cholecystalgia, acute and chronic enterogastritis, etc.

Common Scouring Rush

It is the whole grass of Equisetum hiemale L. (Eguisetaceae).

Effect. Releasing nebula, wind-heat, enhancing visual acuity, and ceasing bleeding.

Indication. Bloodshot eyes, cataract and nebula owing to exopathogenic wind-heat, nebula, hematochezia, hemorrhoidal bleeding, etc.

Common Securidaca Root

It is the root of Securidace inappendiculata Hassk. (Polygalaceae).

Effect. Enhancing blood circulation, removing blood stasis, swelling, pain, heat and inducing diuresis.

Indication. Acute enteritis and gastritis, traumatic injuries, etc.

Common Selfheal Fruit-spike

It is the spike of Prunella vulgaris L. (Labiatae) with flower.

Effect. Releasing heat from the liver, dispersing masses and lowering blood pressure.

Indication. Bloodshot, swelling and painful eyes, photophobia, cataract and nebula, delacrimation, headache, dizziness.

Common Sonthistle Herb

It is the whole herb of Sonchus brachyotus DC. (Compositae).

Effect. Removing cough, heat, detoxicating, restoring qi.

Indication. Bacillary dysentery, laryngitis, cough of deficiency type, internal hemorrhoid with prolapse of rectum and leukorrhagia.

Common Tetragonia Herb

It is the whole herb of Tetragonia tetragonioides (Pall.); O. Ktze. (Aizoaceae).

Effect. Releasing heat, toxic substances, wind and enhancing subsidence of swelling.

Indication. Enteritis, blood poisoning, flushed swollen furuncle, bloodshot eyes resulting from wind-heat, etc.

Common Three-wingnut Root

It is the root, leaf and flower of Tripterygium wilfordii Hook. f. (Celastraceae).

Effect. Killing parasites, removing inflammation and detoxicating.

Indication. Rheumatic arthritis and cutaneous pruritus.

Common Turezaninowia Herb

It is the whole herb or root of Turczaninowia fastigiatus (Fisch.) DC. (Compositae).

Effect. Warming the lung and reducing phlegm, adjusting the middle-energizer and inducing diuresis.

Indication. Cough, dyspnea, borborygmus, diarrhea, dysentery, scanty and painful urine, etc.

Common Turmeric

It is the rhizome of Curcuma longa L. (Zingiberaceae).

Effect. Enhancing blood circulation, flow of qi, releasing pain and obstruction in the meridians.

Indication. Distending pain in the chest and hypochondrium, amenorrhea and rheumatic arthralgia owing to the stagnation of qi and blood stasis.

Common Vetch Herb

It is the whole herb of Vicia sativa L. (Leguminosae).

Effect. Releasing blood stasis, heat, enhancing diuresis, adjusting blood circulation.

Indication. Jaundice, edema, malaria, palpitation, emission, irregular menstruation.

Compatibility of Eight Points on Eight Meridians

Referring to one of the needling methods, the prescription of arranging the related eight points on the eight Extra Meridians into four pairs in accordance with their functions: Compatibility of Neiguan (P 6) with Gongsun (Sp 4), for the diseases in the heart, chest and stomach; Waiguan (TE 5) with Zulinqi (G 41) for the diseases in the eye, cephalic region and cheek; Houxi (SI 3) with Shenmai (B 62), for the diseases in the neck, nape and scapular region; and Lieque (L 7) with Zhaohai (K 6) for the diseases in the throat and thorax diaphragm.

Comprehensive Analysis of Complexion and Pulse

Referring to a diagnostic method. It is a method of making the correct diagnosis based on the patient's changes of complexion and pulse. For examples, the flushed face, and full large pulse with strength indicating an excessive syndrome. Pale complexion, and deep slow pulse without strength indicating the syndrome of cold of insufficiency type.

Concentrated Mind

It is a term in Qigong.

Method. During Qigong practice, trying to get rid of distracting thoughts, concentrating mindwill on a certain part of the body (usually on lower Dantian), reaching into a tranquil state.

Concentrated Mind to Send Qi into Dantian

It is a term in Qigong.

Method. During Qigong practice, trying to get rid of distracting thoughts, concentrating mindwill on lower Dantian, thus achieving a tranquil state of mind and enhancing the essence qi to produce and to be vigorous.

Conch Shell

It is the fresh meat of Rapana thomasiana Crosse (Muricidae), or of other aquatic products with the same kind of conch.

Effect. Enhancing the eyesight.

Indication. Painful eyes.

Confusion

It is a disease.

Symptoms. Mental confusion with visual hallucination.

Pathogenesis. Owing to weakness, invasion of nape by pathogenic factors due to weakness, tenseness of ocular connectors.

Therapeutic Principle. Nourishing qi and blood.

Confusion due to Injury

Symptoms. Vague mind, unconsciousness, pale complexion, clammy limbs, shallow breathing, etc.

Pathogenesis. Owing to serious trauma, exhaustion of blood and qi and mental derangement.

Therapeutic Principle. Giving the emergency treatment, with the combination of Chinese medicine and Western medicine, and removing blood stasis.

Congenital Basis

It refers to the kidney. The kidney takes charge of growth and development, playing an important role in preventing and resisting diseases, being the foundation of the life, the zang-fu organs, yin and yang.

Congenital Cataract

Referring to the ophthalmopathy of lens opacity.

Symptoms. Seen in both eyes with the lens opacity in different positions and different patterns.

Pathogenesis. Owing to parental heredity, or congenital disposition, deficiency of the spleen and kidney, or excessive constitutional rest of the pregnant women or administration of some drugs that affect the fatal development.

Therapeutic Principle. Tonifyign yin, yang, the spleen, enhancing the flow of qi. Operation is applicable to patients with only light sensation and average lens opacity.

Congenital Essence

Referring to the reproductive essence stored in the kidney, coming from the reproductive essence of the parents, opposite to the acquired essence, the congenital essence possessing the ability of generation of offspring and related to the growth, development and aging.

Congenital Vitality

Referring to brain vitality, the root of life, owing its origin to the congenital essence.

Conger Pike

It is the meat of Muraenesox cinereus (Forskal) (Muraenesocidae).
Effect. Detoxicating.
Indication. Malignant boil on the skin, scabies and hemorrhoid with anal fistula.

Congestive Pterygium

It is a symptom.
Symptoms. Membrane on the eyeball with small, thin, red and dense blood streak, lacrimation and photophobia.
Pathogenesis. Caused by wind-head in the liver and lung and stagnation of meridians and collaterals.

Conjoint Invasion of Pathogenic Wind-dampness

Referring to invasion of wind-cold-dampness pathogen into the muscle and joints of the body, thus leading to the occurences of diseases.

Conjunctival Congestion

Referring to hyperemia of bulbar conjunctiva.
Symptoms. Swelling and pain, owing to the invasion of wind-fire and pathogenic toxin; congestion of the white, or crimson eyeball, owing to the upward attack of liver heat; pale red on the white and blurred vision, owing to the yin deficiency of the liver and lung.
Therapeutic Principle. Treatment based on overall analysis of the patient's condition.

Constant Crying of Newborn

Symptoms. The newborn infant crying from time to time, red face, dry lips, yellow urine, etc.
Pathogenesis. Heat in the heart and liver.
Therapeutic Principle. Removing heat and purging fire.

Constipation

Symptoms. Hard stool difficult to be defecated.
Pathogenesis. Mostly owing to accumulation of heat, incoordination of emotions or debility, yin deficiency, insufficiency of blood and qi.

Constipation after Injury

Symptoms. Constipation often in serious injury.
Therapeutic Principle. Elimination of extravasated blood by catharsis; for constipation with dryness of intestines due to deficiency of blood, removing heat and moistening intestines; for constipation due to deficiency of qi, nourishing qi and moistening the intestines.

Constipation due to Cold

Symptoms. Constipation.
Pathogenesis. Owing to pathogenic cold of excess type or deficiency type.
Therapeutic Principle. For the excess type, adjusting qi and the stomach, releasing dampness and relaxing the bowels. For the deficiency type, warming yang, and relaxing the bowels.

Constipation due to Deficiency of Blood

Symptoms. Constipation, pale face, dizziness, dim eyesight, palpitation.
Pathogenesis. Mainly owing to bodily weakness of the aged or deficiency of qi

and blood after delivery, severe or chronic illness.

Therapeutic Principle. Tonifying blood and intestines.

Constipation due to Intestine Heat

Symptoms. Fullness in stomach, constipation, pressing pain with mass in abdomen.

Pathogenesis. Accumulation of heat in the large intestine.

Therapeutic Principle. Removing heat, maintaining fluid, moisturizing the intestine.

Constipation due to Phlegm Stagnation

Symptoms. Dry stool, fullness in chest, dyspnea with chest fullness, dizziness, and bombus, etc.

Pathogenesis. Owing to stagnation of phlegm in the intestine and stomach.

Therapeutic Principle. Releasing phlegm, adjusting the function of fu organs.

Constipation due to Qi Disorder

It refers to two kinds of constipation, qi stagnation of qi deficiency.

1. For the type of qi stagnation.

   Symptoms. Distending fullness of stomach and abdomen, pricking pain in the chest and hypochondrium, etc.

   Pathogenesis. Mental depression due to emotional stress leading to desturbance of the dispersing and discending function and failure in transportation.

   Therapeutic Principle. Adjusting the adverse flow of qi, promoting qi to disperse stagnation and relax the bowel.

2. For the type of qi deficiency.

   Symptoms. Dysphoria, languor, feeble speech, etc.

   Pathogenesis. Internal injury due to overfatigue, bodily weakness of the aged, insufficiency of the lung qi and failure in transmission of the large intestine.

Therapeutic Principle. Nourishing qi and moistening the intestine.

Constipation due to Spleen Deficiency

Symptoms. Constipation, debility of defecation and lassitude of limbs, etc.

Therapeutic Principle. Nourishing the spleen and qi, loosening of the bowel, moistening the intestine.

Constipation due to Wind

Symptoms. Dry stool hard to evacuate, mostly found in the old or those suffering from disease due to pathogenic wind.

Pathogenesis. Attack of pathogenic wind on the lung, involving large intestines.

Therapeutic Principle. Removing wind adjusting blood flow, moistening the intestine.

Constipation of Cold Type

It is a type of constipation, also named yin-accumulation or cold-accumulation.

Symptoms. Dyschesia, proctoptosis, cold pain in the abdomen, pale complexion, cold limbs, pale tongue.

Pathogenesis. Mainly owing to yang deficiency of both the spleen and the kidney, accumulation of severe pathogenic cold.

Therapeutic Principle. Strengthening the kidney and yang.

Constipation of the Aged

Symptoms. Difficulty in defecation, fatigue after defecation or accompanied by shortness of breath, dizziness, dim complexion, etc.

Pathogenesis. Mainly caused by insufficiency of blood and qi or deficiency of kidney or accumulation of heat in stomach and intestinal track.

Therapeutic Principle. Nourishing qi and blood, moisturizing intestines, clearing away heat and warming yang and lowering the adverse flow of qi.

Constriction of Vulva

Symptoms. Subjective sensation of vulval contraction, and even unbearable pain involving the chest, hypochondrium, breast and lower abdomen.

Pathogenesis. Mainly owing to cold invasion into Jueyin Meridian during menstruation or after delivery, or by trauma due to sexual activity.

Therapeutic Principle. Removing cold from the meridians.

Consuming Blood

Referring to heat pathogen deeply invading into the blood system, thus consuming the yin fluid of blood.

Consumption

1. Referring to a disease, the abbreviation for consumptive disease.
2. Referring to one of pathogenic factors, the overstrain.

Consumption due to Prolonged Estrus

Referring to the consumption syndrome.

Pathogenesis. Owing to first awakening of love, the strong sexual desire, thus leading to long-term consumption of fluid and essence of the kidney.

Consumption of Kidney-yin by Heat

Symptoms. Low fever, heat sensation in palms and soles, dry mouth and purple tongue.

Pathogenesis. Usually at the later stage of epidemic febrile disease, the kidney-yin consumed by pathogenic heat.

Consumption of Two Yang Factors in Combination

It is a pathogenesis. Wind and heat both belong to yang pathogen. Combination of wind and heat will certainly exhaust body fluid resulting in symptoms such as dryness in mouth and nose, thirst, etc.

Consumption of Yin due to Yang Excess

Referring to a series of syndromes belonging to heat of excess type.

Pathogenesis. Owing to yang excess, which consumes yin fluid, leading to the lack of the body fluid and yin essence, thus causing the syndromes of the yin consumption due to excessive heat.

Consumptive Disease

Referring to the general term of many chronic asthenic diseases owing to various factors. The main pathogenesis is impairment of zang-fu organs and deficiency of qi, blood, yin, and yang. Including qi, blood, yin, and yang deficiency of zang-fu organs, with longer duration of the diseases.

Therapeutic Principle. Nourishing qi, blood, yin and warming yang.

Consumptive Disease due to Qi Stagnation

Referring to the disease of qi stagnation among the consumptive diseases.

Symptoms. Dysphagia of the chest and diaphragm, vomiting, flatulence of the stomach and abdomen, indigestion, diarrhea, withered and yellowish complexion, weak limbs, gradual emaciation, etc.

Pathogenesis. Mostly owing to deficiency and weakness of zang-fu organ, disharmony of yin and yang.

Therapeutic Principle. Reinforcing the middle-energizer and enhancing qi circulation.

Consumptive Disease in Children

Referring to the infant suffering from tuberculosis.

Pathogenesis. Mainly owing to congenital deficiency.

Consumptive Disease of Pregnant Woman

Symptoms. Cough, hectic fever, or hematemesis, or sexual intercourse in the dream, etc, for a pregnant woman.

Pathogenesis. Owing to insufficiency and loss of the lung yin and hyperactivity of fire due to yin deficiency.

Therapeutic Principle. Nourishing yin and tonifying the kidney; for the case with qi obstruction due to phlegm stagnation, and continual cough with dyspnea, removing phlegm, and cough.

Consumptive Fever

Symptoms. Low unrelieved fever, emaciation, weakness, lassitude, etc.

Pathogenesis. Owing to consumptive disease.

Therapeutic Principle. Releasing heat and hectic fever, tonifying qi and yin.

Consumptive Lung Disease

1. Heat deficiency type.

   Symptoms. Cough with pituitary sputum, shortness of breath, thirst, emaciation, etc.

   Pathogenesis. Mostly due to the lung deficiency, the malnutrition of the lung fluid.

   Therapeutic Principle. Tonifying yin, removing heat, moistening the lung and enhancing the production of the body fluid.

2. Cold deficiency type.

   Symptoms. Cough with thin frothy sputum, aversion to cold, without thirst, etc.

   Therapeutic Principle. Warming the lung and supplementing qi.

Consumptive Fever

Symptoms. Hectic fever due to yin deficiency, tidal fever, dysphoria with feverish sensation in the chest, palms and soles, etc.

Pathogenesis. Mostly caused by deficiency of qi and blood, deficiency of yang and yin.

Therapeutic Principle. Nourishing yin and extinguish fire, tonifying the lung and replenishing qi.

Contact Dermatitis

Symptoms. In the affected area, xerosis, red purple spots, swelling, burning pain, even sores and pus.

Cause. Owing to the contact with insect secretion of the mantis, etc.

Therapeutic Principle. Removing heat and toxic materials.

Continuous Lifting-thrusting Technique

Referring to one of the auxiliary techniques of acupuncture.

Method. With the needle in a certain depth, continuously lift and thrust the needle with a relatively larger amplitude, be sure of keeping the same direction, same depth and same force on the needle. Lifting and thrusting the needle with a small amplitude and high frequency, called vibration needling. Its purpose is to strengthen the needling sensation.

Continuous Menstruation

Symptoms. Continuous and prolonged menstruation.

Pathogenesis. Mainly owing to impairment of the uterine collaterals by blood-heat, or internal injury of Vital and Front Middle Meridians by strain.

Therapeutic Principle. Cooling and nourishing blood.

Contra-acupuncture Point

Referring to the points, most close to the important organs or artery, to which the needling is forbidden.

Contracture

Symptoms. Uncomfortable tugging of limbs or subjective sensation of contraction, thus affecting normal movement.

Pathogenesis. Owing to impairment of muscles by six pathogenic factors, or stagnation of the liver-qi, blockage of meridians or insufficiency of the kidney-yang, dysfunction of the urinary bladder in qi transformation.

Contraindications of Needling

Referring to the precautions to be obeyed during acupuncture. These precautions are forbidden areas, e.g. important organs, great blood vessels, brain and spinal cord, and forbidden times, e.g. starving, over-eating, or violent mood changes.

Contralateral Prick

Referring to a needling technique. For the pathogenic factors attacking the collaterals, using the crossing method of dispersing collaterals, that is, selecting right point for disorder in the left, and left point for disease in the right. Contralateral means crossing.

Contramoxibustion Point

Referring to the points, most close to the important organs or artery, to which the moxibustion is forbidden with moxa cones.

Contusion

Referring to soft tissue injury.

Symptoms. Pain in affected spot, swelling, cyanosis, intense pain on pressure, but no wound on skin, laceration of muscle or deep hematoma, and even injury of internal organs if serious.

Cause. Trauma, pressure and bruise.

Therapeutic Principle. Enhancing blood circulation, removing blood stasis, swelling and pain.

Convergence of Vessels in Lung

Through the circulation, the blood all over the body flowing to the lung via the blood vessels, and through the respiratory function exchanging gases, and transporting the gas throughout the body.

Convulsion due to Blood Deficiency

Symptoms. Dizziness, stiffness of the nape and back, convulsion of limbs, hand and foot, shortness of breath, spontaneous perspiration, lassitude, etc.

Pathogenesis. Mainly due to failure of blood to nourish the tendons and muscles owing to the deficiency of yin blood.

Therapeutic Principle. Nourishing qi, blood, and tendon, removing convulsion.

Convulsion due to Damp-heat

Symptoms. Lockjaw, spasm of limbs in traction test, and opisthotonos, etc.

Pathogenesis. Owing to the progress of disease caused by damp-heat.

Therapeutic Principle. Enhancing diuresis, removing wetness from the lower-energizer, the wind and heat.

Convulsion due to Excessive Summer-heat

Symptoms. Serious vomiting and diarrhea, fever of forehead with sweating and cold limbs and convulsion of the infantile.

Pathogenesis. Owing to excessive summer-heat.

Therapeutic Principle. Nourishing qi and yin, removing heat and wind.

Convulsion due to Pathogenic Heat Entering the Nutrient-blood

Symptoms. Unconsciousness with high fever, dizziness, distending headache, lockjaw, clonic convulsion, or vexation and irritability.

Pathogenesis. Owing to pathogenic heat invading the nutrient-blood.

Therapeutic Principle. Removing wind, pathogenic heat in the nutrient-blood, ceasing convulsion.

Convulsion due to Phlegm-fire

Symptoms. Deviation of the eye and mouth, shaking or convulsion of the limbs, fever, cough with phlegm, slippery and rapid pulse, etc.

Pathogenesis. Owing to the obstruction of excessive phlegm-fire.

Therapeutic Principle. Removing heat, fire and phlegm, and ceasing convulsion.

Convulsion due to Protracted Disease

Symptoms. Fever, hectic complexion, emaciation, convulsion-like state, frequent fainting and deficiency of qi.

Pathogenesis. Owing to long time chronic disease and deficiency of qi and blood.

Therapeutic Principle. Nourishing the spleen, qi and blood, removing convulsion.

Convulsion due to Summer-heat

Symptoms. High fever, sudden coma, tic of limbs, trismus, stiffness of nape and back, or opisthotonos.

Pathogenesis. Owing to suffering from summer-heat.

Therapeutic Principle. Releasing pathogenic heat from the liver, and calming the endopathic wind.

Convulsion Paralysis

Referring to the paralysis after convulsion.

Symptoms. Swelling and pain all over the body and inability to move limbs.

Pathogenesis. Owing to pathogenic wind entering the meridians and collaterals and bone joints.

Therapeutic Principle. Removing wind and enhancing eruption of virus.

Convulsion Syndrome

Symptoms. Lockjaw, convulsion of limbs, opisthotonos.

Pathogenesis. Mainly owing to malnutrition of tendons, muscles and meridians, due to deficiency of blood and body fluid.

Convulsion with Up-lifted Eyes

Symptoms. High fever, convulsion, upward staring eyes for baby.

Pathogenesis. Usually owing to phlegm and heat involving the heart orifice due to exterior affection of wind and heat, or improper milk and food.

Therapeutic Principle. Removing phlegm, heat, calming wind and inducing resuscitation.

Convulsive Disease

Symptoms. Stiffness of the neck and back, clonic convulsion of the extremities and opisthotonos, including tonic convulsion and rigidity with sweating.

Convulsive Seizure Induced by Terror in Children

Symptoms. Incessant crying in children, changes in complexion and fright sensation, with vomiting, diarrhea, and abdominal pain, convulsion and faint if serious.

Pathogenesis. Owing to sudden terror by something.

Therapeutic Principle. Calming the mind and excitement.

Convulsive Syndrome due to Impairment of Yin Caused by High Fever

Referring to a type of convulsive disease.

Symptoms. Persistent high fever, lockjaw and teeth grinding, stiffness of the nape and back, opisthotonus, contracture of hands and feet.

Pathogenesis. Owing to excess consumption of body fluid due to high fever.

Therapeutic Principle. Removing heat, wind, calming the liver.

Cool-dryness Syndrome

1. Referring to one of exopathogenic dryness.

   Symptoms. Cough, stuffy nose, headache, aversion to cold and dry throat and mouth.

   Pathogenesis. Owing to the impairment of lung defending qi, by coolness in autumn.

Therapeutic Principle. Moisturizing dryness-heat and ventilating the lung and removing phlegm.

2. Referring to a therapeutic method to treat the impairment of the lung by the exopathogenic dryness and heat, i.e. removing dryness, and moistening the lung.

Cool-dryness Syndrome Treated by Warm-damp Drugs

Referring to a therapeutic method. In the method, by using drugs pungent in flavor and warm in property for inducing diaphoresis, and enhancing the dispersing function of the lung; drugs of sweet flavor and damp in nature, for nourishing yin essence and moisturize the viscera. The method is good at cool-dryness pathogen in the lungs.

Cool Filthy Disease

Referring one type of filthy diseases
Symptoms. Abdominal pain, cold limbs, etc.
Pathogenesis. Owing to affecting the six natural factors, filth and turbidity or hunger, overeating and overworking.
Therapeutic Principle. Removing turbidity with aromatics.

Coordination of Mindwill and Breathing

It is a term in Qigong.
Method. Through adjusting the mind and breathing to reach to a state of concentrating the mind, getting rid of distracting thoughts and entering a tranquil state.

Coordination of Physique and Qi

It is a diagnostic method.
Referring to the relative balance between physique of man and function of viscera or pathogenic qi.

Coptis Root

It is the rhizome, root and leaf of Coptis chinensis Franch. C. deltoidea C. Y. Cheng et Hsiao, or C. teetoides C. Y. Cheng (Ranunculaceae).

Effect. Removing heat, dampness, fire and toxins.

Indication. Diarrhea, dysentery, vomiting due to damp-heat; high fever, unconsciousness and delirium, dysphoria insomnia, bloodshot eyes, canker sore in the mouth, dark urine, hematemesis, epistaxis due to febrile diseases; suppurative infections on the skin, such as sores, carbuncles, furuncles, eczema, scalds, swollen and sore throat, etc.

Coral

It is the calcariuria skeleton secreted from a coral insect Corallium japonicum Kishinouye (Melitodidae).

Effect. Enhancing eyesight, calming the mind and relieving convulsion, and nebula.

Indication. Oculopathy, epilepsy induced by terror, hematemesis and epistaxis.

Coral Ardisia Root

It is the root of Ardisia crenata Sims (Myrsinaceae).

Effect. Releasing toxic substances, blood stasis, pain and heat.

Indication. Exterior syndromes caused by exopathogens, swollen and sore throat, diphtheria, erysipelas, subcutaneous nodule, hematemesis, owing to overstrain, pain in the chest and abdomen, rheumatic arthralgia, traumatic injuries.

Cordate Pinellia Rhizome

It is the stem tuber of Pinellia cordata N. E. Br. (Araceae).

Effect. Removing pain, blood stasis, swelling and detoxicating.

Indication. Headache, stomachache, abdominal pain, lumbago, traumatic injuries, acute mastitis, pyogenic infection, etc.

Cord-like Mass beside Umbilicus

Generally referring to the cord-like mass in the abdominal cavity.

Symptoms. Distention, tightness and pain in the hypochondrium.

Pathogenesis. Commonly owing to improper diet, impairment of the spleen and stomach, accumulation of cold-phlegm and stagnation of qi and blood.

Therapeutic Principle. Adjusting the functions of the spleen and stomach and enhancing the functional activities of qi.

Coriander Harb

It is the whole herb of Coriandrum saivum L. (Umbelliferae).

Effect. Inducing diaphoresis and enhancing eruption, stimulating appetite and digestion.

Indication. Measles in the early stage, measles without adequate eruption and dyspepsia.

Corktree Bark   ⊛ C-16

It is the bark of Phellodendron amurense Rupr. and P. chinense Schneid. (Rutaceae) without cork.

Effect. Removing heat, dampness, fire, toxins.

Indication. Dysentery, jaundice, leukorrhea, swelling pain in the knees and feet, infections on the skin, such as boils, sores, swelling, ulcers, eczema, hemorrhoids, hemafecia; deficiency of the kidney-yin such as fever, hectic fever, tidal fever, emission, etc.

Corneal Scars and Opacities

It is one kind of nebula.

Symptoms. Formation of turbidity in the black after recovery from an oculopathy related to the black, surface smoothness and clear periphery.

Therapeutic Principle. Removing nebula, improving visual acuity.

Corniculate Spurgentian Herb

It is the whole herb of Halienia corniculata (L.) Cornaz. (Grentranaceae).

Effect. Detoxicating, removing pathogenic heat from the blood and ceasing bleeding.

Indication. Hepatitis, angiitis, fever owing to traumatic infection and traumatic bleeding.

Corn Stigma   ⊛ C-17

It is the style of Zea mays L. (Gramineae).

Effect. Enhancing diuresis, removing heat, calming the liver and normalizing functioning of the gallbladder, lowering blood pressure.

Indication. Edema, dysuria, hyperactivity of the liver-yang, dizziness, jaundice, hypertension, stranguria due to the passage of urinary stone, diabetes, acute mastitis.

Coromadel Coast Falsemallow Herb

It is the whole herb of Malvastrum coromandelianum (L.) Garcke (Malvaceae).

Effect. Enhancing diuresis, releasing heat, blood stasis, and swelling.

Indication. Jaundice, dysentery, malaria, infantile indigestion with food retention, cough due to lung-heat, laryngitis, carbuncle, furuncle, traumatic injuries with swelling and pain, etc.

Corpsy-like Syncope

Symptoms. Suddenly fainting and cold limbs, as if dead, sometimes with bluish complexion, trance, paraphasia, ravings, lockjaw, slight and discontinuous respiration.

Therapeutic Principle. Recovering consciousness.

Correspondence between Man and Universe

Referring to the compatibility of the human body with the nature. The human body is affected directly or indirectly by the changes of the nature, the body responds to these changes.

Corresponding Point Selection

Referring to one of the methods of point selection.

Method. Selecting points in remote areas corresponding to the diseased region, including the front versus the back, upper versus lower and left versus right, etc. For example, choosing Fengchi (G 20) for nasal stuffiness, Chengjiang (CV 24) for stiffness of the neck, Yongquan (K 1) for parietal headache and Chize (L 5) for knee pain, etc.

Corrosive Agent

Referring to corrosive drugs. These drugs are good at treating such symptoms as those with too small opening of a ulcer to dispel pus, inability of ulcerating after the formation of pus in painful swelling on the skin.

Corydalis Tuber

It is the stem tuber of Corydalis turtschaninovii Bess. f. yanhusuo Y. H. Chou et C. C. Hsu (Papaveraceae).
Effect. Enhancing blood circulation, flow of qi and removing pain.
Indication. Pain in the chest, abdomen and the extremities resulting from stagnation of qi and blood stasis.

Cotton

It is the cotton fibre of Gossypium herbaceum L. (Malvaceae).
Effect. Ceasing bleeding.
Indication. Hemoptysis, hematuria, hemafecia, metrorrhagia and cutting wounds with bleeding.

Cottonrose Hibiscus Flower

It is the flower of Hibiscus mutabilis L. (Malvaceae).
Effect. Removing heat, cooling blood, detoxicating and enhancing subsidence of swelling.

Indication. Suppurative infections on the skin, for example, sore, carbuncles, furuncles and boils, cough due to lung dryness, hematemesis, metrorrhagia and metrorrhagia, leukorrhagia, etc.

Cottonrose Hibiscus Leaf

It is the leaf of Hibiscus mutabilis L. (Malvaceae).
Effect. Detoxicating, releasing swelling, pain, and heat from the blood.
Indication. Carbuncles and other suppurative infections on the skin, erysipelas, scalds, traumatic injuries, etc.

Cotton Seed

It is the seed of Gossypium herbaceum L. (Malvaceae).
Effect. Warming the kidney, restoring qi and ceasing bleeding.
Indication. Impotence, painful and swollen testis, enuresis, hemorrhoidal bleeding, proctoptosis, metrorrhagia, metrostaxis and leukorrhea.

Cough

It refers to three types: cough with sound but without phlegm, cough with phlegm but without sound, cough with phlegm and sound.
Pathogenesis. Caused by 1. invasion of the lung by exopathogen; 2. internal impairment of zang-fu with the lung involved.
Therapeutic Principle. For exopathogen case, dispelling pathogen and ventilating the lung. For internal impairment, regulating zang and fu.

Cough and Shortness of Breath

Symptoms. Cough, shortness of breath, asthma and interrupted breathing, etc.
Pathogenesis. Owing to the deficiency of the lung-qi, also owing to the impaired liver-kidney essence.
Therapeutic Principle. Nourishing the lung, the kidney, the kidney-qi, and removing the pathogen.

Cough before Dawn

It refers to cough at early morning or severe cough at dawn.

Pathogenesis. 1. For the excess type, usually due to retention of food in the stomach and attack of fire on the lung. 2. For the deficiency type, mainly due to deficiency of the spleen.

Therapeutic Principle. Strengthening the stomach to promote digestion removing fire from the lung for the excess type. Nourishing the spleen and removing phlegm to relieve cough.

Cough due to Accumulation of Excessive Fluid

Referring to the cough due to the stagnation of pathogenic fluid in the lung.

Symptoms. Cough with clear and thin phlegm, nausea and oppressed feeling in the chest, anorexia and loose stool, etc.

Pathogenesis. Owing to the spleen deficiency and excessive fluid, or kidney deficiency and bold fluid, lung deficiency and fluid accumulation.

Therapeutic Principle. Warming and removing the accumulation of excessive fluid.

Cough due to Blood Deficiency

Symptoms. Cough, tidal fever, dizziness, dysphoria with feverish sensation in the chest, palms and soles, weak constitution.

Pathogenesis. Owing to failure in recuperative medical care after severe and chronic illness, or over-fatigue, physical weakness, insufficient yin blood, deficiency of the lung and kidney.

Therapeutic Principle. Releasing heat in the lung, and nourishing blood, qi, the lung.

Cough due to Cold

Symptoms. Cough with whitish, clear and thin sputum, cold limbs.

Pathogenesis. Owing to attack of pathogenic wind cold, or improper diets of cold and raw food.

Therapeutic Principle. Warming the lung, removing phlegm and cough.

Cough due to Common Cold

Symptoms. Cough, aversion to wind and spontaneous sweating, stuffy nose, heavy voice, or fever etc.

Pathogenesis. Owing to the invasion of cold wind to the lung, affecting the functions of the lung.

Therapeutic Principle. Enhancing the dispersing function of the lung, removing wind, phlegm and cough.

Cough due to Dampness

Referring to cough due to exogenous dampness.

Symptoms. Cough and much phlegm, heaviness in the body, annoying pain in the joints, swollen face and limbs, difficulty in urination, etc.

Pathogenesis. Owing to dampness injuring the spleen and liver.

Therapeutic Principle. Nourishing the spleen, removing phlegm and dampness in the body.

Cough due to Depression

Symptoms. Cough, restlessness and spontaneous, sweating, dry throat, hemoptysis, etc.

Pathogenesis. Owing to overexertion and depressed emotion.

Therapeutic Principle. Tonifying the heart, calming mind and removing cough.

Cough due to Disorder of Liver Meridian

Symptoms. Cough with hypochondriac pain, even inability to turn around, etc.

Pathogenesis. Owing to hyperactive depressed anger, the stagnation of the liver-qi and impairment of lungs by upward invasion of the hyperactive liver-qi.

Therapeutic Principle. Smoothing the liver and enhancing the dispersing function of the lung.

Cough due to Disorder of Qi

Symptoms. Cough, oppressed fullness in the chest with short breath, sticky phlegm or catkin-like phlegm, even spitting pus and blood, etc.

Pathogenesis. Owing to the lung deficiency and obstruction of pathogenic qi, or the impairment of the spleen and lungs by the stagnation of seven emotions.

Therapeutic Principle. Adjusting the lung, reinforcing the body resistance, removing phlegm, pathogen, or removing stagnation and phlegm.

Cough due to Dryness-heat

Referring to cough owing to affection of exopathogenic wind-heat and dryness-heat.

Symptoms. Hot sensation, aversion to cold, dry cough with no phlegm or a little mucous sputum, dryness in the nasal cavity and pharynx, severe cough with tractive pain in the hypochondrium, reddish tongue with little saliva, etc.

Pathogenesis. Owing to seasonal pathogenic heat, pungent food overeaten and consumption of body fluid by pathogenic dryness-heat.

Therapeutic Principle. Releasing heat from the lung and moistening.

Cough due to Exogenous Cold

Referring to the syndrome.

Symptoms. Cough, lower voice, whitish sputum, headache, heaviness sensation of the body, etc.

Pathogenesis. Owing to the exopathic cold.

Therapeutic Principle. Inducing diaphoresis, removing cough, coldness, enhancing the flow of the lung qi.

Cough due to Fire Wrapped by Cold

Symptoms. Cough with yellow phlegm, fever and aversion to cold, dry mouth, yellow urine, constipation, etc.

Pathogenesis. Owing to accumulated heat in the interior complicated by the exposure to exogenous cold.

Therapeutic Principle. Removing cold, and the heat in the interior.

Cough due to Heat Accumulation

Symptoms. Cough, flushed face, dysphoria, insomnia, sputum in the morning, dark urine with difficulty, etc.

Pathogenesis. Owing to accumulated heat of rich fatty diet, alcohol, affection of Yangming Meridian by heat, impairment of the lung by heat.

Therapeutic Principle. Removing the stomach heat.

Cough due to Impairment of Seven Emotions

Symptoms. Cough with sputum, stuffiness and fullness in the chest, dyspnea and eructation, nausea, hypochondriac distention, etc.

Pathogenesis. Owing to vital-qi of viscera impaired by seven emotions, upward adverse flowing of pathogenic qi, leading to retention of phlegm and the failure of the lung to disperse and descend.

Therapeutic Principle. Enhancing the dispersing function of the lung to smooth circulation of lung-qi, and removing cough and sputum.

Cough due to Indigestion

Symptoms. Cough with excessive phlegm, feeling of stuffiness in the chest, eructation with fetid odor, acid regurgitation, diarrhea, etc.

Pathogenesis. Owing to chronic indigestion, injuring the spleen and stomach, impairment of the activity and digesting function.

Therapeutic Principle. Removing phlegm, food stagnancy, reinforcing the spleen and adjusting the stomach.

Cough due to Internal Injury

Referring to cough resulting from deficiency and weakness of the lung, and pathologic changes in other visceral organs with the lung involved.

Symptoms. Insidious onset, often with the symptoms of deficiency and impairment of other visceral organs, and symptoms due to insufficiency and deficiency of qi and blood. In accordance with the features of the internal injury and the differences between the pathologic changes in the visceral organs, the cough includes cough with the Lung Meridian involved, cough with the Heart Meridian involved, cough with the Liver Meridian involved, cough with the Kidney Meridian involved, cough due to qi deficiency and cough due to blood deficiency.

Therapeutic Principle. Adjusting the visceral function mainly.

Cough due to Involvement of Heart Meridian

Symptoms. Cough with precordial pain, blockage in the throat, swelling of the tongue, sore throat, etc.

Pathogenesis. Owing to heating the lung by the stirring heart-heat or the deficiency of the lung-yin due to the insufficiency of the heart blood and the deficiency of the heart-qi, leading to impairment of purifying and descending function of the lung.

Therapeutic Principle. Removing cough, heart-heat, the nourishing the lung.

Cough due to Lung Affection

Referring to one type of cough.

Symptoms. Loud cough or even blood in the sputum.

Pathogenesis. Owing to deficient lung affected by pathogenic factors.

Therapeutic Principle. Removing pathogenic factors, nourishing the lung and ceasing bleeding.

Cough due to Lung Distention

Symptoms. Shortness of breath, fullness and distention in the chest, pain radiating to supraclavicular fossa, or cough with bloody and purulent sputum, etc.

Pathogenesis. Mostly owing to affection of the lung by exopathogen, or the obstruction of the lung by phlegm, etc.

Therapeutic Principle. Adjusting qi and the lung, releasing phlegm, heat in the lung.

Cough due to Lung Dryness

Symptoms. Dry cough with frequent choking, dryness of throat, lips and nose with hoarseness, dry cough or with less sticky phlegm difficult of spit, or with blood stained sputum, etc.

Pathogenesis. Owing to deficiency of the lung, the loss of body fluid or the impairment of the lung by pathogenic dryness.

Therapeutic Principle. Nourishing the lung, moistening the lung dryness, ceasing cough.

Cough due to Lung-heat

Symptoms. Frequent cough with thick yellowish phlegm, flushed face and dryness of the throat, or fever and thirst, child becomes cyanotic collaterals of the index finger, etc.

Pathogenesis. Owing to the invasion of pathogenic heat into the lung.

Therapeutic Principle. Removing the pathogenic heat from the lung.

Cough due to Overstrain

Symptoms. Dull pain in the chest, weak cough, shortness of breath, mental fatigue, etc.

Pathogenesis. Owing to overstrain or dysphoria resulting in the consumption and impairment of qi and blood of the zang-fu organs.

Therapeutic Principle. Nourishing qi and blood, reinforcing the spleen and reducing phlegm.

Cough due to Phlegm Accumulation

Symptoms. Cough with much phlegm, loss of appetite, etc.

Pathogenesis. Owing to injury to the spleen due to retention of food, dysfunction of the spleen in transportation.

Therapeutic Principle. Removing heat, phlegm, dampness in the body and accumulation.

Cough due to Phlegm-dampness

Symptoms. Cough with profuse phlegm, pituitary and white sputum, oppressive feeling in the chest and stomach, lassitude.

Pathogenesis. Owing to the accumulation phlegm-dampness in the lung, and obstruction of the lung-qi.

Therapeutic Principle. Nourishing the spleen, adjusting the lung, removing dampness and functional disturbance of the lung-qi.

Cough due to Phlegm-retention

Symptoms. Cough and abundant whitish or frothy expectoration. For the deficiency of the kidney-yang, aversion to cold, cold limbs, edema, etc.

Pathogenesis. Owing to phlegm stagnation due to pathogenic cold in the lungs and stomach.

Therapeutic Principle. Warming yang and alleviating water retention.

Cough due to Qi Deficiency

Symptoms. Cough with low sound, spontaneous perspiration, shortness of breath, frequently suffer from common cold, mental fatigue and weakness, anorexia, thin sputum, etc.

Pathogenesis. Owing to overstrain and impairment of lung-qi, improper diet and impairment of qi in the middle-energizer.

Therapeutic Principle. Nourishing the lung, the spleen and qi.

Cough due to Retention of Phlegm

Symptoms. Cough and shortness of breath with low sound, fullness in the chest, dizziness, etc.

Pathogenesis. Mainly owing to the retention of phlegm in the chest, blocking the air passage.

Therapeutic Principle. Adjusting the lung, the flow of qi, removing phlegm and the retention of fluid.

Cough due to Sexual Strain

Symptoms. Cough, fever, lumbago, backache, etc.

Pathogenesis. Mainly owing to impairment of the kidney due to sexual strain, and deficiency of the kidney essence.

Therapeutic Principle. Nourishing the kidney and moistening the lung.

Cough due to Summer-heat

Symptoms. Cough, nausea and heaviness sensation of the limbs, dizziness with blurred vision, mental fatigue and lassitude, etc.

Pathogenesis. Owing to the invasion of pathogenic summer-heat, leading to upward flowing of unclean lung-qi.

Therapeutic Principle. Removing the summer-heat, and cough.

Cough due to Wind-cold Pathogen

Symptoms. Cough with watery and white sputum, stuffy nose and watery nasal discharge, chill, anhidrosis, headache.

Pathogenesis. Owing to the invasion of wind-cold pathogen into the lung leading to the obstruction of the lung-qi.

Therapeutic Principle. Removing wind and cold pathogens; regulating the flow of lung-qi.

Cough due to Wind-heat Pathogen

Symptoms. Cough with thick or yellow sputum, thirst, sore throat, yellow nasal discharge, fever, aversion to wind, sweating, headache.

Pathogenesis. Owing to wind-heat attacking the lung, affecting the function of the lung.

Therapeutic Principle. Removing wind, heat and functional disturbance of the lung-qi.

Cough due to Wind-phlegm

Symptoms. Cough when there is sputum, fullness sensation in the thoracic diaphragm, profuse phlegm and saliva, or even cough with the vomiting of food, phlegm and saliva for the serious case, etc.

Pathogenesis. Owing to obstruction of the lung-qi due to sufficiency of wind-phlegm.

Therapeutic Principle. Removing wind and phlegm.

Cough due to Yin Deficiency

Symptoms. Dry cough without phlegm, or with a little thick phlegm mixed with blood, dry and sore throat, fever in the afternoon.

Pathogenesis. Owing to deficiency of lung-yin, affecting the functions of the lung and leading to dryness of the lung and reversed flow of qi.

Therapeutic Principle. Nourishing yin and the lung, removing cough and heat.

Cough during Menstruation

Referring to one type of cough.

Symptoms. Frequent cough during menstruation.

Pathogenesis. Mainly owing to dryness and consumption of the lung essence.

Cough during Pregnancy

Symptoms. Often cough during pregnancy.

Pathogenesis. Owing to phlegm accumulation in the lung, or obstruction of the lung-qi and abnormal upward flow of qi.

Therapeutic Principle. For yin deficiency with lung-heat, tonifying yin, removing heat from the lung; for the phlegm accumulation in the lung, enhancing qi circulation, removing phlegm, and ceasing cough to prevent abortion; for the affection by exopathogen, inducing diaphoresis, enhancing the dispersing function of the lung.

Cough in Children

It is clinically divided into three types.

1. Cough due to exopathy.

   Symptoms. Fever, chills, sore throat, headache.

   Pathogenesis. Mostly caused by the exogenous evils first attack the lung, which leads to the onset of common cold.

   Therapeutic Principle. Expelling wind to relieve superficial syndrome, ventilating the lung to relieve cough.

2. Cough due to phlegm and dampness.

   Symptoms. Cough, wheezing sound in the throat, poor appetite, etc.

   Pathogenesis. Owing to obstruction of lung qi, resulting from indigestion leading to the retention of dampness in the spleen, and stagnation of damp-phlegm in the lung.

   Therapeutic Principle. Nourishing the spleen, releasing dampness and phlegm to relieve cough.

3. Cough due to deficiency of the lung.

   Symptoms. Paroxysmal cough, small amount of mucous sputum, listlessness, flushed face and cheek.

   Pathogenesis. Owing to dysfunction of the lung due to the constitutional deficiency of the body and the damage of body fluid.

   Therapeutic Principle. Enriching yin and invigorating qi, removing cough.

Cough of Deficiency Type

1. **Symptoms.** Cough with whitish frothy sputum or nausea, etc., for qi deficiency.

   Pathogenesis. Owing to the deficiency of qi and blood, etc.

   Therapeutic Principle. Reinforcing the spleen and qi.

2. **Symptoms.** For blood deficiency, night cough, thirst, difficult expectorated sputum or fever, etc.

Therapeutic Principle. Nourishing blood and yin.

Cough Related to Spleen

1. **Symptoms.** Cough with right hypochondriac pain radiating to the shoulder and back, heaviness and even inability to move.

Pathogenesis. Owing to accumulated heat of the spleen and stomach, or phlegm-dampness due to deficiency of the spleen.

Therapeutic Principle. Removing dampness, the lung-heat, invigorating the spleen.

2. **Symptoms.** Constant cough with phlegm and pain radiating to the lower abdomen, etc.

Pathogenesis. Owing to improper diet, excessive eating peppery food, hypofunction of the spleen leading to phlegm to disturb the lung.

Therapeutic Principle. Nourishing the spleen and reducing phlegm.

Cough with Encopresis

Symptoms. Cough with fecal incontinence.

Pathogenesis. Owing to invasion of the Lung Meridian by pathogens, transferred into the large intestine.

Therapeutic Principle. Nourishing the spleen, qi removing, cough.

Cough with Fullness in Epigastrium

Symptoms. Cough, fullness and rigidity in the epigastrium. Pain occasioned by cough.

Therapeutic Principle. Warming the lung, reducing watery phlegm and removing cough.

Cough with Pericardium Involved

Symptoms. Dull pain in the precordial region while coughing.

Pathogenesis. Owing to invasion of exopathogenic factors into the lung, which results in obstruction of the lung-qi, leading to the lung collaterals impeded.

Therapeutic Principle. Removing heat from the heart and enhancing the dispersing function of the lung to relieve cough.

Cough with Vomiting of Bile

Symptoms. Cough vomiting of bile, bitter taste, pain in hypochondrium, etc.

Pathogenesis. Mainly owing to stagnation of heat in Gallbladder Meridian, or excessive gallbladder-heat.

Therapeutic Principle. Removing heat, normalizing the functioning of the gallbladder, and adjusting the flow of qi.

Cough with Wheezing due to Phlegm Retention

Symptoms. Sounding phlegm while coughing, much phlegm and saliva, and fullness in the chest and diaphragm, or the alternate attack of cold and fever, facial dropsy.

Pathogenesis. Usually owing to phlegm-dampness in the stomach going up to the lung.

Therapeutic Principle. Reinforcing the spleen, removing dampness and the phlegm.

Counter-abdominal Respiration

Referring to a breath-regulating method in Qigong.

Method. Draw in the abdomen while inhaling and bulge it while exhaling.

Notice. The method is suitable for the young and the middle aged persons as well as the well-trained Qigong practitioners. But the method is forbidden for the aged and the weak persons or those with hypertension or heart diseases.

Counting Breath

Referring to a term in Qigong.

Method. During practising Qigong concentrating mind on respiration, and silently counting the breath from 1 to 10 or from 1 to 100, again and again, thus adjusting breathing to be thready, soft, even and long, stabilizing the mind and getting rid of distractions to enter a tranquil state.

Coupled Puncture

Referring to a needling technique, one of the Twelve Needling techniques.

Method. With hands hold and push the painful area on the chest and the corresponding area on the back, and puncture these areas obliquely with one needle each. Avoid perpendicular and deep acupuncture to protect the viscera from damage.

Indication. Angina pectoris.

Course of Meridians

Referring to the path and direction of qi and blood of 12 meridians. The path and direction are as follows: the three yin meridians of the hand travelling from the chest to the tips of the fingers; the three yang meridians of the hand from the tips of the fingers to the head and face; from here the three yang meridians of foot to the toe; from which the three yin meridians of the foot to the abdomen or chest.

Cow-bezoare

It is the stone in the gallbladder or biliary ducts of Bos Taurus domesticus Gmelin (Bovidae). The stone is extracted from the bile of ox and pig and then processed, called artificial cow-bezoares.

Effect. Removing heat and toxic material, eliminating phlegm and waking the unconscious patient, expelling wind and relieving spasm.

Indication. Unconsciousness and delirium owing to febrile disease, epilepsy, apoplexy and trismus, infantile convulsion, swollen and sore throat, canker sores in the mouth and on the tongue, carbuncles, boils.

Cow-fat Seed

It is the ripe seed of Vaccaria segelalis (Neck.) Garcke (Caryophyllaceae).

Effect. Recovering menstrual flow, enhancing milk secretion, blood circulation.

Indication. Dysmenorrhea, amenorrhea, postpartum galactostasis, acute mastitis, etc.

Crab

It is the flesh and interior organ of Eriocheir sinensis H. Milne-Edwards (Grapsidae).

Effect. Releasing fever, blood stasis and enhancing reunion of fractured bones.

Indication. Impairment of muscles and bones, scabies, paint dermatitis, scald, etc.

Crab-like Eye

It is a disease, a severe oculopathy.

Symptoms. Diabrosis of the black, then shedding of iris from the diabrotic hole and unbearable pain, with the shape of a crab-like pattern. The pain is alleviated with the leaking out of the pathogenic toxin along with the iris from the hole, but fat-spot nebula is usually left over after its recovery.

Pathogenesis. Owing to sufficiency and flaming of heat toxin in the liver and gallbladder, or untimely treatment of fat-deposit nebula or flower-like nebula.

Therapeutic Principle. Adjusting the liver of pathogenic heat, at early stage of excess type; tonifying the kidney, for a long duration, of the deficiency type.

Crab Shell

It is the shell of Eriocheir sinensis H. Milne-Edwards (Grapsidae).

Effect. Releasing stagnation of qi and lumps.

Indication. Accumulation of blood stasis, costalgia, abdominal pain, acute mastitis, frostbite, etc.

Cramp in Cholera Morbus

It is a syndrome of muscle-spasm of limbs.

Symptoms. Contracture of both legs for the mild case, and abdominal spasm, shrinking scrotum and curling tongue for the serious.

Pathogenesis. Owing to vomiting and diarrhea from cholera, resulting in a sudden loss of body fluid, severe damage of qi and blood, malnutrition of muscles and vessels, or affection of cold.

Therapeutic Principle. Warming middle-energizer, removing cold; in the serious, warming and tonifying the spleen and kidney and recuperating depleted yang, for cholera of cold type; and for cholera of heat type, removing heat and dampness.

Crater Nipple

Symptoms. Sensation of spasm of breast muscles with pain.

Pathogenesis. Owing to walking in the rain and careless sexual intercourse, leading to stagnation of cold and dampness in the Liver Meridian of Foot-jueyin.

Therapeutic Principle. Removing cold from the meridian, and releasing spasm and pain.

Creeping Ceratostigma Root

It is the root of Ceratostigma minus Stapf. (Plumbaginaceae).

Effect. Adjusting and activating the meridians and collaterals and releasing wind-dampness.

Indication. Numbness resulting from wind-dampness, angiitis, etc.

Creeping Dichondra Herb

The whole herb of Dichondra repens Forst (Convolvulaceae).

Effect. Removing heat, detoxicating, inducing diuresis and enhancing blood circulation.

Indication. Jaundice, dysentery, stranguria from urolithiasis, cloudy urine, edema, boils, furuncles.

Creeping Psychotia Twig and Leaf

It is the twig and leaf of Psychotria serpens L. (Rubiaceae).

Effect. Removing pain, swelling, pathogenic wind and dampness, reinforcing muscles and bones.

Indication. Arthralgia due to wind-dampness, swollen and sore throat, subcutaneous swelling and scabies.

Creeping Rostellularia Herb

It is the whole herb of Rostellularia procumbens (L.) Nees (Acanthaceae).

Effect. Detoxicating, releasing heat, pain, dampness, undigested food, enhancing blood circulation.

Indication. Fever due to common cold, cough, sore throat, malaria, dysentery, jaundice, edema due to nephritis, arthralgia and myalgia, infantile indigestion with food retention.

Creeping Waterprimrose Herb

It is the whole herb of Jussiaea repensl L. (Onagraceae).

Effect. Removing swelling, heat, inducing diuresis, and detoxicating.

Indication. Dryness cough, stranguria, measles, erysipelas and suppurative infections on the skin.

Creeping Woodsorrel Herb

It is the whole herb of Oxalis corniculata L. (Oxalidaceae).

Effect. Enhancing diuresis, releasing pathogenic heat from the blood, blood stasis, swelling, toxic substances.

Indication. Diarrhea, dysentery, jaundice, stranguria, leukorrhea with reddish discharge, swollen and sore throat, furuncles, subcutaneous swelling, hemorrhoids.

Crimson and Purple Dry Tongue

Referring to a tongue condition.

Symptoms. The crimson and purple, dry tongue with fissure and prickles.

Pathogenesis. Owing to excessive heat injuring yin and stagnation of qi and blood.

Crimson Tongue with Little Fur

Referring to a tongue condition, dark red tongue with little fur on the surface. Seen in the patient with hyperactivity of heat due to yin deficiency.

Crimson, Withered and Smooth Tongue without Fur

Referring to a tongue condition. The tongue is crimson in color, with smooth surface without fur and withered body, seen in the seriously ill patients with exhaustion of both the stomach-yin and kidney-yin. It is one of critical tongue pictures.

Crispate-leaf Ardisia Root

It is the root or rhizome of Ardisia crispa (Thunb). A. DC. (Myrsinaceae).
Effect. Removing heat, phlegm and inducing diuresis.
Indication. Swelling and sore throat, cough due to the lung-heat unsmooth expectoration, jaundice, edema, toothache.

Crossing Point

Referring to a point where two or more meridians pass by, most in face, head and trunk. For example, Zhongfu (L 1) is the crossing point of the Lung Meridian of Hand-taiyin and the Spleen Meridian of Foot-taiyin. A crossing point can be used to cure diseases belonging to different meridians because different meridians pass by.

Croton Seed   ⊛ C-18

It is the ripe seed of Croton tiglium L. (Euphorbiaceae).
Effect. Removing retention of food by purgation, releasing retained water, swelling, phlegm and sore throat.
Indication. Retention of food due to pathogenic cold, fulminant fullness of abdomen and distending pain, constipation, infantile indigestion, edema and ascites, malaria.

Croton Seed Poisoning

Symptoms. Heat and pain of the mouth and throat, flushed face, severe abdominal pain and diarrhea, even coma, jaundice, the impairment of the kidney and shock.
Pathogenesis. Owing to having eaten or protracted contact with croton seeds.
Therapeutic Principle. Cleaning the stomach with warm water, taking cold milk, egg white and cold rice-water for the early period. Emergency treatment of combination of Chinese traditional and Western medicine shall be used for the severe case.

Croup due to Fire Wrapped by Cold

Symptoms. Rale, asthma, dysphoria, and fullness in the chest.
Pathogenesis. Owing to accumulated heat in the lung complicated by the exposure to exogenous cold.
Therapeutic Principle. Removing the cold in the exterior and the stagnant heat.

Crowndaisy Chrysanthemum Herb

It is the stem of leaf of Chrysanthemum coronarium L. var. spatiosum Bailey (Compositae).
Effect. Adjusting the spleen and stomach, inducing diuresis, enhancing stool and removing phlegm retention.

Crucian Carp

It is the meat or whole body of Carassius auratus (L.) (Cyprinidae).
Effect. Reinforcing the spleen and releasing dampness.
Indication. Weakness of the spleen and the stomach, dysentery, hemafecia, edema, stranguria, subcutaneous swelling, ulcer, etc.

Cry due to Abdominal Pain

Referring to an infant cry due to the abdominal pain.

Pathogenesis. Mostly owing to food stagnancy, parasitosis and cold organs.

Therapeutic Principle. For food stagnancy, enhancing digestion; for parasitosis, killing intestinal parasites; for cold organs, warming middle-energizer to disperse cold.

Crying with Fear

Referring to an infant cry due to fright.

Pathogenesis. Owing to deficiency of qi in the heart and liver, and affection of wind and cold, or immoderate milk, or hearing the strange sound suddenly, or crying and starting due to being frightened occasionally.

Therapeutic Principle. Different treatments based on the different causes.

Crying with Irritability

Referring to the infant's cry at night due to irritability.

Symptoms. Vexation, sleeping unsteadily, and sudden cry while sleeping.

Pathogenesis. Owing to heat syndrome in newborn affecting infant's emotion.

Therapeutic Principle. Removing heat from the heart and tranquilize the mind.

Crystal Sugar

It is rock candy sweet in flavour, neutral in nature.

Effect. Nourishing the middle-energizer, qi, adjusting the function of the stomach and moistening the lung.

Indication. Cough, profuse sputum and saliva, loss of appetite in children, etc.

Cuanzhu (B 2)

A meridian point.

Location. On the face, in the depression on the medial lend of the eyebrow, at the supraorbital notch.

Indication. Headache, dizziness, deviation of the mouth and eye, poor vision, swelling and pain of the eye.

Method. Puncture obliquely downwards 0.3-0.5 cun for ophthalmopathy; puncture to Yuyao (Ex-HN 4) for headache and facial paralysis. Moxibustion is forbidden.

Cudian (Ex)

It is an extra point.

Location. In the depression above the root of penis.

Indication. Sudden onset of depressive psychosis.

Method. Moxibustion.

Cunping (Ex-UE)

It is an extra point.

Location. On the dorsum of the hand, 1 cun above the midpoint of the transverse crease of the wrist, and 0.4 cun lateral to the radial side.

Indication. Cardiac failure, shock, etc.

Method. Puncture perpendicularly 0.3-0.5 cun.

Cupping

Referring to a therapeutic method.

Method. Make an inverted cup or jar closely attach to the skin surface by means of the negative pressure inside the cup or jar. Including fire-insertion cupping, air-pumping cupping, successive flash-cupping, movable cupping, needle-retaining cupping, bloodletting puncturing and cupping etc., for about 10 minutes each time.

Function. This method can cause local hyperemia or passive congestion, thus enhancing the circulation of blood and the flow of qi, removing pain and swelling, etc.

Indication. Common cold, headache, stomachache, abdominal pain, arthralgia due to wind-dampness.

Cupping by Extracting Air

It is a cupping method.

Method. Using specially made cup with a rubber piston fixed at the bottom of the cup, which connects to an air pump to form a negative pressure inside.

Cupping by Pushing the Cup

Referring to a kind of cupping.

Method. After the cup is sucked to the skin, move the cup around the treated area about 6-8 times until the skin of the affected area becoming red, thus enlarging the functioning area. Before cupping, smear some oil, vaseline or paraffin, etc. on the affected area and the edge of the cup. The method is suitable for the lumbodorsal part.

Indication. Rheumatic pain and gastrointestinal diseases.

Cupping with Boiled Cup

Referring to one of the cupping therapies.

Method. Usually boiling a bamboo jar, suction tube in clean water or medical solution for 3-5 minutes, then, picking it out with tweezers, pouring water out and wiping the jar mouth quickly, and immediately making it to cover and adhere to the selected point.

Cupping with Glasses in Alignment

Referring to one of the methods for cupping in cupping treatment.

Method. Arranging several glasses for cupping in alignment along the muscle bundle for treating the muscle bundle strain.

Cupping with Retaining of Needle

Method. Cupping the area where the needle is retained.

Curious Kadsura Root or Stem

It is the root or stem of Kadsura heteroclita (Roxb.) Craib (Magnoliaceae).

Effect. Releasing wind, dampness, enhancing blood circulation and flow of qi.

Indication. Rheumatic arthralgia, abdominal distention and pain, dysmenorrhea, postpartum abdominal pain, traumatic injuries.

Curled-up Tongue

Referring to a tongue condition.

Symptoms. Curved tongue and unable to extend straightly.

Pathogenesis. Owing to flaring-up of the heart-heat, internal disturbance of wind-phlegm, or inward invasion of the pericardium by virulent heat pathogen, or excessive heat in the Liver Meridian.

Curled-up Tongue and Contracted Scrotum

Symptoms. Curved tongue unable to extend straight and ascended scrotum.

Pathogenesis. Mostly owing to internal disturbance of pathogenic heat, exhaustion of body fluid, failure to nourish muscles, or deficiency of yin of cold type.

Curly Bristlethistle Herb or Root

It is the whole herb or root of Carduus crispus L. (Compositae).

Effect. Enhancing diuresis, releasing heat, blood stasis.

Indication. Intermittent headache, vertigo, arthralgia pain due to wind-heat, skin itching, chyluria, hematuria, leukorrhagia, traumatic injuries, boils, furuncles.

Cutaneous Anthrax

Referring to the nail-like boil.

Symptoms. At the beginning, a small red maculopapular eruption, itching but no pain; two days later, the eruption changing into a blister, burning hot, dry, dark and necrotic, with small blisters around it. The patient with fever, headache, etc, ten days later, recovered.

Pathogenesis. Mostly owing to the infection of toxins due to the contact of epidemic livestock, blocked between the skin and the muscle.

Therapeutic Principle. Detoxicating, releasing pathogenic heat from blood, swelling.

Cutting Therapy

Referring to a therapeutic technique.

Method. Cutting the skin in a particular area and removing a little subcutaneous fat, then applying a stimulation in the local area, e.g. the cutting in the thenar eminence, cutting around Danzhong (CV 17), etc.

Indication. Chronic bronchitis, asthma, infantile malnutrition, peptic ulcer, etc.

Notice. Strict sterilization, prevention of accidental injury and careful nursing of the wound.

Cuttle Bone

It is the bone of Sepiella maindroni de Rochebrune, or Sepia esculenta Hoyle (Sepiadae).

Effect. Inducing astringency, ceasing hemorrhage, keeping the kidney essence, curing leukorrhagia, decreasing the production of gastric acid, releasing stomachache, removing dampness.

Indication. Metrorrhagia, metrostaxis, traumatic bleeding, emission, leukorrhagia, stomachache.

Cymose Buckwheat Rhizome

It is the stem and rhizome of Fagopyrum cymosum Meisn. (Polygonaceae).

Effect. Detoxicating, releasing heat from the lung, sputum, reinforcing the spleen and enhancing digestion.

Indication. Pulmonary abscess, carbuncles, sores, furuncles and swelling, scrofula, cough due to the lung-heat, swollen and sore throat, emaciation owing to infantile malnutrition, etc.

D

Dabao (Sp 21)

A meridian point.

Location. On the middle axillary line the lateral side of the chest, in the 6th intercostal space.

Indication. Pain in the chest and hypochondrium, asthma, whole body pain and myasthenia of limbs.

Method. Puncture obliquely 0.5-0.8 cun. Apply moxibustion 5-10 minutes with warming moxibustion.

Dachangshu (B 25)

A meridian point.

Location. On the low back, below the spinous process of the 4th lumbar vertebra, 1.5 cun lateral to the posterior midline.

Indication. Abdominal distention, abdominal pain, borborygmus, diarrhea, constipation, dysentery, lumbago, etc.

Method. Puncture perpendicularly 0.8-1 cun. Apply moxibustion 5-10 moxa cones or 10-20 minutes.

Dacryocystitis

Symptoms. Slight redness and swelling in the local region, discomfort of dull astringency, constant shedding of saliva or pus, and prolonged failure to heal.

Pathogenesis. Mostly caused by invasion of the lacrimal orifice by wind-heat, or by upward attack of the heart-fire and spleen-heat upon the lacrimal orifice.

Therapeutic Principle. Relieving wind, purging fire, clearing away heat and promoting diuresis, at the same time external treatment operation can be used if necessary.

Dacryorrhea

Symptoms. Tearing without emotional excitation, over joying or grief. It can be divided two cases, 1: red eyes, photophobia and painful eyes, 2: no red swelling eyes, more tear against wind and cold tear.

Therapeutic Principle. Case 1: remove wind and clear away heat, cool the blood and improve eyesight. Case 2: promote the blood circulation and remove blood stasis, and promote eyesight by nourish the liver, or apply surgical method to remove the obstruction.

Dadu (Sp 2)

1. A meridian point.

   Location. On the medial border of the great toe, in the depression of the junction of the red and white skin, anterior and inferior to the lst metatarsophalangeal joint.

   Indication. Abdominal distention, epigastralgia, indigestion, hiccups, diarrhea, constipation, febrile disease without perspiration, cold limbs, vexation, etc.

   Method. Puncture perpendicularly 0.3-0.5 cun. Apply moxibustion 3-5 moxa cones or 5-10 minutes.

2. An extra point, one of the Baxie (Ex-UE 9) points.

   Location. At the junction of the red and white skin between the thumb and index fingers.

Dadun (Liv 1)

A meridian point.

Location. On the lateral side of the distal segment of the great toe, 0. 1 cun lateral to the proximal corner of the toe nail.

Indication. Hernia, irregular menstruation, metrorrhagia, hematuria, uroschesis, enuresis, and infantile convulsion.

Method. Puncture obliquely 0.1-0.2 cun or prick to cause bleeding. Apply moxibustion 3-5 moxa cones or 5-10 minutes.

Dagukong (Ex-UE 5)

An extra point.

Location. On the dorsal side of the thumb, at the center of the interphalangeal joint.

Indication. Pain in the eye, pterygium, cataract, marginal blepharitis, epistaxis, vomiting and diarrhea, etc.

Method. Apply moxibustion 3-5 moxa cones, or 5-10 minutes.

Dahe (K12)

A meridian point.

Location. On the lower abdomen, 4 cun below the center of the umbilicus and 0. 5 cun lateral to the anterior midline.

Indication. Hysteroptosis, seminal emission, leukorrhea, irregular menstruation, dysmenorrhea, diarrhea, dysentery.

Method. Puncture perpendicularly 0.8-1.2 cun. Apply moxibustion 3-5 moxa cones or 5-10 minutes with warming moxibustion.

Daheng (Sp 15)

A meridian point.

Location. On the middle abdomen, 4 cun to the center of the umbilicus.

Indication. Diarrhea, dysentery, constipation, pain in the lower abdomen.

Method. Puncture perpendicularly 0.8-1.2 cun. Apply moxibustion 5-7 moxa cones or 10-15 minutes with warming moxibustion.

Dahurian Angelica Root

The root of Angelica dahurica Benth. Et Hook, or A. dahurica (Fich. ex Holtm.) Benth. Et Hook. F. var. formosana (Boiss) Shan. et Yuan. (Umbelliferae).

Effect. Inducing diaphoresis, expelling wind, eliminating dampness, subduing swelling, promoting pus discharge and relieving pain.

Indication. Anodyne for frontal headache in colds, supraorbital neuralgia, toothache, various infections on the body surface with swelling pain, leukorrhea due to cold-dampness, rhinorrhea with turbid discharge, cutaneous pruritus, etc.

Dahurian Buchthorn Bark

It is the bark of Rhamnus davurica Pall. (Rhamnaceae).

Effect. Releasing noxious heat and pathogenic wind.

Indication. Migratory arthralgia, toxic heat on the skin, and cold, heat, toxic arthralgia resulting from skin and external diseases, etc.

Dahurian Buchthorn Fruit

It is the fruit of Rhamnus davurica Pall. (Rhamnaceae).

Effect. Removing heat, enhancing diuresis, ceasing stagnancy and killing parasites.

Indication. Edema with ascites, hernia, abdominal masses, scrofula, scabies, tinea, etc.

Dahurian Rhododendron Leaf

It is the leaf of Rhododendron dauricum L. (Ericaceae).

Effect. Removing cough and dyspnea, ceasing phlegm.

Indication. Acute and chronic bronchitis, bronchial asthma and cough.

Daimai (G 26)

An acupoint.

Location. At the cross vertically 1.8 cun below the front of hypochondrium, or the costal cartilage of the llth rib and horizontally at straight line that starts from the umbilicus.

Indication. Cold lumbago, irregular menstruation, leukorrhea with reddish discharge and pelvic inflammation, etc.

Method. Puncture perpendicularly 0.5-0.8 cun, and apply moxibustion for 5 min to a quarter.

Daju (S 27)

A meridian point.

Location. On the lower abdomen, 2 cun below the center of the umbilicus and 2 cun lateral to the anterior midline.

Indication. Distention of the lower abdomen, oliguria, hernia, seminal emission, premature ejaculation, palpitations caused by fright, insomnia, etc.

Method. Puncture perpendicularly 0.8-1.2 cun. Apply moxibustion 5-7 moxa cones or 10-20 minutes with warming moxibustion.

Daling (P 7)

A meridian point.

Location. At the midpoint of the transverse crease of the wrist, between the tendons of the long palmar muscle and radial flexor muscle of the wrist.

Indication. Cardiac pain, palpitation, stomachache, vomiting, palpitations caused by fright, depression, insanity, epilepsy, pain in the chest, etc.

Method. Puncture perpendicularly 0.3-0.5 cun. Apply moxibustion 3-5 minutes with warming moxibustion.

Damage of Qi

Symptoms. In the case of blockage of qi, unconsciousness, tightness and fullness in chest and hypochondrium with moving pain without a fixed spot, even vexation and shortness of breath can be seen.

Pathogenesis. External injury, fall from a high place or stroke resulting in blockage or stagnation of qi.

Therapeutic Principle. Promoting the circulation of qi and removing obstruction in the collateral, local applying manipulation for relaxing muscles and tendons.

Damen (Ex-HN)

An extra point.

Location. On the head, 3.5 cun above the midpoint of the posterior hairline.

Indication. Hemiplegia.

Method. Puncture subcutaneously 0.3-0.5 cun. Apply moxibustion with a moxa stick for 30 minutes.

Damp

It is one of the six atmospheric pathogenic factors occurring during late summer. Pathogenic dampness is classified into exopathic dampness and endogenous dampness.

1. Exopathic dampness is usually caused by walking in rain, as well as living and working in damp environment.

   Symptoms. Headache as if the head were tightly bound, lassitude, heaviness in the limbs, fullness in the chest, joint pains and swelling with sensation of heaviness.

2. Endogenous dampness usually results from the dysfunction of the spleen in transportation, accumulation, and stagnation of damp.

   Symptoms. Loss of appetite, diarrhea, abdominal distention, oliguria and edema.

Damp Athralgia

Symptoms. Heaviness sensation of limb joints, with aching pain or accompanied by tumefaction, pain in fixed spot, numbness of skin and muscles, whitish and greasy fur, soft and moderate pulse, etc.

Pathogenesis. Invasion of the pathogenic dampness into the body, accumulated in joints is usual.

Therapeutic Principle. Removing dampness and dredging meridians, expelling the wind and dispelling the cold.

Damp Beriberi

Symptoms. Leg edema, numbness and heaviness, weakness, or dysuria, etc.

Pathogenesis. Due to dampness attacking the lower limbs, the meridians fail to remove and activate qi.

Therapeutic Principle. Relieving stagnation and ceasing damp.

Damp cough

1. It refers to cough due to retention of water inside the body.
   Therapeutic Principle. Reinforcing the spleen and eliminating dampness, relieving phlegm and reducing sputum.
2. It refers to cough due to affection by exopathogen of dampness.
   Therapeutic Principle. Enhancing dispersing function of the lung, removing pathogenic factors and ceasing cough.

Damp Diarrhea

Symptoms. Heavy sensation of the body, weakness, depression in the stomach, poor appetite, borborygmus, watery stools, etc.

Pathogenesis. Due to impairment of the spleen and stomach by pathogenic dampness and original weakness of spleen and stomach.

Therapeutic Principle. Reinforcing the spleen and relieving dampness and stopping diarrhea.

Damp-edema

Symptoms. Serious edema of the lower limbs, loose stool, etc.

Pathogenesis. Invasion of dampness into the body and stagnation of dampness. Mostly due to long residence in a damp or cold-damp place.

Therapeutic Principle. Invigorating the spleen and activating yang, and eliminating dampness.

Damp-evil Produced in Interior

Symptoms. Poor appetite, stickiness but not thirsty, nausea, vomiting, loose stool, skin swelling, turbid urine and leukorrhea, etc.

Pathogenesis. Caused by dysfunction of the spleen in transporting and distributing fluid resulting from deficiency of the spleen.

Damp Fever

Symptoms. Sustained fever, perspiration sometimes, stuffiness and tightness in the chest, etc.

Pathogenesis. Resulting from damp-heat pathogen and often occurs in summer and autumn with too much rain.

Therapeutic Principle. Removing dampness and relieving fever.

Damp-heat Accumulated and Evaporated

Referring to the pathological mechanism of damp-heat pathogen and obstruction of functional activities of qi, leading to evaporation upwards or on muscular striae externally during the damp-heat syndrome.

Damp-heat Accumulating in Shaoyang

Symptoms. Chills and fever, like in malaria but more fever, less chills, thirst, vexation, nausea, etc.

Pathogenesis. Due to damp-heat pathogen in shaoyang, and functional activities of qi in tri-energizer stagnating.

Therapeutic Principle. Slightly purging Shaoyang Gallbladder-heat, and removing damp-heat of tri-energizer.

Damp-heat in Spleen and Stomach

Symptoms. Fullness and distention in the abdomen, anorexia, nausea, fatigue, bitter taste in the mouth, scanty and yellow urine, etc.

Pathogenesis. Stagnation of damp-heat pathogens in the spleen and stomach.

Therapeutic Principle. Removing heat and eliminating dampness.

Damp-heat in Urinary Bladder

Symptoms. Frequent micturition, dripping, yellowish and scanty urine and pain in the waist, or hematuria or calculi in urine, etc.

Pathogenesis. Exogenous affection of damp-heat pathogens and improper diet leading to internal production of damp-heat and its invasion into the bladder.

Therapeutic Principle. Removing heat and enhancing diuresis.

Damp-heat Jaundice

Symptoms. Yellow coloration of skin as bright as orange, hot sensation and excessive thirst, or dark and painful micturition, or constipation.

Pathogenesis. Resulting from combat of damp with heat, leading to both stagnation and yellow coloration of the skin.

Therapeutic Principle. Removing heat and enhancing diuresis.

Damp Malaria

It refers to malaria caused by invasion of pathogenic dampness.

Symptoms. Intermittent chills and moderate fever, pantalgia, heavy sensation of the limbs, distress in the epigastrium, vomiting, swollen face and less urine, etc.

Therapeutic Principle. Relieving exterior syndrome to eliminate dampness.

Dampness

Referring to a morbid condition.

Symptoms. Epigastric distress, abdominal distention, anorexia, loose stool, nausea, vomiting tendency, feeling of heavy over the head. etc.

Pathogenesis. Improper diet, over-eating raw or cold food. Being caught in rain and dwelling damp environments.

Dampness and Heat in Liver and Gallbladder

Symptoms. Distending and burning pain in hypochondrium, anorexia, abdominal distention, nausea, loose stool, or scanty dark urine, alternate attacks of chills and fever, jaundice, or eczema of scrotum, itch, or foul yellow-colored leukorrhagia, pruritus of vulva, etc.

Pathogenesis. Owing to stagnation of pathogenic dampness and heat in the liver, gallbladder, the Liver and the Gallbladder Meridians.

Therapeutic Principle. Removing heat and enhancing diuresis, and dredging and smoothing the Liver and Gallbladder Meridians.

Dampness Impairing Spleen-Yang

It refers to a morbid state due to blockade of the spleen-yang by pathogenic dampness.

Symptoms. Mass at spleen, abdominal pain, diarrhea, cold limbs, etc.

Dampness with Heavy and Turbid Nature

It refers to the diseases due to invasion of damp pathogen factors. Usually symptoms are heavy sensations of head and body, aching and sluggishness of the limbs, turbid excreta and secreta, loose stool or mucous stool with blood, turbid urine, excessive leukorrhea and turbid pyogenic fluid, etc.

Dampness with Sticky and Stagnant Nature

It refers two meanings:

1. Symptoms of a damp disease are usually of slimy and greasy feature, e.g. mucous stool and slow urination as well as mucous and turbid secretes or slimy and greasy fur.
2. Damp disease has a long course and is often lingering and difficult to cure, with repeated attacks, such as damp arthralgia, eczema and damp-warm syndrome.

Damp Phlegm

Referring to phlegm generated from turbid fluid retained in the body.

Symptoms. Copious watery phlegm, chest, distress cough with dyspnea, etc.

Pathogenesis. Due to dysfunction of the spleen in transporting and distributing fluid and accumulation and stagnation of dampness.

Damuzhitou (Ex-UE)

An extra point.

Location. At the tips of the thumbs of both hands, 0.1 cun from each thumb nail.

Indication. Edema and nephritis.

Method. Puncture perpendicularly 0.1-0.2 cun. Apply moxibustion 5-7 moxa cones.

Dandelion Herb ⊛ D-1

It is the whole herb of Taraxacum mongolicum Hand. -Mazz. (Compositae) with root and many other species of the same genus.

Effect. Removing heat, detoxicating and inducing diuresis.

Indication. Carbuncle and furuncle, acute mastitis, acute appendicitis, swollen and sore throat, bloodshot eyes, jaundice, snake bite, etc.

Dandelion Herb

Dangrong (Ex-HN)

An extra point.

Location. Lateral to the outer canthus, in the depression on the lateral border of the eye.

Indication. Red eyes with Painful swelling.

Method. Puncture subcutaneously 0.3-0.5 cun. Moxibustion is applicable.

Dangyang (Ex-HN 2)

An extra point.

Location. At the frontal part of the head, directly above the pupil, 1 cun above the anterior hairline.

Indication. Headache, dizziness, common cold, redness, swelling and pain of the eye.

Method. Puncture subcutaneously 0.5-0.8 cun. Moxibustion is applicable.

Dan Jie

1. An acupuncture term. Dan refers to selecting 2 points and Jie refers to selecting a single point.
2. Dan refers to the methods of lifting and reducing; Jie refers to those of pressing and reinforcing.

Dannang (Ex-LE 6)

An extra point.

Location. On the upper part of the lateral surface of the 2 cun directly below the depression anterior and inferior to the head of the fibula e.g. Yanglingquan (G 34).

Indication. Acute and chronic cholecystitis, cholelithiasis, biliary ascariasis, numbness or paralysis of the lower extremities.

Method. Puncture perpendicularly 0.8-1.2 cun. Moxibustion is applicable.

Danshu

An acupoint.

Location. On the back, 1.5 cun below the spinous process of the 10th thoracic vertebra.

Indication. Distention and pain in the chest and abdomen, vomiting, bitter taste, jaundice, pain in the throat, anorexia, epilepsy, etc.

Method. Puncture obliquely 0.5-0.8 cun (avoid deep acupuncture) and apply moxibustion to the point for 5-15 minutes or 3-5 units of moxa cones.

Danzhong (CV 17)

A meridian point.

Location. On the chest at the anterior midline, on the lever of the 4th intercostal space, at the midpoint of the line connecting both nipples.

Indication. Cough, dyspnea, cough with bloody sputum, heart pain, palpitation, irritability, insufficient lactation of parturient, etc.

Method. Puncture subcutaneously 0.3-0.5 cun. Perform moxibustion.

Daoyin (Inducing and Conducting) School Maneuver

Referring to a school of Qigong maneuvers focus on dynamic Qigong. It is featured by closely combining limb movements or self-massage with mindwill and qi.

Daquan (Ex)

An extra point.

Location. At the extreme end of the anterior axillary fold.

Indication. Pain in the shoulder and back, pain in the chest and hypochondrium and measles, etc.

Method. Puncture perpendicularly 0.5-1.0 cun. Obliquely puncture too deep is forbidden.

Dark Complexion

One of ten methods of observation of the patient's complexion. Referring to the dark complexion of the patient, indicating excessive pathogenic factor and stagnation of qi and blood.

Dark Plum

It is the smoked unripe fruit (green plum) of Prunus murne (Sieb.) Sieb. et Zucc. (Rosaceae).

Effect. Astringing the lung and the bowels, increasing body fluid to quench thirst, astringing the lung and relieving cough expelling parasites and arresting bleeding.

Indication. Chronic cough caused by the lung deficiency, chronic diarrhea and dysentery, diabetes caused by heat of deficiency type, abdominal pain and vomiting caused by ascariasis, metrorrhagia and metrostaxis.

Dark Urine

Symptoms. The urine is yellower than usual, even red color.

Pathogenesis. Due to the impairment of yin by interior heat and dampness.

Dark Urine with Difficulty in Micturition

Symptoms. The urine with dark color and difficulty in urination.

Pathogenesis. Due to damp-heat in the urinary bladder, the impairment of the body fluid, the loss of the essence of life and blood, etc.

Dasheen Rhizome

It is the stem tuber of Colocusia esculenta (L.) Schott (Araceae).

Effect. Ceasing scrofula and releasing masses.

Indication. Scrofula, pyogenic infection, hard abdominal masses, neurodermatitis and burns.

Datura Flower   ✿ D-2

It is the flower of Datura metel L. (Solanaceae).

Effect. Relieving cough and asthma, anesthetizing, alleviating pain and relieving convulsion.

Indication. Asthma, chronic bronchitis, cold pain in the chest and abdomen, rheumatic arthralgia, chronic infantile convulsion and epilepsy.

Dayflower Herb

It is the whole plant of Commelina communis L. (Commelinaceae).

Effect. Referring heat, detoxicating and inducing diuresis.

Indication. Common cold of wind-heat type, edema, dysuria, erysipelas, mumps, hematuria, metrorrhagia, swollen and sore throat, boils and pyogenic infections, snake bite, also for common wart, etc.

Daying (S 5)

A meridian point.

Location. In the fovea 1.3 cun anterior to the mandibular angle, where the pulsation of the facial artery is palpable.

Indication. Toothache, facial swelling, mandibular dislocation, scrofula, pain in the neck.

Method. Puncture perpendicularly or obliquely 0.2-0.5 cun. Apply moxibustion 5-10 minutes with warming moxibustion.

Notice. keep away from the blood vessel.

Dazhijiehengwen (Ex-UE)

An extra point.

Location. On the palmar side of each thumb, at the midpoint of the transverse crease of the metacarpophalangeal joint of the thumb.

Indication. Sudden nebula of the eyes.

Method. Moxibustion is applicable.

Dazhijumao (Ex-LE)

An extra point.

Location. On the dorsum of the 1st toe, in the toe hair at the phalangeal joint.

Indication. Apoplexy, headache, vertigo, hernia, testitis, etc.

Method. Puncture perpendicularly 0.1-0.2 cun. Apply moxibustion 3-5 moxa cones or 5-10 minutes with warming moxibustion.

Dazhong (K 4)

A meridian point.

Location. On the medial side of the foot, posterior and inferior to the medial malleolus, in the depression of the medial side and anterior to the attachment of the achilles tendon, 0.5 cun below and slightly posterior to Taixi (k3).

Indication. Coughing up blood, pain in heel, asthmatic breath, idiocy, somnolence, stiffness and pain in the lumbar spine, irregular menstruation.

Method. Puncture perpendicularly 0.3-0.5 cun. Apply moxibustion 3-5 moxa cones or 5-10 minutes with warming moxibustion.

Dazhu (B 11)

A meridian point.

Location. On the back, below the spinous process of the 1st thoracic vertebra, 1.5 cun lateral to the posterior midline.

Indication. Cough, fever, stuffy nose, headache, sore throat, pain in the shoulder and back, stiffness of the neck and nape.

Method. Puncture obliquely 0.5-0.8 cun. Apply moxibustion 3-5 moxa cones or 5-10 minutes with warming moxibustion.

Dazhui (GV 14)

A meridian point.

Location. On the posterior midline, between the spinal process of the 7th cervical vertebra.

Indication. Febrile disease, malaria, cough, dyspnea, stiffness of the nape of the neck and spinal column, pain in the shoulder and back, infantile convulsions, epilepsy, vomiting, jaundice and wind rash.

Method. Puncture obliquely upward 0.5-1.0 cun. Apply moxibustion 3-7 moxa cones or 5-15 minutes with warming moxibustion.

Dead Fetus Delivery

Referring to the death of the fetus in the abdomen at the parturiency.

Pathogenesis. Due to the mother suffering from severe diseases, or taking poisonous medicine, or by the umbilical cord winding itself round the fetal neck.

Therapeutic Principle. Expediting delivery of the dead fetus immediately.

Deadly Tongue

Referring to a black tongue fur, indicating a serious syndrome; black, wet and slippery fur indicating yang deficiency and excessive coldness; black and dry fur indicating excessive fire and exhaustion of the body fluid.

Deaf-mutism

Deafness and mutism are two different symptoms. Mutism resulting from deafness is called deaf-mutism.

Symptoms. Loss of aural ability and failure to speak.

Pathogenesis. Mostly resulting from congenital defect or attacks of warm and heat pathogens, resulting in the deafness of both ears in childhood, inability to learn a language. In addition, some cases are caused by traumatic injury from medicine or vibration resulting from an enormous sound.

Treatment Principle. Removing obstruction in the meridians and opening orifices. Treat deafness before mutism or treating both simultaneously according to general principle.

Deafness

Referring to a disease.

Symptoms. Prolonged subjective sensation of distention and obstruction in the ear, similar to chronic non-suppurative otitis media.

Pathogenesis. Due to retention of pathogenic toxin and stasis of qi and blood.

Therapeutic Principle. Enhancing the flow of qi and blood circulation, clearing the aural passage and orifice, with acupuncture and moxibustion therapy.

Deafness due to Deficiency of Blood

Referring to the deafness.

Symptoms. Deafness, tinnitus, dizziness, lassitude in loin and knees.

Pathogenesis. Owing to deficiency of the liver, kidney, essence and blood.

Therapeutic Principle. Enriching yin and blood.

Deafness due to Kidney Deficiency

Symptoms. Deafness, dizziness, lassitude in loin and legs, feverish sensation in palms and soles, and flushing of zygomatic region, etc.

Pathogenesis. Mainly due to insufficiency of kidney essence, failure of vital essence and energy to moisten ears, and failure in nourishing external acoustic meatus.

Therapeutic Principle. Tonifying the kidney and replenishing essence.

Deafness due to Liver-fire

Symptoms. Tinnitus, deafness, flushed face, bitter taste, hypochondriac pain, etc.

Pathogenesis. Flaming up of the liver-fire leading to the obstruction of the antrum auris.

Therapeutic Principle. Removing heat from the liver.

Deafness due to Qi Deficiency

Symptoms. Deafness which is worsened after restlessness or over-work and lessened after a rest, mental fatigue and sleepiness, asthenia and tastelessness, anorexia, etc.

Pathogenesis. Usually occurs after a severe disease or qi deficiency because aged.

Therapeutic Principle. Invigorating qi, sending up the lucid yang and sending down the turbid qi.

Dearticulation

It refers to slight displacement between both contacted surfaces forming joint resulting from external force.

Symptoms. Pain and dysfunction with inability of self-reposition.

Therapeutic Principle. Manipulations as touching, pressing, holding, lifting, correcting, flexing and extending.

Declination of Five Zang Organs

Referring to declination of the five zang-organs.

1. Swollen hands and feet without lines, indicating declination of the heart; black lips without lines, indicating declination of the lung; darkish complexion with skin and external diseases, indicating declination of the liver; swollen penis and the shrinkage of the scrotum, indicating declination of the kidney; swollen and full umbilical hernia, indicating declination of the spleen.

2. Delirium, indicating declination of the heart; hoarseness and short breath, indicating declination of the lung. Thin and atrophic muscles, indicating declination of the spleen; serious pain in muscle and joint, indicating declination of the liver; continued diarrhea indicating declination of the kidney.

Decocting First

Referring to the method, where some drugs boiled earlier than others. For example, the drugs, such as gypsum, dragon's bone and shell drugs should be boiled first, then 15 minutes, even 30-60 minutes later, the others decocted.

Decocting Later

Referring to a method of some drugs being decocted about 5-10 minutes later than the others. This method is used for light drugs with volatile compositions so as to prevent the volatilization of their volatile active compositions. For example, drugs for treating exterior syndromes and aromatic drugs, such as rhubarb, uncaria stem with hook, should be treated in this way.

Decocting with Wrappings

Referring to a method of some drugs being wrapped with a piece of cloth or gauze for decoction. Some drugs easily form pasty and sticky substances when boiled. Having irritating villus that paste the throat and cause cough and vomiting, such as Asiatic plantain seed, cattail pollen, climbing fern spore, magnolia flower, British inula flower, etc. they should be dealt with this method.

Decoction

Referring to a traditional Chinese medicinal solution obtained by boiling some drugs in water for a certain time, then removing the boiled drugs and taking the solution only. The solution is quick for absorption and effectiveness, also easy to be modified to meet the needs of treatment, and therefore it is most commonly used in the clinical practice.

Decoction-bath

Referring to one of external therapeutic methods.

Method. Soaking or bathing with decoction of medicinal herbs can treat many diseases, hot spring bath for scabies; decoction of camphorwood for rubella.

Decoction Taken Cool

Referring to taking cool decoction. The decoction of prescription cold in nature taken cool is suitable for interior heat syndromes of excess type, enhancing the effect of removing heat; while the decoction of prescription warm in nature taken cool is suitable for the cold syndrome with pseudocold-heat symptoms to prevent the patients from vomiting due to simultaneous occurrence of cold and heat against each other.

Decubitus

Symptoms. Necrotic and ulcerative skin appearing on the pressed body positions caused by lying on the bed for long time.

Therapeutic Principle. Strengthening the body resistance, nourishing qi and blood, clearing away heat and detoxicating. Massage and external treatment is necessary.

Decumbent Bugle Herb

It is the whole plant of Ajuga decumbens Thunb. (Labiatae).

Effect. Clearing away heat and detoxicating, expelling phlegm and arresting cough.

Indication. Swelling and sore throat, carbuncles, sores, cough resulting from the lung-heat, hemoptysis, traumatic injuries, etc.

Deep Complexion

One of ten methods of observation of complexion. Referring to the abnormal complexion of the patient with sunken skin. Mostly seen in the interior syndrome, resulting from stagnation of pathogenic factor in the interior, difficulty of qi and blood in extending in the exterior, deep pathogen and severe disease.

Deep-red Tongue

One of the colors of the tongue. Deep-red tongue refers to invasion of the nutrient system by pathogenic heat of epidemic febrile disease.

Deep-sited Pulse

Referring to pulse felt only on pressing hard to the bone. The pulse status refers to diseases with syncope, severe pains and pathogenic factor in the interior of the body.

Deep-sited Vital Meridian

Name of a meridian, referring to the branch of the Vital Meridian with a deep course through the spinal column of the body. If the disease is at the Deep-sited Vital Meridian, heaviness and pain in the body may result.

Deer Blood

It is the blood of Cervus nippon Temminck or C. elaphus L. (Cervidae).

Effect. Restoring qi and regulating the blood circulation.

Indication. Lumbago, palpitation, insomnia resulting from consumption, hematemesis, metrorrhagia and leukorrhea.

Deer Bone

It is the bone of Cervus nippon Temminck or C. elaphus L. (Cervidae).

Effect. Reinforcing the muscles and tendons.

Indication. Pain of limbs resulting from wind-damp and cold arthralgia of extremities.

Deer Fetus

It is the fetus or placenta of Cervus nippon Temminck or C. elaphus L. (Cervidae).

Effect. Nourishing the kidney and supporting yang, tonifying qi and enhancing vital essence.

Indication. Consumptive disease, tuberculosis, deficiency of vital essence and blood, cold of insufficiency type in women metrorrhagia, metrostaxis and leukorrhea.

Deer Penis and Testes

It is the penis and testicles of Cervus nippon Temminck, or C. elaphus L. (Cervidae).

Effect. Strengthening the kidney, supporting yang and tonifying the vital essence.

Indication. Internal injury resulting from overstrain, lassitude in the waist and knees, deafness, tinnitus, impotence and sterility resulting from uterine coldness.

Deer Tail

It is the tail of Cervus nippon Temminck or C. elaphus L. (Cervidae).

Effect. Warming the waist and knees, restoring vital essence.

Indication. Pain in the loins and back, emission resulting from the kidney deficiency, dizziness and tinnitus.

Defecating before Passing Blood

Symptoms. Hematochezia on the point of defecation with blood following discharging feces.

Pathogenesis. Due to impairment of gastrointestinal function.

Defective Ejaculation

Symptoms. Less amount of ejaculation during sexual intercourse, affecting reproduction.

Pathogenesis. Mainly due to inherent defect, excess of sexual intercourse, or improper diet and overworking.

Deficiency

Generally referring to hypofunction of the body resulting from defect of qi, blood, body fluid and vital substance. It is mainly caused by congenital deficiency, poor nourishment after birth and overwork.

Deficiency and Excess

It refers to the diseases of children appearing as excess syndrome resulting from excessive pathogens, or deficiency syndrome resulting from the insufficient primordial qi, and also, the two syndromes sometimes appear simultaneously.

Deficiency and Failure of Kidney-yang

It is a worse manifestation of deficiency of the kidney-yang, which may affect the function of other organs. For example, it may lead to deficiency of the kidney-yang in the heart or in the spleen. Clinical symptoms include chills, cold limbs and watery diarrhea with undigested food in the stool, impotence, sterility, or edema, etc.

Deficiency Edema

Referring to the edema of deficiency type. **Symptoms.** Slow progress of edema, swelling first on the skin and then distending inward, dark and pale complexion, loose and thin stool, etc. Deficiency edema including: deficiency edema of the spleen and kidney, deficiency edema of the liver and kidney, and edema of lung-deficiency.

Pathogenesis. Due to overwork, overdrinking and excessive sexual intercourse, leading to qi deficiency of the lung and spleen or yang-deficiency of the spleen. **Therapeutic Principle.** Nourishing qi, warming yang and enhancing diuresis.

Deficiency Evil and Harmful Wind

Referring to abnormal weather condition and exterior morbigenous factors harmful to the body exteriorly.

Deficiency-fire Cough

Symptoms. Cough with clear and thin phlegm, flushed face, dyspnea, dryness throat, excessive thirst, etc. **Pathogenesis.** Due to deficiency of primordial qi with the flaming-up of the three-energizer fire, and the lung burned by pathogenic fire. **Therapeutic Principle.** Tonifying yin and the lung.

Deficiency-fire Dizziness

Symptoms. Dizziness, blurred vision, dysphoria with smothery sensation, flushed face with feverish sensation, hectic fever, night sweat, etc. **Pathogenesis.** Due to yin deficiency of the liver and spleen, attacking up of fire of deficiency type. **Therapeutic Principle.** Nourishing the liver, kidney, and yin to cease pathogenic fire.

Deficiency in Both Exterior and Interior

It is one syndrome of diseases involving both interior and exterior. **Symptoms.** Sweating, short breath, dizziness, palpitation, lassitude limbs, poor appetite, loose stools, etc. **Pathogenesis.** Deficiency of both qi and blood after serious disease or constant poor health. **Therapeutic Principle.** Tonifying both qi and blood.

Deficiency in Reality with Pseudo-excess Symptoms

It refers to the diseases caused by deficiency of original energy but exhibits some apparently excess syndrome and signs. Such as patient suffered from abdominal pain, distention, constipation, aversion to cold relieved by pressing, absence of thirst, no desire for hot water. **Therapeutic Principle.** Invigorating qi and enriching blood.

Deficiency Jaundice

Symptoms. Sallow and withered skin, listlessness, palpitation, tinnitus, loose stool, turbid urine, etc. **Pathogenesis.** Mostly caused by the hypofunction of the spleen with the deficiency of blood, or prolonged jaundice and the deficiency of the vital qi. **Therapeutic Principle.** Nourishing qi and blood, reinforcing the spleen.

Deficiency of Blood

Symptoms. Pale complexion, pale lips, tongue and finger nails, dizziness, tinnitus, etc.

Pathogenesis. Due to malnutrition, massive bleeding, hypofunction of the spleen and stomach, dysfunction of hematogenic organ, and impairment of prolonged illness.

Therapeutic Principle. Nourishing blood or qi and blood.

Deficiency of Gallbladder-qi

Symptoms. Fright, anxiety, palpitation, suspicions, insomnia and sighing, etc.

Pathogenesis. Due to qi deficiency during convalescence or hypofunction of biliary qi.

Therapeutic Principle. Warming gallbladder for tranquilization and invigorating qi for those with qi deficiency.

Deficiency of Heart-qi

It refers to a morbid condition due to deficiency of yang-qi of the heart.

Symptoms. Palpitation and shortness of breath, especially more serious after physical activities accompanied with pale face, spontaneous perspiration, fatigue, pale tongue with white coating, and weak pulse.

Pathogenesis. Mostly due to external attack of wind-damp pathogen on the blood to impair yang-qi in the heart.

Therapeutic Principle. Warming yang and tonifying qi.

Deficiency of Kidney-yang

Symptoms. Aversion to cold and cold limbs, listlessness, lumbago, spermatorrhea and premature ejaculation, impotence in man and frequency of nocturia, frigidity or infertility in women, pale tongue, etc.

Pathogenesis. Dysfunction of the kidney.

Deficiency of Kidney-yin

Symptoms. Tidal fever, spontaneous sweating, dizziness and tinnitus, spermatorrhea in man and sexual intercourse when dreaming of women, dry mouth and sore throat, hot palms and soles, etc.

Pathogenesis. Consumption of fluid and essence of the kidney in chronic diseases or due to intemperance in sexual life.

Deficiency of Liver-blood

Referring to a morbid status of shortage of blood in the liver.

Symptoms. Dizziness, tinnitus, pale complexion, impaired vision or night blindness, numb limbs, pale scanty menstruation and even amenorrhea, etc.

Pathogenesis. Resulting from general deficiency, insufficiency of nutrient system blood in the liver, or exhaustion of blood, and too much bleeding.

Therapeutic Principle. Nourishing blood and reinforcing the liver.

Deficiency of Liver-qi

Referring to deficiency of the liver essence and insufficient liver blood.

Symptoms. Pale complexion and lips, blurred vision, contracture in hypochondrium with pain, tinnitus, deafness, etc.

Therapeutic Principle. Reinforcing the liver and the kidney.

Deficiency of Liver-yin

Referring to a morbid status of insufficient essence and fluid of the liver.

Symptoms. Dizziness, tinnitus, dryness of the eyes, trembling of hands and feet, hectic fever and night sweat, dry mouth and throat, dysphoria with feverish sensation in the chest.

Pathogenesis. Because of the deficiency of the liver and the kidney resulting from deficiency of the liver-blood or the kidney essence.

Therapeutic Principle. Nourishing the liver-yin or reinforcing the liver and the kidney.

Deficiency of both Liver-yin and Kidney-yin

Referring to a syndrome due to deficiency of yin essence of the liver and kidney and due to mutual affection.

Symptoms. Dizziness, tinnitus, amnesia, lassitude in the loins and legs, night sweat, pain in hypochondriac region, insomnia, emission and scanty menstruation.

Pathogenesis. Deficiency of the kidney essence often resulting in deficiency of the liver-blood or vice versa.

Therapeutic Principle. Reinforcing the liver and the kidney.

Deficiency of Marrow Reservoir

Referring to a morbid change due to deficiency of the kidney essence and short of nourishment of the marrow reservoir.

Symptoms. Dizziness, tinnitus, limb aching, weakness, blindness and easy to be tired.

Deficiency of Qi and Blood in Vital and Front Middle Meridians

Referring to deficiency of qi and blood due to damage of Vital and Front Middle Meridians resulting from some factors.

Symptoms. Abnormal menstruation, pain of the hypogastrium, uterine bleeding, abortion and infertility.

Deficiency of Spleen with Cold Syndrome

Symptoms. Cold body and limbs, cold and pain in the abdomen with preference for warmth and pressing, chronic diarrhea, dropsy, or dilute leukorrhea.

Pathogenesis. Mostly due to the spleen deficiency and cold or irregular diet, overstrain and over-thinking.

Therapeutic Principle. Warming the middle-energizer and invigorating the spleen.

Deficiency of Stomach-yin

Symptoms. Dryness in the mouth, thirst, preference for cold drinks, fullness and discomfort in gastric cavity, anorexia or ravenous appetite, constipation, etc.

Pathogenesis. Usually due to chronic gastritis or impairment of stomach-yin in the late stage of epidemic febrile disease.

Therapeutic Principle. Nourishing the stomach-yin.

Deficiency Syndrome

Referring to the syndrome due to insufficiency of healthy energy in the body. Including yang, yin, qi, and blood deficiency.

Deficiency Syndrome of Dizziness

Symptoms. Dizziness and blurring of vision, without the feeling of revolving and overturning, lassitude, palpitation, insomnia, liability to a relapse or a serious case induced due to overworking.

Pathogenesis. Usually due to deficiency of both the heart and spleen, insufficiency of both qi and blood, leading to failure to nourish the head and eye; or by deficiency of kidney-yin.

Therapeutic Principle. Invigorating qi and nourishing blood.

Deficiency Syndrome of Impotence

Symptoms. Difficulty or failure of the penis to erect, frequent spermatorrhea, thin and cold sperm, dizziness, tinnitus, palpitation, short breath, pale complexion, lassitude in the loin and knees, chilliness, cold limbs, etc.

Pathogenesis. Mostly caused by excessive sexual intercourse and insufficiency of kidney-yang.

Therapeutic Principle. Warming and supplementing the kidney-yang.

Deficiency Syndrome of Suppurative Otitis Media

Symptoms. Persistent discharge of watery, sticky and thread-like pus, dizziness, lassitude of limbs, poor appetite, shallow complexion, etc.

Pathogenesis. Mostly caused by the accumulation of dampness in the ear resulting from deficiency of the spleen.

Therapeutic Principle. Strengthening the spleen and eliminating dampness.

Deficiency Syndrome of Uroschesis

Symptoms. Difficulty of urination, dribbling urination accompanied with fullness and bulge of the lower abdomen, pale complexion, soreness of the waist and lassitude of the knee joint, loose stools.

Pathogenesis. Mostly due to deficiency of the kidney among aged people, deficiency of qi in the middle-energizer, leading to disturbance in qi transformation of the urinary bladder.

Therapeutic Principle. Warming and invigorating the spleen and kidney.

Deficiency Type of Epilepsy

Symptoms. It appears in the later period of epilepsy: frequent relapses, mild convulsion of the limbs, accompanied with sweating on the forehead, dyspneic respiration with snore, etc.

Pathogenesis. Mostly caused by frequent relapses of epilepsy which lead to deficiency of the heart-blood and kidney-qi, and the imbalance of zang-fu organs and pathogenic changes of qi.

Therapeutic Principle. Nourishing the heart and spleen, reducing phlegm and relieving spasm.

Deficiency Type of Inward Penetration of Pyogenic Agent

Referring to a syndrome of the invasion in the interior by pyogenic agent, during the astringency of carbuncle.

Symptoms. No growth of new flesh on the sore after the end of ulcer, fail to heal with tiredness and anorexia, fever, abdominal pain and diarrhea, etc.

Pathogenesis. Weakness of the spleen and the stomach, and deficiency of both qi and blood.

Therapeutic Principle. Reinforcing the spleen and stomach, nourishing the qi and blood, or recuperating depleted yang.

Deficiency-type Tinnitus and Deafness

Symptoms. Protracted deafness, or discontinuous tinnitus with a low sound and aggravated by overwork. Often accompanied by dizziness, soreness of the lower back, seminal emission, and morbid leukorrhea.

Pathogenesis. Deficiency of kidney essence, causing a failure of the vital essence and energy to reach the ears for nourishment.

Therapeutic Principle. Tonifying the kidney essence.

Deficient Breath

Symptoms. Weak and short rapid breath, lack of strength in speaking.

Pathogenesis. Mostly due to insufficient qi of the spleen, lung and kidney, or turbid phlegm, diet and fluid retention.

Delavay Clovershrub Root

It is the root of Campylotropis delavayi (Franch.) Sehindle (Leguminosae).

Effect. Removing fever.

Indication. Fever caused by common cold.

Delayed Dentition

Symptoms. Delayed dentition in developing.

Pathogenesis. Usually due to deficiency of kidney-qi.

Therapeutic Principle. Tonifying kidney.

Delayed Menstruation due to Blood-Cold

Symptoms. Delayed menstrual period, with scanty discharge of dark and blood clots, colicky pain in the lower abdomen which can be relieved by hot compress, and aversion to cold.

Pathogenesis. Mostly due to the attack of cold during delivery, and the invasion of cold upon the uterus leading to the stagnation of blood and disorder of the blood circulation.

Therapeutic Principle. Warming the meridians to relieve stagnation.

Delayed Menstruation due to Blood Stasis

Symptoms. Menstruation coming after due time with scanty discharge of dark colored blood, accompanied by cold pain in the lower abdomen and tenderness, which is relieved by warmth.

Pathogenesis. Mostly caused by stagnation of qi and accumulation of cold evil.

Therapeutic Principle. Warming the meridians and promoting blood circulation to remove blood stasis.

Delayed Menstruation due to Deficiency of Blood

Symptoms. Occurrence of menstruation over a week later than usual, light flow in pink color, thin menstrual blood, sallow complexion, dizziness and blurring of vision, palpitation and insomnia, pale tongue with thin coating, etc.

Pathogenesis. Mostly due to severe disease or chronic illness, or multiparity, the comsumption and damage of yin-blood.

Therapeutic Principle. Enrich the blood and replenish qi.

Delayed Menstruation due to Emaciation

Symptoms. Delayed menstruation with scanty pale menses, poor appetite and weariness.

Pathogenesis. Owing to the excessive emaciation, qi deficiency and blood insufficiency.

Therapeutic Principle. Supplementing qi and blood.

Delayed Menstruation due to Kidney Deficiency

Symptoms. Delayed menstrual period with scanty menses, dizziness, tinnitus, soreness and weakness of the waist and knees, etc.

Pathogenesis. Commonly caused by congenital deficiency, premature marriage and excessive childbirth, or intemperance in sexual life leading to impairment of the kidney-qi and insufficiency of the essence and blood.

Therapeutic Principle. Tonifying the kidney and nourishing yin.

Delayed Menstruation due to Obesity

Symptoms. Retarded menstruation with scanty pale menses, tiredness and edema.

Pathogenesis. Owing to the obese figure, the spleen deficiency, the small amount of blood, and the phlegm-dampness stagnation.

Therapeutic Principle. Reinforcing the spleen, removing dampness, removing phlegm and dispelling stagnation.

Delayed Menstruation due to Qi Stagnation

Symptoms. Delayed menstrual period, light flow and dark red menstruation with blood clots, distending pain in the lower abdomen, discomfort in the chest, hypochondrium, thin and whitish tongue coating, etc.

Pathogenesis. Mostly due to impairment of the liver by stagnated anger, impeded circulation of qi.

Therapeutic Principle. Relieving the depressed liver, regulating the flow of qi and promoting blood circulation.

Delirium

It refers to the confusing talks and polylogia with absurd information. It is mostly caused by excess of yang-heat, deficiency of qi and blood.

Symptoms. 1. In the case of excess heat, distention in the heart and abdomen, confusion in speaking, fever, constipation, etc. 2. In the case of deficiency of qi, restless sleep, palpitation, confused talks, etc.

Therapeutic Principle. 1. In the case of excess heat, clearing away heat and purging fire. 2. In the case of deficiency of qi, calming the mind by nourishing the heart.

Delirium during Menstruation

Symptoms. Mental disorder, delirium, even unconsciousness.

Pathogenesis. Mostly due to dysphoria and irritation during menstruation and reversed flow of blood with disorder and upward invasion of the hyperactive liver-qi to attack the heart.

Therapeutic Principle. Soothing the liver and relieving mental stress.

Delivery in Hot Weather

Symptoms. Headache, fever, dizziness, even unconsciousness.

Pathogenesis. Puerperal blood heat in damp midsummer.

Therapeutic Principle. Removing heat from blood.

Delusive Speech

Referring to deranged talk.

Pathogenesis. Resulting from excessive yang, the abnormal rising of qi and blood, phlegm-fire going up.

Dementia

Referring to the mental disease.

Symptoms. Strong constitution with a good appetite as before, but slow in movement and confused in speech, etc.

Pathogenesis. Due to excessive mental upset, depression, great surprise and sudden fear, or inherent defect.

Therapeutic Principle. Smoothing liver and dispersing the depressed qi, calming the mind by nourishing the heart or invigorating the inherent defect.

Dendrobium Stem

It is fresh or dried stem of Dendrobium nobile Lindl. (Orchidaceae), and the stem of many other species of the same genus.

Effect. Nourishing the stomach to promote the production of body fluid, nourishing yin to remove heat.

Indication. Chronic febrile diseases with dry mouth, thirst, diminution of vision, debility of the loins and knees, etc.

Densefruit Dittany Root-bark

It is the root of Dictamnus dasycarpus Turcz. (Rutaceae).

Effect. Detoxicating, removing heat and dampness and itching.

Indication. Dermatitis of damp-heat type, scabies and tinea resulting from damp-heat, jaundice, damp-heat, arthralgia, etc.

Dental Caries

Symptoms. The tooth with an interior cavity, that is decayed and painful, aggravation after exposure to cold, rancidity, gum-erosion or purulence.

Pathogenesis. Mostly due to oral dirt, or wind-phlegm and damp-heat that steam and fumigate the Large Intestine Meridian and the Stomach Meridian.

Therapeutic Principle. Clearing away heat to relieve pain.

Dental Retardation

Symptoms. The infant teeth don't grow until after 10 months of age, or milk teeth don't fall off at six or seven years old, and the permanent teeth don't grow after stalling for a long time.

Pathogenesis. Caused by the insufficiency of the kidney-qi of the infant, and failure to nourish bone for eruption of teeth due to deficiency of marrow.

Therapeutic Principle. Tonifying the kidney and nourishing marrow.

Dependence of Yang on Yin

Based on the theory of the interdependence of yin and yang, yang exists depending upon yin. Yin being a prerequisite for the existence of yang. Yang would not be produced without yin. For the human body, there is an interdependent and coordinate relation between the function belonging to yang and the substance belonging to yin. The production of the functions of the body depends on the substances.

Dependence of Yin on Yang

Based on the theory of interdependence of yin and yang, there would be no yin without yang. For human body, yin is considered as of the substances of essence, blood, and body fluid. The transformation of all these substance depends on yang referring to functional activities, i.e. yin essence depends upon the yang functional activities.

Depression of Liver Causing Heat Syndrome

Symptoms. Vertigo, tinnitus, congested and painful eyes, flushed face, or vomiting, hemoptysis, even amentia if severe.

Pathogenesis. Due to the depression of liver qi causing the heat syndrome.

Depressive Psychosis

Symptoms. Emotional depression, silence, dementia, fantasy paraphasia, poor appetite, dim complexion, etc.

Pathogenesis. Mostly caused by the stagnation of phlegm and qi.

Therapeutic Principle. Resolving phlegm by regulating the flow of qi and tranquilizing by clearing away heart-fire.

Derangement of Qi and Blood

It refers to that the coordinative relationship between qi and blood is in disorder. It usually brings on prolonged pain, cold limbs, irregular menstruation and chronic hemorrhage.

Dermal Needle

Specially made needles, including plum-blossom needle (5 needles), seven-star needle (7 needles), temple-guard needle (18 needles) and clustered needle (unlimited needles), used for tapping and pricking certain areas of the body to treat a wide variety of diseases. These needles have the advantage of a broad stimulation area and even stimulation. They are suitable for children for mild stimulation, and therefore is also called infantile needles.

Dermatitis Herpetiformis

Symptoms. At the beginning it has scalding blisters. After breaking yellowish water infuses, even spreading all over the body.

Pathogenesis. Rash action of heart-fire of the affection of the intense pathogenic heat of summer or the damp-heat.

Therapeutic Principle. Removing heat and toxic material, and eliminating dampness.

Dermatitis Rhus

Symptoms. The contact skin suddenly red, swelling, burning hot, itching, small papule and blisters, scratched out, they will ulcerate and flow with water, spreading all over the body with cold physique, fever, headache, etc., in the severe case.

Pathogenesis. Congenital fearing of paint and affection by paint air, occurring on the exposed positions.

Therapeutic Principle. Clearing away heat and toxic material.

Dermatrophia

Symptoms. Withered skin and hairs, flaccidity, cough with choking, rapid breathing.

Pathogenesis. Due to the scorched lung leading to the impairment of the skin and hair.

Therapeutic Principle. Removing the heat, enhancing the production of fluid, nourishing yin to moisten the lung.

Desert-living Cistanche

It is the fleshy stem of Cistanche deserticola C. Ma (Orobanchaceae) with scales.

Effect. Nourishing the kidney, strengthening yang, moistening the bowels to remove constipation.

Indication. Impotence, sterility, cold pain in the loins and knees, lassitude of the muscles, constipation resulting from dryness of the bowel and fluid deficiency, etc.

Deterioration due to Fire

Moxibustion term, referring to the varied symptom-complex caused by misuse of moxibustion.

Deterioration of a Case

It refers to changes in syndromes from a simple to a complicated one and from a mild to a severe one due to severe affection by pathogenic factor, or delay of therapeusis or misdiagnosis and mistreatment.

Determination of Heat Sensitivity

A method of determining the degree of heat sensation of the Jing (Well) points of the Twelve Meridians and the Back-Shu points and comparing the different numerical values of the left and right sides to analyse the deficiency-excess or imbalance of each meridian. Usually it is carried on with an incense burning or a heat sensitivity determination instrument.

Deviation in Qigong Practice

A term in Qigong. In Qigong exercises due to incorrect selection of maneuver or by failure to follow correct directions, occurring serious unusual reactions such as keeping on moving, wrong flowing of qi sensation, flowing of qi sensation up to the head, etc.

Devil-pepper Root

It is the root of Rouwolfia verticillata (Lour.) Baill. (Apocynaceae).

Effect. Relieving the wind-heat and the liver-fire and subduing swelling and detoxicating.

Indication. Common cold, fever, swollen-sore throat, headache and dizziness resulting from hypertension, abdominal pain, vomiting and diarrhea etc.

Dewberryleaf Cinquefoil Herb

It is the whole herb of Potentilla fragarioides L. (Rosaceae).

Effect. Supplementing qi of middle-energizer and yin deficiency.

Indication. Hernia, emaciation caused by blood disorders, etc.

Diabetes

Symptoms. Polydipsia, polyphagia, polyuria and emaciation.

Pathogenesis. Mainly due to overtaking fat and sugar, improper diet, emotional stress and irritability, overwork leading to dryness-heat in zang-fu organs and hyperactivity of fire caused by deficiency of yin.

Therapeutic Principle. Nourishing yin, moisturizing dryness and lowering fire.

Diabetes Involving Lower-energizer

Symptoms. Polydipsia, frequent urination in heavy quantity and turbid quality, dry mouth and tongue, dizziness, blurred vision, easy hunger but no appetite, soreness and weakness of the lumbar back and knees, impotence in men, amenorrhea in women, pale tongue with white coating, etc.

Pathogenesis. Mostly caused by deficiency and consumption of kidney-yin leading to disturbance in qi transformation.

Treatment Principle. Nourishing the kidney to replenish yin.

Diabetes Involving Middle-energizer

Symptoms. Heat in the stomach, excessive eating but enhancement of hunger, lassitude, constipation, urine like rice-water, etc.

Pathogenesis. Phlegm retention, and excessiveness of the stomach-heat.

Therapeutic Principle. Clearing away the stomach-heat, moistening dryness, removing the phlegm and fluid retention.

Diabetes Involving Upper-energizer

Symptoms. Polydipsia and dry mouth and tongue are the main symptoms, accompanied by polyuria, polyphagia, redness of the tip of tongue, thin and yellowish tongue coating, etc.

Pathogenesis. Excessive fire of the heart and lung and dry heat of the upper-energizer.

Treatment Principle. Clear lung-heat, promote the production of body fluid to quench thirst.

Diabetes with Spleen Involved

Symptoms. Urine action immediately after food and drink enter the stomach, eating too much but hungering quickly, emaciation, dry mouth and tongue, praecox ejaculation, emission, etc.

Pathogenesis. Stomach-heat excessiveness, yin deficiency of the spleen and kidney.

Therapeutic Principle. Removing stomach-heat, nourishing the kidney and yin, and promoting the production of body fluid.

Diagnosis by Examining Meridians and Points

A method of diagnosis through examining, detecting and palpating the meridians and acupoints, including superficial palpation on body surface, electric examination of skin, and examination of heat sensibility on the skin of which the former is the main method.

Diagnosis by Palpation

It refers to touching, pressing, or molding method, by which abnormal changes can be found on the acupoints, so as to help make a diagnosis.

Dialectical Point Selection

One of the point selections. According to the principle of syndrome difference, the relevant points are selected by analysing the relationship between the diseases (and syndrome) and the viscera and meridians.

Diaphoresis

Referring to a method for inducing sweating and/or releasing exterior syndrome.

Indication. Exopathy with exterior syndromes, carbuncle, measles and edema severe in the upper body.

Diaphoretics Pungent in Flavour and Cool in Property

Referring to the drugs, diaphoretics pungent in flavour and cool in property, used for dispelling pathogentic wind-heat.

Indication. Affection by exopathogenic wind-heat, such as: fever with slight aversion to cold, dry throat and thirst, yellow thin coating on the tongue, floating and rapid pulse, and eye disease, sore throat, inadequate eruption of measles, cough.

Diaphoretics Pungent in Flavour and Warm in Property

Referring to the drugs, used for dispersing wind-cold.

Effect. Removing pathogenic factors from the exterior of the body by diaphoresis, asthma, pathogenic wind and dampness inducing diuresis.

Indication. Exterior syndrome of excess type owing to exopathogenic wind-cold, such as: fever, headache, pantalgia, anhidrosis, thin and white coating on the tongue, floating and tense pulse; and dyspnea, edema, sore, ulcers and arthralgia owing to wind-dampness with exterior syndromes.

Diaphragm-phlegm Syndrome

Symptoms. Vomiting after eating, constipation.

Pathogenesis. Owing to emotional depression, the retention of phlegm and fluid blocking the diaphragm.
Therapeutic Principle. Removing the dryness with drugs of pungent flavour, dispelling phlegm, and descending qi.

Diaphragm Qi

It is a syndrome.
Symptoms. Difficulty in swallowing, vomiting, fullness in stomach.
Pathogenesis. Depressed feeling, irregular cold and heat harmful diet, imbalance of yin and yang leading to mass formation in the stomach.
Therapeutic Principle. Enhancing flow of qi, releasing obstruction, nourishing yin and blood.

Diarrhea

It is clinically divided into two types: 1. Slow diarrhea marked by loose stool with less urgency. 2. Urgent diarrhea marked by watery stool with greater urgency.
Pathogenesis. Affection by six pathogens, impairment caused by improper diet, over-fatigue, emotional stress, weakness of the spleen and the stomach, and deficiency of the kidney-yang and spleen-yang, etc.

Diarrhea due to Acute Alcoholism

Symptoms. In the damp-heat case, diarrhea; the patient will feel oppressed hot if without diarrhea. In the cold-damp case, gradual reduction of food and emaciation of the body, sleepiness, diarrhea for many days or diarrhea before dawn, or more severe diarrhea during autumn and winter.
Pathogenesis. Owing to the injury of the spleen and the stomach resulting from excessive alcohol-drinking.
Therapeutic Principle. In the damp-heat case, removing heat and dampness. In the cold-damp case, reinforcing and invigorating the spleen and the kidney, and removing cold and dampness.

Diarrhea due to Cold

Symptoms. Cold under the novel, distention and fullness of the abdomen, either yellowish and whitish or clear and black stool, sometimes with indigested cereals, etc.
Therapeutic Principle. Warming the middle-energizer, expelling cold and ceasing diarrhea.

Diarrhea due to Damp-heat

Symptoms. Diarrhea and abdominal pain, burning sensation of the anus, scanty deep-colored urine, yellowish greasy tongue coating.
Pathogenesis. Mostly resulting from accumulation of pathogenic damp-heat or summer-heat in the intestines and stomach, leading to irregular transportation of the large intestine.
Therapeutic Principle. Eliminating dampness and heat, promoting the production of the body fluid and facilitating qi.

Diarrhea due to Deficiency of the Spleen

Symptoms. Intermittent watery stool discharge after taking a little greasy food, loss of appetite, distention, fullness and discomfort in the epigastrium and abdomen, yellow complexion, listlessness of the limbs, pale tongue with whitish coating, thready and weak pulse.
Pathogenesis. Deficiency of the spleen and stomach, dysfunction of the spleen in transportation and production, confusion of nutrition and turbidity.
Treatment Principle. Strengthening the spleen and replenishing qi, elevating the spleen to arrest diarrhea.

Diarrhea due to Fright

Symptoms. Abdominal pain, greenish and sticky stool, annoyance and loss of appetite.
Pathogenesis. Due to the sudden fright, invasion of the hyperactive liver-qi, inability for the functional activities of qi

to go up, and pathogenic dampness to go down.

Therapeutic Principle. Warming liver and expelling dampness.

Diarrhea due to Heat

Symptoms. Borborygmus, paroxysmal diarrhea with abdominal pain, stinking, yellow or watery stool, or with undigested food, burning pain in the anus, thirst with preference for cold drink, dark urine with difficulty, etc.

Pathogenesis. Invasion of the intestine and stomach by heat.

Therapeutic Principle. Removing heat and purging fire; in addition, supplementing qi for those with deficiency of qi with heat, nourishing yin for those with hyperactivity of fire caused by yin deficiency.

Diarrhea due to Impairment of Intestine and Stomach

Symptoms. Diarrhea with pus and blood, difficulty in defecation, tenesmus and pain in the lower abdomen, etc.

Pathogenesis. The impairment of the intestine and stomach due to the stagnation of damp-heat.

Therapeutic Principle. Enhancing diuresis, adjusting qi and removing heat, dampness and stagnation.

Diarrhea due to Improper Diet

Symptoms. abdominal pain and borborygmus, diarrhea with fetid feces, pain abated after diarrhea, sour and rotten eructation, anorexia, etc.

Pathogenesis. Improper diet and food retention blocking the stomach and intestines leading to abnormal transportation.

Therapeutic Principle. Removing food retention, promoting digestion and regulating the function of the spleen and stomach.

Diarrhea due to Kidney Deficiency

A type of chronic diarrhea, also named diarrhea before dawn.

Symptoms. Pain of the abdomen and around the umbilicus at dawn, loose bowels or borborygmus, which is relieved after diarrhea, aversion to cold and cold limbs, soreness and weakness of the lumbus and knees, pale tongue with white coating.

Pathogenesis. Deficiency of kidney-yang resulting in failure to warm the spleen leading to dysfunction of the spleen in transportation.

Therapeutic Principle. Warming the kindey to invigorate yang, strengthening the spleen, controlling discharge of feces to arrest diarrhea.

Diarrhea due to Oxyuriasis

Symptoms. Extreme pruritus and more serious at night, abdominal pain, diarrhea, anorexia, and emaciation, etc.

Pathogenesis. Owing to oxyuriasis living in intestinal tract.

Therapeutic Principle. Killing and expelling intestinal worms.

Diarrhea due to Phlegm Stagnation

Referring to a type of diarrhea.

Symptoms. Occasional diarrhea with white gluey things like albumen, dizziness and nausea, poor appetite, fullness in the chest and abdomen, etc.

Pathogenesis. Due to phlegm stagnation in the lungs and disturbance in the large intestine.

Therapeutic Principle. Dispelling phlegm, strengthening the spleen, clearing away the stagnation, supplementing the intestine and stopping diarrhea.

Diarrhea due to Qi Collapse

Symptoms. Diarrhea with indigested food soon after eating, emaciation, short breath, spontaneous sweating, sleepiness and pale complexion.

Pathogenesis. Qi deficiency of spleen and kidney, the sinking of middle-energizer qi resulting in the failure of the middle-energizer.

Therapeutic Principle. Strengthening the spleen and replenishing qi.

Diarrhea due to Stagnation of Liver-qi

Symptoms. Fullness sensation in the chest and hypochondrium borborygmus, and abdominal pain which is relieved with defecation, attacks again soon afterwards and is aggravated when the patient becomes emotional upset.

Pathogenesis. Emotional upset with improper diet resulting in invasion of the spleen by the adverse flow of the liver-qi

Therapeutic Principle. Promoting the flow of qi, normalizing the function of the stomach and regulating the function of the liver and spleen.

Diarrhea during Menstruation

Symptoms. Regular and frequent diarrhea, during, before or after menstruation.

Pathogenesis. Mostly due to deficiency and consumption of the spleen and kidney.

Therapeutic Principle. Invigorating the spleen for eliminating dampness, or warming the kidney and spleen to reinforce the intestines.

Diarrhea in Children due to Pathogenic Heat

Symptoms. Infantile diarrhea, abdominal pain, borborygmus, restlessness and crying, scanty dark urine.

Pathogenesis. Invasion of the large intestine by summer-heat

Therapeutic Principle. Expelling pathogenic heat and stopping diarrhea.

Diarrhea in Children due to Phlegm

Symptoms. Diarrhea with sticky and thick stool and without definite time, and lassitude.

Pathogenesis. Mostly caused by deficiency and dysfunction of the spleen in transportation and transformation.

Therapeutic Principle. Invigorating the spleen to resolving phlegm.

Diarrhea of Large Intestine

Symptoms. Distress right after eating, whitish stools, borborygmus with pain, etc.

Pathogenesis. Mostly owing to deficiency of the spleen-yang.

Therapeutic Principle. Warming the middle-energizer, removing cold.

Diarrhea with Interior Cold and Exterior Heat

Symptoms. Abdominalgia, borborygmus, watery diarrhea with urgency of defecation, etc.

Pathogenesis. Owing to attack of gastrointestinal tract by heat.

Therapeutic Principle. Removing heat and enhancing diuresis.

Diarrhea with Sticky Discharge

Symptoms. The diarrhea with sticky bloody and purulent stools similar to dysentery resulting from deteriorated cases.

Pathogenesis. Deficiency of both zang and fu organs, the failure of the spleen-qi resulting in the prolapse of the intestine and the stomach.

Notice. It cannot be treated as dysentery.

Dicang (S 4)

A meridian acupuncture point on the Stomach Meridian of Foot-Yangming.

Location. On the face, directly below Juliao (S 3), 0.4 cun lateral to the beside the mouth angle.

Indication. Tremor of eyelids, deviated mouth, toothache, swelling in the cheek, salivation.

Method. Puncture perpendicularly 0.2 cun, or puncture obliquely or horizontally 0.5-1.0 cun, with the tip of the needle directed towards Jiache (S 6). Apply moxibustion 5-10 minutes with warming moxibustion.

Dietetic Restraint

According to patient's condition and therapeutic principle, some sorts of food are prohibited, such as patients with diabetes are prohibited to take sugar, those with edema are prohibited to take salt, those who take traditional Chinese drugs are prohibited to take raw, cold, slimy and greasy food.

Dietetic Therapy

It refers to the cure method of using the different nature and nutrients of the food to regulate qi, blood, yin and yang of zang-fu organs.

Differentiating Meridians and Collateral of Sore

It refers to the diagnostic methods of sores. It can infer which meridian and collateral the sore belongs to, according to the affected position and the circulation, and the distribution of meridians and collaterals. It is based on this method to judge the slight or severe sores, the favourable or unfavourable cases of sores, to choose which drugs for which sores, to guide the drugs to the affected position so that the treatment will be more efficient.

Differentiation of Diseases according to Pathological Changes of Zang and Fu and Their Interrelations

It is one of the basic methods of differentiation of disease.

Differentiating the changes of yin and yang, qi and blood, deficiency and excess, cold and heat in five zang organs and six fu organs, on the basis of the physiological functions and pathological manifestations. It provides the basis for therapy.

Differentiation of Six Meridians

Six meridians mean Taiyang, Yangming, Shaoyang, Taiyin, Shaoyin and Jueyin. They refer to the six different principles applied to the diagnosis of acute febrile diseases at six different stages, but also useful for the syndrome differentiation of other diseases.

Differentiation of Syndromes According to State of Qi and Blood

It refers to a diagnostic method to differentiate syndromes by analysing the pathological changes of qi and blood.

Differentiation of Symptoms and Signs to Identify Etiology

It is a special method to diagnose a disease in TCM, referring analysis, and differentiation of pathological conditions attributable to different kinds of etiological factors for making diagnosis and the principle to use drugs.

Difficulty and Pain in Urination

One of the hernias.

Symptoms. Pain in the lower abdomen dragging the testes and resulting in dysuria.

Pathogenesis. Due to invasion of pathogenic cold into the liver and disturbance of qi transformation of the urinary bladder.

Therapeutic Principle. Dispelling cold, resolving qi and enhancing diuresis.

Difficulty in Sucking

It is a disease.

Symptoms. The newborn infant cannot suck the milk 24 hours after the birth.

Pathogenesis. Due to deficiency of the primordial qi of the infant, deficiency-cold of the spleen and stomach, accumulation of pathogenic heat.

Therapeutic Principle. Reinforcing the primordial energy, the kidney-qi, warming middle-energizer, expelling cold and removing heat.

Diffuse Fluid-retention and Lingering Diarrhea

It is a disease.

Symptoms. Thirst and over-drinking of water. After drinking, diarrhea and more thirst.

Pathogenesis. Due to retention of water in intestine, resulting in diarrhea.

Therapeutic Principle. Invigorating the spleen, warming yang and inducing diuresis.

Digit-pressing Manipulation

A massage method. It refers to pressing the point.

Method. Tap a point on the patient body with the tip of the operator's middle finger while the thumb and index finger are held close to it with force.

Function. Removing cold and dispelling wind, and dredging the meridians and collaterals.

Indication. Contractive pain in epigastrium and aching pain of the waist and leg.

Digua Fig Stem and Leaf

It is the stem leaf of Ficus tikoua Bur. (Moraceae).

Effect. Removing heat, promoting diuresis, activating blood circulation and detoxicating.

Indication. Cough caused by wind-heat, dysentery, edema, jaundice, rheumatic arthralgia, hemorrhoidal bleeding, amenorrhea, leukorrhea, etc.

Dihe (Ex-HN)

An extra point.

Location. Below Chengjiang (CV 24), at the highest point of the process at the midpoint of the lower jaw bone.

Indication. Deep-rooted sore on the face and head, toothache.

Method. Puncture obliquely 0.3-0.5 cun.

Diji (Sp 8)

A meridian acupuncture point.

Location. On the medial side of the leg at the line connecting the medial malleolus and Yinlingquan (Sp 9), 3 cun directly below Yinlingquan.

Indication. Abdominal distention and pain, poor appetite, diarrhea, irregular menstruation, dysmenorrhea, nocturnal emission, dysuria, edema.

Method. Puncture perpendicularly 0.5-1.0 cun. Apply moxibustion 3-5 moxa cones or 5-10 minutes with warming moxibustion.

Diluteyellow Crotalaria Herb

It is the whole herb of Crotalaria albida Heyne. (Leguminosae).

Effect. Removing heat, detoxicating and promoting diuresis.

Indication. Chronic cough with phlegm-dyspnea, urethritis, cystitis, carbuncles and cellulitis.

Dindygulen Peperomia Herb

It is the whole herb of Peperomia dindigulensis Mig. (Piperaceae).

Effect. Removing blood stasis and masses, clearing away heat and toxic materials, and preventing cancers.

Indication. Stomach, liver, mammary and lung cancer.

Dingchuan (Ex-B 1)

An extra point.

Location. On the back, 0.5 cun lateral to the posterior midline, below the spinous process of the 7th cervical vertebra.

Indication. Asthma, cough, bronchitis, torticollis, urticaria, etc.

Method. Puncture perpendicularly 0.5-0.7 cun. Apply moxibustion 3-5 moxa cones or 5-15 minutes with warming moxibustion.

Dingshanghuimao (Ex-HN)

An extra point.

Location. At the midpoint of the hair on the vertex.

Indication. Infantile fright and epilepsy, prolapse of the rectum and bleeding caused by hemorrhoids.

Method. Apply moxibustion 3-7 moxa cones or 10-15 minutes with warming moxibustion.

Diphtheria

Referring to an acute infectious disease.

Symptoms. Swelling and pain in the throat, the more serious pain in swallowing, and pus spots and white thin membrane on the tonsil, with headache, fever, distressed sensation in the chest, and even dyspnea, palpitation, shortness of breath, etc., if serious.

Pathogenesis. Owing to the invasion of the pathogens into the body, in the throat.

Therapeutic Principle. Removing heat and toxic materials.

Diphtheria due to Cold of Insufficiency Type

Symptoms. At the beginning non-fever, normal diet, but pale lips and red face, tiredness, white skin or white mass in the throat, increased at any time.

Pathogenesis. Due to weakness of body and affection of pathogenic cold.

Therapeutic Principle. Expelling cold by warming meridians.

Direct Attack on Three Yin Meridians

It refers to the pathogenic factors of febrile disease attacking directly the three yin meridians, not through transmission of three yang meridians. In the regular pattern of transmission of acute febrile disease between the six pairs of meridians, the three yang meridians are affected first, then the three yin meridians. But when the pathogenic factors are prevailing and qi is undermined, three yin syndrome can be seen at onset and it is called direct attack on the three yin meridians. Clinically, the most common are direct attack on Heart and Kidney Meridians.

Directing Qi Method

A needling technique, while puncturing first slowly thrust and quickly lift the needle for six times. After acquiring qi, make the needle obliquely appoint the affected area. Then let the patient inhale for 5-7 times so as to aid qi getting to the affected area, and then withdraw the needle. It is used for various pain diseases.

Direct Moxibustion

A form of moxa-cone moxibustion, referring to placing a moxa cone directly on a point for moxibustion. According to the different degrees of moxibustion, it is divided into suppurative moxibustion and non-suppurative moxibustion.

Direct Needling

It is one of the twelve methods of needling. It refers to puncture along the subcutaneous diseased part. When pricking, first hold between the fingers the local skin around the point, and then prick into the skin. It is used for numbness and pain of the relatively shallow diseased part.

Disability of Limbs

Symptoms. General aching and weakness of the limbs and inability to move freely.

Pathogenesis. Deficiency of the spleen and its dysfunction in transporting the body fluid to the limbs; or obesity, fire-transmission from excessive phlegm and dampness resulting in the blockage of meridians.

Discolor Cinquefoil Herb

It is the whole herb of Potentilla discolor Bge. (Rosaceae) with root.

Effect. Removing heat, detoxicating, stopping bleeding and relieving swelling.

Indication. Dysentery, bronchitis, pulmonary abscess, mumps, hemaoptysis, hemafecia, hematuria, metrorrhagia and metrostaxis, etc.

Discordance between Water and Fire

Symptoms. Dysphoria, insomnia, lassitude in loin and knees, spontaneous sweat and seminal emission.

Pathogenesis. Excess of the heart yang and deficiency of the kidney yin.

Disease due to Consumption

Symptoms. Lassitude in the loin and knees, night sweat, dribbling urination, moist scrotum, flaccidity, etc.

Pathogenesis. Deficiency of the kidney.

Therapeutic Principle. Invigorating the kidney qi.

Diseases due to External Factors

1. Referring to trauma or injury on the skin, in the muscles, bone, and tendons.
2. Referring to the injury caused by the six exogenous factors opposite to the internal injury of the seven emotions, such as invasion by wind, cold, dampness and summer-heat.

Disease due to Latent Summer-heat

Referring to one type of epidemic febrile diseases in autumn and winter, similar to summer-damp and summer-heat symptoms clinically.

Symptoms. Similar to common cold; at the beginning, chills and fever, then similar to malaria, but irregular; later, higher fever at night without chills, in the morning sweating and body fever subsiding slightly, still with high fever feeling in the chest and the abdomen.

Therapeutic Principle. At onset, removing exterior and interior syndrome, then treating with illness condition, in the case of more dampness applying the method of summer-heat and dampness, in the case of more heat, applying the method of summer-warm.

Disease due to Qi Disorder

It refers to the syndrome caused by functional disturbance of visceral meridians and collaterals, which is divided into the deficiency type and the excess type.

Disease due to Terror

Referring to the syndrome of being frightened easily or the disease caused by terror.

Symptoms. Palpitation, emotional distress, restlessness, trance, urinary and fecal incontinence, etc.

Therapeutic Principle. Reinforcing the kidney, and calming the mind.

Disease Involving both Exterior and Interior

It refers to the co-existence of exterior and interior syndrome or syndrome involving both exterior and interior.

Disease of Large Intestine Meridian of Hand-Yangming

Referring to one of the diseases of twelve meridians.

Symptoms. Toothache of lower teeth, sore throat, epistaxis, clear nasal discharge, dry mouth, yellow eyes, swelling in the neck, etc.

Diseases of Meridian One of the Yinqiao

Referring to one of the pathological symptoms of eight extra meridians.

Symptoms. Drowsiness, uroschesis, difficulty in the movement of the lower limbs.

Disease of Proglottid of Tapeworm

Symptoms. Fullness and pain of abdomen, diarrhea with whitish things in the shape of node and slice, etc.

Pathogenesis. Owing to the affection of the worm, one cun long, a part of taenia by eating raw pork, beef or fish.

Therapeutic Principle. Expelling the taenia till its head is out.

Diseases of Qi System

Symptoms. Edema, fullness and mass in the upper abdomen.

Pathogenesis. Due to obstruction of yang-qi, stagnation of cold-qi and excessive fluid in the body.

Therapeutic Principle. For the patient with internal and external syndrome, warming meridians for activating yang and removing fluid and damp; for the patient with syndrome in middle-energizer enhancing the circulation of qi and releasing stasis, and reinforcing the spleen to induce diuresis.

Diseases of the Back Middle Meridian

Referring to one of the syndromes of the eight extra meridians.

Symptoms. Opisthotonos, stiffness of the neck, manic-depressive disorder, epilepsy induced by terror, dizziness, etc.

Diseases of the Belt vessel

Referring to one of the syndromes of the eight extra meridians

Symptoms. Distention and fullness in the lumbar region and abdomen, leukorrhea with reddish discharge, pain in the navel, lumbar and spinal regions.

Diseases of the Bladder Meridian of Foot-taiyang

Referring to one of the pathological symptoms of the twelve meridians.

Symptoms. Headache, pain of eyes, stuffy nose, epistaxis, lumbago, hemorrhoid, malaria, manic-depressive disorder, flexion dyscinesia of the hip, pain of the calf and foot, swelling and pain of the lower abdomen.

Diseases of the Collateral of Foot-jueyin

Referring to one of the pathological symptoms of the fifteen main collaterals.

Symptoms. Swelling and distention of the testes induced by reversed flow pathogenic qi, sudden onset of hernia; for the excess type, prolonged erection; for the deficiency type, sudden itching at the external genitalia.

Therapeutic Principle. Selecting the Luo (connecting) point of Foot-jueyin to treat these diseases.

Diseases of the Collateral of Foot-shaoyang

Referring to one of the pathological symptoms of the fifteen main collaterals

Symptoms. Excess type, numb and cold feet; deficiency type, paralysis of the lower limbs.

Therapeutic Principle. The Luo (connecting) point of Foot-shaoyang to treat the diseases.

Diseases of the Collateral of Foot-shaoyin

Referring to one of the pathological symptoms of the fifteen main collaterals.

Symptoms. Vexation and oppressive feeling in the chest caused by reversed flow of the meridian qi; in the case of excess type, difficulty in urination and defecation; in the case of deficiency type, lumbago.

Therapeutic Principle. Selecting Luo (connecting) point of Food-shaoyin to treat the diseases.

Diseases of the Collateral of Foot-taiyang

Referring to one of the pathological symptoms of the fifteen main collaterals

Symptoms. For the excess type, stuffy nose, watery nasal discharge, headache, and back pain; for the deficiency type, watery nasal discharge and epistaxis.

Therapeutic Principle. Selecting the Luo (connecting) point of Foot-taiyang to treat the diseases.

Diseases of the Collateral of Foot-taiyin

Referring to one of the pathological symptoms of the fifteen main collaterals.

Symptoms. Cholera morbus caused by reversed flow of qi, vomiting and diarrhea, colicky pain of the abdomen for the of excess type, and flatulence of the abdomen for the deficiency type.

Therapeutic Principle. Selecting the Luo (connecting) point of Foot-taiyin to treat the diseases.

Diseases of the Collateral of Foot-yangming

Referring to one of the pathological symptoms of the fifteen main collaterals.

Symptoms. Sore throat, sudden hoarseness caused by reversed flow of qi; manic-depressive psychosis in the case of excess type; relaxation and myo-atrophy of the leg in the case of deficiency type.

Therapeutic Principle. Selecting the Luo (connecting) point of Foot-yangming Meridian to treat the diseases.

Diseases of the Collateral of Hand-jueyin

Referring to one of the pathological symptoms of the fifteen main collaterals.

Symptoms. Cardiac pain for excess type; dysphoria for deficiency type.

Therapeutic Principle. Puncturing the Luo (connecting) point of Hand-jueyin to treat the diseases.

Diseases of the Collateral of Hand-shaoyang

Referring to one of the pathological symptoms of the fifteen main collaterals.

Symptoms. Contracture of the elbow joint for excess; sluggish of the joint movement for deficiency.

Therapeutic Principle. Selecting the Luo (connecting) point of Hand-shaoyang for treating the diseases.

Diseases of the Collateral of Hand-shaoyin

Referring to one of the pathological symptoms of the fifteen main collaterals.

Symptoms. Distention and fullness in the sustaining region of the chest and diaphragm for excess type; aphasia for deficiency type.

Therapeutic Principle. Selecting the Luo (connecting) point of Hand-shaoyin to treat the diseases

Diseases of the Collateral of Hand-taiyang

Referring to one of the pathological symptoms of the fifteen main collaterals.

Symptoms. For excess type, flaccidity of the elbow; for deficiency type, verruca on the skin.

Therapeutic Principle. Selecting the Luo (connecting) point of Hand-taiyang to treat the diseases.

Diseases of the Collateral of Hand-taiyin

Referring to one of the pathological symptoms of the fifteen main collaterals.

Symptoms. For the excess type, scorching fever of the palm and the wrist region; for the deficiency type, yawn, frequent micturition and enuresis.

Therapeutic Principle. Selecting the Luo (connecting) point of Hand-taiyin to treat the diseases.

Diseases of the Collateral of Hand-yangming

Referring to one of the pathological symptoms of the fifteen main collaterals.

Symptoms. For the excess type, decayed teeth and deafness; for the deficiency type, cold feeling of the teeth and stagnation of the meridian qi.

Therapeutic Principle. Selecting the Luo (connecting) point of Hand-yangming to treat the diseases.

Diseases of the Front Middle Meridian

Referring to one of the pathogenic symptoms of the eight extra meridians.

Symptoms. Pain in the lower abdomen, hernia, leukorrhea, mass in the abdomen, sterility, irregular menstruation, enuresis, emission, pain in the pudendum, etc.

Diseases of the Gallbladder Meridian of Foot-shaoyang

Referring to one of the pathological symptoms of the twelve meridians.

Symptoms. Bitter taste, eructation, aching in the hypochondriac region, grey complexion, migraine, aching of the outer canthus, deafness, swelling and pain of the neck, chills and fever, malaria, etc.

Diseases of the Heart Meridian of Hand-shaoyin

Referring to one of the pathological symptoms of the twelve meridians.

Symptoms. Dry throat, cardialgia, thirst, vexation, short breath, pain of the chest and hypochondrium, yellow eye, etc.

Diseases of the Kidney Meridian of Foot-shaoyin

Referring to one of the pathological symptoms of the twelve meridians.

Symptoms. Anorexia, darkish and dim complexion, cough, phlegm with blood, dyspnea, dry tongue, swelling of the throat, dryness and pain of the throat, palpitation, terror, jaundice, diarrhea, pain of the waist, etc.

Diseases of The Large Collateral of the Spleen

Referring to one of the diseases of the fifteen main collaterals.

Symptoms. If pathogenic changes happens to this collateral, pantalgia in the excess case; and flaccidity and weakness of the joints throughout the body in deficiency type.

Diseases of the Large Intestine Meridian of Hand-yangming

Referring to one of the pathological symptoms of the twelve meridians.

Symptoms. Dry mouth, stuffy nose, epistaxis, toothache, swelling of the neck, pain and swelling of the throat, intestinal colic, borborygmus and diarrhea.

Diseases of the Liver Meridian of Foot-jueyin

Referring to one of the pathological symptoms of the twelve meridians.

Symptoms. Lumbago, hernia, swelling and distention of the lower abdomen, dry throat, dirty and dark, gloomy look complexion.

Diseases of the Lung Meridian of Hand-taiyin

Referring to one of the pathological symptoms of the twelve meridians.

Symptoms. Fullness and tightness of the chest, distention of the lung, cough, dyspnea, vexation, shortness of breath, hot palm, frequent micturition, etc.

Diseases of the Muscle Region of Foot-jueyin

Referring to one of the pathological symptoms of the twelve muscle regions.

Symptoms. Sustaining disturbance of the great toe, aching at the front of the medial malleolus, pain at medial aspect of the knee joint, spasm and pain of the medial aspect of the thigh, dysfunction of external genitalia, impotence caused by consumption of yin-essence caused by excessive sexual intercourse, flaccid constriction of penis resulting from pathogenic cold, prolonged erection of the penis resulting from pathogenic heat, etc.

Diseases of the Muscle Region of Foot-shaoyang

Referring to one of the pathological symptoms of the twelve muscle regions.

Symptoms. Sustaining disturbance of the 4th toe, spasm of the toe connecting to the lateral side of the knee, failure of the knee to flex and stretch; contracture of the muscles of the chest and the neck; contracture in the muscles, and bending from the left to the right, the right eye unable to open.

Diseases of the Muscle Region of Foot-shaoyin

Referring to one of the pathological symptoms of the twelve muscle regions.

Symptoms. Spasm of the sole, pain and spasm along the root of the meridian, pain and spasm of the connected region, epilepsy, convulsion, opisthotonus, dyskinesia.

Diseases of the Muscle Region of Foot-taiyang

Referring to one of the pathological symptoms of the twelve muscle regions.

Symptoms. Uncomfortable sensation in the little toe, pulling pain of the heel, spasm in the popliteal space, opisthotonus, contracture of the neck, dysfunction of the shoulder.

Diseases of the Muscle Region of Foot-taiyin

Referring to one of the pathological symptoms of the twelve muscle regions.

Symptoms. Uncomfortable sensation of the big toe, pulling pain of the medial malleolus, spasm, pain of the knee and the popliteal fossa, torsive pain of the external genitals.

Diseases of the Muscle Region of Foot-yangming

Referring to one of the pathological symptoms of the twelve muscle regions.

Symptoms. Distention, contracture and pain of the middle toe and tibia, rigidity of foot, contracture, pain and swelling in the anterior portion of the thigh, hernia, contracture of abdominal muscles and tendons, sudden occurrence of facial paralysis.

Diseases of the Muscle Region of Hand-jueyin

Referring to one of the pathological symptoms of the twelve muscle regions.

Symptoms. Disturbance in sustaining the connecting region, contracture, spasm along the path of the meridian and at the site where the muscle concentrates, and chest pain or pulmonary mass.

Diseases of the Muscles Region of Hand-shaoyang

Referring to one of the pathological symptoms of the twelve muscle regions.

Symptoms. Disorder in sustaining the circulating parts of the meridian of the regions along the path of the muscles, thus resulting in spasm and contracture and curled-up tongue.

Diseases of the Muscle Region of Hand-shaoyin

Referring to one of the pathological symptoms of the twelve muscle regions.

Symptoms. Contracture in the chest, hard and hidden mass located in the upper abdomen, disturbance of flexion and extension of the elbow, disturbance in sustaining the circulating regions; contracture, spasm and pain along the path of the muscles.

Diseases of the Muscle Region of Hand-taiyang

Referring to one of the pathological symptoms of the twelve muscle regions.

Symptoms. Stiffness the little finger, pain of the posterior border of the ulnar bone, pain along the medial aspect of the arm and upwards to the armpit and its lower posterior side, ache around the scapula radiating to the nape and neck, tinnitus, ear pain radiating to the chin.

Diseases of the Muscle Region of Hand-taiyin

Referring to one of the pathological symptoms of the twelve muscle regions.

Symptoms. Stiffness, contracture and pain in the regions of the path of the muscle region; pulmonary mass, contracture of the hypochondriac region, vomiting, and hematemesis if serious.

Diseases of the Muscle Region of Hand-yangming

Referring to one of the pathological symptoms of the twelve muscle regions.

Symptoms. Stiffness, contracture and pain in the region of the path of this muscle region, failure of raising the shoulder joint high and of turning the neck round.

Diseases of the Pericardium Meridian of Hand-yueyin

Referring to one of the pathological symptoms of the twelve meridians.

Symptoms. Feverish sensation in the center of the palm, contracture of the elbow and arm, swelling of the axilla, suffocating sensation in the chest and hypochondrium, palpitation, red face and yellow eyes, etc.

Diseases of the Tri-energizer Meridian of Hand-shaoyang

Referring to one of the pathological symptoms of the twelve meridians.

Symptoms. Deafness, tinnitus, swelling of the throat, sore throat, pain of the outer canthus, pain of the cheek, spontaneous perspiration, fullness and rigidity of the lower abdomen, flatulence, dysuria, enuresis.

Diseases of the Small Intestine Meridian of Hand-taiyang

Referring to one of the pathological symptoms of the twelve meridians.

Symptoms. Sore throat, acute mumps, deafness, yellow eyes, stiffness of the nape, pain in the shoulder region, difficulty in turning round of lower abdominal pain, diarrhea, loose stool.

Diseases of the Spleen Meridian of Foot-taiyin

Referring to one of the pathological symptoms of the twelve meridians.

Symptoms. Vomiting, gastric pain, abdominal distention, eructation, vexation, jaundice, mass in the abdomen, diarrhea, acute pain in the epigastrium, enuresis, insomnia pain and cold in the region along the path of the meridian.

Diseases of the Stomach Meridian of Foot-yangming

Referring to one of the pathological symptoms of the twelve meridians.

Symptoms. Chills with fever, malaria, stuffy nose, nose bleeding, wry mouth, sore throat, abdominal distention, epigastric pain, nausea vomiting.

Disharmony between Nutrient System and Defence System

Referring to a morbid state of relative excess or deficiency between nutrient system and defence system.

1. Defence system deficiency and nutrient system excess.

   Symptoms. Spontaneous perspiration but no fever.

   Pathogenesis. Due to failure of consolidating superficial resistance induced by defence system deficiency.

2. Defence system excess and nutrient system deficiency.

   Symptoms. Perspiration with fever. Defence system excess referring to a pathologic change induced by resistance to pathogen of defence system-qi, leading to fever; nutrient system deficiency referring to failure of nutrient system-qi to nourish the interior, leading to sweating.

Dishen (Ex-UE)

Referring to a set of extra acupuncture points.

Location. Four points in total on the palmar side of each thumb, at the midpoint of the crease of the metacarpophalangeal point.

Indication. Reinforcing.

Dislocation

It refers to abnormal connection of joints.

Symptoms. Local swelling and pain, deformity and dysfunction.

Cause. Trauma, fall from high place and impact.

Therapeutic Principle. Manual reduction, promoting blood circulation to remove blood stasis, relieving swelling and pain, strengthening muscles, tendons and bones, combination with the Western medicine and functional training.

Dislocation of Ankle Joint

It is a disease.

Symptoms. Local red swelling, pain, deformity and inability to move.

Cause. Mainly due to trauma, torsion and impact.

Therapeutic Principle. Ankle moving reduction and external fixation; activating blood circulation to clear away blood stasis; after the abatement of swelling and pain, by nourishing the liver and the kidney together with passive movements.

Dislocation of Elbow Joint

It is a disease.

Symptoms. Local swelling and pain, dysfunction of movement.

Cause. Mainly caused by trauma, sprain, impact.

Therapeutic Principle. Using the method of pulling-flexing reduction of elbows.

Dislocation of Finger Joint

Symptoms. Local pain, swelling, deformity and restriction of movement.

Cause. Mostly caused by trauma, pressure, sprain, impact, etc.

Therapeutic Principle. Manual reduction and external fixation, promoting blood circulation to remove blood stasis with functional training.

Dislocation of Hip Joint

Symptoms. Local swelling, pain and dysfunction of movement.

Cause. Usually caused by trauma, fall from high place, sprain, ect.

Therapeutic Principle. Manual reduction, promoting blood circulation to remove blood stasis and combination with dirigation.

Dislocation of Knee Joint

Referring to the slight displacement between meniscus and condyle of femur, and tibial plateau.

Symptoms. Dysfunction of extension and flexion of knee joint after injury.

Therapeutic Principle. Manipulation of massage.

Dislocation of Patella

Symptoms. Obvious red swelling in knee region, pain, difficulty in walking, etc.

Cause. Mainly due to trauma and torsion.

Therapeutic Principle. Knee-pushing reduction and fixation with peri-patellapexor; at onset activating blood circulation to clear away blood stasis, removing swelling and pain; after abatement of swelling and pain, supplementing qi and nourishing blood to relax muscle and tendon, together with passive movements.

Dislocation of Phalangeal Joint

Symptoms. Local tumefaction, megalgia, deformity, and restriction of movement.

Cause. Mainly due to trauma.

Therapeutic Principle. Manual reduction, external fixation; internal treatment, by activating blood circulation to clear away blood stasis and functional training.

Dislocation of Radiocarpea

Symptoms. Obvious local tumefaction, megalgia, restriction of movement.

Cause. Due to trauma and sprain.

Therapeutic Principle. Manual reduction and external fixation, promoting blood circulation to remove blood stasis, accompanied with functional training.

Dislocation of Scapula

Symptoms. Pain of the wounded shoulder, tumefaction, deformity and dysfunction.

Cause. Due to trauma, sudden sprain and fall.

Therapeutic Principle. Manual reductions, such as heeling reduction, shoulder-carrying reduction, and carrying reduction.

Dislocation of Wrist Joint

Symptoms. Obvious local tumefaction, pain, deformity, restriction of movement, abnormal sensation of fingers if serious.

Cause. Due to trauma , sprain and fall.

Therapeutic Principle. Manual reduction and external fixation, promoting blood circulation to remove blood stasis accompanied by functional training.

Disorder of Blood

It is a disease, referring to morbid state of blood stasis or hemorrhage caused by trauma.

Symptoms.

1. Blood stasis: Distending pain in a fixed area without moving.
2. Hemorrhage: Bleeding from certain part of the body or orifices from the body, usually accompanied by dizziness, palpitation and dry mouth, etc.

   Cause. Trauma.

   Therapeutic Principle. Promoting blood circulation to remove blood stasis, stopping bleeding. Emergency treatment should be given in combination of Chinese medicine with Western medicine.

Disorder of Gallbladder

Symptoms. Dizziness and tinnitus, palpitation and insomnia, headache, alternate attacks of chills and fever, bitter taste and yellowish eyes.

Pathogenesis. Due to emotional depression, retention of damp-heat in the gallbladder, resulting in the qi and deficiency of gallbladder, or the blockage of the gallbladder fluid.

Therapeutic Principle. Releasing heat from the liver and normalizing function of the gallbladder, calm the mind.

Disorder of Liver-qi

Symptoms. Distending pain of hypochondrium, oppressed feeling in the chest, easy to be anxious, poor appetite or bitter taste, vomiting, etc.

Pathogenesis. Owing to the failure of the liver to control the flow of qi.

Therapeutic Principle. Adjusting the liver and the circulation of qi.

Disorder of Qi

Symptoms. Palpitation, irritability and restlessness, excessive anxiety and fear, etc.

Pathogenesis. Usually caused by sudden fright or emotional depression.

Therapeutic Principle. Adjusting functional activities of qi.

Disorder of Stomach-qi

Symptoms. Anorexia or distention after eating, nausea, insomnia, and disorder of defecation, etc.

Pathogenesis. Due to the deficiency of stomach-yin, the disturbance of the stomach caused by pathogenic heat, or food stagnation in the stomach.

Therapeutic Principle. Treatment based on the pathogenic factors.

Dispelling Heat by Excreting Dampness

Referring to the therapeutic method by using diuretic to remove pathogenic heat through urination.

Indication. The early epidemic febrile disease with dampness.

Dispelling Heat by Mild Diaphoresis

Referring to a therapeutic method of using the drugs pungent in flavor and cool in property to removing external syndromes.

Symptoms. Fever, slight fear of cold, dysphoria, thirst, anhidrosis, etc.

Dispersed Complexion

Referring to the patient's complexion dispersing, mostly seen in new diseases or improved condition, and indicating that the illness is liable to be treated, with favourable prognosis.

Dispersing Exopathogens due to Its Mildness

Referring to the prescription of dispersing diseases due to mild pathogens with superficial lesions, for example, using diaphoretic recipe to dispel superficial pathogens.

Dispersion Helping Remove Obstruction

Referring to a therapy to release stagnancy and obstruction by using drugs with dispersing action, e.g. spleen and stomach qi stagnation in the middle-energizer.

Displacement between Joints of Cervical Vertebrae

Referring to slight lateral displacement between joints of cervical vertebrae.
Symptoms. Dysfunction of cervical vertebrae, local pain and restriction of movement.
Cause. External force produced by torsion.
Therapeutic Principle. Manipulations reduction.

Displacement of Calcaneus-cuboid Joint

Referring to dislocation of the joint formed by distal calcaneus and proximal cuboid bone induced by external forces without self-reposition.
Symptoms. Pain and dysfunction.
Therapeutic Principle. Manipulations reduction.

Displacement of Carpale-metacarpal Joint

Referring to slight displacement of both surfaces between metacarpal and wrist joints.
Symptoms. Serious volardorsal swelling, pain point in carpal-metacarpal joint.
Cause. Owing to external forces.

Therapeutic Principle. Manipulations reduction.

Distal-Proximal Point Association

Referring to a form of point association.
Method. Selecting the points far from the disease region together with those near for the treatment. For example selecting distal Neiguan (P 6) and Zusanli (S 36) and proximal Zhongwan(CV 12) for gastric disease.

Distal Segment Point Selection

Referring to one of the modern point selection methods.
Method. For treating diseases or for acupuncture anesthesia, the points selected in this method, either far from the disease region, or near the spinal segment, for example, selecting points on lower limbs for diseases on the head or operations on the cranium, or points on the upper limbs for lumbocrural problems.

Distant Point Selection

Referring to one of the point selection methods.
Method. Selecting points distal to the region with disease, clinically including selecting points of the same meridian and selecting points of other meridians.

Distending Pain in Hypochondrium

Pathogenesis. Due to qi stagnation, phlegm stagnation, obstruction of meridian and collaterals.
Therapeutic Principle. Adjusting the circulation of qi, calming the liver and releasing phlegm and removing blood stasis and pain.

Distending Pain of Breasts during Menstruation

Symptoms. For a woman with the age of child-bearing, before or during month current, distending pain of the breast or unbearable itching of the nipple and even intangible.

Pathogenesis. Due to stagnation of the liver-qi.

Therapeutic Principle. Smoothing the liver and adjusting the flow of qi.

Distention due to Cold

Referring to a type of distention.

Symptoms. Abdominal distention and fullness, anorexia, vomiting, vexation, cold limbs, etc.

Pathogenesis. Due to the deficiency of spleen-yang, or the stagnation of cold-dampness.

Therapeutic Principle. Warming the middle-energizer, removing cold.

Distention due to Deficiency of Liver and Kidney

Symptoms. Skinny and weakness, pain in lumbar and hypochondrium, oliguria with difficulty and distending cold in the lower abdomen, etc.

Pathogenesis. Due to deficiency of the liver and spleen and dysfunction of the urinary bladder.

Therapeutic Principle. Reinforcing and nourishing liver and kidney, activating the circulation of qi to induce diuresis.

Distention due to Liver Disorder

Symptoms. Distending pain below hypochondrium involving pain in the lower abdomen, and bitter taste.

Pathogenesis. Due to invasion of the Liver Meridian by pathogenic cold.

Therapeutic Principle. Adjusting the liver and expelling cold.

Distention due to Phlegm Stagnation

Symptoms. Feeling of oppression in the chest, abdominal distention, shortness of breath and adverse-rising qi, difficulty in urination and defecation, or even swollen face and limbs, etc.

Pathogenesis. Due to the stagnation of phlegm and qi in the chest and abdomen.

Therapeutic Principle. Adjusting qi and dispelling phlegm.

Distention due to Qi Deficiency

Symptoms. Shapeless stool, alteration of constipation and loose stool, and clear dribbling urination, etc.

Pathogenesis. Owing to the deficiency of the primordial qi.

Therapeutic Principle. Nourishing the spleen and qi.

Distention of Abdomen due to Stagnation of Qi

Symptoms. Fullness and distention of the chest and abdomen, with piercing pain in the abdomen, constipation, etc.

Pathogenesis. Mainly owing to the impairment of the liver caused by anger, the stagnation of the spleen-qi, or blood stasis.

Therapeutic Principle. Adjusting the flow of qi and smoothing depression, or enhancing blood circulation, and removing blood stasis.

Distention of Excess Type

Symptoms. Abdominal distention, rigidity and tenderness, constipation, dark urine.

Pathogenesis. Due to accumulation of damp-heat, stagnation of qi and blood stasis, retention of food in the stomach and spleen.

Therapeutic Principle. Removing heat and dampness, enhancing flow of qi and blood circulation, promoting digestion and dispelling stagnancy.

Distortion of Face due to Pathogenic Wind

Symptoms. Distortion of the eye and mouth, eyelids failure to close tightly, even eversion of lower eyelid, deviation of eyeballs and lips, dizziness, ambiopia.

Pathogenesis. Owing to attack of pathogenic wind on the meridians.
Therapeutic Principle. Removing wind and obstruction in the meridians.

Distracting Thoughts

It is a term in Qigong, referring to the distracting thoughts occurring in practice and making mind unconcentrated and disturbed. So it must be cleared away.

Distressed Dysphagia

Symptoms. Dysphagia once eating, palpitation and coldness of the limbs.
Pathogenesis. Caused by obstruction of qi excessive melancholy and anxiety.
Therapeutic Principle. Relieving mental depression and regulating qi.

Distribution of Complexion

Referring to the areas on the face for representing the viscera and limbs, diagnoses based on the colors and brightness of the areas.

Distribution of Red Vein in Eye

Symptoms. Lots of red veins branching out of the canthi and extending to the white or even to the black eyeball, itching and astringency in the eye, and plenty of secretion and tears.
Pathogenesis. Due to insufficiency and deficiency of the kidney-yin, flaring up of heart-fire or heat accumulation in the tri-energizer.
Therapeutic Principle. Removing heat and purging intense heat.

Disturbance in Ascending and Descending

Referring to a morbid condition.
Symptoms. Abdominal distention, belching, anorexia, and diarrhea.
Pathogenesis. Owing to disharmony between the function of the spleen and stomach with failure of ascending the spleen-qi and descending the stomach-qi.

Disturbance in Qi Transformation

Referring to morbid condition.
Symptoms. Disorders of digestion and absorption, affecting the production of blood, essence, body fluid, qi and excretion of metabolites.
Pathogenesis. Owing to the deficiency of yang-qi.

Disturbance of Defecation

Symptoms. Diarrhea or hard stool, etc.
Pathogenesis. Due to deficiency of the kidney, insufficiency of the spleen-yang.
Therapeutic Principle. Nourishing the kidney and reinforcing the spleen.

Disturbance of Lower Legs due to Cold-dampness

Symptoms. Flaccidity of the feet and knees, difficulty in walking, numbness.
Pathogenesis. Due to the invasion of cold-dampness, the disturbance of meridian-qi and the disorder of blood vessels.
Therapeutic Principle. Warming the meridians, expelling dampness, adjusting blood flow, releasing obstruction in the meridians and relaxing muscles.

Disturbance of Spleen-yang due to Damp

Referring to a morbid condition.
Symptoms. Epigastric distress, abdominal distention, anorexia, loose stool, nausea, vomiting tendency, heavy feeling over the head, etc.
Pathogenesis. Improper diet, overeating raw or cold food, being caught in rain and dwelling damp environments.

Divaricate Knotweed Herb

It is the whole herb of Polygonum divaricatum L. (Polygonaceae).
Effect. Removing heat and stagnancy, treating goiter and stopping diarrhea.
Indication. Large and small intestinal heat accumulation, goiter, abdominal pain caused by heat diarrhea, etc.

Divaricate Saposhnikovia Root   ⊛ D-3

It is the root of Saposhnikovia divaricata (Turcz.) Schischk (Umbelliferae).

Effect. Alleviating exterior syndromes by dispelling pathogenic wind, clearing away dampness, relieving spasm and pain.

Indication. Exterior syndromes resulting from affection caused by wind-cold exopathogens, arthralgia caused by wind-cold-dampness characterized by joint pain, spasm of limbs, tetanus, and exterior syndromes resulting from affection caused by wind-cold exopathogens, etc.

Divaricate Strophanthus Root

It is the rhizome or the leaf of stem of Strophanthus divaricatus (Lour) Hook. et Arn(Apocynaceae).

Effect. Dispelling wind-dampness, clearing and promoting the meridians and collaterals, and detoxicating.

Indication. Rheumatic arthralgia, poliomyelitis sequel, traumatic injuries, carbuncles, scabies and tinea.

Divergent Meridian of Foot-jueyin

Referring to one of the twelve divergent meridians. The Meridian branching from the part of the Meridian of Foot-jueyin on the dorsum of foot, and passing upward to the region of external genitals to converge into and running alongside the divergent Meridian of Foot-shaoyang.

Divergent Meridian of Foot-shaoyang

Referring to one of the twelve divergent meridians. Deriving from the Gallbladder and Meridian of Foot-shaoyang, the meridian passing around the anterior aspect of the thigh, then entering the external genitalia region, emerging with the Divergent Meridian of Foot-jueyin. From the external genitalia region, its branch going into the intercostal space, along the inside of the abdominal cavity to the gallbladder the organ it belongs to and spreading in the liver. Then, the branch passing through the heart and going upwards along the esophagus, and emerging superficially from the middle of the mandible. Continuously, spreading over the face and linking with the posterity of the eye, then running into the cranial cavity. This divergent meridian emerging with the Meridian of Foot-shaoyang at the outer canthus.

Divergent Meridian of Foot-shaoyang and Foot-jueyin

Referring to one confluence of the twelve divergent meridians. The Divergent Meridian of Foot-shaoyang finally joining its own regular meridian in the processes of derivation, entry and emergence. The Divergent Meridian of Foot-jueyin finally joining into its externally-internally related meridian, the Foot-shaoyang Meridian, in the processes of derivation, entry and emergence.

Divergent Meridian of Foot-taiyang

Referring to one of the twelve divergent meridians. Diverging from the Meridian of Foot-taiyang in the popliteal fossa, one branch entering the anus from the region 5 cun below the sacral bone, running into the pertaining organ, the bladder, distributing in and connecting with the kidney, running upwards in the muscles alongside the spine to the heart, and distributing in it; the straight one going continuously upward along the muscle beside the spine, emerging from the neck and returning to the Meridian of Foot-taiyang proper.

Divergent Meridian of Foot-taiyang and Foot-shaoyin

Referring to one confluence of the twelve divergent meridians. The Divergent Meridian of Foot-taiyang finally joining the regular meridian after the circulation of deriving, entering and emerging and the Divergent Meridian of Foot-shaoyin joining the Meridian of Foot-taiyang after the circulation of deriving entering and emerging.

Divergent Meridian of Foot-taiyin

Referring to one of the twelve divergent meridians. From the meridian of Foot-Taiyin, the Meridian arriving at the anterior side of the thigh, meeting the Divergent Meridian of Foot-yangming with it upward to the throat and passing through the root of the tongue.

Divergent Meridian of Foot-yangming

Referring to one of the twelve divergent meridians. From the Meridian of Foot-yangming anterior to the thigh, the said meridian getting into the abdominal cavity, belonging to the stomach organ, and distributing to the spleen, upward to connect with the heart, out from the mouth cavity along the esophagus, upward reaching to the root of the nose and the infraorbital region, and back to link with the tissues posterior to eyes connecting with the brain. The meridian-qi also converges in the Meridian of Foot-yangming.

Divergent Meridian of Hand-jueyin

Referring to one of the twelve divergent meridians. The meridian branching from the Meridian of Hand-Jueyin at 3 cun below the armpit, entering the chest, pertaining to the tri-energizer, passing down along the throat, coming out at the back of the ear and emerging in the Meridian of Hand-shaoyang below the mastoid process.

Divergent Meridian of Hand-shaoyin

Referring to one of the twelve divergent meridians. The meridian branching from the regular Meridian of Hand-shaoyin between the muscles in the axillary fossa, entering the chest, belonging to the heart, going up to the throat, coming out at the face, and joining the Meridian of Hand-taiyang at the inner canthus.

Divergent Meridian of Hand-yangming

Referring to one of the twelve divergent meridians. The meridian branching from Jianyu(SI/4) of the Meridian of Hand-yangming and entering spinal bone of the neck, going down to the large intestine, belonging to the lung; going up to the throat and coming out at the greater supraclaveicular fossa, belonging to the regular Meridian of Hand-yangming.

Diversifolious Buckthorn Root

It is the root or branch leaf of Rhamnus heterophylla Oliv. (Rhamnaceae).

Effect. Removing heat from blood, and ceasing bleeding.

Indication. Hematemesis, hemorrhoidal bleeding, metrorrhagia, metrostaxis, irregular menstruation, dysentery, etc.

Diversifolious Hemiphragma Herb

It is the whole herb or root of hemiphragma heterophyllum Wall. (Scrophulariaceae).

Effect. Invigorating qi, stopping bleeding, clearing away blood stasis, and removing dampness and wind.

Indication. Hematemesis caused by cough, neurosism, lumbago caused by pathogenic wind-dampness, abdominal pain caused by amenorrhea, traumatic injuries, tetanus, etc.

Diversfifolious Patrinia Root

It is the root of Patrinia heterophylla Bunge, and P. scabra Bunge (Valerianaceae).

Effect. Removing heat and toxic materials treating boils, evacuating pus, releasing blood stasis and pain.

Indication. Metrorrhagia, metrostaxis, leukorrhea with reddish discharge, traumatic injuries, suppurative infections on the skin, such as sores, carbuncles, furuncle and boils.

Diwuhui (G 42)

A meridian acupuncture point.

Location. On the lateral side of the instep of the foot, posterior to the 4th metacarpophalangeal joint, between the 4th and 5th metatarsal bones, medial to the tendon of the extensor muscle of the little toe.

Indication. Headache, redness and pain of the eye, tinnitus, deafness, fullness of the chest, pain in the hypochondriac region.

Method. Puncture obliquely or perpendicularly 0.3-0.5 cun. Apply moxibustion 1-3 moxa cones or 3-5 minutes.

Dizziness

Referring to dizziness with blurred vision, feeling of oppression in the chest.

Pathogenesis. Due to exogenous pathogenic factors, the seven modes of emotions caused by internal damages, deficiency of qi and blood, imbalance of yin-yang in the viscera or drug poisoning.

Dizziness Caused by Adverse Flow of Qi

Symptoms. Dizziness dim eyesight, nausea, vomiting, etc.

Pathogenesis. Owing to the dysfunction of ascending and descending of the spleen and the stomach, leading to the adverse flow of the stomach-qi going up to the head.

Therapeutic Principle. Adjusting the stomach and lowering the adverse flow of qi.

Dizziness due to Deficiency of Blood

Symptoms. Subjective feeling of unsteady movement within the head, pale complexion, palpitation, shortness of breath, forgetfulness and insomnia, etc.

Pathogenesis. Caused by the failure of deficiency of yin blood to nourish the brain.

Therapeutic Principle. Supplementing blood and nourishing yin.

Dizziness due to Yang Deficiency

Symptoms. Dizziness and headache, tinnitus and deafness, or shortness of breath and spontaneous perspiration, cold limbs, etc.

Pathogenesis. Due to the deficiency of yang-qi and the failure of lucid yang to rise to the head.

Therapeutic Principle. Warming and promoting yang-qi.

Dodder Seed

It is the ripe seed of Cuscuta chinensis Lam. or C. Japonica Choisy (Convolvulaceae).

Effect. Reinforcing yang and supplementing yin, controlling nocturnal emission and inducing urination, enhancing eyesight and stopping diarrhea.

Indication. Pain in the loins and knees, impotence and seminal emission, frequent urination, leukorrhagia, blurred vision, loose stool, diarrhea, etc.

Dogbane Leaf

It is the leaf of Apocynum venetum L. (Apocynaceae).

Effect. Calming the liver, allaying the mind, removing heat and promoting diuresis.

Indication. Palpitation, insomnia, hyperactivity of the liver-yang, dizziness, relieving cough and dyspnea, headache and edema.

Domination of Dryness Bringing about Deficiency of Fluid

Symptoms. Mouth and nose dryness, skin wrinkles and cracks, throat dryness and itches, dry cough without phlegm, scanty urine, constipation, etc.

Pathogenesis. Due to excessive qi of dryness leading to the impairment of yin fluid.

Domination of Pathogenic Wind Disturbing Body

Symptoms. Shaking, moving of the body, for example, wandering pain of muscles and joints, convulsion of limbs, opisthotonus, deviation of the eye and mouth, falling in a dead faint, etc.

Pathogenesis. Due to pathogenic wind disturbing body.

Domination of Pathogen over Vital-qi

Referring to the deterioration of a disease and even death, owing to the deficiency of the vital-qi or the excess of the pathogenic factors in the course of the struggle between pathogens and the vital-qi.

Donkey-hide Gelatin

It is the dry glue pieces made from the hide of Equus asinus L. (Equidae).

Effect. Nourishing yin blood, ceasing bleeding, and moistening lung.

Indication. Insufficiency of blood dizziness, hemoptysis, epistaxis, hemafecia, metrorrhagia, metrostaxis; vexation, insomnia, dry cough induced by yin deficiency, etc.

Dorsal Position

Referring to the position for acupuncture and moxibustion.

Method. Patient lying on a bed, with the face, chest and abdomen upwards.

Function. Suitable for the acupoints on the head, face, neck, chest, abdomen, upper and lower limbs.

Double-deficiency Combining

Referring to the combination of the two deficiencies, vital-qi deficiency. First, followed by the affecting pathogenic factors, causing diseases; the former being the internal cause, while the latter external one. When vital-qi being deficient, the external pathogenic factor invading and causing disease.

Double Dragons Swaying Their Tails

Operation. Holding the child's elbow with the left hand, pulling and rotating the index and little finger of the child with the right hand.

Function. Induce resuscitation

Indication. Constipation and dysuria.

Double-meridian Febrile Disease

It refers to both yang and yin meridians simultaneous affection by pathogenic cold.

Therapeutic Principle. Recovering yang, warming and promoting yang-qi, enhancing the function of the spleen.

Double Phoenixes Spreading Their Wings

Referring to one of massage manipulations for children.

Operation. With the indexes and middle fingers of both hands holding and lifting the ears of the child for several times, then pressing and nipping Taiyang (Ex-HN 5), Tinghui (G 2), Shuigou (GV 26) and Chengjiang (CV 24) points.

Function. Warming lung.

Indication. Cough induced by wind and cold.

Douzhou (Ex-UE)

It is an extra acupuncture point.

Location. At the lateral aspect of Quchi (LI 11), on the tip of the external humeral epicondyle.

Indication. Neuralgia of the arm and elbow, hemiplegia and neurosism.

Method. Applying moxibustion.

Downward Flow of Damp-heat

Referring to Pathologic changes of downward flow of damp-heat into the lower-energizer.

Symptoms. Scanty and brownish urine, yellow and greasy fur, and anorexia, mucous and bloody discharge with stools, dysentery and diarrhea of damp-heat, turbid urine, leukorrhea and arthralgia of the lower limbs.

Downy Rosemyrtle Fruit

It is the fruit of Rhodomyrtus tomentosa (Ait.) Hassk. (Myrtaceae).

Effect. Tonifying blood, artringing the bowels, strengthening the kidney and preserving the semen.

Indication. Deficiency of blood, hematemesis, hemafecia, dysentery, seminal emission, metrorrhagia, leukorrhea, etc.

Dragonfly

It is the whole insect of Aeshna melanictera Selys (Aeshnidae).

Effect. Supplementing the kidney and yin essence.

Indication. Impotence and seminal emission caused by kidney-yin deficiency.

Dragon's Blood

It is the resinous excretion from the fruit and trunk of Daemonorops draco B1. (Palmae) and many other species of the same genus.

Effect. Externally, stopping bleeding, activating tissue regeneration and wound healing; internally, activating blood circulation to remove blood stasis and alleviating pain.

Indication. Traumatic bleeding, ulcer resistant to healing, pain caused by ecchymoma, dysmenorrhea, postpartum abdominal pain caused by blood stasis, etc.

Dragon's Bone

It is the skeletal fossils of the prehistoric mammals, like hipparion, rhinoceros, deer, elephants, etc.

Effect. Calming the liver, suppressing the sthenica yang, tranquilizing the mind, astringing and invigorating the kidney to preserve essence.

Indication. Intranquillity of the mind, palpitation, insomnia, dreaminess sleep; irritability, and dizziness induced by hyper-activity of yang and deficiency of yin; seminal emission, leukorrhagia, etc.

Dragon-tiger Alternate Prance

Referring to a needling technique, dragon-tiger symbolizing twirling the needle left, right and alternate prance the flow of the meridian qi.

Operation. First, twisting the needle to the left (clockwise), and right (counter clockwise) for 27 times, after getting the needling reaction, twisting and pressing the needle with the thumb moving forward and downward, then vibrating the tail of the needle with the thumb for enhancing the arrival of qi, thrusting and lifting the needle to promote the flow of qi.

Indication. Heat diseases, for example redness of the eye, the carbuncle at initial stage.

Drainage Needling

Referring to a needling technique, one of the nine needling methods, by using a sword needle to cut open the pustule sore to release pus and blood. Today it is used in surgical therapy.

Drainage with Medicated Thread

Referring to a treatment technique.

Method. Draining out the pus by means of inserting into the vomica with powerful bibulous paper in spills with drugs for treating the sore.

Dreamfulness

Referring to excessive dreaming.

Pathogenesis. Due to deficiency and decline of the heart-qi, and mental derangement; imbalance of yin and yang of zang-fu organs affecting mentality.

Dredging Moon from Water

Referring to a massage method.

Operation. Dripping cold water on the palm center and rotate-pushing on it while giving a cold puff.

Function. Removing pathogenic heat.

Indication. Fever. Dried and Withered Hair

Pathogenesis. Due to poor nourishing of the hair induced by deficiency of the kidney and blood-heat, insufficient supply of essence and blood.

Dried Earth and Exhausted Water

Referring to the pathological mechanism of exhaustion of the kidney-yin resulting from excess of Yangming fu-organ and, excessive pathogenic heat attacking the kidney-yin.

Dried Lacquer

It is the desiccated resin of Toxicodendron verniciflua (Stokes) F. A. Barkley (Anacardiaceae).

Effect. Relieving blood stasis with potent drugs, inducing menstruation and killing parasites.

Indication. Amenorrhea and masses in the abdomen resulting from accumulation of blood stasis.

Dried Persimmon Fruit

It is the cake-like food processed by the fruit of Diospyros kaki L. f. (Ebenaceae).

Effect. Moistening the lung, astringing the bowels and ceasing bleeding.

Indication. Hematemesis, hemoptysis, stranguria with hematuria, and dysentery.

Dried Toad

It is the whole body of Bufo bufo gargarizans Cantor or Bufo melanostictus Schneider (Bufonidae).

Effect. Removing the mass in the abdomen, promoting water within the body, removing toxic material, killing parasites and analgesic therapy.

Indication. Furuncles, lumbodorsal cellulitis, scrofula, masses in the abdomen, tympanites, hydrops, malnutrition of children induced by improper feeding.

Dried up Malaria Alba

Symptoms. Hollow, dried and white vesicle, occurrence of confusion in the late stage.

Pathogenesis. Due to malaria alba lasting for a long time and exhaustion of both qi and yin.

Therapeutic Principle. Emergency treatment for qi and fluid.

Dripping with Sweat after Delivery

Symptoms. Dripping with sweat, dizziness, palpitation and shortness of breath.

Pathogenesis. Due to qi-deficiency of the kidney and heart, severe deficiency of the body, after delivery of the women.

Therapeutic Principle. Nourishing the heart and the kidney.

Drooping of Pannus

It is a disease.

Symptoms. Filiform blood hanging down to the black eyeball, xerophthalmia and photophobia, blurred vision.

Pathogenesis. Obstruction of superficial venules induced by sufficiency of wind-heat in the lung and liver.

Therapeutic Principle. Smoothing the liver, removing heat to resolve pannus.

Drug Allergy

Referring to uneasy feeling induced by administration of drugs.

Symptoms. Annoyance and dysphoria with smothery sensation, itching in face and all over the body.

Pathogenesis. Mainly owing to an allergy to the drugs used, and caused by defficiency of stomach.

Therapeutic Principle. Drinking hot ginger decoction.

Drug Contraindication during Pregnancy

Referring to the drugs which are strictly forbidden or are to be used carefully in pregnant women, in order to prevent abortion or harmful to both woman and her fetus. For example poisonous drugs, pungent in flavour and heat in property, and drastic drugs of eliminating blood stasis, emetic, lubricant, etc.

Drugs for Arresting Bleeding

Referring to the drugs used for ceasing the bleeding internally and externally.

Effect. Ceasing bleeding by removing heat from the blood, by astringing, or by warming the meridians.

Indication. Hematemesis, hemoptysis, hemafecia, metrorrhagia, traumatic bleeding, etc.

Drugs for Arresting Secretion

Referring to the drugs used for ceasing and reducing the excessive loss of the vital essence and body fluid.

Effect. Ceasing cough, sweating, diarrhea, keeping the kidney essence, reducing urination, curing leukorrhagia, checking hemorrhage.

Indication. Spontaneous sweating, night sweat, chronic diarrhea, seminal emission, spermatorrhea, enuresis, chronic cough, asthma of deficiency type.

Drugs for Calming Liver and Checking Endogenous Wind

Referring to the drugs used for calming the liver and suppressing hyperactivity of the liver-yang as principal effects.

Effect. Calming the liver to suppress hyperactivity of the liver-yang.

Indication. Dizziness, headache caused by hyperactivity of the liver-yang, and epilepsy caused by terror and convulsion caused by up-stirring of endogenous wind resulting intense heat in the liver, etc.

Drugs for Causing Vomiting

Referring to the drugs used for enhancing, causing, or inducing vomiting as main effect.

Indication. Accidental poisoning of food in the stomach, indigestion and retention of food in the stomach, abdominal distention and pain, difficulty for breathing due to abundant accumulation of phlegm and fluid, etc.

Drugs for Clearing away Heat and Cooling Blood

Referring to the drugs used for clearing away heat and cooling the blood as the main effect.

Effect. Expelling pathogenic heat from the yin and blood systems and nourishing yin.

Indication. Restlessness, unconsciousness, delirium, hematemesis, hemafecia, etc. and febrile diseases, interior heat resulting from yin deficiency, etc.

Drugs for Clearing away Heat and Detoxicating

Referring to the drugs used for removing heat and detoxicating as the main effect.

Indication. Syndromes due to noxious heat, such as sores and carbuncles, erysipelas, maculas and eruptions, swollen and sore throat, mumps, dysentery, and also snake bite and carcinoma.

Drugs for Clearing away Heat and Drying Dampness

Referring to the drugs for removing heat and dampness as the main effect.

Indication. Diarrhea caused by damp-heat pathogen, dysentery, hemorrhoid complicated by anal fistula; damp-heat in the liver and gallbladder, such as distending pain in the hypochondrium, bitter taste in the mouth, jaundice; damp-heat in the lower-energizer, such as dribbling and painful micturition, leukorrhagia, swollen and painful joints, eczema, etc.

Drugs for Clearing away Heat and Purging Fire

Referring to the drugs used for removing heat as the main effect.

Indication. Febrile diseases, such as high fever, sweating, delirium and madness, diabetes, yellow dry coating on the tongue, etc.

Drugs for Clearing away Heat of Deficiency

Referring to the drugs used for removing heat of the deficiency type as the main effect.

Indication. Hectic or tidal fever resulting from yin deficiency, dryness in the mouth and throat, night sweat, red tongue with very little fur, resulting from yin internal heat; epidemic diseases at the later stage, such as fever, nocturnal fever, etc.

Drugs for Eliminating Sputum

Referring the drugs used for eliminating the sputum as the main effect.

Indication. Cough, abundant expectoration, asthma caused by pathologic change of the Lung-Meridian.

Drugs for Eliminating Wind-dampness

Referring to the drugs used for removing pathogenic wind and dampness and relieving arthralgia as the main effect.

Effect. Eliminating wind-dampness, relaxing muscles and tendons, promoting the flow of qi and blood in the meridians and collaterals, relieving pain and reinforcing the muscles and bones.

Indication. Arthralgia owing to wind-dampness, spasm of muscles, numbness and insensitive, hemiplegia, etc.

Drugs for Exterior Syndrome

Referring to the drugs used for removing the pathogenic factors from the superficies of the body and relieving exterior syndrome, clinically including two types: diaphoretic pungent in flavour and warm in property and diaphoretic pungent in flavour and cool in property.

Drugs for Improving Appetite and Digestion

Referring the drugs used for enhancing the digestion and appetite, clearing away the food retention and reinforcing the function of the spleen and stomach as the main effect.

Indication. Abdominal distention and pain belching, acid regurgitation, nausea, vomiting, and indigestion owing to the weakness of the spleen and stomach, etc.

Drugs for Inducing Diuresis and Excreting Dampness

Referring to the drugs used for adjusting liquid passages and relieving water-dampness in the body.

Effect. Releasing swelling, eliminating damp-heat, and inducing diuresis.

Indication. Dysuria, edema, phlegm retention, stranguria, jaundice, etc.

Drugs for Inducing Resuscitation

Referring to the drugs used for covering consciousness for inducing resuscitation.

Effect. Stimulating the sense organs and recovering consciousness.

Indication. Loss of consciousness, sudden coma in the course of terror-induced epilepsy or apoplexy, etc.

Drugs for Moistening Bowels

Referring to the drugs used for softening stool, releasing dryness and enhancing purgation as the main effect.

Indication. Constipation.

Drugs for Nourishing Yin

Referring to the drugs used for nourishing the yin fluid, enhancing the production of the body fluid, moisten dryness, and yin deficiency syndromes.

Drugs for Promoting Blood Circulation and Removing Blood Stasis

Referring to the drugs used for enhancing the blood circulation, releasing blood stasis, and clearing the meridians as the main effect.

Effect. Promoting blood circulation and removing blood stasis, clearing the meridians.

Indication. Various syndromes of blood stasis, for example, amenorrhea, dysmenorrhea, postpartum abdominal pain caused by retention of blood, obstruction of qi in the chest, rheumatic arthralgia, sores, carbuncles, traumatic injuries, etc.

Drugs for Relieving Cough and Asthma

Referring to the drugs used for preventing and/or relieving cough and asthma as the main effect.

Indication. Cough and asthma owing to internal injury and affection by exopathogen.

Drugs for Removing Water Retention

Referring to the drugs used for discharging the retained body fluid with stool as the main effect.

Indication. Edema, hydrothorax and ascites, and dyspnea owing to retention of phlegm and fluid.

Drugs for Replenishing Qi

Referring to the drugs used for replenishing qi and treating qi deficiency syndromes.

Indication. Deficiency of the spleen qi, such as anorexia, loose stool, gastric and abdominal distention, lassitude; deficiency of the lung-qi, such as short breath, hypologia, spontaneous sweating, etc.

Drugs for Restoring Deficiency Syndrome

Referring to the drugs used for supplementing materials needed by the human body, reinforcing the physiological hypofunction of the body, increasing body resistance to diseases and removing weakness syndromes.

Drugs for Tonifying Yang

Referring to the drugs used for nourishing yang-qi in the human body and treating insufficiency of yang-syndromes.

Indication. Cold limbs, lassitude in the waist and knees, impotence, prospermia, sterility owing to uterine coldness, frequent urination during the night, etc.

Drugs for Tranquilizing Mind

Referring to the drugs with the functions of releasing the uneasiness and calming down the mind.

Indication. Irritability, palpitation or severe palpitation, insomnia and dreaminess, and infantile convulsion, epilepsy, mania, etc.

Drugs for Warming Interior

Referring to the drugs with the functions of warming interior, dispelling cold, ceasing pain, etc.

Indication. Interior cold syndromes, such as gastric and abdominal cold pain, vomiting, diarrhea, cold limbs, pale tongue, etc.

Drum-like Ascites

Referring to abdominal distention like a drum.

Symptoms. Abdominal distention with borborygmus, oliguria, etc.

Pathogenesis. Due to over drinking of alcohol, leading to impairment of the spleen and stomach, and retention of fluid dampness.

Therapeutic Principle. Eliminating dampness, promoting diuresis, adjusting the flow of qi, and removing distention.

Dry Abdominalgia

Referring to a syndrome marked by intermittent pain in the abdomen without vomiting and diarrhea.

Symptoms. Intermittent pain in the abdomen without vomiting and diarrhea exacerbation upon movement.

Pathogenesis. Parasitic infestation.

Therapeutic Principle. Killing intestinal parasites.

Dry Asthma

Referring to dyspnea without coughing and phlegm.

Symptoms. Rapid respiration without cough and phlegm.

Pathogenesis. Owing to emotional depression and adverse stagnation of functional activities of qi.

Therapeutic Principle. Lowering the adverse-rising qi, releasing mental depression and ceasing asthma.

Dry Beriberi

Symptoms. Foot and leg weakness, numbness, aching pain, spasm.

Pathogenesis. Due to yang deficiency and interior heat, dampness-heat, impairment of blood and malnutrition of the muscles.

Therapeutic Principle. Dispersing obstruction, removing heat and dampness, adjusting the nutrient system.

Dry Cholera

Symptoms. Sudden attack of gripping pain in abdomen, difficulty in vomiting and defecating. In the serious case, bluish complexion and cold limbs.

Pathogenesis. Mostly caused by improper diet, impairment of the spleen and the stomach and affection by turbid pathogens.

Therapeutic Principle. Clearing away the turbid substance, enhancing the circulation of qi and relieving obstruction.

Dry Cough

Symptoms. Cough, abundant expectoration, thoracic depression, tachypnea, dyspnea and snoring sound from the throat.

Pathogenesis. Owing to qi deficiency resulting in obstruction of the air passage by phlegm and shortness of breath.

Therapeutic Principle. Nourishing primordial qi, and dispelling phlegm and enhancing the flow of the lung-qi.

Dry Hypochondriac Pain

Referring to a continuous slight pain in the hypochondrium.

Pathogenesis. Usually owing to excessive drinking and sexual intercourse.

Therapeutic Principle. Tonifying and replenishing qi and blood, enhancing qi circulation in the meridians and removing pain.

Dry Jaundice

Symptoms. Dysuria, and thirst for drink.

Pathogenesis. Usually owing to stagnation of the accumulated heat.

Therapeutic Principle. Removing heat and dampness.

Dry Mouth during Pregnancy

Symptoms. Subjective sensation of dryness in the mouth and pharynx for a woman during pregnancy.

Pathogenesis. Due to insufficiency and deficiency of the spleen and kidney, and lucid yang and body fluid failing to flow up to moisten the mouth.

Drynaria Rhizome

It is the rhizome of Drynaria fortunei (Kunze) J. Sm. (Drynariaceae), or D. baronii (Christ) Diels. (Polypodiaceae).

Effect. Invigorating the kidney, enhancing blood circulation, ceasing bleeding and enhancing reunion of injuries.

Indication. Lumbago owing to the kidney deficiency, weakness of the limbs, tinnitus, deafness, toothache, chronic diarrhea, traumatic injuries, etc.

Dryness Fire Vomiting

Referring to a disease and syndrome.

Symptoms. Vomiting with dyspnea, dry mouth and lips, excessive thirst, etc.

Pathogenesis. Due to retention of heat in the lung and stomach.

Therapeutic Principle. Releasing heat from the lung, moistening and ceasing vomiting.

Dryness Heat

Referring to a morbid condition.

Symptoms. Pain and swelling of the gums, tinnitus, epistaxis, dry cough, hemoptysis.

Pathogenesis. Owing to consumption of the body fluid by dryness-heat and transformation of it into fire.

Therapeutic Principle. Removing heat and enhancing salivation.

Dryness Heat Dysentery

Symptoms. Hot sensation, vexation, dry tongue and mouth, pain in the abdomen, purulent and bloody stools too sticky to defecate, insomnia and oliguria.
Pathogenesis. Owing to pathogenic dryness-heat.
Therapeutic Principle. Removing heat and detoxicating, for whitish pus stools and severe abdominal pain; for reddish pus and blood stools, cooling the blood, and removing heat and detoxicating; for blood stools and severe pain in the abdomen, adjusting qi and releasing heat from blood and toxic materials.

Dryness Heat Flaccidity

Symptoms. Flaccidity of the hands and feet with parched lips, dry mouth and throat, and wizened skin and hair, etc.
Pathogenesis. Owing to consumption of blood and impairment of body fluid by dryness heat, resulting in malnutrition of muscles and vessels.
Therapeutic Principle. Removing heat and moistening, and enriching yin and blood.

Dryness Transmission

Symptoms. Dry mouth, lips and throat, thirst, dry cough, constipation, oliguria, hemoptysis or nose bleeding.
Pathogenesis. Owing to insufficiency of the body yin fluid and excess of interior heat resulting in consumption of body fluid.

Dry Phlegm Syndrome

There are two meanings:
1. **Symptoms.** Subjective sensation of foreign bodies stuck in the pharynx that can neither be coughed up nor swallowed, distending fullness sensation in the chest and hypochondrium, etc.
Pathogenesis. Stagnation of phlegm in the pharyngeal diaphragm due to emotional stress.

Therapeutic Principle. Consist in soothing the liver and regulating the flow of qi.
2. **Symptoms.** Cough with asthma, or cough with bloody discharge.
Pathogenesis. Anger that impairs the liver, long period disorder of the liver-qi that results in heat-transmission, and impairment of the lung-qi.
Therapeutic Principle. Purging the liver of fire, promoting the dispersing function of the lung, and removing phlegm to relieve cough and asthma.

Dry Throat

Symptoms. Dryness in pharynx and larynx.
Pathogenesis. Due to yin insufficiency of the liver and kidney, flaring up of deficiency fire, or by insufficiency of the lung-yin, for deficiency type; or owing to the heat accumulation in the lung and stomach attacking the pharynx and larynx, for the excess type.

Dry Type of Inward Penetration of Pyogenic Agent

Referring to a syndrome, one kind of the syndromes of invasion of interior by pyogenic agent.
Symptoms. Pus should has been formed, dark grey color of the boil, pain, purple, flat and sunken base, dry and eroded boil top, fever, chills, spontaneous sweating, similar to hematosepsis.
Pathogenesis. Owing to inability to form pus and remove pathogenic factors from the body resulting from the impairment of both qi and blood.
Therapeutic Principle. Tonifying qi and the blood, draining pus and removing pathogenic factors from the interior, removing heart-fire and calming the mind.

Duanhongxue

An Extra acupuncture points.

Location. 1 cun anterior to the 2nd and 3rd metacarpophalangeal articulations of the dorsal hand.

Indication. Dysfunctional uterine bleeding.

Method. Puncture obliquely 0.5-1.0 cun.

Dubi (S 35)

A meridian acupuncture point.

Location. With the knee flexed, on the knee, in the depression lateral to the patella ligament.

Indication. Pain of the knee joint, numbness of the lower limbs, difficulty in flexing and stretching the knee, etc.

Method. Puncture obliquely 0.5-1.2 cun slightly towards the interior of the patellar ligament. Apply moxibustion 5-10 minutes.

Duiduan (GV 27)

A meridian acupuncture point.

Location. On the face, at the labial tubercle of the upper lip, at the junction of the skin and upper lip.

Indication. Coma, psychosis, hysteria, tremble mouth and lip, tremor diabetes with polydipsia.

Method. Puncture obliquely upward 0.2-0.3 cun. Moxibustion is forbidden.

Duji (Ex-B)

An extra point.

Location. On the back.

Indication. Epilepsy.

Method. Performing moxibustion.

Dujiao

Referring to a massage point.

Location. In both sides of the umbilicus 2 cun below the Tianshu (S 25) point.

Operation. Grasping or kneading mainly.

Function. Reinforcing the spleen and stomach, adjusting qi and releasing stagnancy.

Indication. Abdominal pain, fullness of abdomen, diarrhea, etc.

Duodenum (MA-SC 1)

An ear point.

Location. At the lateral 1/3 of the superior aspect of the helix crus.

Indication. Duodenal ulcer, pylorus spasm, cholecystitis and cholelithiasis.

Duoming (Ex-UE)

An extra point.

Location. In the biceps muscle of arm, at the midpoint of the line connecting Jianyu (LI 15) and Chize (L 5).

Indication. Syncope, pain in the forearm, erysipelas, etc.

Method. Puncture perpendicularly 0.5-1.0 cun.

Dushu (B 16)

A meridian acupuncture point.

Location. On the back, below the spinous process of the 6th thoracic vertebra, 1.5 cun lateral to the posterior midline.

Indication. Cardiac pain, abdominal pain and distention, borborygmus, hiccups.

Method. Puncture obliquely 0.5-0.8 cun. And apply moxibustion 3-5 moxa come or 5-15 minutes.

Dutchmanspipe Root

It is the root of Aristolochia debilis Sieb. et Zucc. and Aristolochia contorta Bge. (Aristolochiaceae).

Effect. Enhancing flow of qi, clearing away toxic materials and removing pain and swelling.

Indication. Distention and fullness of chest and hypochondrium, gastric and abdominal pain, snake bite, etc.

Dutchman's Pipe Vine

It is the stem and leaf of Aristolochia debilis Sieb. et Zucc. (Aristolochiaceae).

Effect. Enhancing blood and flow of qi circulation, removing dampness, and ceasing bleeding.

Indication. Stomachache, abdominal pain because of hernia, abdominal pain after childbirth, edema during pregnancy, pain because of pathogenic wind-dampness, etc.

Duyin (Ex-LE11)

An extra Point.

Location. On the plantar side of the second toe, at the midpoint of the distal interphalangeal joint.

Indication. Pain in the abdomen, vomiting, hiccups, hemoptysis, dead fetus resulting from difficult labor, hernia, etc.

Method. Puncture perpendicularly 0.1-0.2 cun and perform moxibustion to the point for 5-10 minutes or 3-5 units of moxa cones.

Dwarf Galangal Rhizome

It is the rhizome of Alpinia pumila Hook. F. (Zingiberaceae).

Effect. Clearing away dampness, relieving swelling, activating flow of qi and stopping pain.

Indication. Rheumatic arthralgia, stomachache, traumatic injuries, etc.

Dwarfism

Symptoms. Extreme shortness and slightness of stature, growing very slowly during the childhood, 30% lower than normal, more severe of the shortness with the increasing age, but the development of intelligence is normal.

Pathogenesis. Due to dyscrinism.

Dwarf Lilyturf Tuber Root

It is the root tuber of Ophiopogon japonicus Ker-Gawl or Liriope spicata Lour (Liliaceae) in the fibrous root.

Effect. Nourishing the lung and yin, invigorating the stomach, enhancing the production of body fluid, removing heart-fire and resolving vexation.

Indication. Dry cough with sticky sputum, phthisic cough with hemoptysis; deficiency of the stomach-yin syndromes as dry tongue, thirst, vexation, insomnia, constipation, etc.

Dwarf Wax Myrtle Root Bark

It is the root bark, stem bark or fruit of Myrica nana Cheval (Myricaceae).

Effect. Inducing astringency, ceasing bleeding, removing inflammation, stopping diarrhea, expelling stagnancy, invigorating the stomach and clearing away wind-dampness.

Indication. Dysentery, diarrhea, dyspepsia, metrorrhagia, metrostaxis, rectum bleeding, proctoptosis, traumatic injuries, etc.

Dye Yam

It is the stem tuber of Dioscorea cirrhosa Lour. (Dioscoreaceae).

Effect. Activating blood circulation, stopping bleeding, adjusting flow of qi and removing pain.

Indication. Postpartum abdominal pain, irregular menstruation, metrorrhagia and metrostaxis, hematemesis caused by visceral injury, arthralgia caused by wind-dampness, dysentery, furuncle, boil, snake bite, traumatic bleeding, etc.

Dying Sweating

Referring to a case that yin and yang depart from each other and yang-qi is exhausted.

Symptoms. Hidrosis like pearls or oil, sticky and greasy and not flow, often short and rapid respiration, cold limbs, etc.

Therapeutic Principle. Recovering depleted yang and rescuing the patient from collapse.

Dyschesia

Symptoms. Protracted interval defecation, or difficulty in bowel movement.

Pathogenesis. Mostly owing to heat in large intestine, or stagnation of qi, or accumulation of pathogenic cold, or insufficiency of both qi and blood, leading to dysfunction of the large intestine in transport.

Therapeutic Principle. First, nourishing blood and removing heat, and then relaxing bowels by purgation.

Dysentery

Referring to one of acute infectious diseases commonly seen in summer and autumn.

Symptoms. Abdominal pain, frequent excretion with less mucus, pus and blood.

Pathogenesis. Usually caused by the invasion of noxious damp-heat in the exterior, the interior injury caused by raw and cold food in the intestine.

Therapeutic Principle. Clearing away heat and dampness, removing pathogenic heat from blood and toxic materials from the body, promoting digestion and removing stagnated food.

Dysentery due to Cold-Dampness

Symptoms. White mucus in stool with a little blood, or watery stool, cold limbs, slight fever, absence of feeling of tenesmus.

Pathogenesis. Owing to the stagnation of qi and disordered transportation.

Therapeutic Principle. Removing the cold and dampness, adjusting the intestines and stomach, warming the middle-energizer.

Dysentery due to Damp-heat Pathogen

Symptoms. Frequent discharge of ropy bloody mucus stool, heavy and distending pain of abdomen, tenesmus, burning sensation of the anus, fever, thirst, yellowish greasy tongue coating.

Pathogenesis. Due to the accumulation of damp-heat pathogen in the intestines resulting in the stagnation of blood and qi and irregular transportation of the large intestine.

Therapeutic Principle. Clearing away heat and dampness, regulating qi circulation and promoting blood circulation.

Dysentery due to Deficiency Accumulation

Symptoms. Abdominal pain, tenesmus, and uncontrolled dysentery.

Pathogenesis. Due to the protracted accumulation resulting from the delicate and the weak spleen and stomach of children, and excessive indulgence in delicacies.

Therapeutic Principle. Invigorating the spleen and strengthening stomach, promoting digestion.

Dysentery due to Over-strain

Referring to chronic dysentery in the state of consumptive disease.

Symptoms. Chronic in the state of consumptive, tidal fever, fatigue, emaciation, etc.

Pathogenesis. Mostly caused by exhausting and injuring qi and blood, deficiency of intestines and stomach.

Therapeutic Principle. Nourishing yin and clearing away heat from the intestines.

Dysentery due to Seven Emotions

Symptoms. Indigested food in intestines and stomach, then unshaped, frequent and protracted watery stool gradually with pus and blood, etc.

Pathogenesis. Owing to impairment of the liver by emotional depression and anger, or the impairment of the spleen by melancholy, grief and anxiety, and indigestion.

Therapeutic Principle. Reinforcing and invigorations the spleen, warming the middle-energizer.

Dysentery with Indigested Food in Stool

There are three meanings:

1. Referring to dysentery caused by deficiency of the stomach and spleen and indigestion.

   Therapeutic Principle. Nourishing the spleen and warming middle-energizer.

2. Referring to dysentery caused by being unaccustomed to the new environment.

3. Referring to lienteric diarrhea.

Dysentery with Mucus or Purulent Discharge

Symptoms. Abdominal pain, tenesmus, dysentery with mucus or purulent discharge.

Pathogenesis. Due to the impairment of qi system by pathogenic damp-heat.

Therapeutic Principle. Removing the heat and the dampness; for the stagnation of cold-dampness, and the impairment of the spleen yang, warming the middle-energizer and eliminating dampness.

Dysfunction in Essence Storing

Symptoms. Spermatorrhea, involuntary emission, prospermia, incontinence of urine, frequent urination at night, diarrhea before dawn, etc.

Pathogenesis. Due to the kidney dysfunction of storing essence energy and controlling urine and feces.

Therapeutic Principle. Strengthening the kidney and controlling nocturnal emission.

Dysfunction of Limbs due to Yang Excess

Referring to a the abnormal activities of the limbs and abnormal gait due to excess of pathogenic yang.

Dysfunction of Liver-qi

Symptoms. Irritability, distending pain in hypochondrium, and breast or mass in breasts before menstrual cycle, and irregular menstruation.

Pathogenesis. Owing to excess or insufficiency of the liver function in adjusting the flow of qi and blood.

Therapeutic Principle. Smoothing the depressed liver and adjusting the circulation of qi.

Dysfunction of Middle-energizer

There are two meanings: 1. Physiological dysfunction due to qi disorder and disturbance in qi transformation of the spleen, stomach, and intestine and that of the liver and gallbladder; 2. The dysfunction of the spleen and stomach to enhance water, transport, distribute, and transform nutrients.

Dysfunction of Mind

Symptoms. Trance of mind, difficulty in turning over, heaviness sensation in the limbs, etc.

Pathogenesis. Due to domination of heat disturbing mind, qi failing to circulate.

Dysfunction of Qi Activity

Qi is enclosed within the body due to blockage of its passage, which results in disturbance of qi function and a morbid state.

Dysfunction of Six Fu-organs

It refers to pathologic mechanism due to disorder of the six fu-organs normal physiological function. Six fu-organs mean a collective term for the gallbladder, the stomach, the small intestine, the large intestine, the urinary bladder and the triple-energizer.

Dysfunction of Spleen in Transport

Symptoms. Abdominal distention, loose stool, poor appetite, listlessness emaciation, edema of limbs.

Pathogenesis. Irregular diet, over-thinking, over-strain and by the consumption of spleen-qi caused by the diseases of other organs.

Dysmenorrhea

It refers a disease in women with lower abdomen and lumbosacral portion pain or even severe and unbearable pain during, before, or after menstruation. Clinically, the diseases are divided into dysmenorrhea caused by qi stagnation; dysmenorrhea caused by blood stasis; dysmenorrhea caused by deficiency of qi and blood; dysmenorrhea caused by impairment of liver and kidney.

Dysmenorrhea due to Blood Stasis

Symptoms. Pricking pain in the lower abdomen with tenderness, occurring before or during the menstruation with little menstrual discharge. The pain is usually relieved by the discharge of blood clots.

Pathogenesis. Unfinished discharge of menses after delivery or menstrual cycle followed by the attack of cold or from internal impairment in emotion.

Therapeutic Principle. Reinforcing blood circulation to remove blood stasis and dredging the collaterals to arrest pain.

Dysmenorrhea due to Cold-dampness

Symptoms. Cold sensation and pain in the lower abdomen with tenderness before menses or during the menstrual cycle, and relieved by warmth, light flow menstruation, dark menses with clots.

Pathogenesis. Mostly resulting from the attack of external pathogenic cold or intake of cold drinks, sitting or sleeping in damp places during menstrual period.

Therapeutic Principle. Dispersing pathogenic cold and dampness, dredging the meridians to relieve pain.

Dysmenorrhea due to Deficiency of Qi and Blood

Symptoms. Lingering light pain in the lower abdomen, relieved by warmth and pressing, light flow, light-colored and thin menstruation, pale tongue.

Pathogenesis. Frequently caused by constitutional deficiency, or a deficiency of qi and blood.

Therapeutic Principle. Invigorating qi and nourishing the blood; supporting the spleen and alleviating pain.

Dysmenorrhea due to Impaired Liver-kidney Essence

Symptoms. Lingering light pain relieved by pressing in the lower abdomen during or after the menstrual period, thin, pink and scanty menses, soreness and pain in the loin and back, dizziness, tinnitus, pale complexion, lassitude, pale tongue.

Pathogenesis. Mostly caused by premature marriage or multiple childbirth, delicate constitution, resulting in impairment of the liver and kidney, deficiency of vital essence and lack of blood.

Therapeutic Principle. Tonifying the liver and kidney; enriching blood to regulate menstruation.

Dysmenorrhea due to Qi Stagnation

Symptoms. Distending pain in the lower abdomen before or during menstruation, with distention and fullness sensation in chest and breast, light menstruation by blood clots, dark tongue with ecchymosis, thin and reddish coating.

Pathogenesis. Mostly caused by the stagnation of liver-qi, impeded blood circulation.

Therapeutic Principle. Relieving the depressed liver and regulating the circulation of qi to promote menstrual discharge.

Dyspepsia

Symptoms. Fullness sensation in stomach, abdominalgia and tenderness, poor appetite, nausea, eructation with fetid odor and acid regurgitation, constipation.

Pathogenesis. Mainly due to dysfunction of both the stomach and spleen in transport, retention of indigested food.

Therapeutic Principle. Invigorating stomach and spleen and activating digestion to remove retention and stagnancy.

Dyspepsia due to Spleen Dysfunction

Symptoms. Abdominal distention and depressed pain, vomiting and acid regurgitation, etc.

Pathogenesis. Dysfunction of the spleen in transportation, food stagnation.

Therapeutic Principle. Enriching the spleen to promote digestion.

Dyspepsia during Pregnancy

Symptoms. Distention and fullness in the stomach and abdomen, or vomiting and diarrhea.

Pathogenesis. Mostly due to pregnant weakness of the spleen and stomach, and improper diet impairing the spleen and stomach.

Therapeutic Principle. Activating the spleen to enhance digestion.

Dysphagia

Symptoms. Difficulty swallowing to different degrees, distention and pain feeling in the chest, obstruction while eating solid food, instant vomiting after food intake, accompanied by progressive emaciation of the patient, lassitude. As severe obstruction, even difficulty in swallowing liquid diet, severe decrease of food intake, over consumption of the body fluids.

Pathogenesis. Mostly caused by severe melancholy and anxiety, leading to stagnation of qi, phlegm-coagulation and blood stasis, or resulting from over-eating and -drinking, resulting in the impairment of body fluid, exhaustion of essence and blood. Also caused by cancer of the esophagus.

Therapeutic Principle. Adjusting the spleen and stomach, tonifying yin and lower the adverse flow of qi.

Dysphagia due to Improper Diet

Symptoms. Retention of food and fullness sensation in stomach, emaciation, mental fatigue or listlessness, pain in the stomach and chest, etc.

Pathogenesis. Mainly due to stagnation of qi and excessive fire, dysfunction of the spleen in transport, retention of indigested food.

Therapeutic Principle. Adjusting the flow of qi, removing pathogenic fire, supplementing the spleen and enhancing digestion, etc.

Dysphagia due to Melancholy

Symptoms. Chocking feeling on swallowing, oppressed feeling in the stomach and chest, emotional stress, anorexia, dry throat and mouth, etc.

Pathogenesis. Impairment of the spleen resulting from excessive anxiety, accumulation of qi resulting from impairment of the spleen, failure to distribute body fluid, simultaneous accumulation of phlegm and qi in esophagus.

Therapeutic Principle. Clearing the liver and regulating qi, resolving phlegm and moistening dryness.

Dysphagia due to Visceral Injury

It is divided into two types, the excess type, and deficiency type.

The excess type:

Symptoms. Deglutition obstruction, thoracic diaphragmatic fullness or pain, eructation, hiccups, or vomiting.

Pathogenesis. Mostly due to stagnation of qi, blood stasis and obstruction of turbid phlegm in the stomach.

Therapeutic Principle. Relieving stagnation to promote the circulation of qi and reducing phlegm to resolve stagnation.

The deficiency type:

Symptoms. Dysphagia, odynophogia, but normal intake of water.

Pathogenesis. Mostly due to pathogenic fire invasion of emotional stress and consumes the body fluid.

Therapeutic Principle. Nourishing the body fluid and eliminating heat to resolve qi stagnation.

Dysphasia

Symptoms. Inflexibility of the tongue-movement with difficulty in speaking.

Pathogenesis. Attack of the wind and accumulation of phlegm and saliva.

Dysphonia due to Broken Metal

Symptoms. Hoarseness of voice caused by impairment of the lung-qi.

Pathogenesis. Mostly due to impaired function of the lung. Deficiency of lung yin or yin of the lung and kidney resulting in the throat is malnourished, thus hoarseness of voice.

Dysphoria and Fullness

Symptoms. Oppressed and full sensation in the chest due to vexation.

Pathogenesis. Internal sufficient pathogenic heat, or stagnation by accumulation of phlegm, or prolonged edema and retention of blood stasis.

Dysphoria due to Blood Deficiency

Symptoms. Fever, dysphoria, thirst, etc.

Pathogenesis. Mostly caused by the failure of blood to nourish the heart.

Therapeutic Principle. Nourishing blood and heart to calm mind.

Dysphoria during Pregnancy

Symptoms. For a pregnant woman, restlessness, depression, fearfulness, irritability, etc.

Pathogenesis. Mainly owing to the invasion of pathogenic heat into the heart.

Therapeutic Principle. Tonifying yin, removing pathogenic heat, and calming the mind, for the yin deficiency type; clearing away heat and phlegm, for upward disturbance by phlegm-heat.

Dysphoria with Feverish Sensation in Chest, Palms and Soles

Symptoms. Fever or feverish sensation in the palms and soles, and dysphoria with feverish sensation in the chest.

Pathogenesis. Mainly owing to hyperactivity of fire resulting from yin deficiency, or unrelieved fever of deficiency type after disease and internal stagnancy of fire and heat, etc.

Therapeutic Principle. Tonifying yin, releasing heat from the liver and adjusting the spleen, etc.

Dysphoria with Smothery Sensation

Symptoms. Dysphoria with subjective hot sensation or restlessness with depressed hot sensation.

Pathogenesis. Sufficient liver-fire, excessive heat caused by yin-deficiency, etc.

Dyspnea due to Anger

Symptoms. Shortness of breath, palpitation, fullness and pain in the chest, bitter mouth.

Pathogenesis. Injury of the liver by anger.

Therapeutic Principle. Alleviating mental depression, lowering the adverse flow of qi and relieving dyspnea.

Dyspnea due to Pathogenic Dryness Fire

Referring to restless dyspnea.

Symptoms. Out of breath cough caused by reversed flow of qi, thick sputum difficult to be coughed up, thirst, hot sensation, dark urine, etc.

Pathogenesis. Due to consumption of body fluid and impairment of the lung caused by dryness-heat.

Therapeutic Principle. Clearing away heat from the lung, and ceasing asthma.

Dyspnea due to Phlegm Retention

Symptoms. Alternation of cough with vomiting, dyspnea once in the lying position, pale complexion, etc.

Pathogenesis. Retention of phlegm going up to the lung due to drinking too much water and dysfunction in transportation and transformation.

Therapeutic Principle. Warming the lung and dispelling phlegm, removing heat and dispelling phlegm and relieving asthma.

Dyspnea due to Stagnancy of Pathogenic Fire in Lung

Symptoms. Shortness of respiration, suffocation, dyspnea, cold limbs, restlessness.

Pathogenesis. Pathogenic fire stagnating and blocking the circulation of lung-qi, and failure of lung-qi to practice the function of dispelling.

Therapeutic Principle. Dispelling the stagnated heat.

Dyspnea of Deficiency Type

Symptoms. Short breath and dyspnea, the frequency of more exhalation and less inhalation, asthmatic breath with low weak sound.

Pathogenesis. Due to the weakness for aging, prolonged asthma disease, or the impairment of the primordial qi during the convalescence, qi deficiency of the lung and spleen, and the failure of the kidney to receive qi.

Therapeutic Principle. Strengthening the lung and kidney.

Dyspnea of Excess Type

Symptoms. Rapid breathing, forceful and coarse breathing with acute onset.

Pathogenesis. Mainly due to stagnation of pathogen in the lung, dysfunction of lung-qi in dispersing and clarifying and sending-down, and obstruction of air passage.

Therapeutic Principle. Eliminating pathogenic factors and promoting circulation of qi.

Dyspnea of Kidney Type

Symptoms. Short breath aggravated on horizontal position, excessive phlegm stuffiness of the chest, expectorated easily, etc.

Pathogenesis. Invasion of the lung by upward rising of pathogenic water in the kidney.

Therapeutic Principle. Warming the liver and removing diuresis, eliminating heat from the lung and relieving asthma.

Dyspnea with Chest Distention

Symptoms. Cough, dyspnea, palpitation, edema of face and lower limbs, stuffiness of chest, distending abdomen, oliguria, etc.

Pathogenesis. Usually due to dysfunction of the lung and the spleen, resulting in accumulation of water, obstruction of air passage.

Therapeutic Principle. Warming the kidney and replenishing the spleen.

Dyspnea with Elevated Shoulders

Symptoms. Cough, dyspnea with mouth open and elevated shoulders, abundant phlegm and fluid.

Pathogenesis. Mostly due to impairment of clearing-up and descending function of the lung, and abnormal rising of the lung-qi.

Therapeutic Principle. Facilitating the lung-qi to relieve asthma, and sending down abnormally ascending qi.

Dystocia due to Blood Deficiency

One of the symptom complexes of dystocia.

Pathogenesis. Owing to difficult fetal rotation during delivery induced by blood deficiency of the parturient.

Therapeutic Principle. Nourishing qi and blood to induce expulsion of the fetus.

Dystocia due to Qi Stagnation

Symptoms. Difficult give birth to the fetus.

Pathogenesis. Parturient   anxiety and fearfulness during the prolonged labour process and qi stagnation.

Therapeutic Principle. Adjusting the circulation of qi and calming the mind.

Dystocia due to Reverse Flow of Qi

It refers to delayed prolonged process of delivery.

Pathogenesis. Mostly due to weakness of the rotating movement and slow descending of the fetus to the pelvis caused by disorder and reverse flow of qi because of the parturient mental stress, fearfulness and long staying in the labor room.

Therapeutic Principle. Reinforcing the circulation of qi and calming the mind.

Dystocia Prevention

It refers to the therapeutic method by strengthening the mother-qi to prevent dystocia and restraining the fetus for smooth delivery in the third trimester of pregnancy.

Dysuria

Symptoms. Oliguria and difficulty in urination.

Pathogenesis. Owing to dysfunction of qi in transforming the body fluid, the retention of water dampness or the stagnation of damp-heat.

Dysuria due to Bladder Dysfunction

Symptoms. Distention and fullness of hypogastrium, dysuria or uroschesis.

Pathogenesis. Mostly caused by disturbance in qi transformation of the lung, kidney and the tri-energizer.

Dysuria with Milky Urine

Symptoms. Difficult urination with pain, cloudy rice water like urine with floating oil or blood filaments, blood clots, dry mouth, etc.

Pathogenesis. Caused by dysfunction of both the spleen and the kidney resulting in inability to separate the refined essence and turbid urine.

Therapeutic Principle. Supplementing the spleen and eliminating dampness; nourishing the kidney and reinforcing the astringency.

E

Eagle Wood

It is the black resinous wood of Aquilaria agallocha Roxb. and A. sinensis (Lour) Gilg. (Thymelaeaceae).

Effect. Promoting the circulation of qi, removing pain, warming the kidney and improving inspiration, adjusting the middle-energizer, warming the spleen.

Indication. Cold retention in middle-energizer, distention and pain in the chest and abdomen, vomiting due to cold in the stomach, and asthma of deficiency type due to failure of the kidney in receiving qi.

Ear Acupuncture

Referring to puncturing certain reaction spots (points) on the auricle to treat disease.

Ear Acupuncture Anesthesia

Referring to one kind of acupuncture anesthesia. Puncturing particular ear points to induce analgesia during surgery.

Early Columbine Herb

It is the whole plant with root of Aquilegia parviflora Ledeb. or Aquilegia oxysepala Trautv. et. Mey (Rapunculaceae).

Effect. Dispelling obstruction of the menstrual flow and promoting the blood circulation.

Indication. Irregular menstruation, gynecopathy, etc.

Early Graying Hair

Referring to premature graying of hair, mainly due to deficiency of the kidney and insufficiency of blood.

Ear Nodule

Referring to the syndrome of bacteria-like nodules growing in the ear.

Symptoms. Forming in the acoustic meatus bacteria-like nodules, with big heads but small bases and slight swelling, pain on touching, blocking the orifice of the ear if serious.

Pathogenesis. Due to condensation of fire-toxin in the liver and kidney.

Therapeutic Principle. Clearing the liver and removing heat.

Earth

This term has two meanings: 1. Referring to one of five elements. Among five elements, fire generating earth, wood restricting earth, and earth generating metal. 2. A synonym of the spleen, usually called the spleen (earth).

Earth Being Source

1. Referring to the earth being the basis of all things, all things generate and develop on earth. 2. Referring to the spleen and stomach of the human body.

Earth Failing to Control Water

Based on the theory of the restraint relation of the five elements, under the normal condition, the spleen (earth) controls water and makes water transportation normally. When the spleen is too weak to control the kidney (water), water overflows to result in such disorders as fluid retention and edema.

Earth Preferring Warmth and Dryness

Earth refers to the spleen. Warmth and dryness are beneficial to the digestive and transporting function of the spleen, while coldness and dampness or over-eating of cold food may disturb the function of the spleen in transporting, distributing and transforming.

Earth Producing Myriad Things

Based on the theory of five elements, the spleen and stomach belong to earth. Based on this theory, the spleen and stomach can be treated as the source for generation and transformation of qi and blood. The stomach controls receiving, digesting and transforming food. The spleen controls absorbing and transporting food essence to provide the material foundation for generation and function of viscera, organs and tissues.

Earth Region

Referring to the upper and lower eyelids, relating to the stomach, which is mainly in charge of holding and digesting water and foodstuff. Observing changes in this part, one can examine the pathological process in the spleen and stomach.

Earthworm E-1

It is the whole body of Pheretima aspergillum (Perrier), or Allobophora caliginosa (Savigny) trapezoides (Ant, Duges) (Megascolecidae).

Effect. Removing heat from the lung, relieving asthma, spasm, clearing and activating the meridians and collaterals, inducing diuresis for treating stranguria.

Indication. High fever, epilepsy induced by terror, spasm and infantile convulsion; arthralgia-syndrome with arthralgia, joints with difficulty in flexion and extension, hemiplegia resulting from apoplexy, cough with dyspnea resulting from heat in the lung, heat stranguria, dysuria, etc.

East-liaoning Oak Fruit

The fruit of Quercus liaotungensis Koidz. (Fagaceae).

Effect. Reinforcing the spleen, ceasing diarrhea, bleeding.

Indication. Abdominal diarrhea resulting from hypofunction of the spleen, hemorrhoidal hemorrhage and proctoptosis.

Easy Cold and Easy Heat

Referring to the status of young yang and yin of an infant. Yin damaged and yang increased a lot, then heat is produced, and also, yang reduced and yin increased a lot, then cold is produced easily, once an infant caught a disease.

Eczema

Symptoms. Common dermatosis.

Pathogenesis. Owing to the attack of pathogenic wind, heat and dampness resulting in the blockage of the dermal meridians.

Eczema due to Blood Deficiency

Referring to one type of eczema.

Symptoms. Rough and thick skin with itching sensation and white-bits coming off, dark brown color of the impaired skin, difficult to cure and frequently attack.

Pathogenesis. Due to prolonged eczema and postponed treatment, blood deficiency resulting from wind and dryness, leading to the failure to nourish the skin.

Therapeutic Principle. Enriching the blood and moistening the dryness.

Eczema due to Damp-heat Pathogen

Referring to a type of eczema.

Symptoms. Beginning with inflammation of local skin, small purple vesicles, and then ulceration with yellowish fluid.

Pathogenesis. Due to attack of the pathogenic factors of wind, dampness and heat, resulting in the blockage of the dermatic meridians.

Therapeutic Principle. Removing dampness and heat.

Edema

Referring to a disease due to retention of fluid dampness in the body.

Symptoms. Facial, limbs, thoracic, abdominal or even general edema, including the excess type and the deficiency type.

Pathogenesis. For the excess type by invasion of exopathic factors, and functional irregularity of qi in transport. For the deficiency type, yang deficiency of the spleen and kidney, failure of transfer of fluid dampness.

Therapeutic Principle. For the former, enhancing the dispersing function of the lung, releasing dampness by diuresis, retained fluid as well as pathogenic factors. For the latter, warming the kidney, nourishing the spleen, enhancing the flow of qi, activating yang etc., with strengthening the body resistance.

Edema Caused by Infantile Convulsion

Symptoms. Swollen limbs and fever.

Pathogenesis. Resulting from repeatedly fright, excessive heart-fire, over-drinking, the failure of spleen-qi.

Therapeutic Principle. Reinforcing the spleen, and enhancing diuresis.

Edema due to Blood Stasis

Symptoms. Edema of limbs, string-like blood stasis on the skin, or edema after menstruation, lower abdominal pain and tenderness, long and thin urine, etc.

Pathogenesis. Retention of blood stasis combined with fluid and dampness.

Therapeutic Principle. Enhancing blood circulation, releasing blood stasis, enhancing diuresis, removing edema.

Edema due to Cold-dampness

Symptoms. Bodily edema, severe bodily pain, oppressed feeling in the chest, cold feet, etc.

Therapeutic Principle. Removing cold by warming up the meridians.

Edema due to Damp-heat

Symptoms. Fever with yellowish eyes, swollen body, reddish urine, difficulty in micturition, distention and fullness in the chest and abdomen.

Pathogenesis. Damp-heat retained on the skin for a long time.

Therapeutic Principle. Removing dampness, heat, enhancing diuresis.

Edema due to Disease of Large Intestine

A disease and syndrome referring to the edema due to disease of large intestine.

Symptoms. Frequent edema and alternation of loose stool and constipation.

Pathogenesis. Due to the disorder of large intestinal transportation, the disfunctional activities of qi, the retention of fluid and dampness in the body, gathering and spreading irregularly.

Therapeutic Principle. Removing dampness and enhancing diuresis.

Edema due to Menstruation

Symptoms. Cyclic edema in the limbs and face during, before or after menstruation.

Pathogenesis. Mostly due to flooding and retention of water in the body resulting from deficiency of both the spleen and kidney.

Therapeutic Principle. Reinforcing the spleen, warming up the kidney and enhancing diuresis.

Edema due to Pathogenic Dryness-fire

Symptoms. Edema of face and the whole body, dyspnea, prickly sensation in hypochondriacs, restlessness, insomnia, dry mouth and lips, reddish and uneven urine, and rapid pulse.

Pathogenesis. Due to dry weather, shortage of water, impairment of the clearing function of lung, and the blocking of air passage.

Therapeutic Principle. Removing heat, nourishing the lung, enhancing diuresis, relieving edema.

Edema due to Qi-stagnation

Symptoms. Dyspnea with the sensation of swollen fullness, vexation and stuffiness of the chest, cough with expectoration of sputum, scanty urine, etc.

Pathogenesis. Due to impairment of purifying and descending function of the lung, deficiency of the kidney yang, disturbance in qi transportation, stagnation of water-dampness in skin.

Therapeutic Principle. Enhancing the dispersing function of the lung, nourishing the kidney, and inducing diuresis to remove edema.

Edema due to Spleen Deficiency

Symptoms. Tired and heavy limbs, loose stool, yellowish and withered complexion, swelling all over the body now and then, etc.

Pathogenesis. Resulting from weakness and deficiency of the spleen.

Therapeutic Principle. Warming up and nourishing the spleen-qi.

Edema due to Unacclimatization

A disease and syndrome, referring to the edema due to unacclimatization.

Symptoms. Swollen face and body, or diarrhea, inability to eat, oppressed feeling, shortness of breath, etc.

Pathogenesis. Due to the spleen deficiency or interior dampness.

Therapeutic Principle. Reinforcing the spleen and removing dampness.

Edema due to Yang Deficiency

Symptoms. Disfunction of metabolism and the metabolic disturbance of water, leading to the water invasion on the muscles and skin, chronic edema as a result.

Pathogenesis. Resulting from yang insufficiency of the kidney, or both the spleen and kidney.

Therapeutic Principle. Warming yang for diuresis or warming the kidney for enhancing diuresis.

Edema during Convalescence

Pathogenesis. Due to the spleen deficiency and the failure of the spleen to regulate water passages and to transfer water-dampness.

Therapeutic Principle. Reinforcing the spleen and inducing diuresis.

Edema during Metrorrhagia

1. Referring to women suffering from edema after amenorrhea.
2. Referring to a disease in the blood system and opposite to the disease of qi system.

   Therapeutic Principle. Restoring menstrual flow for diuresis.

Edema in Children due to Small Intestinal Disease

A disease and syndrome referring to a type of infantile edema due to the small intestinal disease.

Symptoms. Edema, the lower abdomen fullness.

Pathogenesis. Due to the stagnant heat and damp striking each other flowing downward into lower-energizer.

Therapeutic Principle. Removing heat and damp.

Edema of Limbs

Symptoms. Edema and distention of the four limbs.

Pathogenesis. Due to invasion of exo-pathogen, abnormality of qi-transmission, deficiency of qi and blood, yang deficiency of the spleen and kidney and failure to transport dampness leading to floods into the skin.

Therapeutic Principle. Enhancing the dispersing function of the lung, warming the kidney, reinforcing the spleen, replenishing qi and removing wind, dampness by diuresis.

Edema of Lower Limb

Symptoms. Edema from knees to feet in a woman 1-4 months into the pregnancy, with clear and profuse urine.

Pathogenesis. Mostly due to qi stagnation resulting from depression, obstructing its qi from rising and falling, or from downward flow of body fluid and dampness due to yang deficiency of the spleen and kidney.

Therapeutic Principle. Enhancing qi circulation, removing stagnation and dampness for the former; warming yang, reinforcing the spleen and removing dampness for the latter.

Edematization

1. Referring to edema.

   Symptoms. Skin and limbs overfilled with body fluid.

   Pathogenesis. Due to qi deficiency of the kidney and spleen.

2. Only referring to abdominal distention.

Edematous Granulation

Referring to the granulation tissue growing above the skin after ulceration, i.e. granulation edema.

Symptoms. Hyperplasia of granulation tissue on the skin, easily bleeding when touched, remaining unhealed for a long time.

Therapeutic Principle. Checking and reducing edematous granulation.

Edema with Heart Involved

Symptoms. Distention and heaviness of the body, shortness of breath, palpitation, inability to lie on the back, even edema of the genitals.

Pathogenesis. Resulting from the failure of the heart to control water due to the insufficiency of the heart-yang, the reversed flow of water into the heart.

Therapeutic Principle. Warming yang, relieving dampness by diuresis, tonifying qi and the heart.

Edema with Lung Involved

Symptoms. General anasarca, oliguria, shortness of breath, cyanosis of lips and tongue, etc.

Pathogenesis. Pulmonary failure to descend, to dredge water passages to the urinary bladder.

Therapeutic Principle. Enhancing the dispersing function of the lung and inducing diuresis.

Edema with Spleen Involved

Referring to a kind of five Zang edema.

Symptoms. Abdominal distention, heaviness of limbs, deficiency of qi and oliguria with difficulty, etc.

Pathogenesis. Due to the failure of the spleen in transporting water-dampness resulting from deficiency of the spleen-yang.

Therapeutic Principle. Warming up yang and activating the spleen.

Edible Birds Nest

It is the nest built with saliva or saliva mixed with villi by Collocalia esculenta (Apodidae), and many other swallows of the same breed.

Effect. Tonifying qi, moistening dryness, strengthening the function of the spleen and stomach.

Indication. Cough with phlegm-dyspnea, hemoptysis, hematemesis, protracted dysentery, chronic malaria, etc.

Edible Yam Rhizome

It is the stem tuber of Dioscorea eseulenta (Lour.) Burkll. (Dioscoreaceae).

Effect. Reinforcing the middle-energizer, supplementing qi and tonifying the kidney.

Indication. Insufficiency of spleenogastric qi, anorexia, diarrhea and lumbago due to kidney deficiency.

Eel

It is the whole body or flesh of Monopterus albus (Zuiew).

Effect. Treating deficiency syndromes, removing pathogenic wind and dampness, reinforcing muscles and bones.

Indication. Arthralgia resulting from pathogenic   wind-cold-dampness, postpartum, stranguria, dysentery with pus and blood in the stools, piles, ecthyma, etc.

Eel Blood

It is the blood of Monopterus albus (Zuiew).

Effect. Removing the wind, enhancing blood circulation and reinforcing yang.

Indication. Facial hemiparalysis, earache, epistaxis, tinea, fistule, etc.

Effects of Qi Sensation

A term in Qigong terminology referring to various sensational reactions resulting from the qi sensations, gained by a Qigong practitioner during Qigong practice. The reactions of qi sensation: borborygmus; a hot sensation at Dantian; cold, hot, expanding, and tingling. Sensations of the acupoints Laogong (P8) and Yongquan (K1).

Egen (Ex-HN)

An extra acupuncture point.

Location. At the lower area of jaw, 1 cun in the front of the angle of mandible.

Indication. Acute or chronic tonsillitis, laryngopharyngitis, etc.

Method. Puncture 0.5-1 cun perpendicularly.

Egg

The egg of Gallus gallus domesticus Brisson (Phasianidac).

Effect. Moisturizing dryness by nourishing yin, nourishing the blood and preventing abortion.

Indication. Febrile disease with vexation, cough due to dryness, celostomia, sore throat, threatened abortion, postpartum thirsty, dysentery and scalds.

Egg Moxibustion

Referring to a type of indirect moxibustion.

Method. Put half of a boiled egg on the affected area (without the yolk), and apply moxibustion with a moxa cone on the eggshell until the patient filling the sensation of heat and itching.

Indication. Lumbodorsal cellulitis, carbuncle and cellulitis at early stage, etc.

Eggplant Disease

A type of prolapse of uterus.

Symptoms. In women, reddish or whitish eggplant-like object projecting from the vagina.

Pathogenesis. Due to dampness heat, and qi deficiency.

Therapeutic Principle. Removing heat and enhancing diuresis for the case with red color and due to dampness; and replenishing qi, elevating the spleen-qi, for one with whitish color, and due to qi deficiency.

Egg Shell

It is the egg shell of Gallus gallus domesticus Brisson (Phasianceae).

Effect. Detoxicating and ceasing bleeding.

Indication. Gastric abscess resulting from fluid retention, regurgitation, infantile rickets, various bleeding, nebula, furuncles on the head or on the skin and ulcer.

Egg White

It is the egg white of Gallus gallus domesticus Brisson (Phasianidae).

Effect. Moistening the lung to arrest cough, removing heat and detoxicating.

Indication. Sore throat, conjunctival congestion, dry cough, dysentery, malaria, burn, and painful swelling due to noxious heat.

Egg Yolk

It is the yolk of Gallus gallus domesticus Brisson (Phasiaridae).

Effect. Tonifying yin, moisturizing the viscera, and nourishing the blood to cease wind.

Indication. Irritability, insomnia, infantile convulsion due to febrile disease, hematemesis due to consumption, vomiting, dysentery, scalds, and infantile dyspepsia.

Eight Confluence Points

Referring to a category of points. Indicating the points at which the qi of the eight extra meridians are connecting the qi of the 12 regular meridians, including Gongsun (Sp 4), Neiguan (P 6), Houxi (SI 3), Shenmai (B 62), Zulinqi (G 41) Waiguan (TE 5), Lieque (L 7), Zhaohai (K 6). The effects of the points may lead to their connected extra meridians from their own meridians, for treating various diseases of the head and body.

Eight Deficiencies

Referring to the eight positions easily attacked by pathogens: elbow, axilla, thigh and popliteal fossa on both sides. These portions are the vital pathways for circulation of qi and blood. If pathogenic qi retains there, the muscles and joints show the symptoms such as difficulty in flexion and extension.

Eighteen Incompatible Medicaments

Referring to the incompatibility of traditional Chinese drugs in a prescription. The following eighteen traditional Chinese drugs with the serious side effects of incompatibility: pinellia tuber, trichosanthes fruit, fritillary bulb, ampelopsis root and bletilla tuber being incompatible with aconite root; seaweed, knoxia root, kansu rot and genkwa flower, incompatible with liquorice; ginseng, glehnia root, red sage root, scrophularia root, asarum root and peony root, incompatible with veratrum root.

Eight Essentials

Referring to the eight key points of diagnosis and treatment, they are: deficiency, excess, cold, heat, pathogenic factor, vitality, interior, and exterior.

Eight Influential Points

Referring to the eight influential acupoints closely related to Zang, Fu, qi, blood, tendon, blood vessel, bone and marrow. i.e. Zang is associated with Zhangmen (Liv 13), Fu with Zhongwan (CV 12), qi with Danzhong (CV 17) blood with Geshu (B 17), bone with Dazhu (B 11) and marrow with Juegu Xuanzhong (B 39).

Eight Liaos

A general name of eight points on both sides of meridian, namely: Sangliao (B 31), Ciliao (B 32), Zhongliao (B 33) Xialiao (B 34).

Eight Methods for Needling Manipulation

Referring to a general term for acupuncture manipulations. The eight methods are: fathoming, clawing, twisting, flicking, shaking, pressing, massaging along meridians, and twirling.

Elbow (MA-SF 3)

Referring to an ear point.
Location. If dividing the scapha area into six equal parts, the third from the top is the right point.
Indication. Diseases in the elbow area, external humeral epicondylitis and diseases of the thyroid gland.

Elbow-dorsum Tumor

Symptoms. If benign tumor, generally no constitutional symptom, only local prominence and slight pain. If malignant tumor, obvious local areola and swelling, severe pain with general symptom, such as anorexia, listlessness, emaciation, and anemia, etc.
Therapeutic Principle. For the benign one, external application of medicine, or removal of local focus for the malignant one.

Elecampane Inula Root ⊛ E-2

It is the dried root of Inula helenium L. or Inula racemosa Hook f. (Compositae).
Effect. Reinforcing the spleen and stomach, enhancing the flow of qi, removing stagnancy, pain and preventing abortion.

Indication. Distention and pain in the chest, hypochondrium and abdomen, vomiting, diarrhea, pain in the chest and hypochondrium, and threatened abortion.

Eliminating Dampness with Aromatics

Referring to the treatment of diseases.

Symptoms. Heaviness in the head and the body, fullness in the stomach, abdominal distention, nausea, vomiting, loose stool and greasy fur.

Pathogenesis. Owing to damp stagnancy.

Therapeutic Principle. With the drugs of aromatics, releasing dampness.

Eliminating Dampness with Drugs Bitter in Flavor and Warm in Nature

Symptoms. Heaviness of the head and the body, tastelessness without thirst, fullness in the stomach and abdominal distention, nausea, vomiting, clear loose stool, white and greasy fur, and soft quick pulse.

Pathogenesis. Owing to accumulation of dampness and incoordination between the spleen and the stomach.

Therapeutic Principle. With the drugs of bitter in taste and warm in nature, to remove dampness pathogens.

Eliminating Heat of Ying System through Qi System

Symptoms. High fever at night, dysphoria, insomnia, or faint skin rashes, deep-red and dry tongue, thready and quick pulse.

Pathogenesis. Owing to heat in the ying system, toxication, pathogenic heat spreading into yinfen system.

Therapeutic Principle. Removing heat, and detoxicating.

Elongated Nipple

Symptoms. Elongation of the nipple.

Pathogenesis. Due to attack by excessive wind-heat of the Liver Meridian.

Therapeutic Principle. Treating by meditation of diseases belonging to Triple Energizer and Gallbladder Meridians.

Emaciation due to Blood Disorders

Referring to consumptive disease with stasis and deficiency of blood in women.

Symptoms. Oligomenorrhea or amenorrhea, emaciation, poor appetite, hectic fever, and darkish complexion.

Pathogenesis. Due to impairment by five kinds of consumptive diseases, unremoved blood stasis, difficulty in producing new blood, and failure of blood and fluid to nourish yin.

Therapeutic Principle. Enhancing blood circulation, releasing heat, blood stasis, nourishing yin.

Emaciation due to Emotional Upset

1. Referring to the syndrome with fever and emaciation.

   Symptoms. Female with amenia and hematochezia; in male hemorrhage, emission, etc.

   Pathogenesis. Resulting from mental depression and disturbance, overanxiety and mental exhaustion.

   Therapeutic Principle. Smoothing the liver and adjusting the circulation of qi, the mental activities and function of the spleen.

2. One type of diabetes referring to diabetes due to dryness-heat.

Emaciation in Children

Referring to the infantile weakness and emaciation.

Symptoms. High fever and yellowish skin. The infant has loss of appetite, is even unable to eat and drink, and becomes emaciated.

Pathogenesis. Weakness of the spleen and stomach of infant due to improper feeding, dysentery.

Therapeutic Principle. Removing heat, reinforcing the spleen and stomach in the patient having heat; warming middle-energizer, reinforing the spleen, and stomach in the patient having cold.

Emaciation Sterility

Symptoms. Flush of zygoma, dryness in the pharynx, tidal fever, night sweat, emaciation, irregular menstruation, sterility, etc.

Pathogenesis. Resulting from emaciation, insufficiency of essence and blood, and fire hyperactivity due to yin deficiency leading to malnutrition of the Vital and the Front Middle Meridians and the uterus.

Therapeutic Principle. Tonifying yin and the kidney, enriching blood, adjusting menstruation.

Emerging Purgation

Referring to the effect of the drugs used, with sour and bitter taste, on inducing vomiting and purgation.

Emission due to Consumption

Symptoms. Emission due to consumption occurred in the diseases.

Pathogenesis. Due to spleen deficiency, unsteady seminal fluid, hyperactivity of heat due to yin deficiency.

Emission due to Hearing Disease

Symptoms. Palpitation, dizziness, insomnia, emission, etc.

Pathogenesis. Due to hyperactivity of fire resulting from deficiency of yin, and exhaustion of blood.

Therapeutic Principle. Removing the heart-heat and consolidating the kidney.

Emission due to Lung-qi

A kind of emission.

Symptoms. Emaciation, dry cough with less phlegm or blood stained sputum, afternoon fever, night sweat, emission in dream, etc.

Pathogenesis. Due to the failure of the lung-qi, or the hyperactivity of fire resulting from yin deficiency of the lung, etc.

Therapeutic Principle. Nourishing the lung-qi, yin fluid and releasing the heat of deficiency type.

Emission due to Splenic Disease

Symptoms. Emission, yellowish complexion, emaciation, lassitude of limbs, etc.

Pathogenesis. Due to splenic disease.

Therapeutic Principle. Nourishing the spleen, benefiting the kidney and stopping nocturnal emission.

Emission of Kidney Type

Symptoms. Freqent emission, lassitude in loin and legs, dry throat, vexation, tinnitus, amnesia, etc.

Pathogenesis. Because of spermatorrhoea due to kidney deficiency, and failure in ceasing essence.

Therapeutic Principle. Nourishing the kidney, arresting essence.

Emotional Disorder

Symptoms. Low spirit, listlessness, fullness in the diaphragm, lassitude, poor appetite,

Pathogenesis. Due to excessive sadness.

Therapeutic Principle. Nourishing the heart and spleen, adjusting the emotions.

Emotional Dysphagia

Symptoms. Difficulty in swallowing, emaciation, weakness, dysphoria and shortness of breath.

Pathogenesis. Due to melancholy and qi-stagnation.

Therapeutic Principle. Adjusting qi, removing mental depression.

Empirical Selection of Points

Referring to method for selecting points. Based on the clinical experiences to select effective points, usually extra acupuncture points (magical points). For instance, puncturing Sifeng (Ex-UE 10) for infantile malnutrition, and selecting Yiming (Ex-HN 14) for poor vision, etc.

Endocrine (MA IC-13)
Referring to an ear point.
Location. At the bottom of the cavum conchae in the intertragic notch.
Indication. Dysmenorrhea, impotence, irregular menstruation (menopausal), climacteric syndrome, abnormality of endocrine function, acne, intermittent malaria.

Endogenous Cold
Referring to a syndrome.
Symptoms. Vomiting, diarrhea, abdominal pain, cold limbs or edema and phlegm retention. The phlegm, saliva, nasal discharge, and urine are clear and stool is loose.
Pathogenesis. Insufficiency of yang-qi and dysfunction of the Zang-fu organs leading to disturbance of fluid transportation and the retention of turbid yin.
Therapeutic Principle. Warm the interior and remove cold.

Endogenous Cold but Exogenous Heat
Symptoms. Real cold in the interior with pseudo-heat in the exterior.
Pathogenesis. Owing to the excessive yin in the interior and checking yang in the exterior.
Therapeutic Principle. Recuperating depleted yang and rescuing the patient from collapse.

Endogenous Dampness
Referring to the retention of water inside the body.
Symptoms. Poor appetite, abdominal distention, diarrhea, oliguria, yellow face, edema, pale tongue, greasy fur, soft and slow pulse.
Pathogenesis. Due to yang deficiency of the spleen and kidney and functional disturbance in water transportation.

Therapeutic Principle. Warming up for releasing dampness.

Endogenous Dryness
Referring to a syndrome of dryness.
Symptoms. Hectic fever, restlessness, thirst, dry tongue and lips, pachylosis, withered hair, thin muscles, constipation and oliguria.
Pathogenesis. Due to consumption of the yin-fluid and lack of moisturizing of the tissues, organs and their openings.
Therapeutic Principle. Nourishing yin, moisturizing dryness.

Endogenous Wind
1. Referring to a disease.
   Symptoms. Aversion to wind, sweating, etc.
   Pathogenesis. Owing to the invasion of pathogenic wind after sweating due to sexual strain.
   Therapeutic Principle. Removing wind and supplementing qi.
2. Referring to the syndromes of shaving, convulsion, and vertigo in pathogenic change.
   Symptoms. Vertigo, convulsion, tic of limbs, tremor, numbness, sudden fainting, facial hemiparalysis, upward turning of the eyeball, etc.
   Pathogenesis. Due to the exhaustion of essence and blood, the failure of kidney to nourish liver, hyperactivity of the liver-yang, or excessive heat and fire, deficiency of blood and insufficiency of yin, and disorder of qi and blood.
   Therapeutic Principle. Removing wind calming the liver, invigorating yin and checking exuberance of yang.

Endogenous Wind due to Shortage of Blood
Referring to a syndrome of endogenous wind.
Symptoms. Dry skin, or dry muscles and nails with itching or desquamation.
Pathogenesis. Because of exhaustion of blood due to prolonged disease, or short-

age of blood due to aging or prolonged malnutrition and insufficient blood formation, or stasis in the interior, and disturbance of blood formation.

Therapeutic Principle. Moistening and ceasing the endopathic wind.

Endopathic Factors

Referring to the seven emotional factors: joy, anger, anxiety, worry, grief, fear and fright. If an emotional stimulus of the seven occurs beyond the adaptability, they will become pathogenic factors and injure internal organs and cause the functional disorder.

Endopathic Wind due to Blood Deficiency

Referring to the syndrome of deficiency wind to stir inside.

Symptoms. Numbness of extremities and the body, muscular twitch, and even spasm and stiffness of hand and foot.

Pathogenesis. The blood is too deficient to nourish tendons and meridians or massive bleeding or impairment of ying blood by prolonged illness and deficiency of the liver blood.

Therapeutic Principle. Nourishing blood to cease wind.

Endopathogen

It refers to the course of the pathogenic factor coming out from the interior to the surface of the body. For instance infant measles, at the beginning it has such interior syndromes as interior heat dysphoria, cough of dyspnea and fullness of chest, etc. Then fever and sweat, gradual appearance of measles on the skin and followed by alleviation of the dysphoria. It is a sign of recovery.

Endotherapy for Relieving Ulcer

Referring to one of the treatment methods to cure sores by reinforcing the body resistance, removing toxins inside the body.

Indication. For sores not removed at the beginning, patient's body resistance weakened while pathogenic factors prevailing, and patient's ulcer resistant to healing.

Therapeutic Principle. Mainly by using the drugs for invigorating qi and enriching blood while keeping the drugs for enhancing blood circulation and detoxicating subsidiary.

Enhancing Deficiency and Promoting Excess

Referring to an erroneous therapeutic method, weakened body resistance to be weaker while excessiveness of pathogen to be more excessive.

Entering Tranquility

A Qigong terminology. Referring to a highly tranquil, relaxed and comfortable state gained by a Qigong practitioner, that is the mindwill concentrated and the distracting thoughts disappeared.

Entering Tranquility by Irradiation

Qigong terminology. Referring to directly "irradiating" the distracting thoughts with mindwill in order to reach tranquility. During Qigong practice, distracting thoughts come one after another, the practitioner should have an interval of silence without any distracting thought, and concentrate the mind firmly on the interval as long as possible to reach tranquility consciously.

Enterositosis

Referring to the syndrome with abdominal mass due to the parasites in the abdomen.

Symptoms. Abdominal pain around the navel, happening now and then, or soft mass in the abdomen, and move when pushing, accompanied by emaciation with yellowish complexion, vomiting bitter or clear fluid, salivating in sleep, distention in the stomach and abdomen, etc.

Pathogenesis. Due to the parasites in the intestine.

Therapeutic Principle. Killing the parasites and removing the abdominal mass.

Entire Micromelum Root

It is the root, bark or leaf of Micromelum integerrimum (Buch.-Ham.) Roem (Rutaceae).

Effect. Removing wind, dampness, warming up the middle-energizer and eliminating blood stasis.

Indication. Common cold, malaria, rheumatic arthralgia and traumatic injuries, etc.

Enuresis

1. Referring to the inability to control urination leading to spontaneous micturition.

   Pathogenesis. Due to bad eating habit, too fond of play or over-exertion, happens mostly to the infant.

   Therapeutic Principle. Developing good habits of personal hygiene and diet.

2. Referring to unconscious micturition during sleep.

   Pathogenesis. Due to deficiency and cold of the kidney and unconsolidation of kidney-qi, or due to qi-deficiency of the spleen and kidney.

   Therapeutic Principle. Warming the kidney and strengthening it to take in qi in the first case, and supplementing qi and invigorating the spleen in the latter.

Enuresis due to Internal Injury

Symptoms. Spontaneous micturition with normal consciousness, feeble speech, poor appetite, loose stool, cold extremities, etc.

Pathogenesis. Owing to the deficiency of the liver-yin and internal disturbance of the liver-heat or due to the deficiency of spleen and kidney.

Therapeutic Principle. Nourishing the spleen and kidney in the first case, and nourishing yin and removing heat in the latter.

Ephedra

It is the herbaceous stem of Ephedra sinica Stapf, or E. equisetina Bunge. and E. intermedia Schrenk et Mey. (Ephedraceae).

Effect. Induce sweating to expel the exogenous evils from the body surface, promoting diuresis, diaphoresis, and removing asthma, alleviating itching.

Indication. Exterior syndrome of excess type due to exopathogenic wind-cold; edema with exterior syndrome; arthralgia due to wind-dampness, etc.

Ephedra Root

It is the root or rhizome of Ephedra sinica Stapf, or E. equisetina Bge. (Ephedraceae).

Effect. Ceasing sweating.

Indication. Spontaneous and night sweating.

Epidemic cholera

Symptoms. Sudden vomiting and diarrhea, thick and turbid vomit without abdominal pain, cold limbs, profuse drinks due to thirst, continuous vomiting, etc.

Pathogenesis. Due to failure of the stomach and spleen in their functions of descending, and transporting, distributing and transforming.

Therapeutic Principle. Drugs of normalizing the stomach and spleen in the acute case, supplementing qi, enhancing the body fluids production, blood circulation, releasing toxic substances in the chronic case.

Epidemic Cold Syndrome

There are two meanings: 1. Referring to an epidemic disease in spring and early summer, due to catching cold. 2. Referring to cold sensation of the genitalia.

Symptoms. Abdominal pain, cold limbs, vomiting and diarrhea with discharge of cold clear fluids, etc.

Pathogenesis. Owing to seasonal pestilence.

Epidemic Cough

Symptoms. Fever with aversion to cold, headache and stuffy nose and constant cough.

Pathogenesis. Due to the affection of seasonal pathogenic factor being epidemic.

Therapeutic Principle. Adjusting the lung and removing exterior syndrome.

Epidemic Disease of Yang

Referring to a disease.

Symptoms. Red face, eruptions on the face, sore throat and salva with pus and blood.

Pathogenesis. Due to excessive heat in the blood system.

Therapeutic Principle. Detoxifying, removing heat and stagnation.

Epidemic Disease of Yin

Symptoms. Pale appearance, severe pain on the body and sore throat.

Pathogenesis. Due to invasion of pathogens into the blood system, blood stasis, obstruction of meridians and infections of the throat.

Therapeutic Principle. Removing heat and detoxifying and enhancing blood circulation, releasing blood stasis.

Epidemic Disease with Incubation

It refers to epidemic febrile diseases, such as pathogen of summer-heat and dampness, which incubate in the body, and attacks with the inducement of new pathogen in autumn or winter.

Epidemic Disease with Rash

Symptoms. Rash with loose, float, red, and movable, in the case of slight illness, and rash with tight, fixed, violet and gloomy, in the serious case.

Pathogenesis. Due to affection by external epidemic pathogen and excessive toxic heat inside invading nutritional qi, defensive qi and the skin.

Therapeutic Principle. Removing heat, cooling blood and detoxicating.

Epidemic Dysentery

Referring to the serious dysentery with strong infectivity.

Symptoms. Sudden onset, high fever and headache, dysphoria and thirst, severe pain in abdomen, dysentery with pus and blood with violet red or bloody water, even coma and convulsion with cold limbs, etc.

Pathogenesis. Due to the impairment of qi and blood by the obstruction of excessive pathogenic factors in the intestine.

Therapeutic Principle. Releasing pathogenic heat from blood.

Epidemic Eruptive Disease

Symptoms. Aversion to cold with fever, swollen head and face, abdominalgia or oppressed feeling in chest, satiety of chest or diarrhea with pus and blood stool, etc.

Pathogenesis. Because of the stagnation of qi due to accumulation of pathogenic cold lasting until spring, or because of summer-heat stagnation lasting until autumn.

Therapeutic Principle. Pricking blood therapy and removing epidemic eruptive factors.

Epidemic Febrile Disease

Referring to one type of Taiyang meridian syndromes.

Symptoms. Fever, pain of the neck, and thirst, fearless of cold.

Therapeutic Principle. Removing the exterior syndrome with drugs pungent in flavor and cold in property.

Epidemic Febrile Disease Occurring Immediately after Attack of Exopathogen

Referring to epidemic febrile disease with immediate onset after invasion by warm-pathogen, different from epidemic febrile disease with incubation period. The onset of the illness is similar to the features of the disease due to the main climate then, e.g. wind-warm, summer fever, damp-warm, autumn-dryness disease, etc.

Epidemic Headache

A disease and syndrome.

Symptoms. Headache, fever and chill, flushed swollen face and head, infecting the whole family, etc.

Pathogenesis. Due to attack by noxious dampness.

Therapeutic Principle. Removing heat and toxic materials and ceasing pain.

Epidemic Jaundice

Referring to a serious syndrome in jaundice due to epidemic pathogens.

Symptoms. Sudden attack, yellow body and eyes, coma with high fever, abdominal distention with hypochondriac pain, dark urine like tea color, and even epistaxis and bloody urine, etc.

Pathogenesis. Due to affection of epidemic exopathogens or epidemic pathogenic damp-heat, burning of ying blood, excessive noxious heat, cholorrhagia seen on skin.

Therapeutic Principle. Removing toxic materials, heat from blood and inducing resuscitation.

Epidemic Keratoconjunctivitis

Referring to a rapid infectious disease being epidemic in summer and autumn, usually involving both eyes.

Symptoms. A sudden onset of redness on the white of the eye, with pain, itching, photophobia, lacrimation and profuse mucoid secretion.

Pathogenesis. Due to affection of epidemic pathogenic factors, with heat in the lung and stomach, and both interior and exterior pathogenic factors attacking the eyes.

Therapeutic Principle. Removing pathogenic factors, eliminating wind-heat, toxic substances, intense heat, and enhancing visual acuity with external treatment and prevention.

Epidemic Malaria

Referring to an epidemic, infectious and serious malaria.

Symptoms. Alternate attacks of chills and fever, high fever, much perspiration, thirst, oppressed feeling in the chest, etc.

Pathogenesis. Due to damp-heat and filthy turbidity invading pleural diaphragmatic interspace.

Therapeutic Principle. Releasing filth and dampness, taking the season into consideration.

Epidemic Parotitis

Another name for mumps. Referring to the redness, swelling, heat and pain in the parotid.

Symptoms. Aversion to cold, fever, etc.

Pathogenesis. Due to invasion of epidemic virus in the parotid.

Therapeutic Principle. Detoxicating and removing the swelling.

Epidemic Pathogenic Factor

Referring to a strong infectious pathogenic factor in causing disease. Its occurrence and prevalence are related to the factors of famine, war chaos, and drought for a long time, extremely hot, etc. It spreads by air and contact, and may lead to pestilence.

Epididymitis and Orchitis

Symptoms. Swelling and pain in one testis, and also in spermatic cord, or reddish swelling scrotum, and body fever. Sometimes, a chronic disease, or with hydrocele.

Pathogenesis. Due to stagnation of qi and blood, traumatic injury or additional affection of pathogenic factors, blockage of meridians and collaterals, accumulation of damp-heat due to downward flow.

Therapeutic Principle. Removing swelling, blood stasis, heat toxic material, enhancing diuresis, removing swelling, activating blood flow.

Epigastralgia due to Ascariasis

Symptoms. Repeated onsets of epigastralgia with serious pain, pale complexion, cold limbs, or vomiting with ascaris, sallow complexion and emaciation, diet normal after pain; or white spots on the face.

Pathogenesis. Due to the disturbance of ascaris blocking the functional activities of qi.

Therapeutic Principle. Removing colic due to ascaris and releasing pain.

Epigastralgia due to Blood Stasis

Symptoms. Fixed pain in the stomach like being stabbed with needle or cut with knife, or pain with mass, severe in cold and night, vomiting blood, blackish stool, purplish tongue, etc.

Pathogenesis. Due to qi stagnation and blood stasis, prolonged pain entering the collaterals, or on exerting oneself too strongly.

Therapeutic Principle. Releasing blood stasis and enhancing qi circulation in the meridians, adjusting qi and alleviating pain.

Epigastralgia due to Heat Accumulation

Symptoms. Frequent stomachache, even stabbing pain in hypochondrium, hyperhidrosis, chest, fullness and oppressed feeling, vomiting, thirst, dry lips and constipation, etc.

Pathogenesis. Owing to accumulated heat in the interior.

Therapeutic Principle. Removing the stomach heat and adjusting qi by smoothing mental depression.

Epigastralgia due to Phlegm Accumulation

Symptoms. Epigastralgia, nausea, oppressed feeling, sometimes acid regurgitation, slippery and forceful pulse.

Pathogenesis. Due to the weakness of the spleen and stomach, the accumulation of the water staying inside the body, leading to phlegm in the epigastrium and the obstruction of functional activities of qi.

Therapeutic Principle. Adjusting the flow of qi, removing phlegm.

Epigastralgia due to Yin Deficiency

Symptoms. Repeated burning pain in the stomach, dry mouth, gastric discomfort with acid regurgitation, constipation, etc.

Pathogenesis. Due to a prolonged disease, the yin impairment by stagnated fire and the lack of stomach-yin.

Therapeutic Principle. Nourishing yin, adjusting the stomach, ceasing pain.

Epigastric Pain due to Ascaris

Symptoms. Repeated pain, mass in the epigastrium and abdomen, gastric discomfort with acid regurgitation, clenching with salivation during sleep, even severe pain, restlessness, nausea, vomiting, sometimes with yellow-green, bitter, watery fluid, sometimes with ascaris, etc.

Pathogenesis. Due to the disturbance of ascaris, the stagnation of functional activities of qi and the obstruction of qi in the fu organs.

Therapeutic Principle. Removing colic due to ascaris and killing ascaris.

Epigastric Pain due to Blood Stasis

There are two meanings:

1. It refers to the fixed pain in the epigastrium, serious at night.

   Pathogenesis. Accumulation of the blood stasis in the epigastrium due to traumatic injury and improper diet.

   Therapeutic Principle.

   Enhancing blood circulation to cease pain.

2. The stabbing pain in the heart region, even with cold limbs and coma.

   Pathogenesis. Due to blood stasis disturbing upward to the heart.

   Therapeutic Principle. Promoting blood circulation to dispel blood stasis.

Epigastric Pain due to Heat

Symptoms. Restlessness, burning sensation of palms, thirst, constipation, flushed-sallow complexion, and epigastric pain.

Pathogenesis. Owing to attack of pathogenic heat to the heart.

Therapeutic Principle. Removing heat, ceasing the pathogenic fire, and removing the obstruction, and enhancing blood circulation.

Epigastric Pain due to Improper Diet

Referring to pain in the upper abdomen due to improper diet.

Symptoms. Oppressed feeling and fullness sensation with pain in the chest, eructation with fetid odor and acid regurgitation, anorexia and fullness of abdomen, forceful with slippery pulse.

Pathogenesis. Due to impairment of the spleen and stomach, production of phlegm resulting from the accumulation of meridians blood stasis due to stagnation of qi and inactivating heart-yang.

Therapeutic Principle. Enhancing digestion, releasing stagnancy and retention.

Epigastric Pain due to Stagnation of Phlegm

Symptoms. Nausea, fullness with restlessness, repeated acid regurgitation, and slippery pulse.

Pathogenesis. Due to the stagnation of phlegm and qi.

Therapeutic Principle. Removing heat and phlegm.

Epigastric Pain due to Wind-cold

Symptoms. Borborygmus, obstructive sensation in the esophagus, chest fullness, breath shortness, salivation, etc.

Pathogenesis. Due to wind-cold pathogen.

Therapeutic Principle. Warming up the stomach, removing cold, wind and ceasing pain.

Epigastric Pain with Palpitation

Symptoms. Intermittent epigastric pain and palpitation, preference for pressing, relief of pain after eating, more severe pain if hunger, and feeble pulse, etc.

Pathogenesis. Mostly due to deficiency of qi and blood, resulting in impairment of nourishing function of the heart and spleen.

Therapeutic Principle. Tonifying the heart and spleen.

Epigastric Severe Pain

Found in the pregnant woman.

Symptoms. Pain with vomiting without eating anything, and restless fetal movement, etc.

Pathogenesis. Resulting from blood stasis due to cold.

Epilepsy

Symptoms. During seizures, abrupt onset, sudden loss of consciousness, convulsions of the limbs, pale complexion, staring eyes, spitting white saliva, etc., then normal recovery.

Pathogenesis. Due to congenital or acquired weakness and terror or serious emotional irritation.

Therapeutic Principle. Removing phlegm, wind, inducing resuscitation.

Epilepsy due to Accumulation of Wind-phlegm in Diaphragm

Referring to the attack of epilepsy.

Symptoms. Onset of fainting, unconsciousness, showing the whites of one's eyes, inability to raise limbs, and slobbering, etc.

Pathogenesis. Due to the disturbance of seven orifices by the liver-fire with phlegm.

Therapeutic Principle. Calming wind, releasing phlegm and recovering mind.

Epilepsy due to Blood Stasis

Symptoms. Infant brain injury, accumulation of blood stasis in the heart and fright.

Cause. Due to the operation of dystocia, terror, traumatic injury, etc.

Therapeutic Principle. Removing convulsion and inducing resuscitation, and enhancing blood circulation and relieving epilepsy.

Epilepsy due to Terror

This term has two meanings:

1. Referring to the epilepsy due to fear.

    Symptoms. Sudden onset of epilepsy by fright, falling suddenly, sometimes with scream and unconsciousness, urinary and fecal incontinence, etc.

    Therapeutic Principle. Removing phlegm, enhancing qi circulation, and tranquilizing the mind.

2. Referring to the sequelae with the head, mouth, and eyes after epilepsy, such as deviation of the eye and mouth, or strabismus, tilted head, or shaking head, etc.

Epilepsy during Pregnancy

Symptoms. In the third trimester of pregnancy or during or after delivery, faint due to dizziness, unconsciousness, clonic convulsion of the extremities, and repeated after recovery.

Pathogenesis. Due to yin deficiency with excess of yang and up-stiring of the liver, or by upward disturbance of phlegm-fire due to original yin deficiency of the liver and kidney and severe deficiency of both yin and blood after pregnancy.

Therapeutic Principle. Smoothing the liver to suppress yang, nourishing yin, removing heat, or removing phlegm, wind, ceasing convulsion.

Epilepsy of Deficiency Type

Referring to the epilepsy due to the deficiency in origin and excess in superficiality.

Symptoms. Prolonged epilepsy, amnesia, palpitation, dizziness, lassitude of the loin and knees, listlessness and asthenia, etc.

Pathogenesis. Due to overstrain, depression, the deficiency in origin during the convalescence, or the invasion of the six climatic conditions, the stagnation of qi, blood and phlegm entering into the meridians and collaterals.

Therapeutic Principle. Nourishing the heart and kidney caused by deficiency in origin, eliminating phlegm caused by excess in superficiality.

Epiphora

Referring to epiphora when the patient encountered cold wind.

Symptoms. Often lachrymation without redness and swelling of eye, and clear and watery tears without heat sensation.

Pathogenesis. Resulting from narrow or obstructive lacrimal passage due to deficiency of liver-yin and kidney-yin, affection of exopathogen, and some illness in nose.

Therapeutic Principle. Tonify the liver and kidney.

Epiphora with Warm Tears Induced by Wind

Referring to a type of epiphora.

Symptoms. Red and swelling eyes with burning pain, photophobia, warm and thick tears, serious in the wind.

Pathogenesis. Due to excessive liver-fire, or invasion by exogenous pathogenic wind-heat.

Therapeutic Principle. Removing wind and heat, releasing the depressed liver to enhance acuity of vision.

Episcleritis

Referring to the ophthalmopathy, outward projection of the inner layer of the white forming localized purplish-red node, developing slowly, and recurring easily.

Symptoms. Early stage, itching, astringency, pain, photophobia, lacrimation, poor vision and immovable node. If the patient misses the therapeutic chance or is mistreated, the black and pupil might be harmed. The inner layer of the white eyeballs form localized purplish-red node, developing slowly and recurring easily.

Pathogenesis. Resulting from sufficient heat-toxin in the heart and lung, upward attacking the white.

Therapeutic Principle. Detoxicating, removing heat from blood and releasing node.

Epistaxis

Symptoms. Bleeding from inside the nose or nasal bleeding.

Pathogenesis. Owing to liver fire, retention of pathogenic heat in the lung or stomach-heat.

Epistaxis due to Impairment of Five Zang Organs

Symptoms. Epistaxis due to emotional change, with headache, vertigo, red eyes, dysphoria, easy to anger, palpitation, anorexia, dry cough, lumbar lassitude and distention, etc.

Pathogenesis. Caused by the impaired liver due to irritation, the impaired heart due to being over-delighted, impaired spleen due to keep meditating, the impaired lung due to being upset, and the impaired kidney due to suffering from mental depressing.

Therapeutic Principle. Removing heat, cooling blood and ceasing bleeding.

Epistaxis due to Injury

Referring to bleeding from the nose.

Cause. Owing to external injury, or falling down from a high place.

Therapeutic Principle. Treating by hemostasis with absorbent cotton filled into the nasal cavity.

Epistaxis due to Internal Injury

Generally referring to epistaxis due to non-trauma and affection of exopathogen.

Symptoms. Nasal bleeding, dry mouth and nose, or choking cough, or thirst and halitosis, constipation, or dysphoria, reddish eye, or dizziness and tinnitus, etc.

Pathogenesis. Mainly owing to upward obstruction of the lung-heat, fumigating and steaming of the stomach-heat, upward flaring of the liver-fire, floating of pathogenic fire due to yin deficiency, etc.

Therapeutic Principle. Removing heat from the lung with drugs pungent in flavor and cool in property, releasing heat to descend fire, purging the liver of pathogenic fire, nourishing yin to reduce fire, etc.

Epistaxis due to Liver Fire

Symptoms. Nasal bleeding with headache, dizziness, conjunctival congestion, bitter taste, irritability, red tongue with yellow coating, etc.

Pathogenesis. Owing to the flare up of liver fire.

Therapeutic Principle. Releasing heat from the liver and purging the pathogenic fire to cease bleeding.

Epistaxis due to Lung-heat

This syndrome includes three types:

1. The type of excess.

   Symptoms. Dryness of nose, mouth and throat, epistaxis, fever, cough with less phlegm, etc.

   Pathogenesis. Owing to excess heat in Lung Meridian.

   Therapeutic Principle. Clearing away the lung heat, and removing heat from the blood, ceasing bleeding.

2. The type of deficiency.

   Symptoms. Epistaxis, pink blood, frequent attack by heat and overstrain.

   Pathogenesis. Due to yin deficiency and flaring-up of fire of deficiency.

   Therapeutic Principle. Removing heat, nourishing yin to reduce pathogenic fire.

3. The type due to wind

   Symptoms. Stuffy nose, epistaxis, aversion to wind and fever, etc.

   Pathogenesis. Attack by pathogenic wind-heat into the lung.

Therapeutic Principle. Removing wind and heat.

Epistaxis due to Stomach-heat

Symptoms. Nasal bleeding with fresh red color, thirst, oppressive sensation in the chest, bad smell in the mouth, constipation, red tongue with yellowish coating, quick and forceful pulse.

Pathogenesis. Due to the fumigation of the stomach-heat.

Therapeutic Principle. Removing stomach-heat, ceasing bleeding.

Epistaxis during Menstruation

This disease and syndrome includes two types.

1. Due to stagnation of the liver-qi.

    Symptoms. Accompanied irritability, headache, hypochondriac pain, bitter taste, dry throat, vexation, etc.

    Pathogenesis. Invasion of fire-transmission into the lung due to stagnation of the liver-qi.

    Therapeutic Principle. Smoothing the liver and clearing away heat.

2. Due to injury of collaterals by heat in the lung.

    Symptoms. Accompanied by tidal fever in the afternoon, cough, etc.

    Pathogenesis. Injury of collaterals due to excess heat in the lung because of yin deficiency.

    Therapeutic Principle. Nourishing yin and removing heat.

Epistaxis during Pregnancy

Symptoms. Nose-bleeding of a pregnant woman.

Pathogenesis. Over-eating of pungent food resulting in the fire goes upward to steam the lung affecting the nose collateral branches with pathogenic heat causing bleeding. It is a sign of abortion if endless bleeding.

Therapeutic Principle. Nourishing yin, removing heat, ceasing bleeding and preventing abortion.

Erbai (Ex-UE 2)

An extra acupuncture point.

Location. Two points on the palmar side of each forearm, 4 cun proximal to the transverse crease of the wrist, on each side of the tendon of the radial flexor muscle of the wrist.

Indication. Hemorrhoids and proctoptosis, neuralgia in the forearm.

Method. Puncture 0.3-0.7 cun perpendicularly. Perform moxibustion 3-5 moxa cones or 5-10 minutes with warming moxibustion.

Erchui (Ex-HN)

An extra acupuncture point.

Location. At the midpoint of the anterior aspect of the ear lobe.

Indication. Mouth-blocking boil.

Method. Puncture 0.1 cun perpendicularly or prick to bleeding with a triangular needle.

Erheliao (TE 22)

Location. On the posterior border of the hairline of the temple, at the level with the root of the auricle and superfial temporal artery.

Indication. Headache, tinnitus, lockjaw, deviation of the mouth.

Method. Avoiding the artery, puncture obliquely or subcutaneously 0.3-0.5 cun. Moxibustion is applicable.

Erhoufaji (Ex-HN)

An extra acupuncture point.

Location. Seen at the edge of the mastoid process of the temporal bone behind the ear, on the hairline.

Indication. Goiter and scrofula.

Method. Perform moxibustion 3-5 moxa cones or 5-15 minutes with warming moxibustion.

Erhougaogu

It is a massage point.

Location. In the depression inferior to post-auditory process and superior to retro-auricular hair line.

Operation. Mostly employing kneading and arc-pushing manipulations.

Function. Removing wind, exterior syndrome, calming the mind and dysphoria.

Indication. Headache, infantile convulsion, dysphoria, etc.

Eriocarpous Glochidion Twig and Leaf

It is the twig and leaf of Glochidion eriocarpum Champ. (Euphorbiaceae).

Effect. Removing blood stasis, swelling, and pathogenic wind, promoting diuresis, ceasing bleeding.

Indication. Acute gastroenteritis, dysentery, rheumatic arthralgia, traumatic injuries, traumatic bleeding, dermatitis rhus, eczema, dermatitis, etc.

Erjian (Ex-HN 6)

It is an extra acupuncture point.

Location. At the top of the ear auricle when folding the ear forward.

Indication. Eye redness with swelling and pain, eye nebula migraine, headache, facial furuncle, high fever, acute conjunctivitis, and trachoma.

Method. Puncture 0.1 cun perpendicularly, or prick to little bleeding with a triangular needle.

Erjian (LI 2)

An acupuncture point.

Location. On the radial surface of the index finger, at the junction of the reddish and whitish skin in the procoelous site of the metacarpophalangeal articulation, getting the point while bending finger.

Indication. Swelling sore throat, toothache, epistaxis, blurred vision, dry mouth, submental swelling and fever.

Method. Puncture 0.2-0.3 cun perpendicularly and perform moxibustion to the point for 5-10 minutes.

Ermen (TE 21)

Referring to a meridian point, belonging to the Triple Energizer Meridian.

Location. On the face, anterior to the supratragical notch, in the depression behind the posterior border of the condyloid process of the mandible.

Indication. Deafness, tinnitus, otitis media suppurativa, toothache, pain in the neck and jaw, and stiffness of the lip.

Method. Puncture perpendicularly 0.5-1 cun when the mouth is open. Perform moxibustion 1-3 moxa cones or 3-5 minutes with warming moxibustion.

Ermenqianmai (Ex-HN)

Referring to two extra acupuncture points.

Location. 1 cun above or below the point Ermen (TE 21).

Indication. Throat affection due to spleen-wind, resulting in aphasia.

Method. Perform moxibustion 3-7 moxa cones or 5-15 minutes with warming moxibustion.

Erosion

Symptoms. Localized superficial skin injury with moist surface.

Cause. Due to the breaking of herpes and pustule, the dropping of scabs, or the breaking of papular epiderm. Usually no scar after recovery.

Erosion of Vulva

Symptoms. In the female, erosion of the skin, and mucosa of the vulva and vagina thickened swollen, ulcerated sunk skin even swelling, diabrotic and purulent in the severe case.

Pathogenesis. Caused by toxic bacteria overflooding of damp-heat.

Therapeutic Principle. Removing heat, enhancing diuresis and killing bacteria.

Erotomania

Referring to female sexual hyperfunction with mental derangement.

Symptoms. Overjoyed at sight of a man and angry with a woman, or even stark-naked in the presence of others without any sense of shame.

Pathogenesis. Due to kidney-yin insufficiency and fire hyperactivity of the deficiency type.

Therapeutic Principle. Nourishing the kidney and removing heat from the liver.

Ershang (Ex-HN)

It is an extra acupuncture point.

Location. Three-finger-breadths directly above the tip of the ear.

Indication. Sudden onset epilepsy in children.

Method. Perform moxibustion.

Ershangfaji (Ex-HN)

It is an extra acupuncture point.

Location. On the hairline directly above the ear apex.

Indication. Goiter, epilepsy, etc.

Method. Puncture subcutaneously 0.3-0.5 cun. Perform moxibustion 3-5 moxa cones or 5-10 minutes with warming moxibustion.

Ershizhui Point

An acupuncture point referring to one of the extraordinary points.

Location. At the crossing point of the connecting line between the third posterior sacral foramen and the median sacral crest.

Indication. Hematochezia, bleeding from the seven orifices and metrorrhagia.

Method. Perform moxibustion 5-15 minutes or 3-7 moxa cones.

Eruptive Disease

Symptoms. Dizziness and dim eyesight, nausea and vomiting, purpura in the body, etc.

Pathogenesis. Due to affection by abnormal weather in four seasons, and contaminated food.

Therapeutic Principle. Removing heat and cooling blood.

Eruptive Disease in Children

Symptoms. Seeming cold and heat, sluggish limbs, poor appetite, yin eruptive disease in patients with abdominal pain and cold hands and feet; for abdominal pain and warm hands and feet, it is called yang eruptive disease.

Pathogenesis. Due to the exterior cold pathogens and the interior stasis of qi and blood.

Therapeutic Principle. Enhancing the circulation of qi and blood.

Erysipelas

Symptoms. Early on, malaise of the body and fever with aversion to cold, then red maculae on the skin with local swelling, scorching heat and bright red coloration. The color fades when pressed and returns to its original state when released, spreading quickly. Clinically, it includes erysipelas due to wind-heat pathogens and erysipelas due to damp-heat pathogens.

Pathogenesis. Found on the upper part of the body mainly due to wind-heat pathogen; on the lower part of the body, mainly due to fire transformed from damp-heat pathogen.

Erysipelas due to Damp-heat

Symptoms. Besides the general symptoms of erysipelas, mostly seen on the lower limbs, also with fever, vexation, thirst, choking sensation in the chest, swelling and pain in the joints, dark urine, yellow, greasy tongue coating, soft and rapid pulse.

Pathogenesis. Mainly owing to attack of damp-heat and depression of damp-heat in muscles and skin.

Therapeutic Principle. Removing heat, dampness and detoxicating.

Erysipelas due to the Wind-heat Pathogen

Symptoms. Besides the general symptoms and signs of erysipelas commonly seen on the face, fever and chills, headache, aching in joints, poor appetite, constipation and deep-colored urine, red tongue with thin yellow or thin white coating, surging and rapid pulse.

Pathogenesis. Mainly owing to the failure of superficial-qi to protect the body against diseases.

Therapeutic Principle. Removing wind, heat and toxic material.

Erythema Multiforme

Referring to the polytypic acute infective dermatitis, mainly with erythema, and also with papular eruptions and blisters, etc.

Symptoms. Polytypic skin injury, first with erythema or papular eruptions, and also with urticaria and blisters, symmetrically in scarlet or dark red color. Sudden illness with fever, arthralgia, etc., attacked repeatedly. After healing, pigmentation may be left.

Pathogenesis. Due to congenital deficiency, external affection of wind-coldness, or excessive fire-toxins, or by focal infection, drugs, fish and shrimps, etc.

Therapeutic Principle. Adjusting the nutrient, removing toxic materials, heat from the blood and enhancing diuresis.

Erythema of Newborn

Referring to the pathological phenomenon of newborn.

Symptoms. Tender and red skin, slight cyanosis of hands and feet.

Pathogenesis. Due to affection of toxic heat during pregnancy.

Therapeutic Principle. Removing heat and adjusting blood.

Erzhishang (Ex-LE)

It is an extra acupuncture point.

Location. At the midpoint of the line connecting Neiting (S 44) and Xiangu (S 43).

Indication. Edema, swelling and pain of the gum, epistaxis, redness and swelling on the dorsum of the foot.

Method. Perform the moxibustion 3-5 minutes.

Erzhong (Ex-HX)

It is an extra acupuncture point.

Location. At the midpoint of the helix crus.

Indication. Jaundice, and cases affected by pestilent evils in winter and summer, etc.

Method. Puncture perpendicularly 0.1-0.2 cun. Moxibustion if necessary.

Erzhuixia (Ex-B)

It is an extra acupuncture point, also called Wuming.

Location. On the posterior midline, in the depression of the spinous process of the 2nd thoracic vertebra.

Indication. Mental diseases, epilepsy and malaria, etc.

Method. Puncture obliquely 0.5-1 cun. Perform moxibustion 3-5 moxa cones or 5-10 minutes with warming moxibustion.

Escape of Blood from Vessels and Meridians

Symptoms. Bleeding out of vessels meridians, such as metrorrhagia and metrostaxis, hematemesis, bleeding from the eye, ear, nose, mouth or subcutaneous tissues, hematochezia and hematuria.

Pathogenesis. Due to qi deficiency, reversed flow of qi, blood stasis, and pathogenic heat, leading to the failure of the blood circulation, etc.

Esophagus (MA-IC 6)

It is an ear point.

Location. In the middle 1/3 of the inferior aspect of the helix crus.

Function. Adjusting the esophagus.

Indication. Esophagitis, spasm of esophagus, globus hystericus.

Essence Derived from Food

There are two meanings:

1. Referring to a morbid condition of stasis of liver-qi.

   Symptoms. Pain in the hypochondrium but relief of pain if pressed and easy to recur.

   Pathogenesis. Owing to accumulation of food and obstruction of qi in the spleen and stomach.

Therapeutic Principle. Smoothing the depressed liver and activating the spleen, and adjusting qi to eliminate stagnancy.

2. Referring to nutrients taken into the stomach.

Essence Exhaustion
Symptoms. Emaciation, heart throbbing, dyspnea, dizziness, poor memory, lumbago, fear, etc.
Pathogenesis. Owing to the exhaustion of vital essence in zang-fu organs thus leading to diseases.
Therapeutic Principle. Nourishing and producing essence.

Essence from Foodstuff
Referring to the nutritious essence digested and absorbed from foodstuff taken by humans, it is essential for enhancing body development and maintaining life activities.

Essence Impairment
Symptoms. Emaciation, lumbago, poor memory, mental fatigue, weakness, etc.
Pathogenesis. Owing to illness, leading to the consumption of vital essence and blood.
Therapeutic Principle. Nourishing essence qi.

Essence of Life
In a wide sense, the essence of life indicating, generally, qi, blood, body fluid, and essential substances from foodstuff, refers to essential substance for reproduction, or congenital essence in a narrow sense.

Essence-storing
Referring to the physiological features of the kidney, mainly for storing essence, the kidney is better to be closed and consolidated without purgation abnormally.

Eucommia Bark   ⊗ E-3
It is the trunk bark of Eucommia ulmoides Oliv. (Eucommiaceae).

Effect. Nourishing the liver and kidney, reinforcing tendons and bones, and preventing abortion, lowering blood pressure.
Indication. Aches and lassitude of the loins and knees, impotence, frequent urination due to deficiency of the liver and kidney; threatened abortion and habitual abortion, hypertention, etc.

European Grape Root
It is the root of a tall and big twining plat Vitis vinifera L. (Vitaceae).
Effect. Removing wind-dampness and enhancing diuresis.
Indication. Rheumatic arthralgia, generalized edema with abdominal distention, etc.

European Verbena
It is the whole herb or herb with root. of Verbena officinalis L. (Verbenaceae).
Effect. Removing heat, detoxicating, enhancing blood circulation, releasing blood stasis, and inducing diuresis to alleviate edema, killing parasites.
Indication. Fever due to common cold, jaundice due to damp-heat pathogen, edema, dysentery, malaria.

Even Needling
Referring to a needling method, requiring needling reaction only after the insertion of the needle, but not for certain reinforcing and reducing.

Evergreen Mucuna Root
It is the root and stem leaf of evergreen Mucuna sempervirens Hemsl. (Leguminosae).
Effect. Enhancing blood circulation, enriching blood, clearing and activating the meridians and collaterals.
Indication. Wind-damp pain, numbness of limbs, anaemia, irregular menstruation, etc.

Evil Fetus

1. Referring to female mass in the abdomen.

   Symptoms. Amenorrhea with a pregnant-like abdomen.

2. Referring to hydatid mole.

3. Referring to false pregnancy, including aeriform embryo, sanguinopurulent fetus, and sputum-like fetus.

   Pathogenesis. Owing to insufficiency of blood and qi, and qi stagnation from prolonged depression.

   Therapeutic Principle. Adjusting the flow of qi removing embryo, and enhancing blood circulation to release stasis.

Evil Wind

Generally referring to abnormal climatic changes and external harmful pathogenic factors to the human body.

Excellent Mindwill Method

A Qigong terminology. During Qigong practice, a practitioner imagining beautiful scenery, delightful affairs and satisfactory objects to relax and be happy.

Excess Heat Syndrome of Liver

Symptoms. Rigidity and pain in hypochondrium, irritability, dizziness, bitter taste, redness eyes, yellow urine and constipation or insanity, etc.

Pathogenesis. Fire-transmission due to stagnation of liver-qi or retention of dampheat in the interior, etc.

Therapeutic Principle. Removing the liver-heat and dampness by purgation, etc.

Excess in Both Exterior and Interior

Referring to the pathogenic excess syndrome of the nutrient and superficial defensive system of muscles and skin, and qi and blood of the viscera.

Symptoms. Fever, aversion to cold, anhidrosis, headache, general pain, excessive thirst, abdominal pain, constipation, etc.

Pathogenesis. Due to invasion of pathogenic factors into interior with excess before the subsidence of exterior syndrome, or due to the excess in the interior with the affection of excess exterior by exopathogen.

Therapeutic Principle. Removing the pathogenic factors externally and internally.

Excess in Physique but Deficiency in Qi

Referring to fatty physique with hypofunction.

Symptoms. Obesity, pale and sallow skin, general debility, lassitude, shortness of breath, low voice. etc.

Pathogenesis. Due to insufficient functional aspect of internal organs, deficiency of the spleen.

Excess in Reality with Pseudo-deficiency Symptoms

Referring to a morbid condition due to accumulation of pathogenic factors with pseudo-deficiency syndrome instead.

Symptoms. Listlessness, cold body and extremities, deep and floating or slow and uneven pulse. When carefully observed, such symptoms can be seen as high voice, husky breath, deep and deep-sited pulse or slow and uneven pulse but strong, thin body instead of tiredness, red and crimson tongue or dry yellow fur.

Pathogenesis. Due to blockage of meridians and collaterals, stagnation of qi and blood due to heat accumulation in the stomach and intestine, etc.

Therapeutic Principle. Removing the heat in the stomach and intestine.

Excessive Bleeding during Menstruation

Symptoms. Prolonged bleeding in women, during the monthly period.

Pathogenesis. Due to cold and deficiency of vital Meridian and the Front Middle Meridian and disfunction of the meridian qi in women.

Therapeutic Principle. Reinforcing and warming Vital Meridian and the Front Middle Meridian, nourishing the blood and ceasing bleeding.

Excessive Cold

Opposite to deficient cold.

Symptoms. Abdominal pain, pale urine, diarrhea, constipation, white coating of the tongue, deep and stringy pulse, etc.

Pathogenesis. Due to deficiency of yang in the body, insufficiency of vital energy, external accumulation of cold pathogen, and detention of cold in the middle-energizer.

Therapeutic Principle. Warming the middle-energizer, removing cold.

Excessive Dampness Bringing about Chronic Diarrhea

Symptoms. Chronic diarrhea (damp diarrhea).

Pathogenesis. Owing to the impairment of the spleen-yang and the dysfunction of transporting, distributing and transforming, resulting from the excess of dampness.

Excessive Dampness Injuring Yang-qi

Symptoms. Pale face, oppressed feeling in the chest, distention of the abdomen, diarrhea, even edema, etc.

Pathogenesis. Owing to the excessive dampness leading to the decline of yang-qi.

Therapeutic Principle. Nourishing yang of the spleen and kidney, removing dampness.

Excessive Fetal Movement

It refers to the sudden and irregular excessive movement of the fetus during the third trimester of pregnancy with the manifestation of pulse, having no sign of parturition.

Excessive Fluid in Hypochondrium and Epigastrium

Symptoms. Oppressed feeling, shortness of breath, gasping cough, inability to lie flat and looking swollen.

Pathogenesis. Due to impairment of purifying and descending functions of the lung, resulting from accumulation of excessive fluid in the hypochondrium and epigastrium and constriction of the lung.

Therapeutic Principle. Warming up the lung, releasing excessive fluid and ceasing asthma.

Excessive Heat in Bladder

There are two meanings:

1. Referring to a morbid state of excessive heat pathogen in the bladder, such as syndrome of bladder damp-heat.
2. Referring to a syndrome in the Bladder meridian.

   Symptoms. Dysuria, pain in the waist, dizziness, headache, dysphoria and fullness sensation in the chest.

   Therapeutic Principle. Promoting diuresis, removing heat.

Excessive Heat of Large Intestine

Symptoms. Abdominal pain and tenderness, constipation, asthmatic cough, flushed face, fever in the body and pharyngeal tonsils.

Pathogenesis. Owing to the excessive heat in the Large Intestinal Meridian.

Therapeutic Principle. Purgation with drugs bitter in taste and cold in nature.

Excessive Heat Syndrome of Heart

Symptoms. Red face, fever, oral ulceration, dysphoria, headache, dry throat, fear, excess joy, abdominal distention and constipation, full and replete pulse, etc.

Pathogenesis. Owing to flaring heart heat.

Therapeutic Principle. Removing heat and calming the mind.

Excessive Hemorrhage

This term has two meanings:

1. **Symptoms.** Hematemesis, epistaxis, hemafecia, hematuria, dim complexion, deep and weak pulse, etc.

   Pathogenesis. Owing to syndrome of insufficiency of qi and blood due to excessive bleeding in blood troubles.

   Therapeutic Principle. Stopping bleeding and enriching the blood.

2. Referring to the syndrome of faint and uneven pulse due to erroneous use of drugs of diaphoresis and administration of purgatives in exogenous febrile disease.

Excessiveness of Stomach-heat

Referring to syndrome of sthenic type occasioned by excessive heat pathogen.

Symptoms. Burning pain in the epigastrium, preference for cold drinks, foul smell in the mouth, ulceration of the mouth, swelling in the gums, constipation, scanty dark urine, etc.

Pathogenesis. Due to attacks of pathogenic heat on stomach, and taking too much pungent, hot and dry food, stagnation of heat in stomach and intestines in epidemic febrile disease.

Therapeutic Principle. Removing the stomach-heat.

Excessive Salivation in Children

Referring to infants always spitting saliva.

Symptoms. For rise in splenic fever, excessive, mucous and foul saliva. For deficiency and cold of spleen-stomach, excessive, clear and thin saliva, anorexia, loose stool.

Pathogenesis. Due to the splenic fever flowing upward, or the deficiency and cold of the spleen-stomach, disturbance in ascending or descending and disfunction in transport.

Therapeutic Principle. Removing the fever in the case of splenic fever, and warming up middle-energizer and reinforcing the spleen in the case of deficiency.

Excessive Syndrome of Coma with Heat Syndrome

Referring to ceasing urination due to fulminating hyperpyrexia.

Symptoms. Swelling abdomen and contracture.

Pathogenesis. Due to excessive organ qi and stagnancy of heat pathogens.

Therapeutic Principle. Removing heat of organs, and promoting diuresis.

Excessive Thirst in Cholera Morbus

Referring to the extreme thirst after vomiting and diarrhea in cholera.

Symptoms. There are two cases: 1. For exopathogenic cold cholera, depressed dysphoria, dry mouth, thirst, deep and slippery or dashing and rapid pulse. 2. For internal injury, thirst but no desire for drinking, dry mouth but wet lips and tongue, deep, fine and soft or floating and rapid or dashing pulse.

Pathogenesis. Owing to vomiting and diarrhea resulting in loss of body fluid in large amounts without immediate supply.

Therapeutic Principle. Nourishing yin and clearing away heat in case l; supplying qi, producing essence, and quenching thirst in case 2.

Excess of Liver-qi

Symptoms. Reddish eyes, aching of hypochondrium down to the lower abdomen, easy to anger, dizziness, ect.

Pathogenesis. Owing to the excessive pathogen in the Liver Meridian.

Therapeutic Principle. Adjusting circulation of qi, removing liver heat, and calming the liver.

Excess of Lung-qi

Symptoms. Cough, asthma, stuffy nose, excess and stagnation of phlegm, distention and fullness in the chest, etc.

Pathogenesis. Due to pathogenic factors of wind, cold and heat, invasion of turbid phlegm to the lung, the impairment of the purifying and descending function of the lung and the abnormal rising of lung-qi.

Therapeutic Principle. Removing pathogenic factors and enhancing the dispersing function of the lung.

Excess of Yin due to Yang-deficiency

Symptoms. Cold body and limbs, diarrhea, edema, phlegm retention, deep and indistinct pulse, etc.

Pathogenesis. Owing to Yang failure to warm zang-fu organs because of its deficiency, causing hypofunction of zang-fu organs, and leading to the syndrome of excess of yin and cold in the interior.

Therapeutic Principle. Warming yang and removing cold.

Excess Syndrome

Referring to sthenia-syndrome.

Symptoms. High fever, abdominal distention and pain with tenderness, coma and delirium, rapid and deep respiration, the accumulation of phlegm and saliva, constipation, and thick and greasy fur, solid pulse, etc.

Pathogenesis. Due to stagnant diseases, such as exogenous pathogen attacking the body, phlegm-fire, blood stasis, fluid retention, dyspepsia, parasitic infestation, ect.

Therapeutic Principle. Releasing the sthenia-syndrome and the pathogenic factors.

Excess-syndrome of Apoplexy Involving Zang and Fu

Referring to one type of apoplexy involving zang and fu.

Symptoms. Unconsciousness, trismus, clenched fist, red face, short breath, rale in the throat, constipation, anuresis, yellow and greasy coating of the tongue.

Pathogenesis. Due to reversed flow of qi and fire, blood stasis in the upper part, hyperactivity of liver-fire and abundant expectoration

Therapeutic Principle. Removing the endopathic wind and recovering consciousness; releasing heat from the heart and phlegm.

Excess Syndrome of Dizziness

Referring to a type of dizziness.

Symptoms. Paroxysmal dizziness, revolving and overturning of vision, distending pain of the head, easy to anger, distention and fullness in the chest and hypochondriac qi region, nausea, vomiting with phlegm fluid, loss of appetite, red tongue with yellowish and greasy coating, wiry or slippery, rapid pulse.

Pathogenesis. Due to slight hyperactivity of liver-yang, disturbing of the wind-yang, or due to disturbing of the orifices caused by wind-yang and phlegm-turbidity.

Therapeutic Principle. Calming the liver and suppressing yang hyperactivity of the liver, adjusting the function of the stomach to remove phlegm.

Excess Syndrome of Five Zang Organs

It refers to large and full pulse, hot skin, distending abdomen, constipation, and dysuria, and blurring of vision with restlessness. They are called five types of excess syndrome.

Large and full pulse shows invasion of heart by exuberant pathogens; hot skin shows invasion of the lung; distending abdomen means invasion of the spleen; constipation and dysuria indicates invasion of the kidney; blurring of vision with restlessness shows invasion of the liver by exuberant pathogenic factors.

Excess Syndrome of Heart

Referring to the syndrome of the heart disease.

Symptoms. Dysphoria, delirium, ulceration in the tip of tongue, even crazing, etc.

Pathogenesis. Owing to exuberant pathogen, heart attacked by excessive heat, phlegm-fire, etc.

Therapeutic Principle. Releasing the heart-heat.

Excess Syndrome of Impotence

Referring to a type of impotence.

Symptoms. Erection but not lasting long, frequent prospermia, aching and heavy sensation of the lower limbs, dark urine, yellowish and greasy tongue coating, soft and rapid pulse.

Pathogenesis. Mainly owing to the downward flow of damp-heat and relaxation of the assembled tendons.

Therapeutic Principle. Removing dampness and heat.

Excess Syndrome of Liver

Referring to the symptom of pathogenic changes of the liver caused by excess of pathogenic factor.

Symptoms. Dryness of the throat, bitter taste, dysphoria, irritability, constipation, yellow urine, distending pain in the hypochondrium and high fever, etc.

Pathogenesis. Owing to stagnation of qi, excessive fire and stasis, etc.

Therapeutic Principle. Releasing heat from the liver and removing the pathogenic factors.

Excess Syndrome of Otitis Media Suppurative

Referring to a type of otitis media suppurative.

Symptoms. Earache with yellowish purulent discharge, hypoacusis, fever, headache, abdominal fullness and constipation, reddened tongue with yellowish coating, wiry and rapid pulse.

Pathogenesis. Mainly owing to stagnation of fire in the liver and gallbladder, and damp-heat in the tri-energizer.

Therapeutic Principle. Removing wind, and damp-heat, detoxicating and opening the orifices.

Excess Syndrome of Stroke

Symptoms. Sudden swooning, unconsciousness with lockjaw and clenched fists, constipation and dysuria, rigidity and convulsion of limbs, etc.

Pathogenesis. Due to the internal occlusion of pathogenic excessiveness.

Therapeutic Principle. Releasing heat from the liver and expelling wind, inducing resuscitation with drugs of pungent flavor and cool property for heat syndrome of stroke, the yang excess.

Excess Syndrome of Uroschesis

Symptoms. Blockage of urination, lower abdominal distention and pain, irritability and thirst, red tongue with yellowish and greasy coating, rapid pulse.

Pathogenesis. Due to the transmission of damp-heat from the middle-energizer to the urinary bladder leading to the blockage of qi transfer of the urinary bladder.

Therapeutic Principle. Removing heat, and dampness enhancing the flow of qi and blood circulation.

Excess Type of Epilepsy

Symptoms. Sudden fall with loss of consciousness, lockjaw, opisthotonos mouth foaming, convulsion of the limbs after the attack, mere dizziness, inertia, and the patient returning to normal after rest.

Pathogenesis. Mainly owing to qi-stagnation of the liver and heart or dampness caused by the deficiency of the spleen.

Therapeutic Principle. Removing heat, the pathogenic wind and phlegm, calming the mind.

Excess-Type Tinnitus and Deafness

Symptoms. Sudden deafness, or distention and choking sensation in the ear. Cases of flaming up of liver and gallbladder heat, mostly with a flushed face, dry mouth, irritability and a wiry pulse; cases of stagnation of phlegm and heat, mostly with an oppressive feeling in chest, profuse sputum and a slippery rapid pulse.

Pathogenesis. Due to emotional upset, leading to the blockage of the Shaoyang Meridian and flaming up of liver and gallbladder heat, or stagnation of phlegm-heat.

Therapeutic Principle. Removing heat from the liver and phlegm, to clear the orifice.

Excitation Menstruation

Referring to regular menstruation with less amount of blood during the early pregnancy, but no harm to the fetus.

Exfoliative Dermatitis of Newborn

Symptoms. Patchy peeling off of fetal epiderm, rosy carnation, the affected part developing gradually and quickly spreading to all directions, peeling off most of the skin, or even becoming skinless of the body.

Pathogenesis. Due to the pregnant woman's over-eating five types of pungent, burned and smoked foods, etc. or due to infection to the fetus because of parents' syphilis.

Therapeutic Principle. Removing heat, fire and detoxicating.

Exfoliative Inflammation of Lips

Symptoms. At onset, red swelling and itching, ulcer with watery discharge, burning pain.

Pathogenesis. Due to wind-fire of the Stomach Meridian.

Therapeutic Principle. At onset, removing wind, heat, to expel the pathogenic factors from both interior and exterior of the body, and then nourishing blood and expelling the wind. Powder of Borncol and Borax for external use.

Exhaustion due to Summer-heat

Under this term, there are two diseases:
1. Due to over-drinking.

Symptoms. Cough, dyspnea, sudden hematemesis, epistaxis, distention, excessive thirst and restlessness, etc.

Pathogenesis. Due to excessive drinking of alcohol, or eating acrid and hot food in hot summer.

Therapeutic Principle. Removing summer-heat and protecting the lung.

2. Summer phthisis, sudden cough, and hemoptysis like tuberculosis.

Symptoms. Dysphoria with smothery sensation and thirst, cough, dyspnea, hemoptysis, lassitude and asthenia, etc.

Pathogenesis. Due to impairment of the lung and the Lung Collaterals by pathogenic summer-heat.

Therapeutic Principle. Removing heat and nourishing the lung, ceasing bleeding.

Exhaustion of Blood with Cold Limbs

Cold limbs due to deficiency of kidney-yang in lower-energizer, at the same time exhaustion of blood from upper orifices due to deficiency of yang-qi, yin blood not being taken in. It is the syndrome of cold transformation in Shaoyin Meridian. The dangerous phenomena of lower yang impairment and upper yin exhaustion the impairment of yang and blood from inducing perspiration.

Therapeutic Principle. Recuperating depleted yang and nourishing yin.

Exhaustion of Flesh

Symptoms. Emaciation, pale complexion, relaxation of muscles and even paralysis.

Pathogenesis. Due to prolonged consumption and emaciation.

Therapeutic Principle. Nourishing the spleen and reproducing the tissue.

Exhaustion of Fluid

Symptoms. Sluggishness of limbs, pallid complexion, dizziness, tinnitus and lassitude in the loin and knee.

Pathogenesis. Owing to excessive consumption of body fluid.

Exhaustion of Heart Function

Referring to the pulse conditions, in case of complete failure of heart genuine qi. Pressed gently, the pulse is hard and restless, while pressed firmly, the pulse is more restless.

Exhaustion of Kidney Function

Referring to the pulse condition of the kidney failure. The pulse is hard when pressed gently and restless when pressed firmly.

Exhaustion of Liver Function

Referring to the pulse condition of the liver failure. The pulse is weak when pressed gently, and when pressed firmly disappears immediately.

Exhaustion of Lung

Symptoms. Arthralgia due to cold and lumbago, epigastric fullness and rigidity, difficulty in urination, numbness of limbs, etc.

Pathogenesis. Due to exhaustion of primordial qi and visceral deficiency.

Therapeutic Principle. Recovering and nourishing primordial qi.

Exhaustion of Lung Function

Referring to the pulse condition of lung failure. The pulse is weak when pressed gently, and feeble when pressed firmly.

Exhaustion of Meridians and Vessels

Referring to the critical condition of blood depletion with wizened blood vessels.

Symptoms. Pale complexion, easy to anger, alopecia, dysphasia, restlessness due to fright, etc.

Pathogenesis. Due to insufficiency of blood and qi, dissociation of yin and yang.

Therapeutic Principle. Nourishing qi, blood, and adjusting yin and yang.

Exhaustion of Nutrient System

There are two meanings:

1. Referring to the consumptive disease due to impairment by emotional stress.

   Symptoms. Vexation of mind, chest pain and asthenia, perspiration and palpitation.

   Therapeutic Principle. Adjusting qi by alleviation of mental depression.

2. Referring to edema syndrome due to emotional depression.

   Symptoms. Slight swelling in the initial stage, no changes in skin color but exacerbation of years of edema, hard like stone, etc.

   Therapeutic Principle. Adjusting qi and releasing swelling and edema.

Exhaustion of Nutrient System and Essence

Symptoms. Emaciated physique, haggard complexion, listlessness, anorexia, intolerance of cold.

Pathogenesis. Due to internal impairment by emotions, loss of nutrient system and essence.

Therapeutic Principle. Nourishing essence, blood and calming the mind.

Exhaustion of Qi

Referring to the syndrome of consumptive disease due to deficiency of yang-qi.

Symptoms. Dyspnea, shortness of breath, abdominal fullness, anorexia, cold limbs or loose stool, etc.

Pathogenesis. Because of severe and long-standing illness or internal injury due to overstrain and general deficiency of qi, insufficiency of the kidney-yang and deficiency of the spleen-qi.

Therapeutic Principle. Warming and nourishing the spleen and the kidney.

Exhaustion of Qi Resulting from that of Body Fluid

Referring to a morbid state of qi exhaustion.

Symptoms. Profuse sweating, cold skin and extremities, weariness and barely palpable pulse.

Pathogenesis. Due to a high fever and excessive perspiration or due to severe vomiting and diarrhea.

Therapeutic Principle. Ceasing yin-fluid discharge and tonifying yang.

Exhaustion of Vital Essence Resulting in Deficiency Syndrome

Referring to a morbid condition of declining deficient and impairing symptoms.

Symptoms. Pale complexion, mental fatigue, palpitation, shortness of breath, spontaneous sweating, night sweating and thready, weak pulse, etc.

Pathogenesis. Due to physiological hypofunction on disfunction of zang-fu organs, meridians and collaterals and tissues, and due to exhaustion of vital essence, blood, and body fluid.

Exhaustion of Yin

Symptoms. Serious hypopsia or anopsia.

Pathogenesis. Due to excessive consumption of yin essence of the liver and kidney.

Therapeutic Principle. Nourishing yin of the liver and kidney.

Exogenous Febrile Disease

1. Referring to the exogenous febrile disease in a wide sense, a collective term for multiple diseases due to pathogenic heat.
2. Referring to exogenous febrile disease in a narrow sense, the pathogenous changes owing to pathogenic cold.

Exogenous Febrile Disease due to Wind-warm Pathogen

Symptoms. Headache, chills and anhidrosis at the early stage, and then fever, cough, excessive thirst, swelling and sore throat.

Pathogenesis. Due to stagnation of pathogenic wind-heat in the lungs, the restraint of the exterior by cold pathogen.

Therapeutic Principle. Removing wind, cold pathogens, pathogenic heat, and adjusting the lung.

Exogenous Febrile Disease in Summer

Referring to the exogenous febrile diseases.

Symptoms. Fever and chills.

Pathogenesis. Owing to latent heat and new cold invasion.

Therapeutic Principle. For the syndrome due to cold before the summer solstice, febrile disease with cold, inducing diaphoresis, removing heat; for the syndrome due to heat, after the summer solstice, febrile disease with heat, removing summer-heat and purging heat, then reinforcing qi and body fluid, and finally tonifying yin.

Exogenous Febrile Disease of Infant

Referring to the acute feverish disease of an infant due to the affection of the cold pathogens.

Symptoms. Fear of cold, fever, not sweating at early stage, fever increased, annoyance, thirst, constipation, yellow and difficult urine.

Pathogenesis. Due to the external cold pathogens; the cold changing into heat and the heat pathogens entering the interior.

Therapeutic Principle. In the patient with exterior cold at first, removing the exterior syndrome with drugs pungent in flavor and warm in property; for the patient exterior cold changed into heat, removing the exterior and interior heat.

Exogenous Febrile Disease with Foot Muscle Dropping

Symptoms. At the beginning, deep-purple, swelling and painful, later, running water between toes.

Pathogenesis. Usually due to sudden washing of feet with hot water after walking on snow in bare feet, or sudden washing of feet with cold water after walking on the sun-burned ground in bare feet.

Therapeutic Principle. Releasing water and dampness, enhancing diuresis or using garlic moxibustion for the patient with cold-damp and swelling feet. Removing heat and toxic material and cooling urine, for the patient with latent toxic heat on the extremities.

Exogenous Febrile Disease with Reddish Diaphragm

Symptoms. Fever with chills, headache and pain all over at onset, later, bright red coloration of the chest diaphragm, even violent blisters occurring in exterior, serious pain in the chest. Mostly found in spring season.

Pathogenesis. Owing to wind-warm seasonal noxious agents.

Therapeutic Principle. In mild cases, treating both exterior and interior. In serious cases, removing the lung-qi, and stagnated heat.

Exogenous Febrile Disease with Yellowish Ears

Symptoms. Yellowish ears similar to the exogenous febrile disease.

Pathogenesis. Due to, usually in spring season, seasonal noxious agent because of wind-warm invading Large Intestine Meridian, followed by attack of sudden cold.

Therapeutic Principle. With drugs of pungent flavor, releasing toxic substances, clearing away heat internally, and taking drugs to remove toxic substances and pain externally.

Exopathic Cold

Referring to the pathogenic cold factor from the exterior.

Symptoms. Aversion to cold, fever, etc.

Pathogenesis. Due to invasion of the body surface by the pathogenic cold and the consequent obstruction of yang-qi.

Exopathogen

It is a cause of a disease referring to the general term for the environmental pathogenic factors (wind, cold, summer-heat, dampness, dryness and fire) and other epidemic factors.

Expelling Toxin from Within the Body

Referring to a method, with drugs for nourishing the blood and removing pus, for reinforcing the body resistance and releasing the toxins from the inside of the body.

Indication. External sore in mid-stage, etc.

Expelling Wind and Nourishing Blood

Referring to a therapy method of treating damp arthralgia and sluggishness of blood circulation by using the prescription with the action of removing dampness, wind and nourishing blood and enhancing the blood flow.

Indication. Chronic rheumatism, deficiency of the liver and kidney and insufficiency of blood and qi, such as lumbago and knee pain due to cold, limited movement of the joints, and numbness.

Expiration and Inspiration

Referring to expiration and inspiration in Qigong terminology, getting rid of something stale and taking in something fresh, combining the deep respiration with voluntarily controlled concentration for tranquilizing the mind, and for health care and treatment.

Exterior Cold and Interior Heat

Referring to the exterior syndrome together with the interior heat syndrome.

Symptoms. Aversion to cold, fever, pain all over the body, thirsty, constipation, etc.

Pathogenesis. Mainly due to internal harmful heat, invasion of exopathic cold and wind or heat transmission because of exogenous pathogenic factors into the interior or unrelieved exterior cold.

Therapeutic Principle. Releasing superficial syndrome with the help of diaphoresis, removing heat.

Exterior Cold Syndrome

Symptoms. Severe aversion to cold, slight fever without sweat, pain all over the body, thin white coating of the tongue, and floating and taut pulse.

Pathogenesis. Due to wind-cold pathogens invading the skin.

Therapeutic Principle. Using drugs pungent in flavor and warm in property to remove the external syndrome.

Exterior Heat and Interior Cold

Symptoms. Exterior heat: fever, headache, and slight aversion to wind and cold; interior cold: loose stool, copious clear urine, and cold limbs.

Pathogenesis. Owing to cold in the interior and affection by pathogenic wind and heat or no relief of exterior heat and impairment of yang-qi of the spleen and stomach by misusing purgation.

Therapeutic Principle. Removing exterior heat and warming interior cold.

Exterior Pathogen

Referring to the pathogen affecting the superficial portion of the body mainly from the skin, most such diseases belonging to the exterior syndrome.

Exterior Syndrome

Symptoms. Headache, chills, fever, stuff nose, cough, white coating of the tongue and floating pulse, etc.

Pathogenesis. Owing to the invasion of exopathogen to the muscles and skin, the affection of the defensive function by pathogen, the struggle between the vital energy and pathogenic factor.

Therapeutic Principle. Removing exterior syndrome.

Exterior Syndrome Entering Interior

Referring to a pathogenesis.

Symptoms. No aversion to wind and cold, but aversion to heat, excessive thirst, dark urine, yellow and dry tongue coating, etc.

Pathogenesis. Owing to exterior syndrome changing into heat, and progressing toward interior.

Exterior Syndrome of Deficiency

Symptoms. Aversion to wind, spontaneous sweat, slow pulse, etc.

Pathogenesis. Mostly due to the deficiency of offensive qi, invasion of the pathogenic factor, inharmony of the nutrient, and superficial defensive system.

Therapeutic Principle. Releasing pathogenic factors from the superficial muscles, removing wind, and adjusting the functions of the nutrient, and superficial defensive system.

Exterior Syndrome of Excess

Referring to the invasion of exopathogen in the muscles and skin, the blockage of striae of skin, muscles and viscera.

Symptoms. Besides the exterior syndromes, chills, anhidrosis, pain in the head and body, and floating and strong pulse.

Pathogenesis. Owing to yang-qi gathering in the muscles and skin due to invasion by exopathogen.

Therapeutic Principle. Removing exterior syndrome and inducing diaphoresis.

Exterior Syndrome of Heat

Referring to the exterior syndromes.

Symptoms. Fever, headache, dry mouth, or sweating, red tip and edge of the tongue and rapid floating pulse.

Pathogenesis. Owing to affection of the skin by pathogenic heat.

Therapeutic Principle. By using drugs pungent in flavor and cool in property to remove external syndromes of heat type.

Exterior-syndrome Relieved but Interior-Syndrome Unrelieved

Symptoms. Perspiration, regular attack headache, pains in epigastrium, retching, short breath, etc.

Pathogenesis. Owing to phlegm retention in the interior, indigestion, blood stasis, impairment of yin, etc.

Therapeutic Principle. Removing excessive fluid.

External Carbuncle

Symptoms. Headless, local reddish swelling, heat and pain, clear boundaries and contractile root base, easy to swell, to form pus, to ulcerate and to heat; fever, thirst, yellowish fur, wiry and rapid pulse, etc if serious.

Therapeutic Principle. Removing blood stasis, heat, toxic material, enhancing blood circulation.

External Cold Syndrome due to Yang Deficiency

Symptoms. Aversion to cold and rigor.

Pathogenesis. Owing to cold exopathogens affecting the body and the lung, and making the lungs unable to disseminate yang-qi.

External Ear (MA)

Referring to an auricular point, also called ear (MA).

Location. On the supratragi notch close to the helix.

Function. Tonifying the yin of the kidney; checking hyperactivity of the liver-yang.

Indication. Inflammation of the external auditory canal, otitis media, tinnitus, dizziness.

External Genitalia (MA-H 4)

Referring to an auricular point.

Location. On the helix at the same level as the upper border of the inferior antihelix crus.

Indication. Dermatosis of the perineum, impotence, acute orchitis, epididymitis.

External Nose (MA-T 1)

Referring to an auricular point.

Location. On the center of the tragus.

Indication. Stuffy nose, nasal vestibulitis, rhinitis, simple obesity.

External Oculopathy

Referring to the general term of pathologic changes in the eyelid.

Symptoms. Pain, itching, astringency, redness, swelling, erosion, lacrimation, profuse mucoid secretion.

Pathogenesis. Owing to the affection of six external etiological factors or traumatic injury, or food retention, damp-toxin, phlegm-fire, etc.

Therapeutic Principle. Medicinal herbs based on symptoms, and external treatment and operation if needed.

External Posture Changes of Body (External Moving)

Referring to the changes from the static into the dynamic external postures of the body during practice Qigong.

External Scene

Referring to a Qigong practitioner concentrating on an external scence, e.g. a garden with blossom flowers, beautiful rural scenery, bright and clear moon, and/or the blue sea, to enter a tranquil state.

External Stillness and Internal Motion

Referring to the phenomena when practising static Qigong; the external physique looks still while the internal qi circulates actively.

Extra Points

1. Referring to a category of acupoints.
2. Referring to the points, not found in the Fourteen Meridians, but having wonderful clinical effect, also called extraordinary points, magical points or magical acupoints.

   Indication. Special effects for certain diseases.

Extravasated Blood

Symptoms. Necrotic blood overflowing from the vessels and accumulating among the tissues.

Pathogenesis. Mainly owing to stagnated blood accumulated inside due to the coldness of the uterus, blocking the qi circulation.

Extremely Poisonous Drugs

Referring to drugs with strong toxicity and potent action. Treatment of the disease with extremely poisonous drugs should stop immediately when the disease has been reduced to half, otherwise overdosage would injure the human body.

Extremely Shallow Puncture

Referring to one of the five needling techniques, very superficial puncture and quick withdraw, similar to the shallow needling of the nine needling methods, and leading to the current cutaneous needle from this method.

Exuberant Qi

Referring to the qi of five zang-organs in its exuberant period, they are: liver-qi exuberant in spring, heart-qi in summer, and lung-qi in autumn.

Exudative Dermatitis

Referring to one of tinea.

Symptoms. Reddish broken skin, erosion, endless itches, fluid flowing out when scratched off, as if worms creeping on the skin. Similar to the acute eczema and skin rash in Western medicine.

Pathogenesis. Due to the attacking of wind-dampness and heat into the skin and muscle.

Therapeutic Principle. Releasing dampness and killing parasites.

Eye (MA)

It is an ear point.

Location. On the anterior and posterior side of the intertragi notch.

Indication. Glaucoma and pseudo-myopia.

Eyebrow Sore

Symptoms. Sore between the eyebrow like tinea and itching all the time.

Pathogenesis. Ascending neonatal fever.

Therapeutic Principle. Drugs for removing itching, heat and detoxifying, calming wind, Chinese gall and alum into fine powder with sesame oil for external use.

Eye Disorder

Symptoms. The dull ocular movement and blurring of vision.

Pathogenesis. Due to pathogenic heat in Yangming Meridian steaming up.

Eye Dryness and Astringency

Symptoms. Uncomfortable feeling of dryness and astringency of the eyes.

Pathogenesis. Insufficient lung-yin, flaring up of deficiency heat of yin deficiency of both the liver and kidney, deficiency of the liver and lack of blood, etc.

Eye Expression

Referring to an expression of eyes reflecting the vital essence and energy of the zang-fu organs inside the body. Clinically helpful in the diagnosis and prognosis of a disease.

Eye Hemorrhage

Symptoms. Bleeding from eyes. In the servere case the blood sprays out directly from the eyes, accompanied by thirst for drinks, constipation, dry mouth and nose etc.

Pathogenesis. Mostly caused by dryness-heat in Yangming Meridian or liver fire exess, forcing blood to flow up.

Therapeutic Principle. Removing stomach heat and cooling the nutrient system to stop bleeding.

Eye Itching

Symptoms. Unbearable itching like worm crawling and squirming inside in serious cases.

Pathogenesis. Suffering from too much cold or intense heat, dampness-heat, blood deficiency, and also free flowing of qi and blood.

Eyelid Adhesion with Qi Orbiculus

Symptoms. Adhesion of the medial side of the eyelid with the white, affecting ocular activities.

Pathogenesis. Due to suffering from acute trachoma, or erosive substances entering the eye.

Therapeutic Principle. Detoxicating, releasing wind, adhesion, and blood stasis, dredging collaterals. Operation for severe adhesion.

Eye Pain during Menorrhea

Symptoms. During the month, dryness and pain in the eyes, headache and dizziness.

Pathogenesis. Due to great loss of menstrual blood, deficiency of the liver and blood, and malnutrition of the eyes and the head.

Therapeutic Principle. Strengthening the blood and tonifying the liver.

Eye Tinea

Symptoms. Itch and pain around the eye orbits.

Pathogenesis. Owing to stagnation of heat in the liver channels.

Therapeutic Principle. Smoothing the liver and removing heat.

F

Faber Bauhinia Twig and Leaf

It is the twig leaf or root of Bauhinia faberi Oliv. (Leguminosae).

Removing heat and moistening the lung, astringing yin fluid and calming the mind, relieving dampness and poisoning parasites.

Indication. Whooping cough, palpitation, insomnia, night sweat, emission, scrofula, eczema, scabies and tinea, etc.

Face Acupuncture

One of the needling therapies, referring to the method of needling some specific acupuncture points on the face for therapeutic purposes and acupuncture anesthesia.

Face Acupuncture Anesthesia

Referring to a method of the acupuncture anesthesia with certain points on the face needled to induce analgesia for operation.

Face-like Sore

Symptoms. Sores on the elbow and the knee, with a few holes left after ulceration, just like a man's face.

Therapeutic Principle. Reinforcing the body resistance and removing pathogenic factors. Medicated threads for external use, and with an operation if necessary.

Face Pityriasis Simplex

Symptoms. Small painful and itching swellings on the face or between eyebrows, sores, pain or itching at times, and accompanied by white scabs if scratched out.

Pathogenesis. Exopathogen of wind and heat in spring.

Therapeutic Principle. Spreading the tinctura of goldenlarch bark over them.

Facial Edema

1. **Symptoms.** Edema in the face.
   Pathogenesis. Invasion of wind after meal, or wind and heat fighting against each other going upward and attack the head and face.
2. **Symptoms.** Wind syndrome of the stomach.
   Pathogenesis. Invasion of poisonous wind-heat into the meridians and collaterals of Foot-Yangming.
   Therapeutic Principle. Mainly removing heat, detoxicating and relieving dampness by diuresis.

Facial Hemiparalysis

Symptoms. Deviation of the eye and mouth in the face to one side without the manifestation of apoplexy in hemiparalysis, corresponding to facial paralysis or peripheral facial paralysis.

Pathogenesis. Deficiency of the body's vital-qi, and invasion of pathogens into meridians and collaterals.

Therapeutic Principle. Removing the wind and dredging the meridians, and nourishing blood and adjusting the nutrient system.

Facial Hemiparalysis due to Purulent Ear

A kind of apoplexy (windstroke syndrome).

Symptoms. Deviation of the eye and mouth to one side.

Pathogenesis. Incurability of purulent ear, corresponding to otogenic facial paralysis.

Therapeutic Principle. Cf. The term of Apoplexy.

Facial Pain

Spasm and pain on the face.

Symptoms. Paroxysmal radial, lightning and sharp pain with feelings of tearing, stabbing and scorching. Generally, pain occurs from one point by wind attacking, face washing, speaking and eating.

Pathogenesis. Wind-cold pathogen attacking the meridians of Yangming or by wind-heat pathogen attacking the face, mostly occurring on one side and seen on the upper part of the face and the lower jaw.

Therapeutic Principle. Relieving the muscles and meridians of Yangming, Taiyang and Shaoyang.

Facial Paralysis

Symptoms. Facial stiffness, numbness and paralysis on one side, the deviated mouth sloping to the healthy side, disappearance of the wrinkles and nasolabial groove on the ill side, incomplete closure of the eyelid, lacrimation induced by irritation of the wind.

Pathogenesis. Wind-cold, wind-heat pathogens take advantage of the deficiency and attack the muscles and meridians on the face, leading to stagnation of qi and blood stasis and muscular flaccidity.

Therapeutic Principle. Removing wind, releasing the meridians and collaterals.

Fading Murmuring

Referring to a patient's critical sign at the advanced stage.

Symptoms. Unconsciousness, murmuring of low voice, broken and repeated words resulting from the vital-qi deficiency and exhaustion, asthenia cardiac qi and mental confusion.

Failure in Descending of Stomach-Qi

Referring to dysfunction of the stomach in transporting food downward.

Symptoms. Anorexia, distention and pain of the stomach, belching, hiccups, vomiting, etc.

Pathogenesis. Improper diet, adverse rising of the stomach-fire or stagnation of phlegm-damp or insufficiency of the stomach-qi.

Failure in Sending down Turbid Yin

Referring to failure normally in digestion and absorbing the essence of food and water and in excreting the wastes thereof.

Symptoms. Fullness in the chest, abdominal distention, loss of appetite, anorexia.

Pathogenesis. Insufficiency of qi in the spleen and stomach and functional disorder of elevating the lucid yang and lowering the turbid yin.

Failure of Blood to Nourish Muscles

Referring to a morbid state of spasm of muscles due to deficiency of the liver blood.

Symptoms. Numbness of the extremities, spasm of the tendons and tremors of the hands and feet, sluggishness of the joint movement and even clonic convulsion.

Pathogenesis. Malnutrition of the tendons caused by deficiency of the liver blood.

Failure of Defense-Qi to Protect Body against Diseases

Referring to a morbid condition.

Symptoms. Aversion to wind, spontaneous perspiration, etc.

Pathogenesis. Deficiency of yang-qi guarding the surface of the body, failure to consolidate the superficial resistance and leading to the skin and the muscular striae relaxed.

Failure of Heart

One of five cases of failure of five zang organs.

1. Referring to the crisis pulse syndrome.

    Symptoms. Black complexion, no cun pulse in left hand, black and yellow skin, straight sight with shaving head, etc.

    Pathogenesis. The failure of heart-qi.

Therapeutic Principle. Hemostasis by invigorating qi.

2. One kind of prostration syndrome of apoplexy.

    Symptoms. Apoplectic fainting, dysphasia, opening mouth with hands relaxed, urinary and fecal incontinence, etc.

    Therapeutic Principle. Recuperating depleted yang and arresting prostration.

Failure of Kidney

Referring to the severe and critical syndrome of exhaustion of kidney-qi.

Symptoms. Spontaneous emission of seminal fluid, ravings, straight eyesight, yellowish complexion, etc.

Pathogenesis. Mostly owing to general debility in the old age, weakness after chronic disease, intemperance in sexual intercourse. The exhaustion of kidney essence, deficiency of kidney-yang.

Therapeutic Principle. Nourishing kidney and warming yang.

Failure of Lucid Yang to Rise

Referring to the lucid yang transformed from water and food fails to moisten and nourish the head, skin, and limbs.

Symptoms. Dizziness, dim eyesight, tinnitus, deafness, aversion to cold and cold limbs, sleepy, fatigue, tastelessness, poor appetite, loose stool.

Pathogenesis. Insufficiency of yang-qi in the spleen and stomach, dysfunction of ascending clear-qi and descending turbid-qi.

Failure of Lung to Distribute Fluid and Qi

1. The impairment of the lung-yin by heat may affect the function to transport and distribute the fluid over the body, and lead to loss of moisture and nourishment for the skin and internal organs.

2. The tightening of the lung by cold pathogen may cause edema resulting from retention of water and fluid, or sputum, cough and asthma.

Failure of Middle-energizer Yang

Symptoms. Vomiting, diarrhea, loss of appetite, indigestion, tiredness, cold extremities, yellow face, dizziness.

Pathogenesis. Pathological change marked by weakening middle-energizer and function of the spleen-yang stomach in absorption and digestion.

Failure of Qi to Keep Blood Flowing within Vessels

Symptoms. All the syndromes of bleeding.

Pathogenesis. Dysfunction for qi to keep blood flowing within the vessels.

Therapeutic Principle. Nourishing qi and controlling blood.

Failure of Spleen

1. Referring to serious meridian syndrome. One of the fatal cases of the five zang organs.

    Symptoms. Bluish complexion with blackish color around the mouth, feeling cold in the mouth, abdominal heat, unconsciousness of diarrhea, swollen feet, no Guan pulse on the right hand.

    Pathogenesis. The disappearance of spleen-qi.

2. Referring to one of the collapse syndromes of apoplexy.

    Symptoms. Apoplexy with the symptoms of open mouth and loose hands.

    Pathogenesis. Due to the loss of spleen-qi.

    Therapeutic Principle. Warming yang and strengthening the spleen, supplementing the vital energy and rescuing the collapse.

Failure of Vaginal Orifice to Close

Referring to be unable to close of vaginal orifice after delivery.

Symptoms. Swelling of vaginal orifice, shortness of breath, unwillingness to speak, pale complexion and spontaneous sweating.

Pathogenesis. Malnutrition before delivery, postpartum deficiency of qi and blood.

Therapeutic Principle. Nourishing qi and blood.

Failure of Yin in Keeping Yang

Referring to pathologic changes of yang floating, because of yin deficiency or repellence of yang by excessive yin, due to the failure of yin to keep yang-qi.

Failure to Control Blood and Fluid due to Qi Deficiency

1. Referring to the failure of qi to keep blood flowing within the vessels.
2. Referring to the failure of the visceral qi to control blood and the body fluid.

   Symptoms. Spontaneous perspiration, emission, diarrhea, enuresis, metrorrhagia and metrostaxis and hemafecia.

   Therapeutic Principle. Ceasing discharge and invigorating visceral qi.

Failure to Suck in Newborn

Referring to the newborn infant that cannot suck milk 12 hours after birth without congenital defect.

Symptoms. 1. Shallow breath and weak sound; 2. Pale face, cold limbs, crying with body curled up.

Pathogenesis. In the first case, lack of primordial qi; in the second, deficiency cold of the spleen and stomach.

Therapeutic Principle. 1. Tonifying the primordial qi; 2. Warming middle-energizer and the spleen.

Faint

Symptoms. Dizziness with dim eyesight, syncope and coma but restoration afterwards.

Pathogenesis. Malnutrition of meridians and collaterals with the affection of wind-cold to the head.

Therapeutic Principle. Removing wind and obstruction in the meridians and tonifying qi and nourishing blood.

Faint due to Acupuncture

Referring to a fainting phenomenon caused by needling.

Symptoms. Dizziness, blurred vision, dysphoria, nausea, pale complexion, palpitation, profuse cold sweat and drop of blood pressure.

Therapeutic Principle. Withdraw the needle at once and make the patient lie down and have a rest.

Faint during Moxibustion

Symptoms. Referring to a patient becoming faint during moxibustion.

Pathogenesis. Mainly because of delicate constitution, nervous tension, or excess fire or too big a moxa cone.

Therapeutic Principle. Cf. Faint due to Acupuncture.

Faintness due to Metrorrhagia

Symptoms. Muddled eyes or unconsciousness.

Pathogenesis. Too much loss of blood resulting from the metrorrhagia.

Therapeutic Principle. Ceasing bleeding and nourishing blood.

Faint with Cold Limbs

Symptoms. Falling because of sudden dizziness, delirium, and unconsciousness with cold limbs.

Pathogenesis. Mostly owing to sudden confusion of qi, imbalance of rising and falling qi, and dysfunction of qi and blood in circulation.

Therapeutic Principle. Induce resuscitation, or recuperating the depleted yang and rescuing the patient from danger.

Faji

An extra acupuncture point.

Location. On the midline of the forehead at the midpoint of the anterior hairline.

Indication. Migraine, overall headache, vertigo and acute infantile convulsion.

Method. Needling along the skin from 0.5-1 cun, and apply moxibustion for 10-15 minutes.

Falling due to Faint

Symptoms. Falling due to dizziness.
Pathogenesis. Resulting from the deficiency of qi and blood, and imbalance between yin and yang in the zang-fu organs.

False Chinese Swertia Herb

It is the whole herb of Swertia pseudochinensis Hara (Gentianaceae).
Effect. Removing heat, reinforcing the spleen and promoting diuresis.
Indication. Dyspepsia, acute conjunctivitis, toothache, canker sore, etc.

Falsehellebore Rhizome

It is the rhizome of Veratrum nigrum L. (Liliaceae).
Effect. Inducing vomiting endopathic wind-phlegm and killing parasites.
Indication. Apoplexy, epilepsy, inflammation of throat with abundant accumulation of phlegm and fluid, scabies, tinea and tinea capitis.
Notice. It is an extremely toxic substance. It should be used with great care.

False Labor

It is a terminology in gynecology.
Referring to early amniorrhea during full-term or incomplete pregnancy, or amniorrhea without delivery.

False Labor Pain

It is a terminology in gynecology. Referring to clinical false labor pain of a woman of term-pregnancy.
Symptoms. Inconstant abdominal pain without lumbago; or inconstant abdominal pain with fetal movement, or amniorrhea without severe lumbago during the third trimester of pregnancy.

False Pregnancy

Symptoms. Amenorrhea with a swollen pregnant-like abdomen, making women feel like pregnancy.
Therapeutic Principle. Adjusting the flow of qi and enhancing menstrual discharge.

Fanshaped Corallodiscus

It is the whole herb of Parmelia saxatilis Ach. (Parmeliaceae).
Effect. Nourishing blood, acuity of vision, tonifying the kidney, enhancing diuresis, removing heat and detoxicating.
Indication. Blurred vision, hemoptysis, metrorrhagia, pain in the loins and knees, heat stranguria, gonorrhea, leukorrhea, burns and scalds.

Fanshaped Corallodiscus Herb

It is the whole herb of corallodiscus flabellata (Franch) B.L. Burtt. (Gesneriaceae).
Effect. Detoxicating, removing swelling, enhancing blood circulation, and relieving pain.
Indication. Irregular menstruation, leukorrhea with reddish discharge, traumatic injuries, sores, carbuncles, etc.

Fascicular Keratitis

Symptoms. The red-bean-like projection surrounded with blood filaments on the black eyeball. It is often seen in infants, repeated attack, pain, photophobia and lacrimation. After recovery, a scar left over, affecting visual acuity.
Pathogenesis. Heat accumulation in the Liver Meridian, or deficiency of the spleen-qi.
Therapeutic Principle. Mainly removing heat from the liver for the excess type, and adjusting the spleen and stomach for the deficiency type.

Fasting Dysentery

Symptoms. Dysentery, anorexia, nausea and vomiting, in severe cases, emaciation and listlessness yellowish and greasy tongue coating.
Pathogenesis. The retention of damp-heat in the large intestine, excess pathogens impaired stomach-yin and the failure of the stomach-qi to descend, or the impairment of both the spleen and stomach due to prolonged illness and qi-deficiency in the middle-energizer.

Therapeutic Principle. Relieving pathogenic factors and descending the adverse-qi, adjusting the stomach and intestine.

Fat Deposit Nebula

It is an acute ocular disease.

Symptoms. Nebula overspread with fat deposit in the black, beastly headache, acute ophthalmalgia and visual disturbance, and certainly resulting in upward attack of pus, even blindness or exophthalmos.

Pathogenesis. Mostly owing to outward attack of wind-toxin and internal accumulation of excess fire in the liver and gall-bladder, and combination of interior and exterior pathogenic factors to attack upward upon the black.

Therapeutic Principle. Removing wind and detoxicating, purging fire, strengthening body resistance and eliminating pathogenic factors. External treatment is also applicable.

Fatigue

Symptoms. Lassitude, emaciation, disinclination to talk.

Pathogenesis. Usually owing to deficiency and injury of the liver and the spleen, and insufficiency of essence and blood.

Therapeutic Principle. Nourishing the liver and kidney, and replenishing essence qi and reinforcing blood circulation.

Favus

Symptoms. At the beginning, small papula eruptions or small pustules in the root part of the hair on the head skin, in the shape of millets. If they are broken, yellow water flows out, gradually forming tray-like yellow crusts in the sulphur color.

Pathogenesis. The steaming of the head skin by the damp-heat of the spleen and the stomach, or affected by contact infection.

Therapeutic Principle. The external treatment is essential, and to pull out the sick hair with its root is more important.

Fear Causing Sinking of Kidney-Qi

Symptoms. Urinary and fecal incontinence, emission, spermatorrhea and lingering diarrhea.

Pathogenesis. Sinking of kidney-qi.

Fear Dysphagia

Symptoms. Hunger but inability to eat due to the food blocked between the throat and diaphragm, or vomiting of phlegm together with food before the food entering the stomach.

Pathogenesis. Due to grief and qi accumulation resulting in the obstruction of phlegm; lack of kidney-yin caused by alcohol and over sexual intercourse; the obstruction of stagnant heat caused by yin deficiency and fire excess.

Therapeutic Principle. Relieving mental depression and resolving phlegm, nourishing kidney-yin, removing fire, promoting blood circulation by removing blood stasis, replenishing qi and nourishing the spleen.

Fear Melancholia

Symptoms. Pale complexion, aching pain of the waist and weakness of legs, dizziness and tinnitus, impotence, frequent urination, pale tongue with whitish coating and deep and weak pulse, etc.

Pathogenesis. Fear impairs the kidney with exhaustion of the kidney essence.

Therapeutic Principle. Warming the kidney and nourishing the essence.

Feather Cockscomb Seed

It is the ripe seed of Celosia argentea L. (Amaranthaceae).

Effect. Removing nebula, enhancing eyesight, clearing away liver fire.

Indication. Bloodshot eyes with swelling pain and dizziness resulting from the liver-fire, oculopathy, blurred vision, cutaneous pruritus resulting from pathogenic wind-heat, etc.

Febrile Disease due to Drowning

Symptoms. Fever, headache, and pains in joints of all over the body.

Pathogenesis. Affection of wind-cold owing to drowning.

Therapeutic Principle. Eliminating diaphoresis to remove cold, and simultaneously, reinforcing the heart and the kidney.

Febrile Disease of Cold Type

1. Referring to Taiyang febrile syndrome.
2. Referring to epidemic febrile disease with latent pathogen and cold.

   Symptoms. For exterior syndrome, headache, fever, body pain, aversion to cold, etc, at onset, for interior syndromes as vexation, bitter taste, foul breath.

   Therapeutic Principle. Exterior and interior diseases should be treated at the same time.

Febrile Disease with Accumulation of Blood

1. Referring to the blood accumulation of Taiyang meridian.

   Symptoms. Manic state, blood stool, rigidity and distention in the lower abdomen.

   Pathogenesis. Unrelieved Taiyang disease, the pathogenic heat entering the fu-organ through the meridian and the stagnated heat in the lower-energizer.

   Therapeutic Principle. Removing exterior syndrome, the heat and the stagnation.

2. Referring to the accumulation of Yangming meridian due to the accumulation of blood stasis and the pathogenic heat transported into Yangming meridian.

   Symptoms. Rigidity and pain in the lower abdomen and easy defecation with dark hard stool.

Therapeutic Principle. Relieving the heat, reinforcing blood circulation by clearing away blood stasis.

Febrile Disease with Fluid-retention

Symptoms. Thirst, fullness of the lower abdomen, slight fever, difficulty in urination, vomiting immediately after drinking water, etc.

Pathogenesis. Prolonged Taiyang disease, heat following the meridians going into the fu-organs and combining with fluid, leading to the stagnation of the qi circulation.

Therapeutic Principle. Activate yang and promote the activity of qi, expelling pathogenic factors from exterior the body and promoting diuresis.

Febrile Perspiration

Symptoms. Sweating, night fever and excessive thirst, etc.

Pathogenesis. Usually owing to excessive heat in the interior of the body or steaming of fire heat.

Therapeutic Principle. Tonifying yin and relieving fire.

Fecal Impaction in Rectum

Symptoms. Feces impacted in the rectum and difficult in defecation.

Therapeutic Principle. Applying honey and soap powder in the anus, for cold type, adding the powder of wild aconite root to relieve cold and the constipation; for heat type, using pig bile to relieve heat and relax the bowels.

Feech

It is the whole body of Whitman, Hirudo nipponica Whitman and Whitmania acranulata Whitman (Hirudinidae).

Effect. Dissipating blood stasis to eliminate mass.

Indication. Amenorrhea owing to stagnation of blood masses in the abdomen and traumatic injuries.

Feeling of Depression and Dysphoria

Symptoms. Referring to the feeling of depression and dysphoria.

Pathogenesis. The deficiency of vital essence in the lower-energizer or blood deficiency with hyperactivity of yin fire.

Therapeutic Principle. Nourishing the heart, the spleen, reinforcing the kidney to replenish vital essence, and nourishing the blood to calm the mind.

Feeling of Distention and Fullness in Chest

Symptoms. Painless distention and fullness in the chest.

Pathogenesis. The upward obstruction of damp pathogen, phlegm accumulation and qi stagnation and the obstruction of yang-qi in the chest.

Therapeutic Principle. Adjusting the stomach and resolving phlegm.

Feimu (Ex-CA)

An extra acupuncture point.

Location. On the chest, in the 2nd intercostal space, about 1.5 cun lateral to the anterior midline.

Indication. Sudden onset of infantile epilepsy, fullness in the chest, shortness of breath, etc.

Method. Moxibustion is applicable.

Feishu (B 13)

A meridian acupuncture point.

Location. On the back, below the spinous process of the 3rd thoracic vertebra, 1.5 cun lateral to the posterior midline.

Indication. Cough, dyspnea, fullness in the chest, pain in the spine and back, tidal fever, night sweating, hemoptysis, sore throat, nasal obstruction, etc.

Method. Puncture obliquely 0.5-0.8 cun, apply moxibustion to the point with 3-5 moxa cones or 5-15 minutes.

Notice. Deep puncture is forbidden.

Feiyang (B 58)

A meridian acupuncture point.

Location. On the posterior side of the leg, 7 cun directly above Kunlun (B 60) and 1 cun lateral and inferior to Chengshan (B 57)

Indication. Headache, dizziness, stuffy nose, epistaxis, pain in the loins and back, myasthenia of legs, hemorrhoids with pain and swelling, manic-depressive psychosis.

Method. Puncture perpendicularly 1-1.5 cun. Apply moxibustion if needed.

Feiyang Meridian

A meridian, referring to the collateral of the Food-taiyang Meridian in the leg. Beginning at Feiyang (B 58), 7 cun above the lateral malleolus, going to the area anterior to Fuliu (K 7) of the Foot-shaoyin Meridian, and then going up to meet Zhubin (K 9), the Cleft point of the Yinwei meridian.

Felon

A general term for furuncle on fingers.

Symptoms. Reddish, swelling, severely painful, the disease is not serious, if it is easy to ulcerate. If the swelling spreads upwards, even impair the muscles and bones of the palm and finger, or carbuncle complicated by septicemia, it is a deteriorating case.

Pathogenesis. Due to traumatic infection or the attacking of fire-toxin from the zang-fu organs.

Therapeutic Principle. If the skin of the affected finger is hard, use fresh pig bile to cover the affected finger. After the pus is formed, used a needle to stab it and cut it open and drain it.

Female Abdominal Mass

Symptoms. Hard and movable mass in the abdomen of a woman, at beginning like an egg, then a cup, with normal menstrual cycle.

Pathogenesis. It is similar to ovarian cyst. Usually owing to qi obstruction and blood stasis leading to the mass.

Therapeutic Principle. Resolving the mass and removing the cold, reinforcing the flow of qi and blood circulation.

Female Amenorrhea after Edema

Symptoms. Amenorrhea following edema of extremities.

Pathogenesis. Mostly owing to internal retention of body fluid spreading to the skin resulting from deficiency of the spleen that fails to control water, and weakness of the bladder-qi transformation, leading to stasis of menstrual blood.

Therapeutic Principle. Tonifying the spleen and inducing diuresis to recover normal menstruation.

Female Cloudy Urine

Symptoms. Putrid, pus-like discharge from the female urethra, subjective sensation of astringent pain in the urethra, with difficult in micturition.

Pathogenesis. Mostly due to heat from dampness accumulation in the bladder.

Therapeutic Principle. Removing heat and enhancing diuresis.

Female Dream-Intercourse

Symptoms. Intercourse in the dreamland, trance, insomnia and dreaminess, dizziness, headache, and tiredness.

Pathogenesis. Resulting from the malnutrition of mentality caused by qi and blood deficiency, and heart blood insufficiency owing to the impairment of the seven violent emotions.

Therapeutic Principle. Tonifying the heart to calm the mind, or nourishing the kidney.

Female Itching Eruption due to Wind-heat in Blood

Symptoms. Painful and itchy pimple-like lumps on the body skin, persistent dripping of pussy water, irregular menstruation and urine, nocturnal fever and sweat, fear of cold and heat, laziness, and anorexia.

Pathogenesis. Pathogenic wind-heat in the liver and spleen, fire stagnation, and pathogenic blood dryness.

Therapeutic Principle. Smoothing the liver, adjusting the spleen, removing wind and heat, and nourishing blood.

Female Leukorrhagia

Symptoms. Sudden onset of whitish mucus flowing out of the female vagina when she has excessive sexual desire.

Pathogenesis. Mostly owing to failure of the kidney function to consolidate resulting from sexual overstrain.

Therapeutic Principle. Nourishing the kidney to restore its normal function.

Female Talon-like Spasm

Symptoms. Clonic spasm of the female extremities in the shape of talons with pain and difficulty in stretching out.

Pathogenesis. Postpartum blood insufficiency, under nourishment of the tendon and, also due to wind-cold.

Therapeutic Principle. In the case without sweating, tonifying blood and removing wind to adjust the defensive function of the vessel; in the case with sweating, tonifying blood and replenishing qi to harmonize the vessel with its defensive function.

Fengchi (G 20)

A meridian acupuncture point.

Location. On the nape, below the occipital bone, on the level of Fengfu (GV 16), in the depression between the upper ends of the sterno-cleido-mastoideus and trapezius muscles.

Indication. Headache, dizziness, pain and stiffness of the neck and nape, conjunctival congestion with pain, lacrimation, rhinorrhea with turbid discharge, etc.

Method. Puncture obliquely 0.5-0.8 cun toward the nose with the tip of the needle slightly downwards, or subcutaneously through Fengfu (GV16). Apply moxibustion 3-17 moxa cones or 5-15 minutes with warming moxibustion.

Fengchitong (Ex-UE)

An extra acupuncture point.
Location. 2.5 cun above the transverse crease of the wrist.
Indication. Toothache resulting from the wind pathogen.
Method. Moxibustion if needed.

Fengfeixue (Ex-CA)

A set of acupuncture points.
Location. Total 3 points, one point is 0.5 cun below Zhongwan (CV 12); the other two are 1.5 cun lateral to Zhongwan.
Indication. Aphonia and hemiplegia after apoplexy, etc.
Method. Apply moxibustion 3-5 moxa cones or 5-10 minutes with warming moxibustion.

Fengfu (GV 16)

A meridian acupuncture point.
Location. On the nape, 1 cun directly above the midpoint of the posterior hairline, below the external occipital protuberance, in the depression between the trapezius muscle of both sides.
Indication. Manic-depressive psychosis, epilepsy, hysteria, apoplexy with aphonia, palpitations because of grief, fear and fright, dizziness, pain and stiffness of the neck and nape, etc.
Method. The patient sitting with the head bending forward slightly and relaxed, the doctor puncturing slowly and perpendicularly or obliquely downward 0.5-1 cun toward the mandible. Moxibustion is applicable.
Notice. Forward, upward and deep puncture is forbidden.

Fengguan

A point for infantile massage.
Location. The palmar surface of the 1st, 2nd and 3rd segments of the index finger.
Indication. Infant convulsion. Chiefly used for inspection, diagnosis, and mas-

sage. If superficial collaterals can be seen in the first segment, it indicates the infant patient is not seriously ill.

Fenglong (S 40)

A meridian acupuncture point.
Location. On the anterior-lateral side of the leg, 8 cun above the tip of the external malleolus, lateral to Tiaokou (S 38), and two finger breadths (middle finger) from the anterior crest of the tibia.
Indication. Profuse sputum, asthma, cough, pain in the chest, headache, dizziness, sore throat, constipation, manic-depressive psychosis, epilepsy, pain and paralysis, flaccidity, swelling and pain of the lower limbs.
Method. Puncture perpendicularly 0.5-1.2 cun. Apply moxibustion 5-7 moxa cones or for 5-15 minutes.

Fengmen (B 12)

A meridian acupuncture point.
Location. On the back, below the spinous process of the 2nd thoracic vertebra, 1.5 cun lateral to the posterior midline.
Indication. Cough owing to pathogenic wind, fever, headache, vertigo, profuse nasal discharge, stuffy nose, neck rigidity, pain in the chest and back, lumbodorsal carbuncle and cellulitis, hot sensation in the chest.
Method. Puncture obliquely 0.5-1 cun. Apply moxibustion 3-5 moxa cones or 5-15 minutes with moxibustion.
Notice. Deep puncture is forbidden.

Fengshi (G 31)

A meridian acupuncture point.
Location. On the lateral midline of the thigh, 7 cun above the popliteal crease, or at the place touching the tip of the middle finger when the patient stands erect with the arms hanging down freely.
Indication. Hemiplegia owing to apoplexy, muscular atrophy of the lower limbs with pain and numbness, general pruritus, beriberi.

Method. Puncture perpendicularly 1-2 cun. Apply moxibustion 3-5 moxa cones or 5-10 minutes with warming moxibustion.

Fengxi (MA)

It is an auricular point.
Location. At the midpoint between Finger (MA-SF 1) and Wrist (MA-SF 2).
Indication. Urticaria, cutaneous pruritus, asthma, allergic rhinitis.

Fengyan (Ex-HN)

It is an extra acupuncture point.
Location. At the part 0.5 cun anterior to the midpoint of the line connecting the midpoint of the posterior hairline and the lower border of the earlobe.
Indication. Mania, hysteria, headache, neurosis, etc.
Method. Puncturing perpendicularly 1-1.5 cun.

Fengyan (Ex-UE)

It is an extra acupuncture point.
Location. On the radial border of the thumb, at the junction of the red and white skin, and at the end of the crease of the phalangeal joint of hand.
Indication. Irritability, fullness of the abdomen, vomiting, hiccups, pain in all fingers, difficult bending and extending fingers, night blindness, nebula, etc.
Method. Puncture perpendicularly 0.1-0.2 cun. Apply moxibustion 3-5 moxa cones or 5-10 minutes with warming moxibustion.

Fennel Root

It is the root of Foeniculum vulgare Mill. (Umbelliferae).
Effect. Warming the kidney and adjusting the stomach, reinforcing flow of qi and removing pain.
Indication. Periumbilical colic owing to invasion of cold, vomiting owing to cold in the stomach, abdominal pain and arthralgia owing to pathogenic wind-dampness.

Fennel Stem and Leaf

It is the stem and leaf of Foeniculum vulgare Mill. (Umbelliferae).
Effect. Removing pathogenic wind, adjusting upward adverse flow of the lung and the stomach-qi and ceasing pain.
Indication. Eruptive disease, hernial pain and subcutaneous swelling.

Fenugreek Seed

It is the ripe seed of Trigonella foenumgraecum L. (Leguminosae).
Effect. Warming the kidney-yang and removing wind-dampness.
Indication. Deficiency cold in the kidney, abdominal pain due to gastrointestinal spasm, beriberi owing to pathogenic cold and dampness, cold pain in the loins and knees, pain in the lower abdomen with testis, etc.

Fetal Restlessness

Symptoms. Pregnant woman tenesmus owing to abnormal fetal activities with abdominal pain and soreness in the waist, or with a modicum of vaginal bleeding.
Pathogenesis. Due to debility of the vital and the front meridians for blood collection to nourish the fetus resulting from the deficiency of qi, blood and kidney, blood heat and trauma, etc.
Therapeutic Principle. Treating in accordance with the differentiation of causes and signs.

Fetching Water from Tianhe

Referring to a massage manipulation, one of massage manipulations for children.
Operation. Push from Chize (L 5) on the hand bend to Laogong (P 8) with the hands dipped with some water.
Function. Removing pathogenic heat.
Indication. Febrile diseases.

Fever Accompanied by Fear

Referring to fever with restlessness, usually found in the infants.

Symptoms. Lower fever, blue complexion sometimes, sweat on the body, dysphoria at night, palpitation with fright.

Pathogenesis. Fright caused by fever, resulting from the internal heat in the heart and liver.

Therapeutic Principle. Removing heat and purging fire.

Fever due to Blood Deficiency

Symptoms. Lower fever, dizziness, dim eyesight, fatigue, palpitation and restlessness, etc.

Pathogenesis. Mostly due to improper diet and over-fatigue, impairment of the spleen and stomach, or hematemesis, hemoptysis, hematochezia, or metrorrhagia and metrostaxis after delivery, and insufficiency of yin blood, failure of consolidating yang.

Therapeutic Principle. Tonifying yin, blood, qi and removing fever.

Fever due to Blood Stasis

Symptoms. Fever in the afternoon or at night, or feeling cold and hot alternatively, dry mouth and throat without desire for drinking water, pain fixed in certain part, dry skin, withered and yellowish or dark complexion, purplish tongue with spots of blood stasis, etc.

Pathogenesis. Mostly owing to trauma, emotional disturbance, blood stasis stagnating the meridians, obstruction in circulation of qi and blood.

Therapeutic Principle. Reinforcing blood circulation to eliminate blood stasis and clear the meridians.

Fever due to Consumption

Referring to the fever owing to consumption.

Symptoms. Protracted fever alternately, low in the morning and high in the evening, relieved after rest and severe after strain and vexation.

Therapeutic Principle. The same as that of consumptive disease, adjusting and tonifying yin-yang and invigorating the spleen and replenishing qi.

Fever due to Improper Diet

Symptoms. Fever in the evening, vomiting, eructation with fetid odour and acid regurgitation, fullness in the epigastrium, abdominal pain and distention, poor appetite diarrhea, etc.

Pathogenesis. Owing to improper diet, and internal accumulation of food inside.

Therapeutic Principle. Reinforcing digestion, removing stagnation and dispelling the heat.

Fever due to Lung Deficiency

Symptoms. Low fever at night, hypersalivation, emaciation, dry cough without phlegm, or with less sticky phlegm, even hoarseness, etc.

Pathogenesis. Usually owing to protracted illness, the impairment of both qi and yin in the lung meridian by the remaining heat in the lung during the late period of febrile disease.

Therapeutic Principle. Tonifying the lung and yin.

Fever due to Phlegm

Symptoms. Often having a fever at night, nausea and anorexia, weakness, tiredness, etc.

Pathogenesis. Mainly owing to splenic deficiency leading to the inability to transporting and transforming nutrients, the accumulation of wetness producing phlegm, the stagnation of phlegm turning into heat.

Therapeutic Principle. Tonifying spleen and removing phlegm, eliminating distention and expelling heat.

Fever due to Qi Deficiency

1. Generally referring to fever of deficiency type to qi deficiency in the spleen and stomach or in the spleen and lung.

   Symptoms. Fever and anxiety, spontaneous perspiration, aversion to cold, headache and tiredness, etc.

Pathogenesis. Mainly owing to improper feeding, overstrain and internal injury to the spleen and stomach resulting in qi deficiency and fire excess.

Therapeutic Principle. Reinforce and invigorate qi in the middle-energizer.

2. It refers to Summer-dampness, which injures qi.

Symptoms. Fever with tiredness of the limbs, vexation and restlessness short breath, thirst spontaneous perspiration, yellowish urine

Therapeutic Principle. Removing summer-heat and tonifying the vital energy.

3. It refers to summer-heat which consumes qi and body fluid.

Symptoms. Fever, hyperhidrosis, upset and thirst.

Therapeutic Principle. Clearing away summer-heat enhancing the vital energy to promote the production of body fluid.

Fever due to Yin Deficiency

Symptoms. Tidal fever, night sweat, vexation and restlessness, flushing of zygomatic region, etc.

Pathogenesis. Mostly owing to deficient blood failing to astringe yang, flaring of fire deficiency type, excessiveness of yang resulting from deficiency of yin, water failing to astringe fire.

Therapeutic Principle. Tonifying yin and blood, and eliminating fever resulting from deficiency of qi.

Fever in Muscles and Skin

Symptoms. Feverish sensation in muscles and skin, or burnt sensation by pressing, or local red swollen and pain, etc.

Pathogenesis. Usually owing to the invasion of exopathogen, pathogenic heat stagnated in Yangming which reaches to muscles and skin, or deficiency of qi and blood, stagnation of heat of deficiency type in muscles and skin.

Therapeutic Principle. In the case with excessiveness of pathogen, removing pathogenic heat of Yangming; in the case with

qi-deficiency, replenishing qi to remove heat; and in the case with blood deficiency, tonifying spleen and enhancing the production of blood to reinforce qi.

Fever Resulting in Dissipation of Yang

Referring to a pathogenesis, heat enabling the sweat pores open and striae of skin loosen, leading to the hyperhidrosis and excretion of yang-qi result.

Fever with Chill

Referring to fever and aversion to cold, a common symptom often seen in many febrile diseases.

Symptoms. Fever with headache, spontaneous perspiration and intolerance of cold, indistinct and weak pulse, etc.

Pathogenesis. Owing to by exopathogen, such as common cold, exogenous febrile disease, epidemic febrile disease, and internal injury caused by overstrain.

Fewflower Lysionotus Herb

It is the whole herb of Lysionotus panciflora Maxim (Gesneriaceae).

Effect. Removing heat, phlegm, pathogenic heat from blood, ceasing bleeding, eliminating dampness, curing leukorrhagia, eliminating obstruction in the meridians and relieving pain.

Indication. Pulmonary tuberculosis, hemoptysis, leukorrhea, bacillary dysentery, rheumatic arthralgia and traumatic injuries.

Fidgetiness

Referring to one of restlessness caused by heat stagnation in various diseases.

Symptoms. Due to exogenous pathogenic factor, restlessness without sweat generally belonging to excess, while restlessness after sweating mostly belonging to deficiency. For various diseases due to internal damage, more vexation than restlessness.

Pathogenesis. Owing to internal damage and exogenous pathogenic factor.

Fidgetiness due to Deficiency

Referring to the syndrome of oppressed feeling in the chest because of the heat of deficiency type.

Symptoms. Feverish sensation in the chest, oppression and insomnia, dry mouth and throat, and poor appetite, etc.

Pathogenesis. Usually owing to yin deficiency and internal heat, the disturbance by the fire of deficiency type, or the remaining heat of exopathogenic disease after sweating, vomiting and purging, and the impairment of the heart by anxiety.

Therapeutic Principle. Tonifying yin, removing heat and fidgetiness.

Fidgetiness due to Phlegm-fire

Symptoms. Cough, stagnation of qi in the chest, sleeplessness due to restlessness, uneasiness, etc.

Pathogenesis. Owing to fire phlegm disturbing the heart.

Therapeutic Principle. Purging pathogenic fire and eliminating phlegm, and tranquilizing the mind by tonifying the heart.

Field Horsetail

It is the whole herb of Eguiselum arveuse L. (Equisetaceae).

Effect. Removing heat and cough, ceasing bleeding and inducing diuresis.

Indication. Hematemesis, epistaxis, hemafecia, retrograde menstruation, cough with dyspnea and stranguria.

Field Thistle Herb

It is the whole herb or tuber of Cephalanoplos segetum (Bge) Kitam or C. Setosum (Bieb.) Kitam (Compositae).

Effect. Dispelling pathogenic heat from blood, ceasing bleeding, removing toxic substances, lower the blood pressure, and curing carbuncles.

Indication. Hemoptysis, epistaxis, hematemesis, hematuria, metrorrhagia and metrostaxis, carbuncles, sores and other pyogenic infections on the skin owing to noxious heat, etc.

Fig

It is the dried succulent receptacle of Ficus carica L. (Moraceae).

Effect. Improving the function of the stomach and enhancing bowel movements, subduing swelling and detoxicating.

Indication. Enteritis, dysentery, constipation, laryngalgia, carbuncle, sore, scabies, etc.

Figwortflower Picrorrhiza Rhizome

It is the rhizome of Picrorrhiza scrophulariaeflora Pennell (Scrophulariaceae).

Effect. Relieving heat of deficiency type, treating infantile malnutrition with fever and removing damp-heat pathogen.

Indication. Fever owing to yin deficiency, acute dysentery and jaundice owing to damp-heat pathogen, swelling pain of hemorrhoid, abdominal distention owing to infantile malnutrition, etc.

Figwort Root

It is the root of Scrophularia ningpoensis Hemsl. (Scrophulariaceae).

Effect. Removing heat and toxic material, relieving pyogenic inflammation and tonifying yin, purging the sthenic fire.

Indication. Febrile diseases with diabetes, dry mouth, deep-red tongue, maculas, unconsciousness and delirium, hematemesis, epistaxis, swollen and sore throat, suppurative infections on the skin, scrofula, etc.

Filiorm Cassytha Herb

It is the whole herb of Cassytha filiformis L. (Lauraceae).

Effect. Removing pathogenic heat from the blood, detoxicating and inducing diuresis.

Indication. Cough resulting from the lung-heat, jaundice, dysentery, epistaxis, stranguria with blood, carbuncles, swellings, sores, furuncle, scalds, etc.

Filthy Disease with Opisthotonus

Symptoms. Backwardness of nape and head, severe distention and oppressed feeling in the heart and chest, physique in opisthotonus.

Pathogenesis. Filthy toxin invading interior and corruption of zang and fu, and poor prognosis.

Therapeutic Principle. Tranquilization and alleviation spasm, scaling the neck, chest or back, and detoxicating.

Fimbriate Orostachys Herb

It is the whole of herb of Orostachys fimbriatus (Turcz.) Berger, or Orostachys erudescens (Maxim.) Ohwi (Crassulaceae).

Effect. Removing pain, subduing swelling, detoxicating, and promoting diuresis.

Indication. Hemoptysis, inflammation of lung, epistaxis, dysentery, hepatitis, heat stranguria, hemorrhoid, eczema, suppurative infections on the skin, burns and scalds, etc.

Finger (MA-SF 1)

An auricular point.

Location. Divide scaphoid fossa into six equal parts, from up to down, the 1st equal part is the finger.

Indication. Paronychia, pain and numbness of fingers.

Finger Citron Fruit

It is the fruit of Citrus medica L. var. sarcodactylis Swingle (Rutaceae).

Effect. Soothing the liver, adjusting flow of qi and stomach and resolving phlegm.

Indication. Stagnation of qi of the liver and stomach, epigastric and abdominal distention, stomachache, poor appetite, nausea, vomiting, and cough with profuse sputum.

Finger-kneading Manipulation

It is a massage manipulation.

Operation. Pressing and moving to and fro or circularly on an acupoint or affected area with the whorl surface of the finger, the manipulation applicable to all parts of the body.

Finger-needle Therapy

Referring to the therapeutic method.

Operation. Hold the terminal segment of the middle finger with the thumb and the index finger, lightly and then heavily press and massage the point with the tip of the middle finger to the extent of the subjective sensation of aching, numbness and distention, the operation time depends on the patient's condition.

Effect. Relaxing muscular tendons and enhancing the flow of qi and blood in the meridians and collaterals, removing blood stasis and stagnation of qi, inducing resuscitation and ceasing pain, replenishing qi and calming the mind, etc.

Indication. Shock, syncope, heatstroke, epilepsy, gastropathy, toothache, etc.

Finger Poking Technique

Referring to a acupuncture manipulation.

Method. Hold the needle with the thumb and index finger and pluck the body of the needle gently with the middle finger, thus enhancing the needling sensation.

Finger Pressing

Referring to a needling technique in acupuncture.

Operation. Pressing the point with the thumb of the left hand, and inserting the needle into the skin right against the surface of the thumb. This technique is usually used to puncturing with short needles.

Finger-pressing Manipulation

It is a massage manipulation.

Operation. Push and press the body surface with the tip or the whorl surface of the thumb.

Effect. Relaxing muscles, enhancing the blood circulation and removing pain.

Indication. Stomachache, headache, aching pain and numbness of the extremities, etc.

Finger Pulling

It is an acupuncture manipulation, referring to lifting the needle to the subcutaneous level, waiting until feeling of the needling qi subsides and no tight or heavy feeling in the hand, and finally withdrawing the needle. So as to make nutrient and defensive qi spread and not escape.

Finger-rubbing Manipulation

It is a massage manipulation.

Operation. Keep the index, middle and ring finger on the certain part. Rotate rhythmic along with the palm and fingers, with the wrist joint as the center.

Effect. Adjusting the function of the stomach and spleen, relieving dyspepsia.

Indication. Epigastralgia, indigestion with distention, stagnancy of qi.

Finger Tip Kneading-pinching-pressing Technique

It is a type of treatment.

Method. Press on and pinch up the skin adjacent to the point with the thumb and index finger of the left hand to help the insertion of the needle with the right hand. It usually uses for the horizontal puncture on the face points, such as Yintang (HN 3), Zanzhu (B 2), Dicang (S 4), etc.

Fire

1. One of the five elements. Referring to yang-heat, heat things in nature or excessive condition.
2. Referring to vital-qi and the power of life activities.
3. Referring to a cause of disease. Fire is one of the six climatic conditions in excess as pathogenic factors, same as warm, summer-heat and heat pathogens in nature without marked seasonal change.

Fire and Heat in Interior

Referring to a pathologic manifestations of interior disturbance of fire pathogen and hyperfunction of body due to yang excess, or yin deficiency, or stagnation of blood and qi or pathogenic factors.

Fire and Wind Stirring Up Each Other

A pathological change causing high fever with convulsions and unconsciousness in febrile disease.

Symptoms. High fever, coma, convulsions, neck stiffness, dizziness.

Pathogenesis. Up-stirring of the liver owing to impairment of the liver by excessive heat pathogen.

Therapeutic Principle. Removing heat and the endopathic wind, enriching the body fluid.

Fire Boil

Symptoms. On the lips and the mouth, the palms and between the finger joints, small red and yellow vesicles, with painful, itching and numb, even alternate attack of fever and chill, dysphoria and stiff tongue.

Pathogenesis. Due to the noxious heat in the heart meridian.

Therapeutic Principle. The same as Furuncle.

Fire Cough

Symptoms. Protracted cough with less phlegm or bloody phlegm, extreme thirst and flushed face, pain in the hypochondrium and constipation, etc.

Pathogenesis. Caused by the impairment of the lung by pathogenic fire.

Therapeutic Principle. For the fire of excess type, removing the fire from the lung; for fire of deficiency type, tonifying yin to reduce pathogenic fire.

Fire Cupping

Referring to one of the cupping methods.

Method. Burn fire in the cup, driving away the air to create a negative pressure inside, thus producing suction of the cup to the skin.

Fire Failing to Generate Earth

It refers to that the yang of kidney (fire) fails to warm the spleen and stomach (earth). Thus causing the dysfunction of digestion, absorption and transformation of water and dampness.

Symptoms. Waist soreness, cold knee, aversion to cold, dyspepsia, urine incontinence, general edema and diarrhea before dawn.

Therapeutic Principle. Warming the kidney and reinforcing the spleen.

Fire Formation due to Accumulation of Pathogenic Factors

Referring to a morbid state of stagnation of yang-qi, and fire syndrome caused by the pathogenic factors.

1. It refers to the yang is transformed into heat and fire, due to exopathic wind, cold, dampness and dryness invade the interior and are stagnated in the body
2. The pathologic metabolic products in the body, such as phlegm dampness and blood stasis, or parasitic infestation tend to be stagnated and transformed into fire.

Fire from Gate of Life

Referring to the kidney-yang. It is very essential for the functions of the zang-fu organs and the ability of reproduction, as well as warming and nourishing five zang organs and six fu organs and being the source of heat energy.

Fire Invasion

Referring to one kind of the syndromes of invasion of interior by pyogenic agent.

Symptoms. Boils in dark purple color, wide base, dry opening without pus, burning pain, or high fever, thirst, constipation, etc.

Pathogenesis. The invasion of pathogenic fire into nutrient blood resulting from inadequate yin blood, excessive pathogenic fire, loss of treatment, wrong treatment, squeezing and pressing, etc.

Therapeutic Principle. Relieving pathogenic heat from blood and detoxicating.

Fire Needling

It is an acupuncture method.

Effect. Expelling cold by warming the meridians and removing cold, clearing and activating meridians and collaterals.

Method. Puncturing a point quickly with a red-hot needle.

Indication. Carbuncle and furuncle with pus-pocket not ulcerate, scrofula, nevus verruca, polyp, etc.

Fire of Deficiency Type

Symptoms. Flushing of cheeks, afternoon fever, restlessness, heat sensation in palms and soles, insomnia, night sweat, dry mouth and throat, dizziness, tinnitus, etc.

Pathogenesis. Due to insufficiency of essence, blood and yin, serious impairment of yin fluid and excess of yang.

Fire of Excess Type

Symptoms. Bloodshot eyes, high fever, flushed face, thirst, bitter in the mouth scanty deep colored urine, constipation, aphthous stomatitis, in serious case, coma and delirium, or restlessness.

Pathogenesis. Excessive pathogenic fire.

Fire Stagnancy

Symptoms. Bitter taste, anxiety, chest tightness, distention in hypochondriac region, acid regurgitation, constipation, scanty dark urine, headache, bloodshot eyes.

Pathogenesis. Pathogenic fire and heat caused by emotional and liver-qi stagnation.

Fire toxin

1. It refers to a noxious pathogenic factor formed by accumulated fire, which causes boils, ulcers, red burning heat,

bright swelling, easiness to form pus, fever, thirst, etc.

2. Burns and scalds complicated with infection.

Fish-brains-like Dysentery

Symptoms. Dysentery with fish-brains-like excreta, fullness in the chest, dysphoria, tenesmus and abdominal pain, etc.

Pathogenesis. Usually owing to the internal excess of the turbid dampness, or the impairment of the body fluid by fire-toxin.

Therapeutic Principle. Removing the turbid dampness, and intense heat and detoxicating.

Fish Mass

Symptoms. The mass in the abdomen sometimes disappearing, eructation, nausea and abdominal distention, etc.

Pathogenesis. Usually owing to the general weakness of the spleen and stomach, the improper diet of raw fish, leading to the stagnation of the cold in the stomach and abdomen.

Therapeutic Principle. Enhancing the spleen and warming the middle-energizer, removing the accumulation of pathogen and the mass.

Fish-scale-like Furuncle

1. A kind of lingual pustule. Referring to furuncle on the tip of the tongue.

   Symptoms. Pustule on the tongue, purplish, nail-head-like, hard and painful, with subjective sensation of fever and aversion to cold.

   Pathogenesis. Fire-toxin in the Heart Meridian.

   Therapeutic Principle. Removing pathogenic fire and detoxicating.

2. Anther designation of ichthyosis.

   Symptoms. Skin of the infant turns greyish, dry and rough with fish-scale-like scabs, marginal areas are sticking up, and tightly attached to the skin surface soon after his/her birth.

Pathogenesis. Blood deficiency, wind-dryness and malnutrition.

Therapeutic Principle. Nourishing blood and moistening dryness.

Fish Spine Carbuncle

Referring to the syndrome of the carbuncle like the fish spine grown between the ribs.

Symptoms. The carbuncle only on the skin, hard and painful white vehicles at the beginning, gradually like a fish spine, when broken, yellow water flowing out, but forming pus quite slowly.

Pathogenesis. The stagnancy caused by the cold of insufficiency of yang-qi and the obstruction of damp-heat.

Therapeutic Principle. Apply moxibustion with garlic slices at first to activate yang.

Fissured Tongue

Symptoms. Vexation, dryness in the mouth, fissures, furuncle and pain of tongue.

Pathogenesis. Mostly owing to flaming up of the hear-fire, impairment of body fluid because of dryness-transformation, or by excessive heat because of deficiency of yin.

Fist-hitting Manipulation

It is a massage manipulation.

Operation. The wrist straightened to strike the body surface with the back of the fist or the empty fist clenched.

Fist-pressing Manipulation

It is a massage manipulation.

Operation. Clench the solid fist to press the point or part with the backs of all the proximal interphalangeal joints and push-press or poke in a narrow range.

Effect. Enhancing blood circulation, adjusting muscles and tendons, and removing contracture of meridians.

Indication. Aching pain of the shoulder and back, pain of the waist and legs, etc.

Fistular Onion Stalk

It is the bulb near the root of Allium fistulosum L. (Liliaceae).

Effect. Expelling pathogenic factors from the muscles and skin by means of inducing diaphoresis, expelling cold from the body surface and enhancing the flow of yang-qi, clearing toxic substances and masses.

Indication. Light affection by exopathogenic wind-cold, diarrhea, infections on the body surface, etc.

Five Colors

Referring to blue, red, yellow, white and black corresponding to the five zang organs (the liver, heart, spleen, lung and kidney) respectively based on the theory of the five elements. The five colors correspond to the five zang-organs reflecting on certain part of the face. The blue color suggests cold, pains, convulsion, or blood stasis. The color changes on the corresponding parts indicate the zang-fu organ diseases.

Five-element Function

Referring to the five most fundamental element: wood, fire, earth, metal, and water with their characteristic properties; an ancient philosophical concept to explain the composition and phenomena of the physical universe and later used in traditional Chinese medicine to expound the unity of the human body and the natural world, and the physiological and pathological relationship between the internal organs.

It refers to the qi functional activities of the five elements, they are against one another, and at the same time they are for one another and set in a state of constant motion and change. Also referring to the five evolutive phases: generating, growing, changing, collecting, and storing.

Five-element Generation

The five materials, wood, fire, earth, metal and water inherently posses the relations of production and promotion, i.e. the generation relation among them. The order of generation is as follows: wood generates fire, fire generates earth, earth generates metal, metal generates water, and water in its turn, generates wood.

Five-element Restriction

Referring to the relation of control or restraint among the five elements, (wood, fire, earth, metal and water). Each one has the function of restricting and inhibiting the other one, such as wood restricts earth, earth restricts water, water restricts fire, fire restricts metal and metal restricts wood.

Five Emotions

The five kinds mental changes (joy, anger, anxiety, melancholy and fear) are closely related to the functions of five zang organs. The joy, anger, anxiety, sorrow, and fear assigned to the heart liver, spleen, the lung and kidney respectively.

Five Excesses

It is an acupuncture manipulation, referring to over-reinforcing or over-reducing in acupuncture. Over-reinforcing enhancing pathogen, and over-reducing exhausting vital qi are called the five excesses.

Five-kind Flavors

Referring to the tastes of the drugs: pungency, bitterness, sweetness, sourness, and saltiness. Different flavors of the drugs have different actions. The action of pungent flavor is used to disperse and relieve; the action of sour to astringe; the action of sweet to tonify and slowly act; the action of bitter to purge and dry; and the action of salty to soften and cause laxation.

Five-Shu Points

Referring to five points on the twelve regular meridians distributing distal to the elbow and knees, varying in their condition of the flow of qi and blood. The size of water flow is an analogy used to describe the characteristics of the qi in meridians moving from the small to the large, from the shallow to the deep and from far to near. They are well, spring, stream, river, and sea points.

Five Zang-Organs' Charges

The five zang-organs (heart, lung, liver, spleen and kidney) are in charge of the vessels, skin, tendons, muscles, and bones respectively.

Five Zang-organs Exerting Their Qi on Six Fu-organs

It is one of the theories of the close relation of zang and fu, referring to their coordination of physiological actions kept by the meridians connecting zang and fu. The functions of six fu organs to transform food-stuff are performed with the cooperation of the qi of five zang-organs. For example, stomach digestion needing spleen transportation and transformation, and bladder's urination depending on kidney-qi transformation, etc.

Fixed Mass due to Water Retention

Symptoms. Abdominal masses, hypochondriac distention and fullness, general edema, dysuria and constipation, etc.

Pathogenesis. Usually owing to the obstruction of meridians and collaterals, the water retention in the abdomen.

Therapeutic Principle. Adjusting the flow of qi and removing retained water.

Flaccidity

Symptoms. Muscular flaccidity of the limbs, inability to clench the hands and walk, and particularly weakness of lower limbs.

Pathogenesis. Mainly owing to heat of the five zang organs, especially the heat of the lungs leading to the consumption of body fluid, invasion of dampness-heat, deficiency of qi and blood, and deficiency of the liver and kidney.

Therapeutic Principle. For the consumption of body fluid resulting from lung-heat, remove heat and treat dryness syndrome by moisturizing; for the invasion of damp-heat, remove heat and dry up the dampness; for the deficiency of qi and blood, to replenish qi to nourish blood and yin; for deficiency of the liver and kidney, to nourish the liver and kidney.

Flaccidity Confluence

Symptoms. Flaccidity of foot, impotence, etc.

Pathogenesis. Sexual strain and masturbation, etc.

Therapeutic Principle. Nourishing the kidney and enhancing the muscles.

Flaccidity due to Damp-heat

Symptoms. Flaccid and slightly swollen feet, numb toes, with severe feeling of oppression in the chest, reddish urine, difficulty in micturition.

Pathogenesis. Damp-heat invading and damaging the muscles and tendons.

Therapeutic Principle. Removing heat and dampness, invigorating the spleen.

Flaccidity due to Deficiency of Blood Supply

Symptoms. Weak extremities with a sensation of joint breaking, difficulty to raise extremities, and even failure to stand.

Pathogenesis. Often owing to flaring-up of heart fire, abnormal rising of blood qi, deficiency of blood in the lower part, or absence of blood nourishment in meridians after loss of blood.

Therapeutic Principle. Removing the fire of heart, and tonifying blood and qi.

Flaccidity due to Injury

Symptoms. Softness and asthenia of bone and muscle, muscular emaciation, dyscinesia and inability of free movement.

Pathogenesis. Owing to traumatic paralysis, flaccid atrophy, articular contracture and hyperosteogeny due to spine injury.

Therapeutic Principle. Acupuncture and moxibustion, massage and oral administration of medicine. For the type of blockage of meridians, removing blood stasis and activating meridians;for the type of deficiency of blood and qi, by invigorating blood qi and activating meridians; for the type of flaccidity of bone and muscle, by enhancing muscle, tendon and bone.

Flaccidity due to Invasion of Damp-heat Pathogen

Symptoms. Flaccidity of limbs, heavy sensation of the body, numbness, mild edema mostly in the lower extremities, or upward heat-qi from the feet and legs, fever, feeling of stuffiness in the chest and epigastrium, scanty deep colored urine.

Pathogenesis. Mostly owing to the invasion of dampness in meridians, leading to the blockage of the circulation of nutrient and defensive systems, stagnation of heat, injury of the body fluids and malnutrition of the tendons and muscles.

Therapeutic Principle. Clear and activate the meridians and collaterals, remove and enhance diuresis.

Flaccidity due to Kidney-heat

Symptoms. Flaccidity of lower limbs, lassitude in loin and spinal column, inability to stand or with giddiness, tinnitus, dry throat, emission, etc.

Pathogenesis. Usually owing to deficiency of the kidney, or excess of sexual intercourse, difficulty in recuperating lost essence, or overstrain, insufficiency of yin-essence leading to insufficiency of water and excess of fire in the kidney and failure to nourish muscles.

Therapeutic Principle. Nourishing the kidney essence, yin and removing heat.

Flaccidity due to Lung-heat

Symptoms. Flaccidity of the hair and skin, cough, shortness of breath, dry pharynx, scanty and deep-colored urine, dry stool, etc.

Pathogenesis. The scorched lung involving hair and skin.

Therapeutic Principle. Removing heat and enhancing salivation, nourishing yin and moistening the lung.

Flaccidity of Extremities

Symptoms. Slow weak movement of hands and feet.

Pathogenesis. Resulting from the injury of body fluid owing to the lung heat, or the deficiency and weakness of the spleen and stomach.

Flaccidity of Limbs due to Qi Deficiency

Symptoms. Weakness of limbs, feeble movement of limbs, with short breath, pale and swollen face, etc.

Pathogenesis. Mainly owing to the internal injury resulting from over-fatigue, improper diet, or qi deficiency of the spleen and stomach resulting from long illness, failure of the nourishing the limbs and body.

Therapeutic Principle. Mainly nourishing the spleen and qi.

Flaccidity of Mouth in Infant

Symptoms. For infant, pale lips, weakness of oral muscles and sometimes slobbering.

Pathogenesis. Owing to lack of milk and food and deficiency of qi in the spleen and stomach.

Therapeutic Principle. Reinforcing the spleen and the stomach.

Flaccidity of Neck

Symptoms. The weak neck failure to arise the head.

Pathogenesis. Usually infant's congenital defect and weakness of marrow resulting from the deficiency of kidney, or acquired injury, deficiency of the spleen and stomach, failure of clear yang to ascend, etc.

Therapeutic Principle. Warming the kidney, nourishing the spleen, the marrow and enhancing yang to ascend.

Flaccidity Syndrome due to Deficiency of Liver-Kidney Yin

Symptoms. Weakness of the lower limbs, difficulty to stand long, and even difficulty to walk, progressive muscular atrophy of the legs, often with dizziness, baldness, dry throat, tinnitus, emission, enuresis, irregular menstruation.

Pathogenesis. Deficiency of liver blood and kidney essence, leading to failure to nourish muscles, tendons, bones and meridians.

Therapeutic Principle. Clear and activate the meridians and collaterals; nourish the liver and kidney.

Flaccid Tongue

Symptoms. Retracted and curled tongue and flaccidity of its muscles. Color of the tongue is not fresh with dryness and flaccidity.

Pathogenesis. Mostly owing to deficiency of the spleen unable to supply essence qi or consumption of yin fluid leading to malnutrition of the muscle.

Therapeutic Principle. Reinforcing the middle-energizer and enriching the blood.

Flaccid Tongue with Aphasia

Symptoms. In chronic disease, the syndrome with pale and flaccid tongue, thin shape of the tongue and weakness, failure in speaking.

Pathogenesis. Owing to wind phlegm in fulminating disease or endopathic wind caused by blood deficiency.

Therapeutic Principle. Nourishing the heart and spleen.

Flaming of Heart-fire

Symptoms. Mental irritability, insomnia, palpitation and even delirium, mania, and ceaseless laughing.

Pathogenesis. Owing to the excessive heart-fire and dysfunction of taking charge of mental activities.

Therapeutic Principle. Removing the heart-fire, nourishing the heart, tranquilizing the mind.

Flaming-up of Liver-fire

Symptoms. Dizziness, flushed complexion, blood shot eyes, bitter taste, dry throat, restlessness and irritability, burning pain in hypochondrium, constipation, yellow urine, or hematemesis and epistaxis.

Pathogenesis. The stagnation of the liver-qi, or impairment of the liver by anger, upward invasion of the hyperactive liver-qi or overacting of five emotions or excess of dampness and heat in the liver and gallbladder, transformed into fire.

Therapeutic Principle. Purging the liver of pathogenic fire.

Flaring-up of Deficiency Fire

Symptoms. Dry and sore throat, dizziness, restlessness and insomnia, tinnitus, amnesia, feverish sensation in palms and soles, conjunctival congestion, oral ulcers, etc.

Pathogenesis. Owing to the deficiency of the kidney-yin, leading to the failure of water to control the heat-fire, and causing yin-fire rising up.

Therapeutic Principle. Tonifying yin to reduce pathogenic fire.

Flash-fire Cupping

Method. Insert a long burning slip of paper or burning ball of alcohol-cotton held with forceps into the cup; go along the inside the cup for one turn and then, take the flame away and cover the part to be cupped immediately with the cup upside-down.

Flat-pushing Manipulation with Fist

Referring to a massage manipulation, one of pushing manipulations.

Operation. Clench one's fist and push with the processes of interphalangeal joints of the index, middle, ring and little fingers.

Effect. Promoting the blood circulation, removing spasm, wind, dampness and pain.

Indication. Internal impairment owing to overstrain in the waist, back and extremities, old injury, arthralgia owing to pathogenic wind-dampness and dyserethesia.

Flatstem Milkvetch Seed

It is the ripe seed of Astragalus complanatus R. Br. (Leguminosae).
Effect. Warm and nourish the liver and kidney, arrest spontaneous emission, and improve eyesight.
Indication. Lumbago owing to the kidney deficiency, impotence and seminal emission, enuresis, frequent micturition, leukorrhagia, blurred vision, dizziness and dim eyesight, etc.

Flatulence due to Qi Deficiency

Symptoms. Abdominal distention and discomfort, anorexia or loose stool, etc.
Pathogenesis. The abdominal distention and fullness due to qi deficiency.
Therapeutic Principle. Reinforcing the spleen and nourishing qi.

Flatulence of Large Intestine

Symptoms. Fullness and distention of the stomach and intestine, and abdominal pain with borborygmus.
Pathogenesis. Due to the invasion by pathogenic cold into the large intestine.
Therapeutic Principle. Removing cold, stagnancy by tonifying the spleen and adjusting qi.

Flatulence of Small Intestine

Symptoms. Distention and fullness of the lower abdomen, leading to pain in the waist.
Pathogenesis. Cold in the small intestine.
Therapeutic Principle. Adjusting qi and removing cold.

Fleece-flower Root ⬡ F-1

It is the root tuber of herb Polygonum multiflorum Thunb. (Polygonaceae).
Effect. Tonifying the liver and kidney, nourishing the vital essence and blood, blacken the hair and beard, removing constipation, toxins, moistening the intestine.
Indication. Dizziness, blurred vision, early graying of hair, lassitude of the loins and legs, seminal emission, chronic malaria carbuncles, cellulitis and scrofula, constipation etc.

Fleece-flower Stem

It is the stem of Polygonum multiflorum Thunb. (Polygonaceae).
Effect. Tranquilizing the mind by nourishing the heart, expelling the obstruction of the collaterals and wind.
Indication. Insomnia, hyperhidrosis, pain in the extremities resulting from the blood deficiency; and skin eczema and pruritus as a lotion, etc.

Fleshy Goiter

Symptoms. Single lump on one side or either side of the right middle of the prominentia laryngeal. The lump is in the form of a hemisphere smooth, soft, painless, which moves up and down during swallowing. It shows no body symptoms. It may have such secondary diseases as hyperthyroidism and cancer.
Pathogenesis. Caused by depression and anger, the accumulation of damp phlegm.
Therapeutic Principle. Regulating the flow of qi to alleviate mental depression, removing phlegm, and softening hard masses, or treating with an operation.

Fleshy Tumor

Symptoms. Swelling up of the tumors from muscle, in different numbers and sizes, soft, easy to be pressed flat, movable when pushed, in normal skin color, painless.
Pathogenesis. Over-thinking, improper diet and phlegm stagnancy, etc.
Therapeutic Principle. Reinforcing the spleen, adjusting qi by alleviation of mental depression and removing phlegm, or operation if needed.

Flicking Manipulation

1. Referring to a massage manipulation.

   Operation. Press the finger-nails of one hand heavily with the print surface of the other hand fingers and flick the fingers out in heavy force, continuously, 120-160 times per minute.

   Effect. Relaxing muscles and tendons, clearing collaterals, removing wind and cold.

   Indication. Stiffness of the neck and headache.

2. Referring to a type of auxiliary acupuncture technique. (1) Flick the skin around the point before the insertion of the needle with fingers. (2) Gently flick the needle handle after the insertion of the needle for enhancing the needle sensation.

Floating Yang

A disease and syndrome.

Symptoms. Flushed cheeks, dry mouth bleeding from the mouth and nose, adverse cold from feet tibia-region.

Pathogenesis. Usually consumption of the primordial qi in the lower part and kidney-yang floating to the upper.

Therapeutic Principle. Nourishing primordial qi, reinforcing yang and removing prostration syndrome.

Fluid Deficiency in Large Intestine

Symptoms. Constipation or difficulty in discharging stool, emaciation, dry skin and throat, red tongue with less coating.

Pathogenesis. Yin-blood deficiency or consumption of body fluid due to febrile disease.

Therapeutic Principle. Tonifying the bowel to release constipation.

Fluid Distention

Symptoms. Facial and limb edema with severe palpitation, dyspnea, etc.

Pathogenesis. Mostly caused by splenic deficiency failing to transport body fluid, leading to the skin overfilled with the fluid.

Therapeutic Principle. Inducing diuresis, and nourishing the spleen to control the circulation of body fluid.

Fluid-dyspnea

Referring to dyspnea caused by attack of the excessive fluid to the lung.

Symptoms. Dyspnea, fullness in the chest and diaphragm, distention in the abdomen, severe palpitation, swelling of face or limbs, impairment of urination, etc.

Pathogenesis. Mostly owing to impairment of purifying and descending function of the lung, stagnant dampness in the spleen, the dampness up and the fluid retention in the kidney.

Therapeutic Principle. For superficiality, removing the retained fluid to adjust dampness and descending lung-qi; for origin, adjusting the spleen and warming kidney. In the cases of distention followed by dyspnea, regulating the function of the lung; in cases of dyspnea followed by distention, regulating the function of the spleen.

Fluid Retention during Convalescence

Symptoms. Distention and fullness below the waist, difficulty in urination and defecation, etc.

Pathogenesis. Qi disorder resulting in the obstruction of damp-heat, and the failure of retained fluid and accumulated below the waist.

Therapeutic Principle. Removing retained water, clearing away the heat, softening and resolving hard mass.

Flushing of Zygomatic Region

Symptoms. Appearance of bright red color on the zygomatic region.

Pathogenesis. Owing to deficiency of yin in the liver and the kidney, and upward floating of yang in deficiency condition.

Food Obstruction in Diaphragm

Symptoms. The desire for food but vomiting with phlegm and food after eating, etc.

Pathogenesis. Usually due to the impairment of the seven emotions, the phlegm transformed from the stagnated qi and its obstruction in the diaphragm, the block of the middle-energizer qi and the stagnation of functional activities of qi.

Therapeutic Principle. Alleviating the mental depression and eliminating phlegm, and enhancing blood circulation to remove blood stasis.

Food Regurgitation from Stomach

Symptoms. Distention in the abdomen after eating, vomit in the evening what was eaten in the morning, comfort after vomiting, lassitude, dim complexion, etc.

Pathogenesis. Usually owing to improper diet, or the spleen and the stomach impaired by worry and anxiety, or retention of indigested food in the stomach due to deficiency cold in the middle-energizer.

Therapeutic Principle. Warming the middle-energizer, reinforcing the spleen, and lowering the adverse flow of qi to adjust the stomach.

Foot Motor Sensory Area

Referring to the specific stimulation area for scalp acupuncture.

Location. At the two points which locate on the 0.3 cun bilateral sides of the midpoint of the anterior-posterior midline, draw 1 cun long straight lines backwards, parallel to the midline.

Indication. Contralateral lower extremity paralysis, pain and numbness, acute lumbar sprain, nocturia, hysteroptosis, etc.

Foot Numbness

Symptoms. Numbness and pain of foot, difficulty in walking.

Pathogenesis. Usually owing to deficiency of qi and blood leading to malnutrition of muscles and tendons.

Therapeutic Principle. Nourishing qi, blood, muscles and tendons.

Foot-pangguang

It is a massage point.

Location. On the straight line from the superior edge of the knee on the medial leg to the middle point of the groin.

Operation. Pushing manipulation.

Effect. Removing pathogenic heat and enhancing diuresis.

Indication. Dark urine and dysuria, anuria and watery diarrhea, etc.

Foot Perspiration

Symptoms. Subjecting to sweating from feet.

Pathogenesis. Mainly due to damp-heat in the spleen and the stomach, or incoordination between yin and yang, obstruction of meridians in flow of qi, or cold of deficiency in middle-energizer.

Forbes Wildginger Herb

It is the rhizome, root or whole herb of Asarum forbesii Maxim. (Aristolochiaceae).

Effect. Removing wind, cold, inflammation, asthma and pain, inducing diuresis, enhancing blood circulation.

Indication. Common cod resulting from wind-cold, cough with asthma resulting from phlegm retention, edema, rheumatism, traumatic injuries, headache, pain resulting from dental caries and abdominal pain resulting from eruptive disease.

Forehead (MA)

Referring to an auricular point.

Location. At the anterior and inferior corner of the external side of antitragus.

Effect. Calming mind and ceasing pain.

Indication. Headache, dizziness, insomnia, dreaminess sleep.

Forrest Bugle Herb

It is the whole herb of Ajuga forrestii Diels. (Labiatae).

Effect. Removing heat, clearing away toxic materials, ceasing dysentery and killing parasites.

Indication. Dysentery, mastitis, ascariasis, etc.

Fortune Euonymus Stem of Leng

It is the stem of Euonymus fortinei (Turcz.) Hand. Mazz. (Celastraceae).

Effect. Relaxing muscles and tendons, enhancing flow of qi and blood circulation in the meridians and collaterals, ceasing bleeding and removing blood stasis.

Indication. Lumbar muscle strain, rheumatic arthralgia, hemoptysis, metrorrhagia, irregular menstruation, fracture owing to injury and traumatic bleeding.

Fortune Eupatorium

It is the aerial parts of Eupatorium fortunei Turcz. (Compositae).

Effect. Damp-dissolving aromatics, activate the spleen and improve appetite, remove superficial syndrome and relieve summer-heat.

Indication. Disturbance of the middle-energizer owing to the accumulation of dampness, feeling of fullness and oppression in the chest and abdomen, affection by exopathogenic summer-heat and dampness and summer fever at the early stage chillness, fever, etc.

Fortune Firethorn Fruit

It is the fruit of Pyracantha fortuneana (Maxim.) Li (Rosaceae).

Effect. Reinforcing the spleen, releasing stagnancy of indigested food, promoting blood circulation by expelling blood stasis and ceasing bleeding.

Indication. Masses in the abdomen, indigestion, diarrhea, dysentery, metrorrhagia and postpartum retention of blood.

Fortune Windmillpalm Fruit

It is the ripe fruit of Trachycarpus wagnerianus Becc. (Palmae).

Effect. Astringing to arrest bleeding.

Indication. Fresh-bloody stool, metrorrhagia and leukorrhea.

Fortune Windmillpalm Root

It is the root of Trachycarpus wagnerianus Becc. (Palmae).

Effect. Stop bleeding, expel dampness, reduce swelling and remove toxic substances.

Indication. Hematemesis, hemafecia, blood stranguria, metrorrhagia, dysentery, arthralgia, edema, scrofula and traumatic injuries.

Forward-moving manipulation

It is a massage manipulation.

Operation. Put the palm flat on the affected part, rub the body surface slowly but forcibly, hold the muscle lasting for a moment, then move the hand forward and hold the muscle again. Repeat the movement constantly. It is good at treating the diseases of the back and abdomen.

Effect. Enhancing blood circulation and removing the blood stasis, and relieving the stagnancy of the indigested food.

Indication. Local injury of the soft tissues, distention of the epigastrium, stagnancy of the indigested food and abdominal pain.

Fossil Crab

It is the fossil of an ancient arthropod animal Telphusasp and other similar animals.

Effect. Nourishing the liver to improve visual acuity, detoxicating and promoting subsidence of swelling.

Indication. Bloodshot eyes, nebula covering the cornea, inflammation of the throat, carbuncle and swelling and paint dermatitis.

Foulage Manipulation

1. It is a needling technique, supplemental manipulation.

Operation. Hold the needle body with the thumb and index fingers of the right hand, and then twist it towards one way just like twisting thread.

Effect. Enhancing the needle sensation.

2. Referring to a massage manipulation, a relaxation manipulation.

Operation. Hold a certain part with two palms facing each other kneading and pressing it rapidly with relative force, often used to the extremities and the costal regions.

Four-leaf Peperomia Herb or Root

It is the whole herb or root of Peperomia tetraphylla (Forst f.) Hook. et Arn. (Piperaceae).

Effect. Removing heat, and toxic material, dispelling blood stagnation.

Indication. Cough owing to overstrain, asthma, rheumatic arthralgia, dysentery, heatstroke, diarrhea, infantile malnutrition and traumatic injuries, carbuncle, sore, etc.

Four Properties of Drugs

Referring to the drugs having four properties cold, hot, warm, cool. Drugs effective for the treatment of heat symptom complexes are endowed with cold or cold properties, while those effective for cold symptom complexes with warm or hot properties.

Four Sources and Three Tubers

The meridians originate from the ends of the four limbs (the extremities) called the four sources. The meridians also connect with certain portions of the head, chest and abdomen, and the parts of the head, chest and abdomen called three tubers. They illustrate the relationship of the meridians and points indications of the four limbs with those of the head and truck. The fact for selecting points on the limbs clinically to treat diseases of the head, face,

and trunk is related to the relationship between sources and tubers.

Fourstamen Stephania Root

It is the root of Stephania tetrandra S. Moore. (Menispermaceae).

Effect. Promoting diuresis to reduce edema, dispelling wind and relieving pain, eliminating phlegm and relieving asthma.

Indication. Rheumatic arthritis, edema and oliguria, ascites, bronchial asthma, beriberi, etc.

Foxy Mass

Symptoms. Pregnant-like signs as pain in the chest, hypochondrium, lumbar back, good appetite but nausea, preference for sleep and contemplation, with flaccidity of the limbs, vaginal swelling, dysuria, amenorrhea, and sterility.

Pathogenesis. Trauma caused by sadness and fearfulness, or mental confusion and attack by pathogenic cold-damp during menstruation.

Therapeutic Principle. Adjusting the flow of qi to induce diuresis and remove stasis, but incurable at the advanced stage.

Fragrant Melodinus Fruit

It is the fruit of Melodinus suaveolens Champ, ex Benth, (Apocynaceae).

Effect. Arresting pain by activating qi, dispelling dampness and killing parasites.

Indication. Stomachache, hernia, scrofula, sarcoptidosis, pellagra, etc.

Fragrant Solomonseal Rhizome   ⊛ F-2

It is the rhizome of Polygonatum odoratum (Mill.) Druce var. Pluriflorum (Miq.) Ohwi (Liliaceae).

Effect. Tonifying yin, moisturizing the lung, enhancing the production of body fluid and nourishing the stomach.

Indication. Dry cough caused by dryness-heat, dry tongue, sore throat, thirst, inappetence, etc.

Franchet Groundcherry Calyx of Fruit   ✡ F-3

It is the whole herb of Physalis alkekengi L. var. Franchetii (Mast.) Makino (Solanaceae).

Effect. Removing heat, detoxicating and promoting diuresis.

Indication. Heat cough, sore throat, jaundice, dysentery, edema, furunculosis, erysipelas, etc.

Frankincense

It is the gum-resin Boswellia carterii Birdwood (Burseraceae), or other plant of the same genus.

Effect. Enhancing blood circulation, removing pain, reducing swelling, relaxing the tendons and dredging the meridians, and enhancing regeneration of the tissue.

Indication. Dysmenorrhea, amenorrhea, rheumatic arthralgia, traumatic injuries, swelling pain owing to carbuncles and cellulitis, and ulcerated sores.

Freckle

Symptoms. Scattered spots in black and brown color or in light black color on the skin on the face, the neck, the back of the hand, etc. Smaller ones like a needle point, bigger ones like a green gram, different in number, even spreading over the whole face.

Pathogenesis. The stagnation of fire in the minute collaterals of the blood system, and by the additional stagnation of wind, or by blood heat in the lung meridian.

Therapeutic Principle. Smearing the affected parts with freckle-expelling agent externally.

Frequent Nictitation

Symptoms. For mild case, normal appearance of the eyes, slight red of the white, photophobia, itching, astringency and preference for massage if serious, often seen in infants.

Pathogenesis. Resulting from the impairment of the spleen and stomach caused by improper diet, or by flaring up of deficient fire caused by insufficiency of the lung-yin.

Therapeutic Principle. Nourishing the spleen and removing food stagnancy, nourishing yin, removing heat and moistening dryness.

Fresh Ginger

It is the rhizome of Zingiber officinale Rose. (Zingiberaceae).

Effect. Inducing diaphoresis to dispel cold, warming the middle-energizer and ceasing vomiting, eliminating phlegm and removing cough, detoxication.

Indication. Exterior syndromes owing to affection by wind-cold exopathogens with symptoms of vomiting owing to cold in the stomach, cough owing to wind-cold pathogen tightening the lung, etc.

Fresh Ginger Moxibustion

Referring to a type of crude herb moxibustion.

Operation. Put the paste of the fresh ginger on the selected point or affected area, for example on the breast area for acute mastitis. Pound the fresh ginger with a kind of herb for malnutrition, these two herbs into a paste, then apply it to Yongquan (K 1) before sleep and remove it next morning for treatment of infantile malnutrition.

Fresh-water Turtle Meat

It is the meat of Amyda sinensis (Wiegmann) (Triunychidae).

Effect. Nourishing yin and removing heat from the blood.

Indication. Hectic fever owing to yin-deficiency, protracted dysentery, metrorrhagia and metrostaxis, leukorrhea, scrofula, etc.

Fresh-water Turtle Shell

It is the back shell of Amyda sinensis (Wiegmann) (Triunychidae).

Effect. Tonifying yin, suppressing hyperactive liver yang, softening and removing masses and lumps.

Indication. Chronic tidal fever owing to yin deficiency, night sweat, amenorrhea, masses in the abdomen, etc.

Fresh-water Turtle Shell's Gelatin

It is the gelatin decocted from shell of Amyda sinensis (Wiegmann).

Effect. Tonifying yin and blood, removing fever and blood stasis.

Indication. Hectic fever owing to yin deficiency, masses in the abdomen, the swelling and pain of hemorrhoids, etc.

Freyn Cinquefoil Herb

It is the whole herb of Potentilla freyniana Bornm. (Rosaceae).

Effect. Dispelling heat and detoxify, removing blood stasis.

Indication. Bone tuberculosis, stomatitis, scrofula, traumatic injuries and traumatic bleeding.

Fright at Night

Symptoms. Infant sudden wake up and sitting up with staring its eyes at night.

Pathogenesis. Owing to terrible frightening, etc.

Therapeutic Principle. Calming the mind and removing the fright.

Fright Impairing Kidney-qi

Great fright causes fear, leading to impairing the spirit and kidney-qi and making qi sink. The kidney storing the essence of life, impairment of the kidney-qi leading to the patient perplexed and uneasy, and atrophic debility of bones, spermatorrhea and urinary incontinence.

Fringed Iris Herb

It is the whole herb of Iris japonica Thunb. (Iridaceae).

Effect. Detoxicating, removing pain, reducing swelling.

Indication. Hepatitis, laryngalgia, stomachache, etc.

Fritillary Bulb **F-4**

Two variants: Sichuan fritillaria cirrhosa D. Don and Zhejiang fritillaria thunbergii Mig. (Liliaceae).

Effect. Clearing away heat and dispersing, relieving stagnation and eliminating the mass.

Indication. Chronic cough owing to deficiency of the lung, dry cough and scanty sputum, cough owing to pathogenic windheat stagnation of phlegm-fire, acute mastitis lung abscess and scrofula.

Frog Tympanites

Symptoms. Blue and pale complexion, obstruction of pharynx, borborygmus, insect creeping sensation in the skin, dysphoria with feverish sensation of palms and soles, cough with pus and blood, distention and fullness in the abdomen belonging to advanced stage of tympanites caused by parasitic infestation, similar to the stage of hepatosplenomegaly of schistosomiasis.

Pathogenesis. Noxious agents produced by parasites.

Therapeutic Principle. Enhancing blood circulation by removing blood stasis, destroying parasites and removing mass.

Front-Mu Points

It refers to the specific points on the chest and abdomen where the qi of the respective zang-fu organs flows together. Each of the twelve zang-fu organs has one corresponding Front-Mu point. The lung corresponds to Zhongfu (L 1) point, the stomach to Zhongwan (CV 12), the pericardium to Danzhong (CV 17) point, the bile to Riyue (G 24) point, the heart to Jujue (CV 14), the bladder to Zhongji (CV 3), the liver to Qimen (Liv 14), the large intestine to Tianshu (S 25), the spleen to Zhangmen (Liv 13), the tri-energizer to Shimen (CV 5), the kidney to Jingmen (G 25) and the small intestine to Guanyuan (CV 4); they are used for the diagnosis and treatment of the disorders of their corresponding zang-fu organs.

Frost-like Powder of the Watermelon

It is the white crystal obtained from the mixed peel of watermelon and mirabilite.

Effect. Clearing away heat and removing toxic substances and stopping pain.

Indication. Inflammation of the throat, acute throat trouble, canker sore in the mouth, ulcerative gingivitis.

Frost of Dried Persimmon Fruit

It is the white powder on the surface of Diospyros kaki L. f. (Ebenaceae), formed during making a dried persimmon.

Effect. Removing heat, moisturizing the viscera and dispersing phlegm.

Indication. Dryness cough owing to the lung-heat, dry and sore throat, canker sores in the mouth and on the tongue, hematemesis and diabetes.

Fuai (Sp 16)

A meridian acupuncture point.

Location. On the upper abdomen, 3 cun above Daheng (Sp 15), and 4 cun lateral to the anterior midline.

Indication. Abdominal pain, borborygmus, indigestion, constipation and dysentery.

Method. Puncture perpendicularly 1-1.5 cun. Moxibustion if needed.

Fubai (G 10)

A meridian acupuncture point.

Location. On the head, posterior and superior to the mastoid process, at the junction of the middle third and upper third of the curved line connecting Tianchong (G 9) and Wangu (G 12).

Indication. Headache, pain and stiffness of the neck and nape, tinnitus, deafness, toothache, scrofula, goiter, pain when raising the arm, paralytic foot.

Method. Puncture subcutaneously 0.5-0.8 cun. Apply moxibustion 1-3 moxa cones or 3-5 minutes with warming moxibustion.

Fufen (B 41)

A meridian acupuncture point.

Location. On the back, below the spinous process of the 2nd thoracic vertebra, 3 cun lateral to the posterior midline.

Indication. Contracting feeling in the shoulder and back, stiffness and pain of the nape and neck and numbness of the elbow and arms.

Method. Puncture obliquely 0.5-0.8 cun. Apply moxibustion 3-5 moxa cones or 5-15 minutes with warm needling.

Notice. Deep puncture is forbidden.

Fujie (Sp 14)

A meridian paint.

Location. On the lower abdomen, 1.3 cun below Daheng (Sp 15), and 4 cun lateral to the anterior midline.

Indication. Abdominal pain around the umbilicus, hernia and diarrhea.

Method. Puncture perpendicularly 0.8-1.2 cun. Apply moxibustion 3-5 moxa cones or 5-10 minutes with warming moxibustion.

Fuliu (K 7)

A meridians point.

Location. On the medial side of the leg, 2 cun directly above Taixi (K 3), anterior to the achilles tendon.

Indication. Diarrhea, borborygmus, edema, abdominal distention, swelling in the legs muscular atrophy of the foot, night sweating, pain and stiffness along the spinal column.

Method. Puncture perpendicularly 0.8-1 cun. Moxibustion if needed.

Fullness in Chest

Symptoms. The feeling of stuffiness and depressed fullness in the chest without pain and distention, eructation with fetid odor and acid regurgitation, lassitude and asthenia, etc.

Pathogenesis. Usually owing to the deficiency of the spleen-qi, indigestion, the retention of water, the obstruction of yang-qi result from the phlegm accumulation, and the failure of the stagnated qi to flow.

Therapeutic Principle. Adjusting the flow of qi and reinforcing the spleen, removing phlegm, eliminating stagnated food and resolving stagnation.

Fullness of Hypochondrium

Symptoms. Usually with hypochondriac pain, eructation and nausea, sighing and epigastric distress.

Pathogenesis. Usually due to qi stagnation of the liver and gallbladder, accumulation of phlegm and heat and internal blood stasis.

Therapeutic Principle. Smoothing the liver, adjusting of the gallbladder, removing phlegm, clearing away heat, and enhancing blood circulation to remove obstruction in the meridian.

Fulminant Dysentery

Symptoms. Frequent defecation with more pus blood and less stool and an extremely foul smell, sharp pain in the abdomen, tenesmus, thirst, severe pyrexia, dysphoria, even coma and convulsions or falling down.

Pathogenesis. Invasion of epidemic pathogenic factors steaming the intestines and tri-energizer by the dominant heat, leading to the stagnation of qi and blood and disorder in transportation. It is an acute and severe disease.

Therapeutic Principle. Removing heat and detoxicating, regulating the intestines and stomach.

Fumigation

It is one of external treatment techniques.

Method. Burning drugs, using upward steaming drug's potency and heat to enhance dredging striae of skin, muscles and viscera, and to enhance free flowing of qi and blood. The method is good at treating the swelling pyogenic infection, ulcer and dermatosis, etc.

Fumigation and Steaming Method for Hemorrhoid Complicated by Anal Fistula

Method. Using medicine and heat of hot decoction to treat hemorrhoid complicated by anal fistula.

Indication. Internal hemorrhoid, thrombosed external hemorrhoid, inflammatory external hemorrhoid, anal fissure, proctoptosis, fistula and initial perianal abscess.

Functional Activities of Qi

Referring to four basic abilities of functional activities of qi: ascending, descending, exiting, and entering, for indicating the physiological functions and pathologic changes of zang-fu organs, meridians, collaterals and tissues, e.g. harmonious functional activities of qi, disharmonious functional activities of qi, and stagnation of qi functional activities.

Function of Spleen is Like Earth

The spleen belongs to the central part in the five orientations and corresponds to earth in the five elements. The earth producing all things in the world while the spleen possessing the functions of transporting and transforming water and food, and then sending the food essence to nourish zang-organs and fu-organs, and limbs and bones. The spleen is the source of qi and blood, so it is named.

Funneled Physochlaina Root

It is the dried root of Physochlaina infundibularis Kuang (Solanaceae).

Effect. Arresting cough and relieving asthma, calming the mind and ceasing convulsion.

Indication. Cough and asthma diarrhea owing to cold of deficiency type.

Fu-organ Containing Refined Juice

Referring to the gallbladder, among the six fu-organs, the gallbladder simply stores bile and not receives and transforms food content like other fu-organs.

Furor

Symptoms. Mental confusion, mania, derangement, damaging things and ravings, running fit and anger, etc.
Pathogenesis. Usually owing to depression of the seven emotions, and the heart confused by phlegm.
Therapeutic Principle. Relieving phlegm, inducing resuscitation, purging pathogenic fire and resolving accumulation.

Furuncle Complicated by Septicemia

Symptoms. Dark and hollow tip of the furuncle without pus, slow spreading of the swelling, with irritability resulting from high fever, dizziness, vomiting, unconsciousness.
Pathogenesis. Mostly owing to deficiency of the vital qi, excess toxic-heat, or mistaken or delayed treatment result in the spread of furunculosis into the blood system, internally attacking the viscera.
Therapeutic Principle. Removing heat, clearing away toxic material and cooling the blood.

Furuncle Directly Opposite Mouth

Symptoms. Furuncle directly on the middle of the neck (at the pillar bone) opposite the mouth. At the beginning, itching but painless, with a small opening, a small bit like a pockmark on it in red or yellow color.
Therapeutic Principle. Puncturing the points of Dazhui (GV 14) and Weizhong (B 40) at once.

Furuncle of External Auditory Meatus

Referring to swelling furuncle in the external auditory canal.
Symptoms. Local redness and swelling, pain and process like the seed of prickly-ash.

Therapeutic Principle. Dispelling pathogenic wind and bring down the heat, clearing away toxic substances and enhancing subsidence of swelling.

Furuncle of Nose

Symptoms. Itching redness, swelling, distending pain, or a small white vesicle with a hard tip and protruding root blocking the nasal cavity. For serious cases, pain in the forehead, swelling of the checks and lips, pus on breakage, and an internal attack of furunculosis.
Pathogenesis. Usually owing to accumulation of fire-toxin in the Lung meridians.
Therapeutic Principle. Clearing away heat and toxic materials.

Fushe (Sp 13)

It is an acupoint.
Location. In the lower abdomen, 4 cun inferior to the umbilicus, 0.7 cun superior to Chongmen (Sp 12) and 4 cun to the anterior median line.
Indication. Abdominal pain, abdominal mass, and hernia.
Method. Puncture perpendicularly 1-1.5 cun and perform moxibustion 3-5 moxa cones or for 5-10 minutes.

Futokadsur Stem

It is the stem of Piper futokadsura Sieb. et Zucc. and several species of the same genus (Piperaceae).
Effect. Expelling wind-dampness, clearing and activating meridians and collaterals, warming the lung to relieve cough.
Indication. Rheumatic arthralgia, rheumatalgia of joints with muscular contracture, pain in the loins and knees and pain owing to traumatic injuries.

Futonggu (K 20)

A meridians point.
Location. On the upper abdomen, 5 cun above the center of the umbilicus and 0.5 cun lateral to the anterior midline.

Indication. Abdominal pain and distention, vomiting, precordial pain, palpitations, pain in the chest and sudden loss of voice.

Method. Puncture perpendicularly or obliquely 0.5-1 cun. Moxibustion if needed.

Futu (LI 18)

A meridians point.

Location. On the lateral side of the neck, beside the laryngeal protuberance, 3 cun lateral to Adam apple, between the anterior and posterior borders of the sternocleidomastoid muscle.

Indication. Cough, asthmatic breath, sore throat, sudden loss of voice, goiter, scrofula.

Method. Puncture perpendicularly 0.5-0.8 cun. Apply moxibustion 3-5 moxa cones or 5-10 minutes with warming moxibustion.

Futu (S 32)

A meridian acupuncture point.

Location. On the anterior side of the thigh and on the line connecting the anterior superior iliac spine and the superior border corner of the patella, 6 cun above this corner.

Indication. Lumbo-iliac pain, cold lumbar and knee, numbness, beriberi, hernia, abdominal distention.

Method. Puncture perpendicularly 0.6-1.2 cun. Apply moxibustion 3-5 moxa cones or 5-10 minutes with warming moxibustion.

Fuxi (B 38)

A meridian acupuncture point.

Location. At the lateral end of the popliteal crease, 1 cun above Weiyang (B 39), medial to the tendon of the biceps muscle of the thigh.

Indication. Numbness of gluteal and femoral regions, cramp of tendons in the popliteal fossa, constipation.

Method. Puncturing perpendicularly 0.5-1 cun. Moxibustion 3-5 moxa cones or 5-15 minutes with warming moxibustion.

Fuyang (B 59)

A meridian acupuncture point.

Location. On the posterior side of the leg, posterior to the lateral malleolus, 3 cun directly above Kunlun (B 60)

Indication. Heavy sensation in the head, headache, pain in the waist and legs, paralysis of the lower limbs, redness and swelling of the external malleolus.

Method. Puncture perpendicularly 0.5-1.2 cun. Moxibustion is applicable.

G

Galactorrhea

Symptoms. 1. Spontaneous lactation during pregnancy; 2. Galactorrhea during non-breast feeding period.

Pathogenesis. Deficiency of qi and blood, or excessive dispersing of the liver-qi.

Therapeutic Principle. 1. Nourishing qi and blood; 2. Weakening the liver-qi.

Galangal Fruit

It is the dried ripe fruit of Alpinia galanga Willd. (Zingiberaceae).

Effect. Eliminating dampness and expelling cold, enlivening the spleen and promoting digestion.

Indication. Abdominal distention due to retention of food, vomiting, diarrhea, gastric and abdominal cold pain, and alcoholism.

Gall Bladder Collateral

It is one of the fifteen collaterals. It branches at Guangming(G 37) 5 cun above the external malleolus, goes into the Liver Meridian of Foot-jueyin and runs down along the back of foot. The pathological changes along these superficial venules refer to qi, which reversely flows and fails to go down. The excessive syndrome is cold of foot, while the deficient syndrome is lassitude in the legs, difficult walking, and hard to stand up from the sitting position.

Gallbladder Deficiency

Symptoms. Excessive suspicion, frequent sigh, insomnia, or bitter taste and palpebral blotch, bilious vomiting, etc.

Pathogenesis. Insufficiency of gallbladder.

Therapeutic Principle. Warming the gallbladder and restoring qi.

Gallbladder Divergent Meridian

A meridian and collateral. It is one of the twelve divergent meridians, which branches from the Gallbladder Meridian of Foot-shaoyang, passes along anterior thigh, enters vulva, and connects with the Liver Meridian of Foot-jueyin, its branch goes upward between 11th and 12th rib, connect the gallbladder, spread over the liver and passes through the heart, travels along the esophagus, runs to mandible, and throughout the face, connect with the eyes and returns to Gallbladder Meridian of Foot-shaoyang at the outer canthus.

Gallbladder-fire

Symptoms. Fullness in hypochondrium, palpebral blotch and flushed face, bitter taste and upset, restlessness, etc.

Pathogenesis. Stagnation of the liver-qi and accumulation of heat in the Gallbladder Meridian.

Therapeutic Principle. Removing heat from the liver, purging intense heat, removing mental depression and eliminating dampness.

Gallbladder-heat

Symptoms. Pain in hypochondrium, jaundice, yellow and red urine, bitter taste, dry pharynx, alternate attacks of chills and fever, vomiting, poor appetite with abdominal distention, or headache, dizziness, easy anger, deafness, etc.

Pathogenesis. The heat caused by pathogenic factor in Gallbladder Meridian.

Therapeutic Principle. Dissipate and discharge Shaoyang.

Gallbladder Meridian of Foot-shaoyang

It is one of twelve regular meridians. This meridian includes the following points:

Tongziliao	G1	Zhejin	G23
Tinghui	G2	Riyue	G24
Shangguan	G3	Jingmen	G25
Hanyan	G4	Daimai	G26
Xuanlu	G5	Wushu	G27
Xuanli	G6	Weidao	G28
Qubin	G7	Juliao	G29
Shuaigu	G8	Huantiao	G30
Tianchong	G9	Fengshi	G31
Fubai	G10	Zhongdu	G32
Touqiaoyin	G11	Xiyangguan	G33
Wangu	G12	Yanglingquan	G34
Benshen	G13	Yangjiao	G35
Yangbai	G14	Waiqiu	G36
Toulinqi	G15	Guangming	G37
Muchuang	G16	Yangfu	G38
Zhengying	G17	Xuanzhong	G39
Chengling	G18	qiuxu	G40
Naokong	G19	Zulinqi	G41
Fengchi	G20	Diwuhui	G42
Jianjing	G21	Xiaxi	G43
Yuanye	G22	Zuqiaoyin	G44

Gallbladder-sthenia

Symptoms. Distention and pain in hypochondrium, bitter taste and dry mouth, headache, constipation, or jaundice.

Pathogenesis. Accumulated damp-heat, the failure in removing stagnancy and obstruction of gallbladder.

Therapeutic Principle. Clearing away heat by promoting circulation in fu, and dispersing and rectifying the depressed liver energy.

Gamboge

It is the colloidal resin of Garcinia morella Desv. (Guttiferae).

Effect. Detoxicating, stopping bleeding, reducing swelling and destroying parasites.

Indication. Boils and pyogenic infections on the body surface, chronic eczema, malignant sore, traumatic bleeding, ulcerative gingivitis, dental caries, scald and burn, etc.

Ganshu (B 18)

A meridian point on the Bladder Meridian of Foot-taiyang and Back-shu point of the liver.

Location. On the back 1.5 cun lateral to Jinsuo (GV 8) between the spinal processes of the 9th and 10th thoracic vertebrae.

Indication. Jaundice, hypochondriac pain, backache, hematemesis, epistaxis, congestion of the eyes, blurred vision, dizziness, night blindness, manic-depressive disorder.

Method. Puncture obliquely 0.5-0.8 cun. Apply moxibustion 3-5 moxa cones or 5-15 minutes with warming moxibustion.

Gansui (Radix Euphorbiae Kansui) Moxibustion

A term of crude herb moxibustion.

Indication. Apply it to Dazhui (GV 14), for treating malaria, to Feishu (B 13) for asthma and to Zhongji (CV 3) for uroschesis, etc.

Method. Grind the proper amount of dried tuberous root of Gansui (Euphorbiae Kansui) into powder, and apply it on the selected point and then fix it with adhesive plaster, or add the proper amount of flour to the powder of kansui root, and mix them into a paste with warm boiled water, apply the paste to the selected point, cover the paste with oil paper and fix it with adhesive plaster.

Gaogu (EX-UE)

An extra point.

Location. On the high point of the styloid process of the radius.

Indication. Pain of the wrist.

Method. Puncture subcutaneously 0.5-1 cun. Apply moxibustion 3-7 moxa cones or 5-10 minutes with warming moxibustion.

Gaohuang (B 43)

A meridian point on the Bladder Meridian of Foot-taiyang, also named Gaohuangshu.

Location. On the back, below the spinous process of the 4th thoracic vertebra, 3 cun lateral to the posterior midline.

Indication. Pulmonary tuberculosis, cough, dyspnea, hematemesis, transportation, amnesia, emission, loose stool containing undigested food, pain in the scapular region and back.

Method. Puncture obliquely 0.5-0.8 cun. It is not advisable to puncture deep. Apply moxibustion 7-15 moxa cones or 20-30 minutes with warming moxibustion.

Gardea Sorrel Root

It is the root of Rumex acetosa L. (Polygonaceae).

Effect. Clearing away heat, promoting diuresis, eliminating pathogenic heat from the blood and destroying parasites.

Indication. Heat dysentery, stranguria, dysuria, hematemesis, malignant sore, psora, tinea, etc.

Garden Balsam Seed ❀ G-2

It is the seed of Impatiens balsamina L. (Balsaminaceae).

Effect. Removing blood stasis, promoting digestion and softening hard masses.

Indication. Amenorrhea and abdominal masses.

Garden Burnet Root ❀ G-1

It is the root of a perennial herb Sanguisorba officinalis L. (Rosaceae).

Effect. Cooling the blood, arresting bleeding, detoxication and promoting wound healing.

Indication. Hemoptysis, epistaxis, hematemesis, hematuria, hemafecia, hemorrhoidal bleeding, metrorrhagia, metrostaxis, scalds, eczema, skin infection or ulceration, etc.

Garlic

It is the bulb of Allium sativum L. (Liliaceae).

Effect. Diminishing swelling, detoxication and killing parasites.

Indication. Abscesses, scabies, tinea, tuberculosis, paroxysmal cough, dysentery, diarrhea, ancylostomiasis, enterobiasis, influenza and crab poisoning.

Gas Gangrene

It refers to the furuncle.

Symptoms. Mostly appears on the hand and the foot. Symptoms as swelling and pain in the affected area at the beginning, with dark red color around it, blisters, edema in the affected limb, which is severely painful, ulceration in the part, with light brown juice flowing out, with skin color changing into purple black, and with a little sunken furuncle surface. The affected area will give a twirling sound when it is pressed. If it is pressed hard gas bubbles will flow out with offensive odor. In the severe syndrome, it is accompanied by such symptoms as fever, headache, coma and delirium, etc. This disease is similar to gaseous gangrene, which is easy to ulcerate, appears urgently, is easy to become septicemic, and endangers life.

Pathogenesis. Infection of toxin due to the breaking of skin, or the steaming of toxic fire of damp-heat.

Therapeutic Principle. Clearing away heat and detoxicating, and promoting diuresis.

Gas Rushing

Symptoms. Gasp, the uprising gas to the chest, fullness of the chest, rough breath and gas rushing up, cough and choke at times, etc.

Pathogenesis. Rushing up of gas due to evil qi affecting the lung and the reversed flow of qi in meridians.

Therapeutic Principle. Descending qi and relieving asthma.

Gastric Discomfort due to Accumulation of Phlegm

Symptoms. Obscure hunger, loss of appetite, spitting phlegm and salvia, etc.

Pathogenesis. Due to the retention of excessive phlegm.

Therapeutic Principle. Dispelling phlegm, regulating the flow of qi and removing intense heat in the lung.

Gastrodia Tuber

It is the stem of tuber of Gastrodia elata B1. (Orchidaceae).

Effect. Expelling evil wind to relieve convulsion, calming the liver and subduing hyperactivity of the liver-yang, and removing obstruction in the collaterals to relieve pain.

Indication. Endogenous liver wind, infantile convulsion, epilepsy, dizziness and headache due to excessive rise of the liver-yang, rheumatic arthralgia, numbness of the limbs, etc.

Gecko

It is the dried corpus of vertebrate Gekko gecko L. with the viscera removed (Geckonidae).

Effect. Invigorating the lung and nourishing the kidney improving inspiration, relieving asthma and cough and replenishing vital essence and blood.

Indication. Cough due to lung deficiency, asthma due to kidney deficiency, dyspnea with cough due to consumption, impotence due to deficiency of the kidney-yang and consumption of the vital essence and blood, etc.

Geguan (B 46)

A meridian point.

Location. On the back, below the spinous process of the 7th thoracic vertebra, 3 cun lateral to the posterior midline.

Indication. Anorexia, vomiting, eructation, tight and oppressive feeling in the chest, stiffness and pain in the back spine.

Method. Puncture obliquely 0.5-0.8 cun. It is not advisable to puncture deep. Apply moxibustion 3-5 moxa cones or 5-15 minutes with warming moxibustion.

Gemen (EX-CA)

An extra point.

Location. 3 cun lateral to the midpoint of the root of penis, at the male inguinal region

Indication. Hernia, reverse qi attacking the heart.

Method. Puncture perpendicularly 1-1.5 cun. Apply moxibustion3-5 moxa cones or 5-10 minutes with warming moxibustion.

General Aching during Menstruation

Symptoms. General pain during, before or after menstruation, with remission and disappearance following menolipsis.

Pathogenesis. Blood deficiency and body fluid insufficiency, or by blood stasis due to cold.

Therapeutic Principle. Nourishing blood and regulating menstruation, and nourishing the tendon to relieve pain for the former case, as supplementing qi, promoting blood circulation and dispelling cold to alleviate pain for the latter.

General Arthralgia

Symptoms. General pain, numbness with heaviness sensation, spasm of the neck and back, etc.

Pathogenesis. The qi deficiency, the invasion of pathogenic wind, and cold and wetness into the blood vessels and muscles.

Therapeutic Principle. Supplementing qi and regulating nutrients, eliminating the evil factors warming and activating.

General Edema

Symptoms. The edema with the head, limbs, chest, abdomen, and even the whole body involved. It is the main symptom of edema.

Pathogenesis. It is classified into two types. 1. Deficiency type is caused by the exhaustion of the lung, spleen and kidney, retention of fluid spreading in the skin. 2. Excess type is caused by the invasion by exopathogen and the disorder of diet and daily life.

Geshu (B 17)

A meridian point.

Location. On the back, below the spinal process of the 7th thoracic vertebra, 1.5 cun lateral to the posterior midline.

Indication. Distention and pain in the epigastrium, vomiting, hiccups, dysphagia, asthma, cough, hemoptysis, hectic fever, night sweating, stiffness and pain in the back.

Method. Puncture perpendicularly 0.5-0.8 cun. Apply moxibustion 3-5 moxa cones or 5-15 minutes with warming moxibustion.

Gestational Edema

Symptoms. General edema accompanied by abdominal distention and dyspnea.

Pathogenesis. Yang deficiency of the spleen and kidney, retention of body fluid due to disorder of ascending and descending flow of qi, and dysfunction in transport of fluid with the growing of the fetus.

Therapeutic Principle. Warming yang and reinforcing the spleen and regulating the flow of qi to alleviate water retention.

Ghost Malaria

It is one type of malaria.

Symptoms. Irregular onset, falling into a trance, being subject to changing moods, continuous trembling due to felling cold or thirst and dryness when in fever.

Therapeutic Principle. Confer the term of Malaria.

Giant Knotweed Rhizome

⊛ **G-3**

It is the dried rhizome and root of a perennial herb Polygonum cuspidatum Sieb. et Zucc. (Polyonaceae).

Effect. Promoting blood circulation to remove obstruction in meridians, relieving pain, removing heat, promoting diuresis, detoxicating, dispelling phlegm and relieving cough.

Indication. Rheumatic arthralgia, traumatic injuries, jaundice due to damp-heat pathogen, enteritis, dysentery, bronchitis, pneumonia, cough due to lung-heat, scalds and burns.

Giantleaf Ardisia Rhizome

It is the rhizome of Ardisia gigantifolia Stapf (Myrsinaceae).

Effect. Expelling wind and dampness, strengthening the tendon, muscle, bone, promoting blood circulation and eliminating stagnation.

Indication. Arthralgia and myalgia due to wind-dampness, traumatic injuries, postpartum blood stasis, carbuncle, deep-rooted carbuncle and ulcer.

Giant Needle

A type of acupuncture apparatus. It usually is made of stainless steel, the needle body 0.5-1 mm in diameter, 3 cun or 5 cun or 10 cun in length, etc. The needles are used to puncture subcutaneously and puncture the muscles and tendons to treat the diseases of paralysis, muscular spasm, etc.

Giant St. John's Wort Herb

It is the whole herb of Hypericum ascyron L. (Hypericaceae).

Effect. Arresting bleeding, calming the liver, detoxicating, subduing swelling.

Indication. Dizziness and blurred vision due to hyperactivity of the liver-yang, hematemesis, traumatic injuries, dermatopathy and furuncle.

Giant Typhonium Rhizome

It is the dried tuber of Typhonium giganteum Engl. (Araceae).

Effect. Dispelling phlegm, expelling wind, removing dampness, detoxicating and resolving masses.

Indication. Accumulation of excessive wind-phlegm, anti-convulsion for epilepsy or tetanus, migraine, snake bite.

Gingival Abscess

Symptoms. Swelling in the deep part of the gum, distending hardness, redness and burning pain. In the serious case, the swelling extends to the parotid gland and cheek with alternate attacks of fever and chills, ozostomia, constipation.

Pathogenesis. Stagnancy of fire-toxin in the Stomach Meridian that fails to disperse and thus goes up to attack the gum.

Therapeutic Principle. Clearing away fire from the stomach, reducing swelling and removing toxic substances. If pus forms, cut it open to release pus.

Gingival Hemorrhage

Symptoms. Bleeding from gum or space between teeth, gingivitis, ozostomia, loose tooth, etc.

Pathogenesis. Usually ascribable to excessiveness of the stomach heat, insufficiency of the liver-yin and kidney-yin, rising up of premier fire and excessive heat in the blood system.

Therapeutic Principle. Clearing away heat from stomach, nourishing yin purging intense heat.

Ginkgo Leaf   ✿ G-4

It is the leaf of a deciduous arbor Ginkgo biloba L. (Ginkgoaceae).

Effect. Preventing asthma and relieving pain.

Indication. Cough and asthma due to the lung deficiency; hyperlipidemia, hypertension, coronary heart disease, angina pectoris and cerebrovascular spasm.

Ginkgo Poisoning

Symptoms. Fever, vomiting, abdominal diarrhea, convulsion, stiffness of limbs, even coma till death, etc.

Pathogenesis. Overeating of raw ginkgo.

Therapeutic Principle. Emergency treatment of combination of traditional Chinese and Western medicine in severe cases.

Ginkgo Seed

It is the ripe seed of Ginkgo biloba L. (Ginkgoaceae).

Effect. Relieving asthma, arresting of secretion and stopping leukorrhagia.

Indication. Dyspnea with cough and profuse sputum due to adverse flow of qi, gonorrhea, leukorrhea, enuresis, and frequent micturition.

Ginseng

It is the root of Panax ginseng C. A. Mey. (Araliaceae).

Effect. Replenishing the primordial qi, tonifying the spleen and lung, promoting the production of body fluid to relieve thirst, tranquilizing the mind and improving mental power.

Indication. The debility from chronic illness, anorexia caused by deficiency of the spleen-qi, cough due to deficiency of the lung-qi, thirst and diabetes due to impairment of body fluid, irritability, insomnia and dreaminess, palpitation induced by fright, etc.

Ginseng Leaf

It is the leaf of Panax ginseng C. A. Mey. (Araliaceae).

Effect. Relieving summer-heat, promoting the production of the body fluid and reducing fire of deficiency type.

Indication. Thirst due to summer-heat, febrile disease to consume the body fluid, deficiency of the stomach-yin, toothache caused by fire of deficiency type, etc.

Glabrous Crazyweed Herb

It is the whole herb of Oxytropis glabra DC. (Leguminosae).

Effect. Anaesthetic, relieving pain and relieving convulsion.

Indication. Toothache, arthralgia, neurosism, skin pruritus, etc.

Glabrous Greenbrier Rhizome

It is the rhizome of Smilax glabra Roxb. (Liliaceae).

Effect. Detoxicating, removing dampness and easing joint movement.

Indication. Syphilis, carbuncles and dermatopathy due to fire-toxin, beriberi, scrofula and heat strangury.

Glaucousback Three-wingnut Root-bark

It is the whole plant or root-bark of a deciduous twining shrub Tripterygium hypoglaucum (Lévl.) Hutch. (Celastraceae).

Effect. Promoting recover of fractured bones and dispelling blood stasis and obstruction in the meridians.

Indication. Traumatic injuries, fracture and rheumatalgia.

Glehnia

It is the root of Glehnia littoralis F. Schmidt ex Mig. (Umbelliferae).

Effect. Removing heat from the lung, nourishing yin, strengthening the stomach and enhancing the production of body fluid.

Indication. Dryness cough or phthisic cough with hemoptysis due to the lung-heat and yin deficiency; consumption of body fluid due to febrile disease of dry tongue, thirst, anorexia, etc.

Globeamaranth Flower

It is the inflorescence or the whole herb of Gomphrena globosa L. (Amaranthaceae).

Effect. Clearing away heat from the liver, dispersing obstruction and relieving cough and asthma.

Indication. Seborrheic dermatitis, painful eyes, cough with dyspnea, pertussis, dysentery, infantile convulsion, scrofula, dermatopathy. etc.

Globethistle

It is the root of Rhaponticum uniflorum (L.) DC., or Echinops latifolius Tausch (Compositae).

Effect. Clearing away heat and detoxicating, treating carbuncles, dissolv-ing masses and stimulating milk secretion.

Indication. Abscesses, sores and swelling, painful swelling in breast, galactostasis, acute mastitis, hemorrhoidal bleeding, etc.

Globus Hystericus

Symptoms. Subjective feeling of a foreign body in the throat with inability to or cough it up, as if a nut-meat were stuck in, but not interfere with eating and swallow-ing, mental depression, eructation, full-ness sensation in the chest.

Pathogenesis. Stagnation of the liver qi, phlegm accumulated in the throat leading to combination of phlegm and stagnated qi.

Therapeutic Principle. Relieving depressed liver, regulating the circulation of qi and relieving stagnation.

Glossocele

A tongue picture.

Symptoms. Swelling of the tongue usually accompanied by pain.

Pathogenesis. Emotional stress, intense fire in the Heart Meridian, invasion of wind-heat upon deficiency of the spleen and the heart and stagnation of qi and blood stasis.

Glossodynia

Symptoms. Excessive heat, thirst, vexa-tion and scanty dark urine for excessive heat, dryness of the tongue, sore throat and celostomia for deficiency yin.

Pathogenesis. Furuncle appearing on the tongue, the prickly tongue, the fissured tongue and the red thorn on the tip of the tongue.

Therapeutic Principle. Purging intense heat and detoxicating, in the syndrome of excessive heat. Replenishing the vital essence and removing heat in the syndrome of yin deficiency.

Glossy Privet Fruit

It is the ripe fruit of Ligustrum lucidum Ait. (Oleaceae).

Effect. Invigorating the liver and kidney, darkening the hair clearing away heat and improving acuity of vision, tranquilizing the mind.

Indication. Deficiency of liver-yin and kidney-yin, dizziness and dim sight, lassitude in the loins and knees, premature grey hair, fever due to yin deficiency, hypopsia, blurred vision, etc.

Glossy Privet Leaf

It is the leaf of Ligustrum lucidum Ait (Oleaceae).

Effect. Dispelling wind, improving acuity of vision, diminishing swelling and relieving pain.

Indication. Dizziness, painful eyes, bloodshot eyes due to wind-heat, unhealing ulcer and external diseases, scald, etc.

Glutinous Rice Root

It is the root of Oryza sativa L. (Gramineae).

Effect. Reinforcing the stomach and promoting the production of the body fluid, suppressing sweating and removing heat.

Indication. Spontaneous perspiration, night sweat; persistent fever of deficiency type.

Goat Blood

It is the blood of Capra hircus L. (Bovidae).

Effect. Improving blood circulation, dissipating ecchymosis, removing obstruction in the meridians and detoxicating.

Indication. Traumatic injuries, pains of muscles and bones, hematemesis, epistaxis, hematochezia, hematuria, subcutaneous swelling.

Goat Meat

It is the meat of Capra hircus L. (Bovidae).

Effect. Tonifying deficiency and invigorating yang.

Indication. Internal injury due to consumption, lassitude and debility along spinal column, impotence, leukorrhea, etc.

Goiter Disease

Symptoms. Two swelling parts on the both sides of the larynx, dullness in the chest oppressed sensation, cough, difficulty in swallowing. It is similar to local thyroid enlargement.

Pathogenesis. Internal damage caused by emotional stress, improper diet and living in mountain area for a long time or unaccustomed oneself to climate of a new place, which result in stagnation of qi, phlegm accumulation and blood stasis in the front of the neck.

Therapeutic Principle. Regulating circulation of qi and resolving phlegm, and dispersing the goiter and the accumulation.

Goldenlarch Bark

It is the dried root-bark or lower stem-bark of Pseudolarix kaempferi Gord. (Pinaceae).

Effect. Destroying parasites and stopping itching.

Indication. Scabies, tinea and pruritus.

Golden Lycoris Bulb

It is the bulb of Lycoris aurea Herb. (Amaryllidaceae).

Effect. Treating noxious carbuncles, alleviating subcutaneous swelling and destroying parasites.

Indication. Suppurative infections on the body surface, furuncle, subcutaneous nodes, burns and scalds, etc.

Goldenrod

It is the whole herb of Solidago virgaaurea L. var. leiocarpa (Benth.) A. Gray (Compositae) with root.

Effect. Dispelling wind, clearing away heat, arresting cough, preventing attack of malaria, removing blood stasis and subduing swelling.

Indication. Catch cold, cough, swollen and sore throat, pertussis, dysentery, malaria, traumatic injuries, cellulitis due to carbuncle, etc.

Gongsun (Sp 4)

A meridian point.

Location. On the medial side of the foot, antero-inferior to the proximal end of the lst metatarsal bone, at the junction of the red and white skin.

Indication. Stomachache, vomiting, indigestion, borborygmus, abdominal pain, dysentery, diarrhea, frequent drink, cholera, edema, insomnia, infatuation beriberi.

Method. Puncture perpendicularly 0.5-0.8 cun. Apply moxibustion 3-5 moxa cones or 5-15 minutes with warming moxibustion.

Gonorrhoea

Symptoms. Difficulty and pain in urination, frequency and dribbling with burning or ardor sensation during urination, contracture sensation in lower abdomen or immediate onset after overwork, lassitude in loin and legs, mental fatigue and asthenia, etc.

Pathogenesis. Stagnated damp-heat, stagnation of qi, aged debility, sinking of qi of middle-energizer, disturbance in qi transformation due to deficiency of the kidney.

Therapeutic Principle. Eliminating dampness and heat, promoting the circulation of qi or invigorating spleen and supplementing qi, invigorating the kidney and arresting discharge.

Goose Blood

It is the blood of Anser domestica Geese (Anatidae).

Effect. Detoxication.

Indication. Dysphagia, regurgitation, etc.

Goose Gall

It is the gall of Anser domestica Geese (Anatidae).

Effect. Clearing away heat and removing toxic.

Indication. Hemorrhoids at the early stage.

Goose Meat

It is the meat of Anser domestica Geese (Anatidae).

Effect. Benefiting qi, curing deficiency, regulating the stomach and quenching thirst.

Indication. Frailty and diabetes.

Gordon Euryale Seed   ✿ G-5

It is the dried kernel of ripe seed of Euryale ferox Salisb. (Nymphaeaceae).

Effect. Tonifying the spleen, expelling dampness, invigorating the kidney and arresting spontaneous emission.

Indication. Chronic diarrhea due to spleen-deficiency; spontaneous emission due to kidney deficiency, aconuresis, leukorrhagia, etc.

Gout

Symptoms. Redness swelling and severe migratory pain in the joints of the limbs, difficulty in crooking and stretching, the pain removed in the day and aggravated at night.

Pathogenesis. Deficiency of the liver and kidney, invasion of pathogenic wind-cold-dampness in the meridians and collaterals involving joints and the stagnation of qi and blood.

Therapeutic Principle. Mainly tonifying the liver and kidney, dispelling wind and arthralgia syndrome and alleviating pain.

Graceful Jessamine Root

It is the root or the bark of Gelsemium elegans Benth (Loganiaceae).

Effect. Subsiding swelling, arresting pain and knitting bones.

Indication. Boils, furuncles and other pyogenic infections on the body surface, traumatic injuries and fracture.

Gradfly

It is the female insect of Tabanus bivittatus Mats. (Tabanidae).

Effect. Removing stagnated blood, dispersing swellings.

Indication. Amenorrhea due to blood stasis, masses in the abdomen, traumatic injuries, etc.

Grain Jaundice

Symptoms. Distention and fullness in the chest and abdomen, dizziness after eating cold or hot food, yellowish discoloration of the body and eyes, oliguria, etc.

Pathogenesis. Improper diet and accumulation of dampness and heat as a consequence of food retention in the middle-energizer.

Therapeutic Principle. Clearing away heat and removing dampness and regulating the flow of qi to dispel stagnation.

Granular Intradermal Needle

A needling apparatus specially made for subcutaneous embedding of the needle, also called a wheat-shaped intradermal needle. This kind of needle is divided into two kinds, i.e. 0.5 cun and 1 cun in length, the diameter of the needles is like the filiform needle. Its tail is granule-like.

Method. Grip the body of the needle with a pair of tweezers, mildly puncture 0.3-0.8 cun subcutaneously, then fix it with adhesive cloth. The duration of retaining the needle is decided for the concrete condition.

Grape

It is the fruit of a tall and big twining plant Vitis vinifera L. (Vitaceae).

Effect. Invigorating qi and blood, strengthening the bones and muscles and benefiting diuresis.

Indication. Deficiency of qi and blood, cough due to the lung deficiency, heart palpitation, night sweat, rheumatic arthralgia, stranguria, general edema, etc.

Grasping Manipulation

A massage manipulation.

Operation. Lifting and squeezing or lifting and rapidly releasing affected muscles with the thumb, and the index and middle finger, or the thumb and the other fingers. Pinching and lifting are called grasping.

Function. Expelling wind, eliminating cold, causing resuscitation, removing pain, relaxing muscles and tendons, and clearing collaterals.

Indication. Blockage syndrome, injury of soft tissues and local pain.

Grassleaved Sweetflag Rhizome

it is dried rhizome of Acorus gramineus Soland. (Araceae).

Effect. Calming the mind, eliminating phlegm for resuscitation, relieving mental stress, resolving dampness and restoring normal functioning of the stomach.

Indication. Loss of consciousness, insanity and melancholia, distention in the chest and abdomen, poor appetite.

Gravity Abscess

Symptoms. Suppurative disease in the multiple and deep tissues of the limbs. It may appear as caking or stretching swelling of muscular tissue in the deep parts of limbs.

Pathogenesis. Deficiency of qi and blood.

Green Gram Seed

It is the seed of Phaseolus radiatus L. (Leguminosae).

Effect. Clearing pathogenic heat, removing summer-heat and detoxifying metallic and drug poisoning, such as croton seed, prepared aconite root, promoting tissue regeneration etc.

Indication. Excessive thirst due to summer-heat, carbuncles, erysipelas, edema, diarrhea, etc.

Greenish Leukorrhagia

Symptoms. Incessant, sticky, thick, foul and greenish discharge from the vagina.

Pathogenesis. Multiparity injury, attack by damp and turbid pathogens, or retention of dampness and heat of the Liver Meridian in the lower part of the body.

Therapeutic Principle. Clearing heat to induce diuresis, regulating the liver-qi.

Green Tangerine Orange Peel

It is the immature fruit peel of Citrus reticulata Blanco (Rutaceae), or many other species of the same genus.

Effect. Soothing the liver, restoring the normal flow of qi, removing obstruction and eliminating stagnated food.

Indication. Distending pain in the hypochondrium due to stagnation of the liver-qi, gastrointestinal distention and mastitis.

Green Turtle Probing Its Cave

A needling technique.

Operation. Puncture first deeply and then lift it to the shallow layer, then successively move the needle upwards, downwards, leftwards and rightwards; thrusting three times and lifting one time, as if a turtle were digging into the earth in various directions to find its cave.

Function. Promote the circulation of meridian qi.

Greying of Hair

Symptoms. Premature greying of hair.

Pathogenesis. Impairment of the liver and kidney resulting in insufficient supply of essence and blood.

Therapeutic Principle. Benefiting the liver and kidney and nourishing yin blood.

Greyish and Dry Tongue Fur

A tongue picture. The tongue fur is grey and dry, and the tongue is deep red. It is caused by the impairment of body fluid due to internal heat or cold dampness.

Symptoms. Red complexion, restlessness and thirst, constipation and yellowish urine, etc.

Greyish and Slippery Tongue Fur

A tongue picture. The coating is greyish and slippery and the surface is wet with excessive saliva. It is caused by yang insufficiency, cold excess and water stasis.

Symptoms. Aversion to cold, cold limbs, abdomineal pain, vomiting and diarrhea.

Greyish Black and Thorny Dry Tongue Fur

A tongue picture, referring to the greyish black and dry tongue fur with thorns. This is because excess of the viscera heat and consumption of the body fluid.

Symptoms. High fever, fidgeting and thirst, abdominal distention, constipation, etc.

Griantreed

It is the tender lymph of Arundo donax L. (Gramineae).

Effect. Clearing away heat and purging fire.

Indication. Hematemesis due to the lung-heat, hectic fever due to yin-deficiency, dizziness, strangury due to heat and toothache.

Griantreed Rhizome

It is the rhizome of Arundo donax L. (Gramineae).

Effect. Clearing pathogenic heat and promoting urination.

Indication. Mania by calentura, consumption and hectic fever due to yin-deficiency, stranguria, dysuria, toothache due to pathogenic wind-fire.

Griffth Woodsrrel Herb

It is the whole plant or root of Oxalis griffithii Edgew. et Hook. f. (Oxalidaceae).

Effect. Clearing pathogenic heat, inducing diuresis, removing blood stasis and diminishing swelling.

Indication. Nephritic hematochezia, subcutaneous swelling, thrush and traumatic injuries.

Grimy Tongue Fur

A tongue picture. It refers to thick tongue coating with greasy dirt. It is usually seen in dyspepsia or retention of phlegm or dampness.

Symptoms. Gastric and abdominal distention pain, nausea, vomiting, poor appetite or anorexia.

Gripping Pressing Manipulation

A term in acupuncture. It is one kind of the needling pressing manipulation.

Operation. Puncture the needle onto the point with the right hand, hold the lower part of the needle body (pay attention to 1/10 or 2/10 cun of the needle tip exposed) with the thumb and index finger of the left hand, then insert the needle into the point with the cooperative efforts of both hands. It is applicable to insertion by long needles.

Groove on the Back of Auricle(MA)

Name of an ear point.

Location. Through the backside of the superior antihelix crus and inferior antihelix, in the depression as a "Y" form.

Indication. Hypertension and skin pruritus.

Guanchong (TE 1)

A meridian point.

Location. 0.1 cun lateral to the corner of the finger nail on the ulnar side of the ring finger.

Indication. Headache, bloodshot eyes, tinnitus, deafness, inflammation of the throat, stiffness of the tongue, calenture and vexation.

Method. Puncture subcutaneously 0.1 cun, or prick to cause little bleeding. Apply moxibustion 1-3 moxa cones or 5-10 minutes with warming moxibustion.

Guangming (G 37)

A meridian point.

Location. 5 cun directly above the tip of the external malleolus, at the anterior edge of the fibula.

Indication. Eye pain, night blindness, distending pain of the breast, pain of the lower extremities.

Method. Puncture perpendicularly 1-1.5 cun. Apply moxibustion 3-5 moxa cones or 5-10 minutes with warming moxibustion.

Guanmen (S 22)

A meridian point.

Location. On the upper abdomen, 3 cun above the center of the umbilicus and 2 cun lateral to Jianli(CV 11).

Indication. Abdominal pain and distention, diarrhea, anorexia, water swelling, enuresis.

Method. Puncture perpendicularly 0.8-1.2 cun. Apply moxibustion 3-5 moxa cones or 5-10 minutes with warming moxibustion.

Guanyi (EX-LE)

An extra point.

Location. On 1 cun at the level with and 1 cun to the lateral side of the knee.

Indication. Angina in the lower abdomen.

Method. Puncture perpendicularly 0.5-1 cun. Apply moxibustion 3-7 moxa cones or 5-15 minutes with warming moxibustion.

Guanyuan (CV 4)

A meridian point. A point on the Front Middle Meridian, the Front-mu point of the small intestine, the crossing point of the three Yin Meridians of the Foot and Front Middle Meridian, the place where the Vital Meridian starts, also called Cimen, Sanjiejiao, Xiaji, or Dazhongji.

Location. 3 cun below the umbilicus on the abdominal midline.

Indication. Collapse due to apoplexy, consumptive disease, thinness and weakness, pain in the bilateral abdomen, vomiting and diarrhea due to cholera, dysentery, prolapse of anus, hernia, hemafecia, hematuria, dysuria, frequent urination, anuria, spontaneous emission, impotence, praecox ejaculation, irregular menstruation, amenorrhea, dysmenorrhea, external genitalia, persistent lochia, retention of placenta, diabetes, dizziness.

Method. Puncture perpendicularly 0.5-1 cun. Apply moxibustion 3-7 moxa cones or 5-15 minutes with warming moxibustion.

Guanyuanshu (B 26)

A meridian point.

Location. On the low back, below the spinous process of the 5th lumbar vertebra, 1. 5 cun lateral to the posterior midline.

Indication. Abdominal distention and pain, diarrhea, frequent or difficult urination, bed-wetting, diabetes, lumbago.

Method. Puncture perpendicularly 0.8-1 cun. Apply moxibustion 3-7 moxa cones or 5-15 minutes with warming moxibustion.

Guidang (EX-UE)

An extra point.

Location. On the ulnar side of the thumb of each hand, at the junction of the white and red skin proximal to the end of the cross striations of the finger joint of hand.

Indication. Infantile gastrointestina l isease, conjunctivitis, corneal macula.

Method. Puncture perpendicularly 0.1-0.2 cun. Moxibustion is applicable.

Guiding Drug

A term in Prescription. It refers two types: one is known as the medicinal guide which leads the other drugs in the prescription to the location of the disease; the other is known as a mediating drug which harmonizes the effects of various ingredients in the prescription.

Guiding Yang from Yin

A principle for selecting acupoints. When yang meridians are attacked by patho-

genic factors, yin meridians are to be punctured first to guide the factors.

Guiding Ying from Yang

A principle for selecting acupoints. When yin meridians are attacked by pathogenic factors, yang-meridians are to be punctured first to guide the factors.

Guilai (S 29)

1. A meridian point.
   Location. On the lower abdomen, 4 cun below the umbilicus and 2 cun lateral to the anterior midline.
   Indication. Pain in the bilateral lower abdomen, amenorrhea, hysteroptosis, leukorrhea, hernia and pain in penis.
   Method. Puncture perpendicularly 0.8-1.2 cun. Apply moxibustion 5-7 moxa cones or 10-20 minutes with warming moxibustion.
2. An extra point
   Location. 2 cun bilateral to Zhongji (CV 3).
   Indication. Enuresis.

Guixin (Ex-UE)

An extra point.

Location. At the tip of the thumb, 0.3 cun from the nail.

Indication. Edema.

Method. Apply moxibustion to the point with 7 moxa cones.

Guiyan (Ex-UE&LE)

An extra point.

Location. At the corner of the root of the radial (tibia) side of the thumb (big toe).

Indication. Epilepsy, mental disorder and syncope, etc.

Method. Moxibustion is applicable.

Gum Bleeding due to Internal Impairment

Symptoms. Gum bleeding, headache, halitosis, constipation, fever, etc.

Pathogenesis. Mostly due to overeating fat and greasy food, over-drinking alchohol, or liking to eat bitter food, which results in accumulation of heat in the intestines and stomach, fire accumulation in the blood, kidney-yin deficiency, and flaming-up of deficiency fire.

Therapeutic Principle. Clearing away stomach heat and purging fire, nourishing yin and lowering fire, cooling the blood and arresting bleeding.

Gum Hole

Symptoms. Abscess in the gum. Mostly appeared abscess in the gum of upper and lower incisors. At the early stage, there appear yellowish blisters that are severely swelling and painful.

Pathogenesis. Heat accumulation and yin deficiency.

Therapeutic Principle. Nourishing yin and dispersing fire.

Guoliangzhen (Ex)

Name of a group of extra points, referring to the 14 extra points used to treat manic-depressive psychosis and other mental disorders. In clinical application, the depth of puncture should accord with the patient's condition (fat or thin, weak or sthenia). The insertion should not be too deep.

Gynura Herb

It is the leaf or the whole herb of Gynura segetum (Lour.) Merr (Compositae).

Effect. Activating blood circulation, stopping bleeding and clearing away toxins.

Indication. Traumatic injuries, epistaxis, hemoptysis, hematemesis, carbuncles of breast, innominate inflammatory swellings and insect-bite.

Gypsum

It is the soft mineral of Gypsum chiefly composed of hydrated calcium sulphate ($CaSO_4 \times 2H_2O$).

Effect. Clearing away and purging pathogenic heat-fire, removing restlessness and thirst, promoting regeneration of the tissue and healing wounds.

Indication. Epidemic febrile diseases, high fever, cough and asthma due to lung-heat, toothache due to stomach-fire, headache, externally as astringent and hemostatic, slow healing ulcerated carbuncles, furuncles, sores, eczema, burns and scalds, etc.

H

Habitual Abortion due to Blood Deficiency

Symptoms. Mental fatigue and tiredness, yellowish complexion, lumbago and abdominal pain, or even threatened abortion.

Pathogenesis. Blood deficiency with the history of habitual abortion caused by deficiency of both blood and yin resulting in fetal malnutrition.

Therapeutic Principle. Enriching blood to prevent abortion.

Habitual Abortion due to Blood-heat

Symptoms. Repeated abortion.

Pathogenesis. Insidious heat from excess of original yang in Vital and Front Middle Meridians, forcing blood to flow violently and resulting in impairment of the fetal qi.

Therapeutic Principle. Clearing away heat from blood to prevent abortion.

Habitual Abortion due to Qi-deficiency

Symptoms. Repeated abortion.

Pathogenesis. Deficiency and weakness of the spleen and stomach, and insufficiency of qi in the middle-energizer, resulting in malnutrition of the fetus.

Therapeutic Principle. Invigorating the spleen and replenishing qi.

Habitual Abortion due to Trauma

Symptoms. Repeated abortion.

Pathogenesis. Impairment of Vital and Front Middle Meridians and disturbance of the fetus caused by fall, stumble, sprain, overwork and excess sexual intercourse.

Therapeutic Principle. Strengthening qi and nourishing blood and kidney to prevent abortion.

Haichow Elsholtzia Herb

It is the whole herb of Elsholtzia splendens Nakai ex F. Maekawa and Mosla chinensis Maxim. (Labiatae).

Effect. Relieve superficial syndromes by diaphoresis, regulating the stomach, removing dampness, promoting diuresis and subduing swelling.

Indication. Fever, adversion to cold, headache, anhidrosis, abdominal pain with vomiting and diarrhea, edema and dysuria, etc.

Haiquan

One of the extraordinary points.

Location. At the middle point of the frenum of the tongue.

Indication. Vomiting, hiccups, pharyngitis, diarrhea and diabetes.

Method. Puncture perpendicularly 0.1-0.2 cun, or prick with a three-edged needle.

Hairline Boils

Symptoms. Like a millet at the beginning, gradually becoming large, hard and rising up, white top and red base, quite painful and itching, a little pus flowing out after breaking. It is multiple, lingering and difficult to heal.

Therapeutic Principle. Expelling wind and removing dampness, and clearing away heat and toxic material.

Hairy Birthwort

It is the dried rhizome or herb of Aristolochia mollissima Hance. (Aristolochiaceae).

Effect. Expelling wind and eliminating dampness, removing obstruction in the meridians and arresting pain.

Indication. Arthralgia due to pathogenic wind-dampness, numbness of the limbs, carbuncle and swelling, and traumatic injuries.

Hairy Clover Shrub Root

It is the root or whole herb of Myrsine africana L. (Myrsinaceae).

Effect. Activating blood circulation, dispelling pathogenic wind and dampness.

Indication. Subduing arthralgia due to wind-dampness, diarrhea, dysentery, hematuria, cough caused by consumption, etc.

Hairy flower Actinidia Root

It is the root of Actinidia eriantha Benth. (family Actinidiaceae).

Effect. Clearing away heat, inducing diuresis, promoting blood circulation, removing swelling and detoxicating.

Indication. Aphonia caused by retention of pathogenic heat in the lung, dysentery, leukorrhagia, breast carbuncle, hernia, arthralgia, dermatitis, cancer, etc.

Hairy Holly Root

It is the root of Icex pubescens Hook. et Arn. (family Aquifoliaceae).

Effect. Clearing away heat, detoxicating, promoting qi and blood circulation to remove blood stasis, eliminating phlegm and relieving cough and asthma.

Indication. Common cold caused by wind-heat, asthma and cough caused by lung-heat, laryngeal edema, tonsillitis, dysentery, hemiplegia, thromboembolism erysipelas, central choroidoretinitis, uveitis, hypertension, hypercholesterinemia, skin infection, burn and wound-infection, etc.

Hairy Leaf Chonemorpha Root or Stem

It is the root, stem, or stem bark of Chonemorpha valvata Chatt. (Apocynaceae).

Effect. Relieving bleeding, promoting regeneration of tissue, relaxing muscles and activating the tendons.

Indication. Traumatic bleeding, fracture, rheumatism, etc.

Hairy-vein Agrimony Bud

It is the winter bud of Agrimonia pilosa Ledeb. (Rosaceae).

Effect. Killing parasites.

Indication. Cestodiasis.

Hairy-vein Agrimony Herb

✿ **H-1**

It is the whole herb of Agrimonia pilosa Ledeb. (Rosaceae).

Effect. Arresting bleeding by astringency, relieving pain and killing parasites.

Indication. Hemoptysis, epistaxis, hematuria, metrorrhagia diarrhea, skin infection, etc.

Hairy Waxmyrtle Bark

It is the bark or root bark of Myrica esculenta Buch.-Ham. (Myricaceae).

Effect. Subduing inflammation, inducing astringency, stopping diarrhea, relieving the blood and arresting pain.

Indication. Dysentery, enteritis, stomachache, metrorrhagia and metrostaxis.

Hance Rosewood Stem

It is the stem or root of Dalbergia hancei Benth. (Leguminosae).

Effect. Promoting qi circulation to relieve pain and eliminating stagnancy.

Indication. Pain caused by disorder of qi in the chest and stomach, flatulent dyspepsia and epistaxis.

Hankow Willow Leaf and Twig

It is the twig and leaf of Salix matsudana Koidz. (Salicaceae).

Effect. Expelling pathogenic wind and dampness, and clearing away damp-heat.

Indication. Hepatitis with jaundice, rheumatic arthritis and eczema.

Hanyan (G 4)

A meridian acupuncture point.

Location. On the head, in the hair above the temples, at the junction of the upper quarter and lower three quarters of the curved line connecting Touwei (S 8) and Qubin (G 7).

Indication. Headache, dizziness, pain of outer canthus, toothache, tinnitus, epilepsy induced by terror, clonic convulsions.

Method. Puncture subcutaneously and backward 0.3-0.4 cun. Moxibustion is applicable.

Hare Dung

It is the dried feces of Lepus toail Pallas (Leporidae) and other hares.

Effect. Killing parasites and improving eyesight.

Indication. Blurring of vision, infantile malnutrition, and anal fistula.

Harlequin Glorybower Leaf

It is the twig and leaf of Clerodendrum trichotomum Thunb. (Verbenaceae).

Effect. Removing wind-dampness, lowering blood pressure, antimalaria, eliminating sputum, relieving cough and dyspnea.

Indication. Rheumatic arthralgia, numbness of extremity, hemiplegia, hypertension and chronic bronchitis.

Harmonization of Yin and Yang

Keep yin and yang in a harmonious state is one of the basic principles of treating diseases in TCM. The imbalance of yin and yang turns out to be the fundamental pathogenesis of diseases. Therefore, harmonizing yin and yang so as to restore the relative balance between them will be necessary.

Hawksbill Shell

It is the shell of Eretmochelys imbricata (L.) (Chelonidae).

Effect. Calm the liver to stop convulsion and clearing away heat and toxic material.

Indication. Acute febrile diseases with high fever, restlessness, unconsciousness, delirium, apoplexy, noxious pox and furuncle.

Hawthorn Fruit   ✿ H-2

It is the fruit of Crataegus cuneata Sieb. et Zucc. or C. Pinnatifida Bge. var. major N. E. Br. (Rosaceae).

Effect. Strengthening the stomach and improving digestion, removing food stagnancy, promoting blood circulation and removing blood stasis, lowering blood pressure and the level of blood lipids.

Indication. Indigestion, abdominal distention, abdominal pain and diarrhea, postpartum abdominal pain due to blood retention, and lochiorrhea, hernia, hypertension and hyperlipoidemia, etc.

Haziness

A symptom referring to unconsciousness and mental confusion as if being covered up.

Pathogenesis. Evil affecting the seven orifices, and impairment of the mind due to exogenous febrile disease, apoplexy, syncope, epilepsy, etc.

Headache

The pain all over the head, or in the front part, the rear part or just on one side of the head.

Pathogenesis. The six exogenous factors or various diseases due to internal damage.

Headache due to Blood Deficiency

Symptoms. Tic pain in the part from the tip of eyebrow to the forehead angle, or dull pain of head, usually accompanied by dizziness, pallor, blurring vision, propensity to be frightened, palpitation, lassitude, etc.

Pathogenesis. The failure of blood.

Therapeutic Principle. Enriching the blood and invigorating qi.

Headache due to Blood Stasis

Symptoms. Stabbing headache which is fixed to a certain part of the head, appearing and fading at frequent intervals for a long time, poor vision, hypomnesis, dark and sluggish complexion, spots of blood stasis on the tongue, uneven pulse, etc.

Pathogenesis. Surgical trauma on the head, prolonged pain entering the meridians, and blood stasis stagnating the meridians.

Therapeutic Principle. Promoting the blood circulation to remove blood stasis and alleviate pain.

Headache due to Cold

Symptoms. Rigid and painful head and neck, fever with aversion to cold, heaviness sensation of the body, etc.

Pathogenesis. Wind-cold attacking the superficial part of the body from the outside, stagnancy of defensive yang, failure of the lucid yang to spread, and disorder in collaterals.

Therapeutic Principle. Dispelling wind and cold from the body.

Headache due to Cold-dampness

Symptoms. Headache often occuring in the cloudy and rainy conditions, stuffiness in the chest, sluggish extremities, etc.

Pathogenesis. Stagnancy of yang-qi due to cold and damp, sluggishness of blood circulation, and contracture of the blood vessels.

Therapeutic Principle. Removing cold and dispelling dampness.

Headache due to Common Cold

Symptoms. Headache, stuffy nose, spontaneous perspiration and aversion to wind, etc.

Pathogenesis. Invasion of external noxious factors into the body.

Therapeutic Principle. Dispelling the wind and relieving the exterior syndrome.

Headache due to Damp-heat

Symptoms. Severe headache, restlessness, heaviness of the body, swollen face and limbs, restless arthralgia of limbs, etc.

Pathogenesis. Attack of damp-heat blocking up the five orifices.

Therapeutic Principle. Clearing away heat and dispersing dampness.

Headache due to Deficiency of both Qi and Blood

Symptoms. Headache with dizziness, more severe ache when overstraining, intermittent pain, palpitation and restlessness, shortness of breath and fatigue, pale complexion.

Pathogenesis. Asthenia of qi and blood.

Therapeutic Principle. Nourishing qi and blood.

Headache due to Excessive Drinking

Symptoms. Nausea and vomiting, dizziness and vertigo, serious headache, etc.

Pathogenesis. Unfavourable disturbance of qi and blood caused by excessive drinking.

Therapeutic Principle. Regulating stomach and relieving the alcoholic harm.

Headache due to Excessive Heat and Reversed Qi

Symptoms. Protracted headache, dysphoria, pain relieved in cold, more severe in heat.

Pathogenesis. Upward pathogenic heat and reversed meridian qi.

Therapeutic Principle. Clearing away heat and purging fire.

Headache due to Improper Diet

Symptoms. Headache, oppressed feeling in the chest and epigastrium, eructation with fetid odour and acid regurgitation, loss of appetite, occasional fever.

Pathogenesis. Improper diet injuring the spleen and stomach, and failure of lucid yang to rise.

Therapeutic Principle. Promoting digestion and relieving stasis, lifting lucid yang and lowering turbid yin.

Headache due to Internal Injury

The syndrome mainly found in various chronic diseases.

Symptoms. Slow attack and remittent pain that appear by fits and starts.

Pathogenesis. Impairment of qi and blood in the visceral organs, or upward disturbance of pathogenic qi. It can easily break out while the patient is overtired and emotionally stimulated.

Headache due to Invasion by Wind

Symptoms. Aversion to cold and fever, stuffy and running nose, headache, etc.

Pathogenesis. The external attacking of wind pathogens.

Therapeutic Principle. Relieving the exterior syndrome to stop pain.

Headache due to Kidney Deficiency

Symptoms. Headache with empty feeling, dizziness, tinnitus, lassitude in loin and legs, aversion to cold, cold limbs, etc.

Pathogenesis. Debility, long deficiency of the kidney-essence, or sexual overstrain, failure to nourish the brain caused by insufficiency of marrow, or deficiency of yin affecting yang.

Therapeutic Principle. Nourishing the kidney-yin, warming and tonifying the kidney-yang.

Headache due to Pathogenic Fire

Symptoms. Cephalea, beating or distending pain of head involving cheeks and teeth, accompanied by dysphoria, thirst, dry mouth, red eyes, constipation, etc.

Pathogenesis. Upward offense of fire in the Stomach Meridian.

Therapeutic Principle. Clearing away heat and purging intense fire.

Headache due to Phlegm Syncope

Symptoms. Headache and dizziness, distress of the chest and vomiting, restlessness, cold limbs, heavy sensation of the body, etc.

Pathogenesis. Improper diet, or impairment of activity and digesting function of the spleen, interior phlegm dampness produced inside, and phlegm rising adversely with qi.

Therapeutic Principle. Depress the abnormal rising of qi, dispelling phlegm and warming the middle-energizer.

Headache due to Phlegm Turbidity

Symptoms. Headache, dizziness with a tightening feeling in the forehead, fullness in the chest and stomach, nausea, vomiting with phlegm-salivation, loose stool.

Pathogenesis. Head confused by phlegm-dampness.

Therapeutic Principle. Resolve phlegm and lower turbidity, remove the obstruction in the collaterals to relieve pain.

Headache due to Qi Deficiency

Symptoms. Headache with empty sensation, tinnitus and lassitude, shortness of breath, anorexia and loose bowel, etc.

Pathogenesis. Qi deficiency and the failure of lucid yang to rise, weakness of the spleen and stomach, incapability of formation and transformation of qi.

Therapeutic Principle. Strengthening the spleen and replenishing qi.

Headache due to Qi Disorder

Symptoms. Headache which is serious on both sides and top of head, vertigo with blurred vision which deteriorates in a rage, abdominal distention and vomiting of gastric juice, etc.

Pathogenesis. Emotional depression, the stagnation of the liver-qi and adverse flow of qi, and the upward liver fire disturbing the seven orifices.

Therapeutic Principle. Smoothing the liver and regulating the circulation of qi.

Headache due to Summer-heat

Symptoms. Distention of head and fever, thirst and much sweat, vexation, dirty complexion, greasy or yellowish greasy fur, light and rapid pulse, etc.

Pathogenesis. Pathogenic summer-heat invading meridians and going up to the head, obstructing the clear yang, leading to the impairment of the flow of qi and blood, and blocking the passage of collaterals.

Therapeutic Principle. Clearing away summer-heat by eliminating dampness.

Headache due to Wind

Symptoms. Aversion to cold of the nape and the back, extremely cold sensation of Naohu (GV 17), severe headache, etc.

Pathogenesis. Attacks of wind pathogen on the head.

Therapeutic Principle. Warming and expelling cold.

Headache due to Yang Deficiency

Symptoms. Dull headache with aversion to light, chills with cold limbs, tiredness and weakness, inappetence and pale tongue.

Pathogenesis. Deficiency of yang-qi, the failure of lucid yang to rise.

Therapeutic Principle. Replenishing qi and supporting yang.

Headache due to Yin Deficiency

Symptoms. Headache, especially severe in the afternoon, accompanied by emaciation, dry mouth and lips, etc.

Pathogenesis. Deficiency of yin, and deficient fire disturbing upward.

Therapeutic Principle. Nourishing yin, alleviating fire and nourishing blood.

Head Needle

1. An acupuncture point apparatus. It is used for needling specific stimulation areas of the scalp, usually a filiform needle in No. 28-30 or 4.5-6.0 cm in length.
2. Therapy of head acupuncture. A therapeutic technique to puncture specific stimulating zone, which is used chiefly to treat encephalopathy.

Head Stephania Root

It is the root tuber of Stephania cepharantha Hayata (Aristolochiaceae).

Effect. Clearing away heat and expelling phlegm, cooling blood, detoxicating and relieving pain.

Indication. Sore throat, cough, hematemesis, epistaxis, traumatic bleeding, hydroperitoneum, dysentery, gastroduodenal ulcer, subcutaneous abscess caused by noxious heat and articular pain.

Head Wind

Symptoms. Excessive sweat in the head and face, adversion to wind, headache, etc.

Pathogenesis. Wind attacking the body after taking a shower.

Therapeutic Principle. Eliminating wind and stopping pain.

Heart Apoplexy

Symptoms. Fever, headache, flushed face, confusion of consciousness, stiff tongue, dry mouth, contracture of the chest and back, trance, sweating, etc.

Pathogenesis. Heart meridian attacked by pathogenic wind.

Therapeutic Principle. Expelling pathogenic wind and nourishing the heart to calm the mind.

Heart Blood Deficiency

Symptoms. Palpitation, dysphoria, anxiety, insomnia, amnesia, dzziness, pale face, pale lips and tongue.

Pathogenesis. Blood loss, excessive mental labor and insufficiency production of blood.

Therapeutic Principle. Enriching the blood for tranquilization.

Heart-deficiency Syndrome

Symptoms. 1. The syndromes of deficiency of the heart blood are pale complexion, dizziness, severe palpitation, dysphoria, night sweat, insomnia, excessive dreaming, amnesia; 2. The syndromes of deficiency of the heart-qi are palpitation, shortness of breath, stuffiness in the chest, spontaneous perspiration, amnesia, susceptible to fright.

Pathogenesis. Deficiency of heart blood or insufficiency of heart-qi.

Therapeutic Principle. Tonifying heart blood and nourishing the heart to calm the heart for deficiency of the heart blood; tonifying the heart-qi for deficiency of heart-qi

Heart Disease

The various diseases involving the heart.

Pathogenesis. Deficiency of both the qi and blood, stagnation of blood stasis and qi retardation, heart-yin deficiency or heart-yang deficiency, excessive heart-fire, retention of fluid attacking the heart, etc.

Heart Fright

Symptoms. Palpitation, dysphoria, frightening and mental irritability on encountering sudden events or hearing sudden sounds, etc.

Pathogenesis. Postpartum hemorrhage, hematemesis, or insufficiency of yin-blood and the heart-spleen impairment by excessive anxiety.

Therapeutic Principle. Enriching the blood and nourishing the blood to calm the mind.

Heart Governing Tongue

The function of the tongue is closely related to the heart. The tongue serves as the specific organ. When the heart functions well, the tongue will be red and bright, with taste sensitivity and fluency of speech. When there is something wrong with the heart, the tongue is affected, and diagnosis of the heart will be made through tongue physiological and pathological activities.

Heart Impairment

Symptoms. Reddish face, lassitude of the lower extremities, irritability, fever.

Pathogenesis. Mental overstrain and deficiency of the blood of the heart.

Therapeutic Principle. Invigorating qi and enriching the blood.

Heartleaf Houttuynia Herb

It is the whole herb of Houttuynia cordata Thunb. (Saururaceae).

Effect. Clearing away heat, dissipating phlegm, arresting cough, detoxicating, evacuating pus, inducing diuresis and relieving swelling.

Indication. Pneumonia, phthisis, cough due to heat in the lung, urethritis, appendicitis, cholecystitis, tympanitis, mastitis, edema, hemorrhoids, and difficulty and pain on micturition, etc.

Heart Malnutrition

Symptoms. Palpitation, shortness of breath, lassitude, etc.

Pathogenesis. Heart impaired by anxiety, grief and worry, or the malnutrition of the heart is caused by deficiency of blood circulation.

Therapeutic Principle. Enriching the blood and nourishing the heart.

Heart Meridian Malnutrition

Symptoms. Yellow face with red cheeks, high fever, dysphoria, aphthae, dark and difficult urine and night sweat.

Pathogenesis. Stasis of heat in the Heart Meridians.

Therapeutic Principle. Eliminating pathogenic heat from the heart.

Heart Obstruction

Symptoms. Palpitation, precordial pain, stuffiness in the chest, dyspnea, dry throat, eructation, vexation, insomnia, etc.

Pathogenesis. The obstruction of the heart-qi and the blood vessels due to the heart impaired by worry, deficiency of blood and qi and the invasion of the heart by exopathogen.

Therapeutic Principle. Eliminating pathogenic factor, nourishing the heart, and promoting blood circulation to remove meridian obstruction.

Heart Passes the Evil Heat to the Small Intestine

The heart and small intestine affect each other pathologically because of an exterior and interior relationship between them, e.g. the accumulated heat in the heart can move to the small intestine.

Symptoms. Dark urine, pain in urination, ulcers on the tongue, etc.

Therapeutic Principle. Clearing away excessive heat in the small intestine.

Heart-qi

Referring to: 1. The essence and energy of the heart. 2. The functional activities of the heart and the heart function keeping the blood circulation.

Heart-qi Exuberance

Symptoms. Palpitation, dysphoria, insomnia, excessive dreaming, or even ravings, coma, and all types of hemorrhage, reddened crimson and pricked tongue, rapid pulse.

Pathogenesis. Sthenia of the heart energy.

Therapeutic Principle. Eliminating the heart-fire.

Heart-qi Stagnation

Symptoms. Consciousness, annoyance in the chest, amnesia, etc.

Pathogenesis. Stagnation of the heart-qi.

Therapeutic Principle. Relieving the stagnation, tranquilizing the mind, restoring orifices and resolving filthy pathogenic factors.

Heart-qi Unconsolidation

Symptoms. Listlessness, mental aberration, amnesia, anxiety, palpitation, spontaneous sweating or sweating with action of body.

Pathogenesis. Insufficiency of the heart-qi.

Heart Relating to Joy

Under the normal conditions, joy can promote the heart-qi and blood-qi circulation and make the nutrient with defensive systems in harmony. But excessive joy will lead to relaxation of heart-qi, manifested as mental derangement, trance, or ceaseless laughing.

Heart Spasm

Symptoms. Palpitation, restlessness, shortness of breath, cough, etc.

Pathogenesis. Cold of deficiency type of heart-qi or flaming up of the fire in the gallbladder and tri-energizer involving the heart.

Therapeutic Principle. Invigorating the heart-qi and warming the heart-yang for the patients with deficiency of heart-qi, clearing away fire and arresting the mind for the fire in the gallbladder and triple energizer.

Heart System

Referring to the meridians and collaterals linking the heart with other zang-organs.

Heart-vessel Obstruction

Symptoms. Oppression and pain in the chest, with inconsistent referred pain in the shoulder, upper back and medial side of the arm, and palpitation, sudden pain in the precordium, even cold extremities, profuse perspiration in severe case.

Pathogenesis. Insufficient yang-qi, cold stagnation of blood vessels or accumulation of phlegm.

Heart Wind

1. A disease of the affection of the heart by
   pathogenic wind.

Symptoms. Hyperhidrosis, aversion to wind, dryness of the mouth and tongue, dysphoria, anger, even stiff tongue and dysphrasia, etc.

Therapeutic Principle. Expelling wind, tranquilizing the mind.

2. A kind of epilepsy.

Symptoms. Mental lethargy, irregular happiness and anger, or disorder of verbal communication, etc.

Pathogenesis. Emotional deterioration, the stagnation of the liver-qi, or the deficiency of the heart and spleen, the insufficiency of qi and blood, the obstruction of phlegm and mental derangement.

Therapeutic Principle. Clearing away the heart fire and tranquilizing the mind, tonifying the heart and spleen, relieving the stagnation and resolving phlegm.

Heart-Yin

Referring to the yin fluid of the heart. The physiological and pathological changes are closely related to the heart-yin, and also to the excess or deficiency of the lung-yin and the kidney-yin.

Heart-Yin Deficiency

Symptoms. Palpitation, irritability, insomnia, fright and amnesia, night perspiration, etc.

Pathogenesis. Prolonged ill and fatigue, or emotional frustration or excessive heart-fire and liver-fire.

Therapeutic Principle. Nourishing the heart to calm the mind.

Heat Accumulation in Chest

Symptoms. Fullness and pain in the abdomen, fever, thirst, stuffiness, dry mouth, constipation, etc.

Pathogenesis. Accumulation of heat and recurrent fluid retention in the chest.

Therapeutic Principle. Relieving accumulation and purging heat.

Heat-conducting Moxibustion

Another name for warm needling. An acupuncture point technique of burning the pulp of mugwort on the handle of the needle after inserting the needle into the body.

Heat Constipation

Symptoms. Fever, flushed face, aphthae, dry mouth, thirst, dark brown urine, yellow coating of the tongue, etc.

Pathogenesis. Constipation caused by accumulation of heat in the large intestine.

Therapeutic Principle. Clearing away heat and applying the purgative therapy.

Heat Croup

Symptoms. Dyspnea, wheezing in the throat, chest fullness, thick yellowish sputum, flushed face, sweating, thirst, red tongue with yellow and sticky coating, etc.

Pathogenesis. Exuberance of lung-fire, accumulated phlegm and upward rising of qi.

Therapeutic Principle. Clearing away the lung-heat and expelling phlegm to stop dyspnea.

Heat Diarrhea

Symptoms. Abdominal pain with bombus, diarrhea with pain, sticky or watery stool, thirst, dark urine etc.

Pathogenesis. Invasion of heat into intestines and stomach.

Therapeutic Principle. Clearing away the heat and purging the pathogenic fire.

Heat Dysentery

Symptoms. Fever, abdominal pain, tenesmus, diarrhea with mucous-bloody feces, polydipsia, dark and ardor urine, yellow and sticky tongue coating, etc.

Pathogenesis. Accumulated heat in the stomach and large intestines.

Therapeutic Principle. Removing pathogenic heat from blood and clearing away toxic material.

Heat Dyspnea

Symptoms. Dyspnea, yellowish thick sputum, fullness in the chest and dysphoria, etc.

Pathogenesis. Attack of the lung by pathogenic heat, dysfunction of water metabolism, accumulated phlegm-fire in the air passage.
Therapeutic Principle. Clearing away the lung heat.

Heat Flaccidity
Symptoms. Hectic fever, flaccidity of muscles and bones, and inability to walk, etc.
Pathogenesis. Yin and blood burned and consumed by internal heat, malnutrition of tendon.
Therapeutic Principle. Nourishing yin, clearing away heat, tonifying the liver and kidney, and strengthening the muscles and bones.

Heat in both Exterior and Interior
Referring to the coexistence of exterior and interior syndrome of heat.
Symptoms. Fever and flushed face, aversion to cold, extreme thirst, vexation, yellow and dry tongue coating, rapid pulse, etc.
Pathogenesis. Invasion of pathogenic heat into the interior before the relief of the exterior heat, or pathogenic heat in the interior with the affection by warm pathogen.
Therapeutic Principle. Relieving exterior syndrome and removing obstruction due to interior syndrome, and clearing away heat from interior.

Heat in Gallbladder
Symptoms. Chest distress, hypochondriac pain, and bitter taste in the mouth.
Pathogenesis. Flowing-up of the gallbladder qi due to irresolution.
Therapeutic Principle. Purging away heat and normalizing functioning of the gallbladder.

Heat of Excess Type
Symptoms. High fever, extreme thirst and excessive drinking, constipation, abdominalgia with tenderness, dark urine, yellowish dry fur, etc.

Pathogenesis. Excessive exogenous pathogens enter the interior of the body and transform into heat while the body resistance is undermined.
Therapeutic Principle. Clearing away heat and removing pathogenic factors.

Heat of Liver-qi
Symptoms. Bitter taste in the mouth, tense of the tendons and spasm of the muscles.
Pathogenesis. The exhaustion of the liver-yin due to pathogenic heat and qi excess in the liver, and failure of essence of blood to nourish muscles.
Therapeutic Principle. Clearing away the liver heat and nourishing the liver blood.

Heat Phlegm
Symptoms. Yellowish, thick sputum difficult to cough up, flushed face, fidget, mania, epigastrium, dry mouth and throat, etc.
Pathogenesis. Combination of pathogenic heat and phlegm with prolonged stagnation.
Therapeutic Principle. Clearing away the heart-fire, dispelling phlegm and arresting cough.

Heat-producing Needling
A needling technique.
Indication. Cold syndrome.
Method. The insertion depth is divided into three equal portions: superficial, medium and deep; after insertion of the needle, heavily thrusting and gently lifting, or twirling, the needle for nine times at each portion in a superficial, medium and deep sequence. Repeat the operation to induce the warm sensation.

Heat Stagnation
Symptoms. Dizziness, thirst, dryness of the lips and tongue, yellow and dark urine, or muscular fever, etc.
Pathogenesis. Protracted stagnation transforming into heat.
Therapeutic Principle. Clearing away heat and relieving the depressed liver.

Heat Stranguria

Symptoms. Frequent urination with oliguria, difficulty and pain, lumbago, contracture and distending pain in the lower abdomen, etc.

Pathogenesis. Accumulation of damp-heat in the lower-energizer.

Therapeutic Principle. Clearing away heat and eliminating dampness.

Heatstroke

A acute disease, also named sunstroke.

Symptoms. Dizziness, headache, fever, restlessness, vomiting or sudden collapse, and convulsion of limbs.

Pathogenesis. Attack of pathogenic summer-heat in hot summer.

Heat Syndrome due to Heart Deficiency

1. A kind of heart deficiency syndrome.

   Symptoms. Dyspnea, fatigue, palpitation, restless sleep, etc.

   Pathogenesis. Deficiency and heat of the Heart Meridian.

   Therapeutic Principle. Nourishing yin, clearing away heat and relieving mental stress.

2. One kind of consumptive fever.

   Symptoms. Subjective feverish sensation in the cardiac area, palmar heat, vomiting, poor memory, insomnia, bitter taste, etc.

   Therapeutic Principle. Nourishing the heart and clearing away heat.

Heat-syndrome in Newborn

1. A kind of syndrome appearing in the newborn.

   Symptoms. Infant with flushed face, swelling eyes, high fever, crying, red urine and dry stool after birth.

   Pathogenesis. Infantile affection of newborn by the pathogenic heat of the mother in pregnancy.

   Therapeutic Principle. Clearing away pathogenic heat and toxin.

2. Blindness of pregnant women just before delivery.

Pathogenesis. Eating peppery food excessively.

Therapeutic Principle. Clearing away Heat toxins of the Liver Meridians.

Heat Syndrome of Excess Type

It refers to the syndrome caused by excess of heat or interior and exterior heat.

Symptoms. High fever and restlessness, flushed face and congested eyes, thirst, abdominal pain with tenderness, constipation, scanty and deep-colored urine, reddened tongue with yellowish fur, etc.

Therapeutic Principle. Clearing heat and purging fire.

Heat Syndrome of Spleen-qi

Symptoms. Dry mouth, thirst, numbness, etc.

Pathogenesis. Exogenous pathogenic heat invading the body and staying internally, the heat accumulated in the stomach and intestine, excessive intake of rich fatty and sweet food with dryness and heat in nature.

Heat Syndrome with Pseudo-cold Symptoms

Referring to the real heat existing internally while false cold is appearing externally.

Symptoms. Aversion to cold, cold extremities, watery diarrhea, thirst, dry throat, dark yellow urine.

Pathogenesis. Repellence of yin by excessive yang caused by heat transmission of exogenous pathogenic factors into the interior of the body.

Therapeutic Principle. Clearing heat, which mainly use with drugs cold and cool in nature.

Heat Vomiting

Symptoms. Projectile vomiting after eating, flushed face, preference for cold, polydipsia with desire for drinking, yellow and dark urine, constipation, etc. It can be seen as inflammation of the organs in the abdominal cavity such as acute gastritis, cholecystitis, pancreatitis and hepatitis, etc.

Pathogenesis. Heat accumulated in the spleen and stomach, or the attack of the stomach by pathogenic heat.

Therapeutic Principle. Clearing away the liver-fire, and regulating the stomach to stop vomiting.

Heaviness in Head

Symptoms. The sensation of heaviness in the head, or wrapped sensation.

Pathogenesis. Affection by exogenous or endogenous dampness, or the obstruction of damp-phlegm in the interior, or the lack of primordial essence.

Heaviness in Loin

The symptom with sensation of heaviness in the loin.

Pathogenesis. Deficiency of kidney and stasis of water-dampness.

Heavy Deficiency

It means wrongly using purgation in treating the patient with deficiency syndrome, resulting in impairment of vital-qi, making deficiency syndrome even more deficient.

Heavy Hearing

Symptoms. Poor hearing in a low voice, and hearing a loud one.

Pathogenesis. Invasion of exopathogen of wind to Shaoyang Meridian, the accumulation of the pathogenic factor in ear and obstruction of circulation of qi.

Hectic Fever due to Yin-deficiency

Symptoms. Tidal fever, flushing of zygomatic region, faint breathing, dysphoria and insomnia, etc.

Pathogenesis. Insufficiency of kidney essence, hyperactivity of fire due to yin deficiency.

Therapeutic Principle. Tonifying the kidney and supplementing kidney essence, nourishing yin to eliminate heat.

Hectic Fever of Kidney Type

Symptoms. Hectic fever, weakness, withered ears, etc.

Pathogenesis. Improper diet at the time of initial cure of a febrile disease.

Therapeutic Principle. Restoring qi and promoting digestion.

Hectic Fever of Lung Type

Symptoms. Dryness of mouth and nose, dry cough, thirst, etc.

Pathogenesis. Eating beef, mutton and drinking, or sexual strain, after the lung-heat disease resulting in the remained pathogenic heat.

Therapeutic Principle. Clearing away heat, nourishing yin and moistening the lung.

Hedge Prinsepia Nut

It is the dried ripe fruit of Prinsepia uniflora Batal. (Rosaceae).

Effect. Expelling wind, clearing away heat, tonifying the liver and improving the visual acuity.

Indication. Acute conjunctivitis, swollen and painful eyes, poor vision, photophobia, blepharitis angularis, rhinorrhagia, etc.

Heding (Ex-HN)

An extra acupuncture point.

Location. On the head, 3.5 cun directly above the midpoint of the anterior hairline, the same location as Qianding (GV 21).

Indication. Epilepsy, dizziness, vertigo, pain in vertex.

Method. Puncture 0.5-0.8 cun subcutaneously backwards; apply moxibustion with a moxa stick for 5-10 minutes.

Heding (Ex-LE 2)

An extra acupuncture point.

Location. Above the knee, in the depression at the midpoint of the upper border of the patellar bone.

Indication. Knee pain, weakness of foot and leg, paralysis of lower extremities, beriberi, etc.

Method. Puncture 0.5-0.7 cun perpendicularly; apply moxibustion to the point for 5-7 minutes.

Heel (MA-Ah 1)
An ear point.
Location. At the medial and superior angle of the superior crus of the antihelix.
Indication. Pain in the heel.

Heel Pain
Symptoms. The pain in one or both heels without red and swelling, and difficult walking.
Pathogenesis. Caused by insufficiency of essence and blood due to deficiency of the kidney, or blood-heat and phlegm-dampness.

Hegu (LI 4)
An meridian acupuncture point
Location. On the dorsum of the hand, between the first and second metacarpal bones, along the middle of the second metacarpal bone on the radial side.
Indication. Headache, redness, swelling and pain of the eye, epistaxis, toothache, trimus, deviation of the mouth and eye, deafness, mumps, sore throat, fever, anhibrosis, hidrosis, abdominal pain, constipation, amenorrhoea, dystocia, etc.
Method. Pucture perpendicularly 0.5-0.8 cun. Moxibustion is applicable.

Heliao (LI 19)
An meridian acupuncture point.
Location. On the upper lip, directly inferior to the exterior border of the nostril and parallel to Shuigou (GV 26).
Indication. Wry mouth, lockjaw, stuffy nose, epistaxis, rhinitis, facial paralysis and nasal polyp.
Method. Puncture perpendicularly or obliquely 0.3-0.5 cun and apply moxibustion to the point for 3-5 minutes.

Heliao (TE 22)
An acupuncture point, a point on the Tiple-energizer Meridian.

Location. On the lateral side of the head, at the posterior border of the hair on the temples, parallel to the anterior region of the auricular root, at the posterior border of the superficial temporal artery.
Indication. Heaviness sensation and pain of head, tinnitus, lockjaw, a wry mouth, cervical swelling, and swelling of the submandibular region, etc.
Method. Puncture obliquely or subcutaneously 0.3-0.5 cun, keep away from the artery, and apply moxibustion to the point for 3-5 minutes.

Heliosis during Pregnancy
Symptoms. Fever, thirst, spontaneous perspiration, restlessness, mental confusion, tiredness, excessive fetal movement, etc.
Pathogenesis. Affection of pathogenic summer-heat during pregnancy.
Therapeutic Principle. Eliminating summer-heat to prevent abortion.

Hemafecia
Referring to the discharge of blood through the anus.
Pathogenesis. Failure of the spleen to keep the flow of blood within the vessels resulting from insufficiency of the spleen, or large intestinal damp heat.

Hemafecia due to Cold
Symptoms. Hemafecia, abdominal pain, aversion to cold, lassitude, dim complexion, pink tongue, etc.
Pathogenesis. Splenoasthenic cold, and hypofunction of the spleen due to improper diet of rawness and cold.
Therapeutic Principle. Warming the middle-energizer to dispel cold and arresting hemorrhage.

Hemafecia due to Damp-heat
A kind of hemafecia.
Symptoms. Blood comes first, followed by stool in bright red color; burning pain of anus.

Pathogenesis. Retention and accumulation of damp-heat in the large intestine due to eating acrid food and drinking alcohol, resulting in impairment of superficial venules.

Therapeutic Principle. Clear heat and promote diuresis, regulate Ying to stop bleeding.

Hemafecia due to Deficiency of the Spleen

Symptoms. Discharge of stool followed by blood, dull abdominal pain, pale complexion, fatigue, laziness in speaking, anorexia.

Pathogenesis. Deficiency of spleen-qi and the failure of the spleen to keep blood flowing within the vessels.

Therapeutic Principle. Invigorate the spleen to control the blood.

Hemafecia due to Heat Accumulation

Symptoms. Abdominal pain, hemafecia, etc.

Pathogenesis. Accumulation of heat in the intestines and stomach resulting in injury of meridians.

Therapeutic Principle. Clearing away heat, removing blood heat and stopping bleeding.

Hemafecia due to Injury

Symptoms. Defecated turbid things like blood stasis.

Pathogenesis. Traumatic injury, injuring internal blood vessels to exude blood into intestines.

Therapeutic Principle. Promoting blood circulation and activating meridians and collaterals and arresting bleeding.

Hemafecia in Newborn

Symptoms. The infant's stool and urine with blood within seven days after birth.

Pathogenesis. Excessive heat of original qi of fetus, and bleeding due to blood-heat.

Therapeutic Principle. Clearing away heat and arresting bleeding.

Hematemesis

Symptoms. Vomiting blood without obvious nausea and cough.

Pathogenesis. Drinking and overeating of hot, sweet and fatty foods; sadness, anger and worries, overwork and weakness, leading to stomach-heat excessiveness, fire resulting from liver-stagnation, or dysfunction of the spleen in keeping blood flowing within blood vessels.

Therapeutic Principle. Clearing away fire and checking upward adverse flow of qi, removing pathogenic heat from blood to stop bleeding.

Hematemesis and/or Epistaxis during Menstruation

Symptoms. At the menstruation and before or after menstruation, cyclic and repeated hematemesis and epistaxis.

Pathogenesis. Flaring up of blood-heat pressing adverse flow of blood.

Therapeutic Principle. Clearing away heat from blood and lowering abnormally ascending qi.

Hematemesis due to Adverse Flow of Qi

Symptoms. Hematemesis, dysphoria and hot temper, thirst and bitter taste and vexation, distention and pain of hypochondrium, etc.

Pathogenesis. Disorder of emotion, the liver stagnation and flaming-up of the liver-fire together with qi.

Therapeutic Principle. Removing fire from the liver, descending the adverse flow of qi, stopping hematemesis.

Hematemesis due to Consumptive Disease

Symptoms. Hematemesis, insomnia due to vexation, severe palpitation, amnesia, perspiration caused by fright, dizziness, pain in the waist, lassitude, etc.

Pathogenesis. Overstrain and prolonged illness resulting in deficiency and damage of the five zang-organs, consumption of both qi and yin, leading to hyperactivity of fire and forcing blood to circulate abnormally.

Therapeutic Principle. Invigorating the spleen and nourishing the heart, nourishing yin and supplementing qi, stopping bleeding, etc.

Hematemesis due to Deficiency of Yin

Symptoms. Hematemesis, dry mouth and throat, flushing of zygomatic region, tidal fever, night sweet, lassitude in the loin, restlessness, etc.

Pathogenesis. Deficiency of kidney-yin, or hyperpyrexia of the liver, leading to the injury of meridians.

Therapeutic Principle. Nourishing yin and removing fire; cooling blood and arresting bleeding.

Hematemesis due to Liver-fire

Symptoms. Spitting of bright red or dark purple blood, bitter taste, hypochondriac pain, irritability, red or dark red tongue.

Pathogenesis. Damage of the stomach; resulting from excess liver-fire.

Therapeutic Principle. Remove heat from the liver and regulate the stomach; purge fire and stop bleeding.

Hematemesis during Pregnancy

Symptoms. Hematemesis, distending pain in the stomach and abdomen, bitter mouth, pain in the hypochondrium, vexation, liability to anger, dark colored stool, etc.

Pathogenesis. Excessive fire in the liver and stomach, etc.

Therapeutic Principle. Clearing away heat and arresting bleeding to prevent abortion.

Hematohidrosis

Referring to the syndrome of blood flowing in an abnormal way and overflowing the exterior muscles.

Symptoms. Dark red spots on the skin, dizziness, dysphoria with feverish sensation in palms and soles, fever and thirst, red or pale tongue, etc.

Pathogenesis. Deficiency of qi and blood, or hyperactivity of fire due to blood heat.

Therapeutic Principle. Nourishing qi and blood, nourishing yin to reduce pathogenic fire, and removing heat from the blood to stop bleeding.

Hematoma of Uvula

Symptoms. Sudden swelling of the throat, unable to swallow, nausea and vomiting.

Pathogenesis. The accumulation of heat in the lung and stomach, upward attacking of wind, fire, and phlegm toxins to throat.

Therapeutic Principle. Clearing away heat and toxic materials, subduing swelling and removing heat from the blood.

Hematuria due to Flaring Heart-fire

Symptoms. Hematuria in bright red color, dark and hot urine, irritability and thirst, ulcers in the mouth and tongue, red tongue tip, and rapid pulse.

Pathogenesis. Exuberant heart-fire moving downward to the small intestine.

Therapeutic Principle. Clear heat from the blood, purge pathogenic fire of the heart.

Hematuria due to Yin Deficiency and Hyperactivity of Fire

Symptoms. Hematuria, scanty dark urine, dizziness, tinnitus, tidal fever, night sweat, lassitude in loin and legs, red tongue with little coating, thready and rapid pulse.

Pathogenesis. Deficiency of kidney-yin, and hyperactivity of fire due to yin deficiency.

Therapeutic Principle. Nourish yin, remove heat and reduce pathogenic fire to stop bleeding.

Hemianesthesia

A symptom referring to muscular and dermal numbness on one side of the body.

Pathogenesis. Asthenia both of qi and blood, and stagnation of phlegm-dampness in between the muscular and dermal meridians and collaterals.

Hemihidrosis

Symptoms. Sweating on the upper body or lower body, or on the left side or on the right side instead of sweating all over the body.

Pathogenesis. Deficiency of qi and blood, and cold phlegm blocking the circulation in meridians.

Hemiparalysis

One of the commonly seen symptoms of apoplexy.

Symptoms. Inability to act freely of the limbs on one side of the body, accompanied by deviation of the mouth and eyes and slurred speech, etc.

Pathogenesis. Early debility of the nutrient and superficial defensive system in which qi and blood are lodged, resulting in emptiness of meridians and collaterals, invasion of pathogenic qi into the body, or insufficiency of vital essence and energy due to kidney deficiency.

Hemoptysis

Referring to the cough with blood.

Symptoms. Itching of throat and cough, phlegm with blood, dryness of mouth and nose, or fever and bone soreness due to exopathy for external invasion of pathogenic wind; frequent cough, phlegm with blood or fresh blood, stabbing pain of the hypochondrium, vexation, and hot temper, dry stool, in the cases of attack on the lung by liver-fire.

Pathogenesis. External invasion of pathogenic wind, the transmission of heat and dryness, the impairment of pulmonary vessels, or the attack on the lung by liver-fire.

Therapeutic Principle. Expelling wind and stopping blood for cases of external invasion of pathogenic wind; purging the liver and removing heat from the lung, regulat-ing collaterals and stopping blood in the cases of attack on the lung by liver-fire.

Hemoptysis due to Attack of Liver-fire on the Lung

Symptoms. Cough with blood stained sputum, or expectorating blood with a bright red or dark purple color, chest pain radiating to the hypochondrium, irritability, scanty dark urine, bitter taste.

Pathogenesis. Attack of liver-fire on the lung, resulting in damage to the pulmonary vessels.

Therapeutic Principle. Clear fire from the liver and remove heat from the lung, regulate collaterals and stop bleeding.

Hemoptysis due to Deficiency of the Spleen

Symptoms. Severe spitting of blood with a dim-purple color, and accompanied by a pale complexion, timid breath and lassitude, loss of appetite.

Pathogenesis. Weakness of the spleen and stomach, and failure to keep the blood flowing within the vessels.

Therapeutic Principle. Replenish qi to control blood.

Hemoptysis due to Yin Deficiency and Hyperactivity of Fire

Symptoms. Cough with a little phlegm mixed with scarlet blood, tidal fever and night sweat, dry mouth and throat, flush of zygomatic region.

Pathogenesis. Hyperactivity of fire due to yin deficiency.

Therapeutic Principle. Supplement yin and nourish the lung, clear heat to stop bleeding.

Hemorrhoids

A chronic disease occurring in the anal and rectal region. Clinically, it is divided into internal hemorrhoids external hemorrhoids and mixed hemorrhoids.

Pathogenesis. Long-term sitting or standing; improper diet; protracted dysentery, diarrhea and constipation; or overtiredness, pregnancy and labor, etc, resulting in the derangement of qi and blood in the anal and rectal region, stagnation and stasis in the meridians and retention of damp-heat. It is clinically divided into hemorrhoids due to damp-heat pathogen, and hemorrhoids due to qi-deficiency.

Hemorrhoids Complicated with Fistula

A disease of hemorrhoids dripping with pus, blood, and chronic yellow watery exudation.

Pathogenesis. Without treatment or mistreatment after ulceration of hemorrhoids.

Therapeutic Principle. Supplementing vital energy, administering drugs for external use, using methods of moxibustion, and washing.

Hemorrhoids due to Damp-heat Pathogen

Symptoms. At the beginning, they are small hemorrhoids, or drop by drop bleeding due to friction; developing into the enlargement of the hemorrhoids, leading to dyschezia and difficult urination.

Pathogenesis. Improper diet, pungent and fatty foods and the downward flow of damp-heat, leading to qi and blood disorder, and blood stasis in the collaterals.

Therapeutic Principle. Clear heat and resolve stagation.

Hemorrhoids due to Qi Deficiency

Symptoms. Sallow complexion, prolapse of hemorrhoids, tenesmic and distending sensation of the anus, short breath, poor appetite, weakness.

Pathogenesis. Lingering dysentery, overexertion, delivery or too much bleeding, disorder of qi and blood in the anus and intestine.

Therapeutic Principle. Supplement qi and elevate the sinking qi.

Hemorrhoids with Proctoptosis

Symptoms. Prolapse of rectum in stools excretion, painful with blood, or yellow water flowing out, etc.

Pathogenesis. Long-standing case of hemorrhoids, and the additional affection of damp-heat exopathogen, qi deficiency, and the loss of nourishment.

Therapeutic Principle. Removing damp-heat, replenishing qi and elevating prolapse.

Hemostasis by Removing Blood Stasis

A therapy of administering a prescription with blood-activating and eliminating blood stasis action and that of hemostasis to treat hemorrhage resulting from blood stasis.

Hemp Seed

It is the ripe seed of Cannabis sativa L. (Moraceae).

Effect. Moisturizing the intestine and relaxing the bowels, nourishing yin and restoring vital energy, constipation caused by consumption of fluid and dryness of intestine.

Indication. Febrile disease with consumption of yin and fire hyperactivity, or yin deficiency, constipation of the aged, puerperal and weak patients.

Hemsley Monkshood Root

It is the root tuber of Aconitum hemsleyanum Pritz. (Ranunculaceae)

Effect. Relieving convulsion, decreasing blood pressure, promoting diaphoresis and inducing urination.

Indication. Pain of the lions and lower extremities, innominate inflammatory swelling, traumatic injuries, tinea, carbuncle, etc.

Henbane Blak Seed

It is the seed of Hyoscyamus niger L. (Salanaceae).

Effect. Anesthesia and alleviate pain, expel wind, relieve cough and asthma.

Indication. Mental disorder, dyspnea and cough, stomachache, chronic diarrhea and dysentery, toothache, subcutaneous swelling, malignant boil, etc.

Henggu (K 11)

A point on the Kidney Meridian.

Location. On the lower abdomen, 5 cun below the center of the umbilicus and 0.5 cun lateral to the anterior midline.

Indication. Pain of the pudendum, pain of the lower abdomen, nocturnal emission, impotence, enuresis, retention of urine, hernia.

Method. Puncture perpendicularly 1-1.5 cun. Apply moxibustion with a moxa stick for 3 minutes.

Henry Magnoliavine Stem or Root

It is the stem or root of Schisandra henryi Clarke or Schisandra sphenanthera Rehd. et Wils. (Magnoliaceae).

Effect. Nourishing blood, removing blood stasis, regulating flow of qi and dispelling dampness.

Indication. Hematemesis caused by overstrain, arthralgia, chest and abdominal pain caused by disorder of qi, irregular menstruation and traumatic injuries.

Hepatic Asthenia

There are two meanings:

1. Referring to consumptive disease caused by damage of the liver by overwork.

   Symptoms. Dry black complexion, bitter taste, absence of mind, fright with blurred vision, fullness and distention of hypochondrium, etc.

   Therapeutic Principle. Nourishing the liver and strengthening the body resistance.

2. Referring to the eyestrain caused by prolonged vision and impairment of liver blood.

Therapeutic Principle. Proper balance between work and rest and nourishing the blood and the liver.

Hepatic Mass

Symptoms. Hypochondriac pain involved the lower abdominal, cold foot with edema, hernia, abdominal mass, dribbling urination, withered skin and nails, and spasm of muscle, etc.

Therapeutic Principle. Soothing the liver and regulating the circulation of qi and promoting blood circulation.

Hepatic Shock due to Postpartum Putrid Blood

Referring to spasm of extremities and muscles caused by lochia entering the Liver Meridian.

Therapeutic Principle. Soothing the liver, dispelling wind and nourishing the muscle and tendon to relieve spasm.

Hepatopathy

Referring to all kinds of hepatic disease.

Symptoms. Distending pain in hypochondrium, headache, dizziness, tinnitus, liability to anger or panic, or hematemesis, epistaxis, or numbness of limbs, convulsion with cold limbs, etc. It is classified into four types: cold, heat, deficiency and excess.

Therapeutic Principle. Warming the liver to the cold type, clearing away heat from the liver to the heat type, nourishing the liver to the deficiency type, and purging the liver of pathogenic fire to the excess type.

Herb of Serrulate Brake

It is the whole herb or root of Pteris nultifida Poir. (pteridaceae).

Effect. Enhancing diuresis, releasing heat from blood, swelling, detoxicating and ceasing bleeding.

Indication. Hepatitis with jaundice, enteritis, stranguria with turbid urine, leukorrhagia, hematemesis, epistaxis, hemafecia, hematuria, parotitis, suppurative infections on the skin, etc.

Herbst Bloodleaf Herb

It is the whole herb of Iresine herbstii Hook f. ex Lindl (Amaranthaceae).

Effect. Cooling blood and relieving bleeding.

Indication. Hematemesis, epistaxis, hemoptysis, traumatic bleeding, menalgia and dysentery.

Hernia

There are two meanings:

1. Referring to the outside projection of the object in the body cavity, accompanied by symptoms of pain caused by qi disorder, such as the part of intestine downward into the scrotum from the abdominal cavity.
2. Referring to the symptoms of genitalia, testicle, and scrotum, such as external genitalia ulcer, and swelling with pus, accompanied by abdominal symptoms.

Hernia due to Impairment of Back Middle Meridian

Symptoms. Sudden pain in the lower abdomen, attacking upward to the heart and stomach, downward to the testis, dysphoria and stuffiness.

Pathogenesis. The impairment of the Back Middle Meridian.

Therapeutic Principle. Sending down qi and relieving pain.

Hernial Pain due to Blood stasis

Symptoms. Blood stasis and swelling and stabbing and fixed pain in external genitals.

Pathogenesis. Original blood stasis, further induced by overstrain or coldness.

Therapeutic Principle. Promoting blood circulation to remove blood stasis, and warming and nourishing kidney-qi.

Hernia Qi due to Heat

Symptoms. Pain in the testis, redness and swelling of scrotum with burning sensation, pain in the affected part when pressed, headache and soreness in the limbs, scanty dark urine.

Pathogenesis. Accumulation of pathogenic cold-dampness transmitting into heat or the downward flow of damp-heat in the Liver and Spleen Meridians.

Therapeutic Principle. Clearing heat and eliminating dampness, subduing swelling and dispersing accumulation of the pathogen.

Herpes

Symptoms. It is a kind of dermatosis with lacunae containing water-like or blood-like fluid. The injury with water is white. The injury with blood is slightly red. Their walls are usually quite thin and break easily. After breaking, erosion appears. After drying, thin scabs are formed.

Pathogenesis. Mostly caused by damp-heat or superficial heat.

Therapeutic Principle. Removing fire from the liver, clearing away damp-heat.

Herpes Simplex

Referring to an acute dermatosis appearing after or in the course of a fever.

Symptoms. At the beginning, groups of small blisters appear on the skin, surrounded with red color. After the blisters have broken, there are erosive surfaces on them. After drying and forming of scabs, it will heal with pigmentation. It has a tendency to recur, with natural feeling of itching and burning heat.

Pathogenesis. External affection of wind-heat or the downward flow of dampness and heat in the liver and the gallbladder, the deficiency of yin with interior heat.

Therapeutic Principle. Dispelling wind, clearing away heat and toxic material, or removing dampness by diuresis, or with nourishing yin.

Herpes Zoster

Symptoms. Stabbing pain or slight fever and exhaustion, etc in the affected part (usually on the waist, the side of chest and the face). Then blisters appear in the size of mung beans or soybeans, just like string of beads, arranged in the form of ropes, with red bases. The skin between the piles of blisters is normal. At the beginning, the juice of the blisters is transparent, and then turns turbid.

Pathogenesis. Rash action of the liver-fire, the retention of damp-heat in the interior.

Therapeutic Principle. Removing fire from the liver and clearing away damp-heat.

Heyang (B 55)

A meridian acupuncture point.

Location. On the posterior side of the leg, on the line connecting Weizhong (B 40)and Chengshan (B 57), 2 cun below Weizhong (B 40).

Indication. Lumbar and spinal pain extending to the abdomen, aching pain of the lower extremities, paralysis and arthralgia syndrome of legs, metrorrhagia, metrostaxis and hernia pain.

Method. Puncture perpendicularly 1-2 cun; apply moxibustion for 5-10 minutes.

Hiccups

Symptoms. Continual hiccups, thirst and flushed face.

Pathogenesis. Dysfunction of the spleen and stomach and the retention of food in the stomach causing the stomach-qi adversely rise.

Therapeutic Principle. Regulate the stomach to descend the stomach-qi, and relieve hiccups.

Hiccups Caused by Qi Disorder

The general syndrome of hiccups caused by stagnation of the qi and qi-deficiency.

Symptoms. In the case of stagnation of the qi, the syndrome is cold complexion, frequent hiccups, poor appetite, distention and fullness in the abdomen, borborygmus, etc; in the case of qi-deficiency, the syndrome is weak hiccups, cold hands and feet, inappetence and lassitude, vomiting, diarrhea, etc.

Therapeutic Principle. Regulating qi and dispersing the depressed qi calming the adverse rising energy and regulating the stomach-energy in the case caused by stagnation of the qi; invigorating the spleen and supplementing qi, regulating the middle-energizer and calming the adverse-rising qi in the case caused by qi-deficiency.

Hiccups due to Internal Injury

Pathogenesis. Functional disorders of the visceral organs, emotional abnormity, and disease with improper diet.

Therapeutic Principle. Regulating the function of the stomach to lower the adverse flow of qi and stop hiccups.

Hiccups due to Qi Stagnation

Symptoms. Constant hiccups, worsened by low spirit, accompanied by oppressed feeling in the chest, lack of appetite, distention and oppressive feeling in the stomach and hypochondrium, borborygmus, wind from bowels.

Pathogenesis. Depressed emotions, hyperactive liver-qi attacking the lung and the stomach, adverse rising of the stomach-qi.

Therapeutic Principle. Lower the adverse flow of qi to alleviate mental depression.

Hiccups due to Stasis

Symptoms. Stabbing pain in the heart and chest, prolonged hiccups, slight yellowish eyes, cold hands and feet, loose and black stool, fever in the evening, etc.

Pathogenesis. Blood stasis in the chest caused by prolonged qi stagnation.

Therapeutic Principle. Promoting blood circulation to remove blood stasis, and calming the adverse rising qi to stop hiccups.

Hiccups due to Stomach-cold

Symptoms. Slow and forceful hiccups, distention with cold sensation of the stomach, preference for hot drink, cold hands and feet, profuse clear urine, loose stool, etc.

Pathogenesis. Cold evil attacking the stomach resulting in the failure of stomach-qi to descend.

Therapeutic Principle. Warm the middle-energizer to dispel cold; lower the adverse flow of the stomach-qi to stop hiccups.

Hiccups due to Stomach-heat

Symptoms. Loud and forceful hiccups, smell in the mouth, excessive thirst, preference for cold drink, scanty dark urine, constipation, etc.

Pathogenesis. The accumulation of excess heat in the stomach and intestine resulting in the ascending of stomach fire, mostly due to excessive eating spicy food and warm tonics, over-drinking.

Therapeutic Principle. Clear heat, regulate the stomach.

Hiccups due to Yang Insufficiency

Symptoms. Hiccups with low voice, short breath, pale tongue with whitish coating.

Pathogenesis. Deficiency of the spleen and stomach, adverse up-moving of qi of deficiency type.

Therapeutic Principle. Warm and invigorate the spleen and stomach; regulate the middle-energizer and keep the adverse qi downward.

Hiccups due to Yin Deficiency

Symptoms. Rapid but intermittent hiccups, dry mouth and tongue, dysphoria, red and dry tongue, etc.

Pathogenesis. Deficiency of stomach-yin, resulting in a failure to moisten and the descending of the stomach-qi.

Therapeutic Principle. Promote the production of the body fluid to nourish the stomach and relieve the hiccups.

Hiccup Phlegm

Symptoms. Disturbance of breath, hiccups with phlegm sound, etc.

Pathogenesis. Accumulation of phlegm and the abnormal rising of qi.

Therapeutic Principle. Eliminating phlegm and circulating qi.

High Fever

One of the cardinal symptoms of acute febrile diseases in all clinical branches.

Symptoms. Sudden fever with tremendous force and a body temperature of up to 40 degrees. Accompanied by other symptoms of the primary disease commonly seen in various inflammatory or infectious diseases caused by bacteria or viruses. Also seen in hyperthyroidism, heatstroke and pulmonary tuberculosis, etc.

Pathogenesis. Six pathogenic factors attacking the body.

Therapeutic Principle. Reduce fever and expel pathogenic factors.

High Fever with Dehydration

It refers to the newborn infant has 39-40 degrees fever 2-4 days after birth. It may last several days.

Therapeutic Principle. Clearing away heat and dispelling toxin.

High Pathogenic Factor and Painful Abdomen

Referring to the invasion of Gallbladder Meridian. According to connection of gallbladder with the liver and interrelation of spleen to stomach, the abdomen will be painful in case of subjugation of spleen by liver, and vomiting will occur in case that the fire of the gallbladder invades the stomach. The entry explains the mechanism of vomiting and abdominal pain in Shaoyang disease.

Himalayan Mayapple Fruit

It is the dried ripe fruit of Podophyllum emodi Wall. (Berberidaceae)

Effect. Regulating menstruation and promoting blood circulation.

Indication. Amenorrhea caused by blood stasis, dystocia, and retention of placenta dead fetus.

Himalayan Teasel Root
It is the root of Dipsacus japonicus Miq. Or D. asper Wall. (Dipsacaceae).

Effect. Invigorating the liver and kidney, stopping metrorrhagia, calming the fetus, activating the blood circulation, promoting reunion of fractured bones and strengthening the muscles and bones, expelling wind dampness.

Indication. Arthralgia due to wind-dampness, lumbago, beriberi, emission, metrorrhagia, metrostaxis, vaginal, bleeding during pregnancy, threatened abortion, traumatic injuries, etc.

Hirsute Shiny Bugleweed Herb ⊛ H-3
It is the whole herb of Lycopus lucidus Turcz. or Lycopus lucidus Turcz. var. hirtus Regel (Labiatae).

Effect. Promoting blood circulation to remove blood stasis, inducing diuresis and subduing edema.

Indication. Amenorrhea due to stagnation of blood, dysmenorrhea, postpartum lochiostasis due to retention of blood stasis, edema, traumatic injuries, etc.

Hispid Arthraxon Herb
It is the whole plant of Arthraxon hispidus (Thunb.) Mak. (Gramineae).

Effect. Relieving cough and asthma, and destroying parasites.

Indication. Chronic cough, dyspnea and malignant sore.

Hoarse Cough
Syndrome. Cough with a hoarse voice.

Pathogenesis. Obstruction of phlegm and heat in the lung leading to dysfunction of the lung-qi, or fire enveloped by cold leading to obstruction of the pulmonary qi.

Therapeutic Principle. Removing heat and promoting the dispersing function of the lung, or removing cold and releasing heat; and nourishing yin and moistening the lung for the case of tuberculosis.

Hollyhock Root
It is the root of Althaea rosea (L.) Cav. (Malvaceae).

Effect. Clearing away heat and cold the blood, inducing diuresis and evacuating pus.

Indication. Stranguria, leukorrhea, hematuria, hematemesis, metrorrhagia, acute appendicitis, sore swelling, etc.

Homalomena Rhizome
It is dried rhizome of Homalomena occulta (Lour.) Schott (Araceae).

Effect. Dissipating pathogenic wind and dampness, strengthening muscles and bones, arresting pain and subduing.

Indication. Stomachache, rheumatic arthralgia, cold pain in the loins and knees, muscular contracture, numbness of the legs, carbuncle and boils.

Honey
It is the carbohydrate substances made by the hive-bee Apis cerana Fabricius or A. mellifera L. (Apidae).

Effect. Moistening the lung, relieving cough, moistening the intestines and relaxing the bowels.

Indication. Abdominal pain, chronic cough due to the lung deficiency, and constipation, external use for skin infection, burn, etc.

Honeysuckle Flower ⊛ H-4
It is the flower-bud of Lonicera japonica Thunb. (Caprifoliaceae).

Effect. Clearing away heat, detoxicating and dispelling pathogenic wind and strong antibacterial action.

Indication. 1. For the onset of seasonal febrile diseases or exogenous wind-heat syndrome with high fever and mild chilliness. 2. For the qi system sthenic heat syndrome with high fever, excessive thirst, yellow fur, full and large pulse. 3. For the nutrient system and the blood system heat syndrome with fever, restlessness and insomnia, skin eruption, crimson and dry tongue. 4. For sore throat, skin infections. 5. For dysentery due to intense heat-toxic.

Honeysuckle Stem

It is the stem leaf of Xyloid vine Lonicera japonica Thunb. (Caprifoliacea).

Effect. Clearing away heat, detoxicating and activating collaterals.

Indication. Epidemic febrile disease, fever, skin and external diseases, bloody dysentery due to noxious heat, pain, swelling, redness and heat in the joints, etc.

Hongkong Pavetta Stem and Leaf

It is the whole plant of Sphagnum teres (Schimp.) Angster (Sphagnaceae).

Effect. Clearing away heat, improving eyesight, and subduing swelling.

Indication. Leukoma, acute conjunctivitis, and swollen and painful eyes, etc.

Hoodwinking upward and Flowing downward

Referring to damp-heat pathogen hoodwinking upward and damp-turbid pathogen flowing downward.

Symptoms. Feeling of fullness in the head, vomiting, coma, thirst and less drinking, anuria, etc.

Therapeutic Principle. Inducing resuscitation with aromatics, inducing diuresis.

Hookworm Disease

It refers to the disease due to hookworm parasitized in the small intestine.

Symptoms. Hunger with polyphagia, lassitude, sallow skin, edema of face and foot, etc.

Therapeutic Principle. Strengthening the spleen and killing parasites.

Hordeolum

Symptoms. Sores on the eyelid, even with blood and pus. Painful and reddish eye with swelling of head and face.

Pathogenesis. Stagnation of spleen heat.

Therapeutic Principle. Clearing away heat and toxic materials, dispelling wind.

Horse Bezoar

It is the calculus found in the gastrointestinal tract of Equus caballus orientalis Noack (Equidae).

Effect. Relieving convulsion, resolving phlegm, open the orifice, removing heat from liver and detoxicating.

Indication. Epilepsy caused by terror, accumulation of heat-phlegm, unconsciousness due to heat disease, hematemesis, epistaxis, apoplectic coma, malignant boils, pyogenic infections and oral ulcer, etc.

Horse Milk

It is the milk of Equus caballus orientalis Noack (Equidae).

Effect. Clearing away heat and quenching thirst, tonifying blood, moistening the bowels.

Indication. Dysphoria with smothery sensation caused by blood deficiency, hectic fever caused by consumptive disease, diabetes, ulcerative gingivitis, etc.

Hosie Ormosia Seed

It is the seed of Ormosia hosiei Hemsl. et Wils. (Leguminosae).

Effect. Regulating flow of qi, inducing menstruation and arresting pain.

Indication. Abdominal pain caused by cold hernia and amenorrhea due to the stagnation of blood.

Host-guest Point Selection

A term in acupuncture, referring to the point prescription of selecting a "host" point and a "guest" one in combination with each other, according to the disease that belongs to each meridian: select the primary point of each meridian as the "host", and cooperatively the collateral point, which is exterior-interior related to the primary one, as the "guest". For example, if there is a disease belonging to the Lung Meridian, select the primary point of the Lung Meridian Taiyuan (L 9) in combination with the collateral point of the Large Intestine Meridian Pianli (LI 6).

Hot Moxibustion

A kind of moxibustion, generally referring to all kinds of moxibustion with heat energy, such as moxa-cone and moxa stick moxibustion, burning rush moxibustion, mulberry twig moxibustion, wick moxibustion, electric heating moxibustion.

Hot Sole

The patient feels hot in his soles, or the doctor detects that the patient's soles are hotter than the back of his feet. It is caused by asthenia yin causing excessive pyrexia, which steams in the sole along Kidney Meridian.

Houding (GV 19)

An acupuncture point.
Location. On the head, 1.5 cun directly above Qiangjian (GV18), 3 cun superior to Naohu (GV 17).
Indication. Headache, dizziness, rigid nape, insomnia, psychosis, epilepsy, etc.
Method. Puncture subcutaneously 0.5-0.8 cun and apply moxibustion with a moxa stick for 5-10 minutes.

Houxi (SI 3)

A meridian acupuncture point.
Location. On the posterior ulnar side of the fifth metacarpophalangeal joint, at the junction of the red and white skin of the transverse crease caput. Clench fist to locate this point.
Indication. Pain and rigidity of the head and neck, deafness, redness of the eye, blurred vision, contracture of the elbow, arm and finger, febrile disease, malaria, depressive psychosis, mania, epilepsy,

night sweating, dizziness and vertigo, blepharitis angularis and scabies.
Method. Puncture perpendicularly 0.5-1 cun, apply moxibustion to the point for 3-7 minutes.

Huagai (CV 20)

A meridian acupuncture point.
Location. On the chest and on the anterior midline, the midpoint of the sternal angle, on the level of the first intercostal space.
Indication. Cough, asthma, chest pain, pain in hypochondriac region, inflammation of the throat, and tonsillitis.
Method. Puncture subcutaneously 0.3-0.5 cun; apply moxibustion with a moxa stick for 3-5 minute.

Huangmen (B 51)

A meridian acupuncture point.
Location. On the low back, below the spinous process of the first lumbar vertebra, 3 cun lateral to the posterior midline.
Indication. Epigastric pain, abdominal masses, constipation, female mastoptosis.
Method. Puncture obliquely 0.5-0.8 cun, apply moxibustion with a moxa stick for 5-10 minutes.

Huangmu (Ex-CA)

An extra acupuncture point.
Location. The point is directly below the nipple Ruzhong (S 17), the distance from the nipple to the point is half of the distance from the nipple to the navel.
Indication. Abdominal masses with pain, jaundice, and asthenia after disease, etc.
Method. Apply moxibustion with a moxa stick for 3-7 minutes.

Huangshu (K 16)

A meridian acupuncture point.
Location. On the middle abdomen, 0.5 cun lateral to the center of the umbilicus.
Indication. Abdominal pain, vomiting, abdominal distention, dysentery, diarrhea, constipation, hernia, irregular menstruation, and pain along the spinal column.

Method. Puncture perpendicularly 0.8-1.2 cun; Apply moxibustion with a moxa stick for 5-7 minutes.

Huanmen (Ex-B)

An extra acupuncture point.

Location. On the back, 1.5 cun lateral to the spinous process of the 5th thoracic vertebra.

Indication. Hectic fever, emaciation with sallow complexion, poor appetite, cough, seminal emission, night sweating, chest and back pain, etc.

Method. Moxibustion is applicable.

Huantiao (G 30)

An acupuncture point.

Location. Lateral to the femur, assuming a lateral recumbent lying posture with the thigh flexed, at the junction of the lateral and middle third of the distance of the great trochanter and the hiatus of the sacrum.

Indication. Pain in the lumbar, leg and knee regions hemiplegia, flaccidity of lower limbs, edema, German measles, etc.

Method. Puncture perpendicularly 2-3 cun; apply moxibustion with a moxa stick for 5-10 minutes.

Huanzhong (Ex)

An extra acupuncture point.

Location. At the midpoint of the line connecting Huantiao (G 30) and Yaoshu (GV 2).

Indication. Sciatica neuralgia.

Method. Puncture perpendicularly 1-1.5 cun. Moxibustion is applicable.

Huaroumen (S 24)

A meridian acupuncture point.

Location. On the upper abdomen, 1 cun above the center of the umbilicus and 2 cun lateral to the anterior midline.

Indication. Vomiting, borborygmus, diarrhea, madness, and stomachache.

Method. Puncture perpendicularly 0.8-1.2 cun; apply moxibustion with a moxa stick for 5-10 minutes.

Huiqi (Ex-B)

An extra acupuncture point.

Location. At the point of the sacral vertebra, beneath the "red and white" skin.

Indication. Hemorrhoids, hemafectia, and fecal incontinence, etc.

Method. Apply moxibustion to the point with 5-10 moxa sticks.

Huiyang (B 35)

A meridian acupuncture point.

Location. On the sacrum, 0.5 cun lateral to the tip of the coccyx.

Indication. Pain in the abdomen, pain of the leg, leukorrhea, impotence, dysentery, hemafecia, and hemorrhoids.

Method. Puncture perpendicularly 1-1.5 cun, apply moxibustion with a moxa stick for 5-15 minutes.

Huiyin (CV 1)

A meridian acupuncture point.

Location. On the perineum, at the midpoint between the posterior border of the scrotum and anus in the male and between the posterior commissure of the large labia and anus in the female.

Indication. Drowning, asphyxia, coma, manic-depressive psychosis, epilepsy induced by terror, dysuria, enuresis, perineal pain, pruritus vulva, proctoptosis, prolapse of uterus, hernia, hemorrhoids, seminal emission, and irregular menstruation.

Method. Puncture perpendicularly 0.5-1 cun, careful application in pregnant women; Apply moxibustion with a moxa stick for 3-7 minutes.

Huizong (TE 7)

A meridian acupuncture point.

Location. On the dorsal side of the forearm, 3 cun proximal to the dorsal crease of the wrist, about 1 cun lateral to the ulnar side of Zhigou (TE 6) and on the radial border of the ulna.

Indication. Deafness, epilepsy, pain in the muscle and skin, and pain of the upper extremities.

Method. Puncture perpendicularly 0.5-1 cun, apply moxibustion with a moxa stick for 3-5 minutes.

Hukou (Ex-UE)

An extra acupuncture point.
Location. At the midpoint of the line connecting the small heads of the first and second metacarpal bones, when clenching fists.
Indication. Headache, dysphoria with smothering sensation, dizziness, insomnia, night sweating, precordial pain, toothache, lockjaw in children, and tonsillitis, etc.
Method. Puncture obliquely 0.3-0.5 cun, apply moxibustion with a moxa stick for 3-5 minutes.

Hunchback

Symptoms. High hunching back, projecting spine and bending waist.
Pathogenesis. Kidney deficiency and the lack of essence and blood over a long period of time.

Hunger with Inability to Eat

Referring to inability to eat with hungry sensation.
Pathogenesis. Accumulation of pathogens in epigastric region, exhaustion of stomach and spleen fluid.

Hungry Sensation due to Heat

Symptoms. Hunger immediately after eating, burning heat in the stomach, dysphoria, bitter taste, constipation and dark urine, etc.
Pathogenesis. Stomach burned by pathogenic fire.
Therapeutic Principle. Clearing away the stomach-fire, and nourishing the stomach-yin.

Hunmen (B 47)

A meridian acupuncture point.
Location. On the back, below the spinous process of the 9th thoracic vertebra, 3 cun lateral to the posterior midline.

Indication. Fullness in the chest and hypochondrium, backache, anorexia, vomiting, borborygmus and diarrhea.
Method. Puncture obliquely 0.5-0.8 cun, apply moxibustion with a moxa stick for 3-7 minutes.

Hunshe (Ex-CA)

An extra acupuncture point.
Location. On the abdomen, 1 cun lateral to the center of the umbilicus.
Indication. Dysentery with blood and pus in the stool, enteritis, dyspepsia, and habitual constipation, etc.
Method. Puncture perpendicularly 0.5-1 cun. Moxibustion is applicable.

Hyacinth Bletilla Tuber

It is the tuber of Bletilla striata (Thunb.) Reichb. (Orchidaceae)
Effect. Arrest discharge, relieving bleeding, subduing swelling and promoting tissue regeneration.
Indication. Hemoptysis, hematemesis, traumatic bleeding, skin and external diseases and pyogenic infections, cracked skin of the hands and feet.

Hyacinth Dolichos Flower

It is the flower of Dolichos lablab L. (Leguminosae).
Effect. Removing summer-heat and eliminating dampness, invigorating the spleen and strengthening the stomach.
Indication. Summer-heat and dampness syndrome with feeling of oppression in the chest, fever with diarrhea or dysentery, and leukorrhea with reddish discharge in female, especially suitable for those with dampness-heat in the spleen.

Hyacinth Dolichos Seed

It is the seed of Dolichos Lablab L. (Leguminosae).
Effect. Strengthening the spleen and eliminating dampness.
Indication. Insufficiency of the spleen and stomach with dampness, fatigue, lassitude, poor appetite and loose stool or diar-

rhea, and pathogenic dampness due to the spleen deficiency in women, leukorrhagia, affection of summer-heat and dampness manifested as vomiting, diarrhea, feeling of oppression in the chest, etc.

Hydrocele

Symptoms. Swollen and painful scrotum, the scrotum swollen like crystal, or itching scrotum which produces yellowish fluid when scratched, or lower abdomen with water sound when pressed, etc.

Pathogenesis. Attack of cold-damp into the lower part of the body.

Therapeutic Principle. Eliminating the retention of fluid with the powerful purgatives.

Hydrops Discharge by the Stiletto Needle

One of Five Variant Technique of Acupuncture, referring to puncturing the branches of collateral meridians on joints so as to reduce dampness.

Hyperactivity of Liver-Yang

Symptoms. Dizziness, tinnitus, distending pain in the head and eyes, flushed face, congested eyes, vexation, lassitude in the loins and legs, feeling heavy in the head, palpitation, amnesia, insomnia and dreaminess, red tongue and forceful taut pulse.

Pathogenesis. On the base of deficiency of liver-yin, liver-yin fails to counterbalance yang, yang-qi of the liver rises abnormally.

Therapeutic Principle. Nourishing yin, and calming the liver and suppressing the hyperactivity of the liver-yang.

Hyperactivity of Ministerial Fire

Symptoms. Headache, vertigo, tinnitus, deafness, flushed face, bloodshot eyes, anxiousness, dreaminess, lassitude in loin and knees, spermatorrhea and premature ejaculation.

Pathogenesis. Deficiency of the liver-yin and kidney-yin upward flare of fire.

Hyperphoria

A symptom, referring to the eyeballs turning out with more white than black in color.

Symptoms. Epilepsy, infantile convulsion, convulsive seizure, etc, which belong to serious cases.

Pathogenesis. Exhaustion of essence and vital energy, liver-wind, mental disorder due to phlegm stagnation.

Hypertrophy of Breast

Symptoms. Referring to painful masses appearing in the mammary areola of boys and girls, or in middle- or old-age males, an abnormal mammary development.

Pathogenesis. Insufficiency of kidney-qi for males; imbalance of Vital and Front Middle Meridians, the loss of nourishment in the liver, stagnancy of qi and phlegm for females.

Therapeutic Principle. Warming yang and resolving phlegm in the case of the insufficiency of the kidney-yang; nourishing yin and resolving phlegm in the case of the deficiency of the kidney-yin.

Hyphaema and Vitreous Hemorrhage

Symptoms. A little bit of fresh blood in the pupil due to blood stasis therein, rapid hypopsia.

Pathogenesis. Excessive heat in the liver and gallbladder, or hyperactivity of fire due to yin deficiency or traumatic injury and surgery, etc.

Therapeutic Principle. Clearing away heat from the liver and gallbladder, nourishing yin to reduce pathogenic fire and removing heat from blood to dissipate stasis.

Hypochondriac Lump

Symptoms. Lumps at coastal regions with pain, appearing and fading at frequent intervals. The lumps may not be felt with exceptions in the state of pain.

Pathogenesis. Mostly caused by improper diet, the injury of the spleen and stomach, accumulation of cold phlegm, and conflict and combination of qi and blood.

Therapeutic Principle. Regulating qi and dispelling phlegm, expelling accumulation and removing lumps.

Hypochondriac Nodes

Symptoms. Strip-like lumps below the costal margin, distending or pricking pain, tidal fever, shortness of breath and dyspnea.

Pathogenesis. Accumulation of excessive fluid, stagnation of phlegm and retention of food and pathogenic cold and heat fighting with each other and blocking in the body.

Therapeutic Principle. Dissipating blood stasis, and regulating qi flow and removing food stagnancy.

Hypochondriac Pain due to Anger

Symptoms. Distending pain in the hypochondrium, oppression in the chest, shortness of respiration, more serious after anger, etc.

Pathogenesis. Caused by anger which injures the liver and leads to qi stagnation in the hypochondriac region.

Therapeutic Principle. Relieving depressed liver-qi, and regulating blood and relieving pain.

Hypochondriac Pain due to Blood Stasis

Symptoms. Fixed and persistent hypochondriac pain, with a history of traumatic injury, or a history of chronic hypochondriac pain, distending into the hypochondrium with tenderness or mass.

Pathogenesis. Impairment of hypochondriac meridians and collaterals, leading to the stagnation of qi and blood due to traumatic injury.

Therapeutic Principle. Promote blood circulation to remove obstruction in the meridians and collaterals, promote circulation of qi to relieve pain.

Hypochondriac Pain due to Damp-heat

Symptoms. Pricking or burning pain in the right hypochondriac region; during acute period, accompanied by aversion to cold, fever, bitter taste, nausea and vomiting, aversion to oil.

Pathogenesis. Mostly due to attack of pathogenic factors, retention of damp-heat pathogen and qi-stagnation of the liver and gallbladder.

Therapeutic Principle. Clear heat and eliminate dampness, soothe the liver and normalize the function of the gallbladder.

Hypochondriac Pain due to Liver-fire

Symptoms. Flushed complexion and conjunctiva congestion, restlessness, irritability, burning pain in the hypochondrium, etc.

Pathogenesis. Usually caused by disorder of the liver-qi, fire-transmission from stagnated qi, the liver-fire burning the hypochondriac region.

Therapeutic Principle. Resolving fire from the liver.

Hypochondriac Pain due to Retention

Symptoms. Hypochondriac pain, or mobile pain in the hypochondrium with filtering sound for the serious case, accompanied by cough, dyspnea, etc.

Pathogenesis. Mostly caused by obstruction of visceral function from flowing of the stagnated fluid and turbid sputum into Jueyin Meridians.

Therapeutic Principle. Removing phlegm to dredge the impeded meridians.

Hypochondriac Pain due to Sexual Strain

Symptoms. Dull hypochondriac pain, lassitude in the waist and legs, dizziness and tinnitus, etc.

Pathogenesis. Caused by the impairment of the kidney by sexual strain, deficiency of the essence and blood.

Therapeutic Principle. Tonifying the kidney and regulating the flow of blood.

Hypochondriac Pain due to Stagnated Liver-qi

Symptoms. Distending pain in the hypochondria, without definite part and consistent intensity, less pain in warming and more serious pain after disturbance in mood.

Pathogenesis. Caused by inhibited emotions which results in the inability to dispel and remove liver-qi.

Therapeutic Principle. Relaxing liver and regulating circulation of qi.

Hypochondriac Pain due to Yin Deficiency

Symptoms. Dull and moveable pain in the hypochondriac region without sensation of distention or pressure, which is worsened by tiredness or change of posture; flush of zygomatic region, low fever, spontaneous perspiration, dizziness, palpitation, and rapid pulse.

Pathogenesis. Retention of damp-heat and impairment of yin by stagnated fire resulting in failure to nourish the liver collaterals.

Therapeutic Principle. Nourish yin and blood, regulate collaterals and alleviate pain.

Hypochondriac Pain during Menstruation

Symptoms. Pain in the hypochondrium, and dark-red menstrual blood.

Pathogenesis. Mostly caused by stagnation of the liver-qi.

Therapeutic Principle. Arresting pain by alleviation of mental depression.

Hypochondriac Pain during Pregnancy

It refers to the pregnant woman's pain in the hypochondrium.

Symptoms. Distending pain in the hypochondrium and rib, vexation and liability to anger in one case, oppressed pain in the chest and hypochondrium and accumulation of the phlegm and saliva in another case.

Pathogenesis. Impairment of the liver by depressed anger for the former case, and stagnation the liver-qi, or by stagnation of turbid phlegm for the latter case.

Therapeutic Principle. Soothing the liver and regulating the flow of qi for the former case, and eliminating phlegm for resuscitation and regulating flow of qi for the latter case.

Hypofunction of the Bladder

Referring to loss of control of urination.

Symptoms. Dribbling urination, incontinence of urine, or enuresis.

Pathogenesis. Deficiency of the kidney-yang.

Hypogalactia due to Deficiency of Qi and Blood

Symptoms. Galactostasis or little milk, without distending sensation in the breasts, pale complexion, pale lips and nails, spiritual tiredness, poor appetite, loose stool.

Pathogenesis. Mostly caused by weakness of the spleen and the stomach, lack of formation of qi and blood, or much blood loss with parturient.

Therapeutic Principle. Supplement qi and enrich the blood and promote lactation.

Hypogalactia due to Stagnation of Liver-qi

Symptoms. Lack of lactation after delivery, distending pain in breasts, mental depression, oppressive feeling in the chest, anorexia.

Pathogenesis. A type of hypogalactia due to emotional disorder after delivery, resulting in dysfunction of the liver in maintaining the free flow of qi, and the disturbance of the qi and blood circulation, leading to the obstruction of milk secretion.

Therapeutic Principle. Soothe the liver and regulate the circulation of qi, supported by activating the mammary collaterals.

Hypomenorrhea due to Blood-cold

Symptoms. Obstructed menstruation and scanty menstrual blood.

Pathogenesis. Pathogenic cold invasion into the body, resulting in obstruction of blood circulation.

Therapeutic Principle. Warming the meridians and nourishing blood.

Hypomenorrhea due to Blood Deficiency

Symptoms. Obvious decrease of menstrual blood.

Pathogenesis. Caused by original weakness, blood exhaustion due to prolonged illness; impairment of the spleen due to improper diet, tiredness and sorrow; and blood insufficiency in the stomach and spleen.

Therapeutic Principle. Nourishing blood to regulate menstruation.

Hypomenorrhea due to Blood Stasis

Symptoms. Hypomenorrhea accompanied by purplish black menstrual blood with clots, and pain in the lower abdomen, etc.

Pathogenesis. Caused by blood coagulation due to cold invasion in the uterus, or impeded blood circulation due to qi stagnation, resulting in blood stasis in the uterine collaterals.

Therapeutic Principle. Promoting blood circulation to remove stasis and regulate menstruation.

Hypomenorrhea due to Kidney Deficiency

Symptoms. Menstrual discharge of abnormally small amount pink or dark in color accompanied by lassitude in the waist and knees, heel pain, dizziness, tinnitus, or cold sensation in the lower abdomen, frequent urination at night, etc.

Pathogenesis. Caused by congenital defect, or by early marriage, multiparity and labor strain, all of which impair the kidney with the result of insufficiency of the kidney-qi, essence and blood, and menoxenia due to insufficiency of Vital Meridian.

Therapeutic Principle. Nourishing the kidney and blood to regulate menstruation.

Hypopyon

Symptoms. The acute ophthalmic disease of accumulation of yellowish pus between the black eyeball and iris.

Pathogenesis. Caused by flaring up of fire-toxin in the tri-energizer that burns the iris.

Therapeutic Principle. Purging fire and detoxicating.

Hysteria

Symptoms. Trance, joy and anger without reason, often caused by mental stimulation. In the case of deficiency of blood and spleen: fullness in the stomach, palpitations, insomnia. For the case of deficiency of heart and kidney: vertigo, tinnitus, red complexion, feverish sensation in palms and soles, soreness of waist, amnesia, and insomnia due to vexation.

Pathogenesis. Commonly due to prolonged melancholy, damage of the heart and spleen and consumed blood which lead to failure to nourish the heart.

Therapeutic Principle. Nourish yin and supplement qi, nourish the heart to regulate the mind.

Hysteroptosis due to Kidney Deficiency

Symptoms. Something like a goose egg coming out of the vagina, tenesmus sensation in the lower abdomen, soreness and weakness of the waist and legs, frequent micturition, dry vagina without leukorrhea, dizziness, tinnitus.

Pathogenesis. Commonly due to impairment of the kidney, multiparity and excess of sexual life, resulting in debility of the Vital and Front Middle Meridians, dysfunction of the Belt Meridian in binding meridians and collaterals, leading to failure to keep the uterus high in its normal position.

Therapeutic Principle. Reinforce kidney-qi and strengthen uterine collaterals to elevate the uterus.

Hysteroptosis due to Qi Deficiency

Symptoms. Something like a goose egg coming out of the vagina, tenesmus sensation in the lower abdomen, mental fatigue, lassitude of limbs, short breath.

Pathogenesis. Mostly due to over-exertion in delivery, impairment of qi of the middle-energizer, leading to the sinking of qi in the middle-energizer and flaccidity of the uterus.

Therapeutic Principle. Supplement qi, elevate yang and consolidate the uterus.

I

Illness of Deficiency Type Treated by Tonifying Method

One of the principles of acupuncture treatment. It refers to the application of the reinforcing method in deficiency syndromes to strengthen the body resistance.

Imbricate Mosquito Fern Herb

It is whole herb of Azolla imbricata (Roxb.) Nakai (Azollaceae).

Inducing perspiration, dispelling pathogenic wind and promoting eruption.

Indication. Pain due to wind-dampness, wind skin rash, measles without adequate eruption, tinea, sores, burns, etc.

Immature Bitter Orange

It is the immature fruit Citrus aurantium L. or Citrus wilsonii Tanaka and poncirus trifoliata (L.) Raf. (Rutaceae).

Effect. Relieving the stagnation of qi, promoting digestion and removing stagnated food, resolving phlegm to relieve distention and fullness.

Indication. Stagnation of indigested food, abdominal pain, constipation, tenesmus, stiffness and fullness in the chest, visceroptosis, etc.

Impaired Water Metabolism

It refers to a morbid condition of dysuria and edema.

Pathogenesis. The lung and spleen fail to regulate the water passages, especially the kidney-yang is impaired, the water passage of the tri-energizer will be obstructed and fluid can not be transported into all parts of the body.

Impairment by Alcohol

Symptoms. Dizziness and headache, thoracic fullness, nausea and vomiting, restlessness or lethargy, etc. Severe case can cause abdominal mass, jaundice.

Pathogenesis. Impairment of zang-fu organs by over-drinking.

Therapeutic Principle. Diaphoresis, removing dampness and relieving alcoholism.

Impairment by Drinking Water

Symptoms. Emaciation or dropsy with sallow complexion, abdominal distention, etc.

Pathogenesis. Caused by drinking profuse water.

Therapeutic Principle. Strengthening the spleen and resolving dampness, diaphoresis and inducing diuresis.

Impairment by Fright

Symptoms. Lassitude, asthenia of joints, restlessness, timidness and aptness to be frightened, etc.

Pathogenesis. Caused by extreme fright.

Therapeutic Principle. Tranquilizing the mind and allaying excitement.

Impairment due to Anxiety

Symptoms. Irritability, anorexia and mental fatigue, asthenia of limbs, etc.

Pathogenesis. Caused by over-anxiety.

Therapeutic Principle. Depressing upward reverse flow of qi and relieving stagnation.

Impairment of Consciousness by Turbid Pathogens

Symptoms. Dizziness and heavy feeling in the head, stuffy nose, deaf, dim sight of eyes, sticky and greasy feeling in mouth, etc.

Pathogenesis. Damp-heat pathogen accumulated upwards to obstruct lucid yang and cover seven orifices of head.

Impairment of Heart due to Overstrain

Symptoms. Lassitude, weakness, palpitation, dysphoria, dryness of the mouth and throat, constipation, etc.

Pathogenesis. Impairment of the heart by overstrain.

Therapeutic Principle. Nourishing yin, regulating nutrient, tranquilizing the mind and tonifying the heart.

Impairment of Lung by Dryness

It refers to a morbid condition resulting from impairment of the Lung Meridian by autumn dryness.

Symptoms. Dry cough without sputum, or sputum which is difficult to be expectorated, or bloody sputum, sore throat and chest pain.

Pathogenesis. Autumn dryness invades the lung and consumes the lung fluid through the mouth and nose.

Therapeutic Principle. Moistening dryness, clearing away lung heat and nourishing yin.

Impairment of Lung due to Overstrain

Symptoms. Cough, hemoptysis, tidal fever, sweat, dysphoria with feverish sensation in the chest, gradual emaciation, ect.

Pathogenesis. Mostly caused by inherent defect, intemperance in sexual life, severe or chronic illness, which leads to the impairment of qi, blood and fluid, the deficiency of blood resistance.

Therapeutic Principle. Nourishing the deficiency.

Impairment of Lung-Qi due to Flaring-up of Fire Deficiency Type

It means that hyperactivity of deficient fire and damages lung-qi. It is one of pathogenesis, which causes the fever of deficiency type and the consumptive lung disease or cough and dyspnea.

Impairment of Muscles and Tendons by Heat

Symptoms. Muscular contracture, flaccidity or paralysis of the limbs, etc.

Pathogenesis. Malnutrition of the muscular system and damaged the yin blood resulting from high or long-standing fever.

Impairment of Purifying and Descending Function of Lung

The lung takes charge of respiration and qi descending. If the pathogen including exopathy and internal injury, invades the lung, the lung's normal function of purifying and descending is impaired, which leads to dyspnea, shortness of breath or shallow breath, cough with expectoration, and tightness and fullness in chest.

Impairment of Qi

An abnormal condition in acupuncture treatment, referring to impairment of the vital-qi by incorrect needling methods.

Impairment of Vital and Front Middle Meridians

Symptoms. Abnormal menstruation, pain of the hypogastrium, lumbago, uterine bleeding, habitual abortion and infertility.

Pathogenesis. Malnutrition of the liver, kidney, qi and blood. They also result from sexual strain or frequent gestation and childbirth.

Impairment of Yang

It refers to impairment of yang-qi resulting from attack of cold on meridians, or yang deficiency and interior cold, excess of yin-qi, or overdose of cold-natured drugs, or overuse of diaphoretics and cathartics, or retention of water dampness. In addition, excessive emotional stimulation can impair yang-qi.

Impairment of Yin

It refers to impairment of genuine yin resulting from excessive yang-qi and impairment of yin fluid, especially that of the liver and kidney in advanced cases of febrile diseases.

Symptoms. Lower fever, heat sensation in palms and soles, mental fatigue, dry mouth and tongue or sore-throat, deafness, flushed cheeks, red tongue with thin and dry coating, soft, feeble and rapid pulse.

Impetigo

Symptoms. Mostly appears on the face, the arm and the leg, etc. At the beginning, it has erythema or small vesicles. Soon they become bean-size vesicles and pustule. After breaking they will be dry, form crusts, and heal gradually. There are also cases that attack repeatedly, and persistent for rather a long time. In these cases, they may be accompanied by such body symptoms as fever and thirst, etc.

Pathogenesis. Caused by the steaming of stagnation of damp-heat to the skin, or by the infection of eczema and miliaria.

Therapeutic Principle. Clearing away heat, promoting diuresis and detoxicating.

Impossible Survival with Solitary Yin

The relationship between yin and yang is opposition and interdependence. Solitary yin means that there is only yin without yang. In this case, the abnormal relationship of opposition and interdependence may result in disease and even deadly disease.

Impotence

Symptoms. Incapability of the penis to erect, or the penis is not hard enough in sexual activity.

Pathogenesis. Usually caused by excess of sexual intercourse, the fire of deficiency type of the liver and kidney, the impairment of the heart and spleen, unrelieved fear, and the impairment of the liver by depression.

Therapeutic Principle. Warming the kidney to reinforce the primordial qi, strengthening the spleen and nourishing the heart, nourishing yin and removing fire and soothing the liver and alleviating depression, etc.

Improper Diet with Cold

Symptoms. Headache, fever, aversion to cold, rigidity of the limbs, nausea, vomiting, distention in the stomach, eructation with fetid odor and acid regurgitation, etc.

Pathogenesis. An exogenous disease due to improper diet first, then affection by cold, or affection by cold first, then improper diet.

Therapeutic Principle. Relieving exterior syndrome at first, then promoting digestion, or relieving exterior syndrome combined with promoting digestion.

Improving Measles

It refers to sufficient vital-qi and deficient pathogens of the patients with measles.

Symptoms. Slight fever, cough without dyspnea and measles appears 3 or 4 days after running a fever. Initially measles appear on the head and face, then on the chest, back and limbs, with even red spots and without other complicated symptoms. In three days, measles adequately erupt, and then the fever disappears gradually, the cough gets mild, and the patient finally recovers perfectly from measles.

Impulse of Qi

It possesses two implications:

1. It refers to start of meridian qi in every point.
2. It refers to palpitation around the navel, mostly caused by erroneous sweating and deficiency of the spleen yang.

Inability of Eye Moving

Symptoms. Inability to move the eyeballs often found in serious cases of febrile diseases due to exogenous pathogenic factor, or various diseases caused by internal damage.

Pathogenesis. Caused by the domination of evil-heat which prevents the essence and qi from nourishing the eyes or deficiency of liver blood which can not provide the eyes with enough blood.

Inability to Raise Limbs

Symptoms. Limited activities of the limbs and inability to raise.

Pathogenesis. Usually caused by the invasion of pathogenic wind into the meridians and collaterals, weakness of the spleen and kidney or heat accumulation in the interior, malnutrition of muscles and confluence of tendons.

Inactivity of Yang-qi

Symptoms. Edema of limbs.

Pathogenesis. Usually caused by deficiency of the spleen and its failure to control water.

Therapeutic Principle. Warming the spleen, invigorating qi and subsiding swelling.

Incessant Exudation of Perspiration

Symptoms. Profuse sweating like leaking.

Pathogenesis. Attacked by wind pathogen on the exterior and failure of defensive energy to protect the body against diseases.

Incised Wound

It refers to the wound caused by sharp metallic weapon or tool. It also means the furuncle due to the infected wound.

Inclination for Cold Drinking

Symptoms. Preference of patient for drinking cold water.

Pathogenesis. Consumption of body fluid because of excessive heat, belonging to internal heat syndrome.

Inclination for Hot Drinking

Symptoms. Preference of patient for drinking hot water in order to warm the middle-energizer to dispel cold.

Pathogenesis. Due to internal cold, belonging to internal cold syndrome.

Incontinence of Urine

Symptoms. Frequent and scanty urination with difficulty to control.

Pathogenesis. Usually caused by the impairment of the spleen and lung by overstrain and excessive anxiety, the qi deficiency and its failure to harness water fluid, or the deficiency of the kidney-qi, the consumption of the essence and blood.

Incoordination between Liver and Spleen

Symptoms. Distending pain and oppressed feeling in the chest, anorexia, prolonged abdominal pain and tendency to diarrhea and relieving pain after diarrhea, sighing, restlessness, anger, constipation borborygmus.

Pathogenesis. Caused by incoordination between the liver and the spleen resulting from disorder of hepatic qi and disturbance of the function to smooth and regulate the flow of vital-qi and blood, which affects the normal function of the spleen and stomach.

Therapeutic Principle. Invigorating the spleen and relieving depression of the liver-qi.

Incoordination of Physique and Qi

It refers to imbalance between the physique of man and the function of viscera or pathogenic qi. There are two cases: 1. Excess in physique but deficiency in qi. It can be seen as fatty physique with insufficient function, general debility, shortness of breath and lassitude. 2. Excess in qi and deficiency in physique. It can be seen as emaciation physique with excessive stomach-fire, restlessness and hunger with polyphagia.

Indian Azalea Flower

It is the flower or fruit of Rhododendron simsii Planch. (Ericaceae).

Effect. Promoting blood circulation to remove blood stasis and regulating menstruation, expelling phlegm to arrest coughing, clearing away heat and detoxication.

Indication. Irregular menstruation, amenorrhea, metrorrhagia and metrostaxis, traumatic injuries, rheumatalgia, hematemesis, and epistaxis.

Indian Azalea Leaf

It is the leaf of Rhododendron simsii Planch. (Ericaceae).

Effect. Clearing away heat, detoxicating and arresting bleeding.

Indication. Subcutaneous swelling, furuncle, carbuncle, traumatic bleeding and urticaria.

Indian Azalea Root

It is the root of Rhododenron simsii Planch. (Ericaceae).

Effect. Regulating blood circulation, dispelling phlegm to stop cough, arresting bleeding, expelling wind and dampness.

Indication. Bronchitis, stomachache, hematemesis, irregular menstruation, metrorrhagia and metrostaxis, mastadenitis, dysentery, pain because of wind-dampness and traumatic injuries.

Indian Chrysanthemum Flower

It is the anthodium of Chrysanthemum indicum L. (Compositae).

Effect. Dispelling pathogenic wind and clearing away heat, subduing swelling and detoxicating.

Indication. Influenza, acute conjunctivitis, headache cough due to the lung-heat, sore throat, bloodshot eyes, tuberculosis, hepatitis, dysentery, eczema, cutaneous pruritus, etc.

Indian Epimeredi Herb

It is the whole herb of Epimeredi indica (L.) Rothm. Ktze. (Labiatae).

Effect. Expelling pathogenic wind, removing dampness, detoxicating and relieving spasm.

Indication. Cold with fever, acute nephritis, hypertension, aversion to cold, vomiting, abdominal pain, arthralgia and myalgia, urticaria and hemorrhoid.

Indian Heliotrope Herb

It is the whole herb or root of Heliotropium indicum L. (Boraginaceae).

Effect. Clearing away heat and promoting diuresis, detoxicating and subduing swelling.

Indication. Pneumonia, phthisis, empyema, sore throat, toothache, cough, acute enteritis, bladder stone, acute infantile convulsion, canker sores, skin and external disease, etc.

Indian Iphigenia Bulb

It is the bulb of Iphigenia indica Kunth et Benth. (Liliaceae).

Effect. Arresting cough and asthma, relieving pain and preventing cancers.

Indication. Bronchits, cough, asthma, scrofula, cardiac depression, mastocarcinoma and nasopharyngeal carcinoma.

Indian Jujube Bark

It is the bark of Ziziphus mauritiana Lam. (Rhamnaceae).

Effect. Relieving inflammation and promoting tissue regeneration.

Indication. Burns, scald, etc.

Indian Lettuce Root

It is the root of Lactuca indica L. (Compositae).

Effect. Clearing away heat, cooling blood, detumescence, detoxicating.

Indication. Metrorrhagia, metrostaxis, edema, abscess, acute mastadenitis and traumatic injury.

Indian Madder Root

It is the root of Rubia cordifolia L. (Rubiaceae).

Effect. Cooling blood, arresting bleeding, promoting blood circulation, eliminating blood stasis and activating meridians.

Indication. Hematemesis, bleeding caused by trauma, bleeding due to blood-heat, amenorrhea, pain due to blood stasis and arthralgia of arthralgia-syndrome.

Indian Madder Stem or Leaf

 ❀ I-1

It is the stem or leaf of Rubia cordifolia L. (Rubiaceae).

Effect. Arresting bleeding, removing blood stasis and activating meridians.

Indication. Hematemesis, metrorrhagia, traumatic injuries, lumbago, joint pain, boils and swelling.

Indian Maesa Herb

It is the whole herb of Maese indica Wall. (Myrsinaceae).

Effect. Clearing away heat and detoxicating.

Indication. Hepatitis, diarrhea, stomachache, hypertension and measles.

Indian Mustard Leaf

It is the tender branch leaf of Brassica juncea (L.) Czern. et Coss. (Cruciferae).

Effect. Facilitating the flow of the lung, eliminating phlegm, warming the middle-energizer and promoting flow of qi.

Indication. Cough with stagnation of phlegm fullness and distress in the chest, etc.

Indian Mustard Seed

It is the seed of Brassica juncea (L.) Czern. et Coss. (Cruciferae).

Effect. Warming the middle-energizer, dispelling cold, promoting flow of qi, eliminating phlegm, clearing the meridians and collaterals and subduing poisoning swelling.

Indication. Vomiting due to cold in the stomach, chest and abdominal pain, cough due to lung-cold, arthralgia aggravated by cold, inflammation of the throat, carbuncles of yin nature, traumatic injuries.

Indian Rorippa Herb

It is the whole herb of Rorippa indica (L.) Hiern. (Cruciferae).

Effect. Dispelling phlegm, relieving cough, clearing away heat, detoxicating, inducing diuresis and curing jaundice.

Indication. Cough with phlegm-dyspnea, swollen and sore throat, skin and external diseases and jaundice caused by damp-heat pathogen.

Indian String-bush Root ❀ I-2

The root of Wikstroemia indica (L.) C.A. Mey. (Thumelaeaceae).

Effect. Clearing away heat, detoxicating, removing stasis, inducing diuresis, relieving swelling and destroying intestinal worms.

Indication. Cough with asthma due to of the lung-heat, nephritis hydrops, amenorrhea, mastadenitis, scrofula, pyogenic infections due to skin and external diseases and traumatic injuries.

Indigestion

Symptoms. Distention and fullness in the epigastrium, eructation and acid regurgitation or anorexia, etc.

Pathogenesis. Mainly due to weakness of stomach and spleen, and dysfunction of them in transport.

Therapeutic Principle. Invigorating the spleen to promote digestion.

Indigo Blue Lips and Nails

It results from deficiency of spleen-yang, invasion of Shaoyin meridians by cold, stagnation of phlegm in the lungs, qi stagnation and blood stasis. It belongs to intermingled asthenia and sthenia syndrome, which is considered as severe symptoms.

Indigophant Fruit

It is the fruit of Polygonum tinctorium Ait. (Polygonaceae).

Effect. Removing heat and detoxicating.

Indication. Epidemic eruptive diseases, sore throat, infantile malnutrition, poisoning swellings, sores and furuncles, etc.

Indigo Woad Leaf

It is the leaf or the branch of Isatis indigotica Fort. (Cruciferae).

Effect. Clearing away heat, detoxicating, cooling blood and curing skin eruptions.

Indication. Headache with fever due to the exogenous pathogenic wind-heat, high fever with unconsciousness, parotiditis maculas, sore throat, jaundice, dysentery, carbuncle and cellulitis.

Indigo Woad Root

It is the root of Isatis indigotica Fort. (Cruciferae).

Effect. Clearing away heat, detoxicating, cooling the blood and relieving sore-throat.

Indication. Headache and sore throat with fever caused by the exogenous pathogenic wind-heat, mumps, suppurative infections on the body surface, coma, hematemesis, epistaxis, infection with swollen head, etc.

Indirect Moxibustion

A form of moxa-cone moxibustion. Place certain barriers between the acupuncture point and moxa-cone, to prevent the fire from burning the skin and make use of the effects of both moxa and the barrier chosen.

Indisposition of Throat

Symptoms. Pain, dryness, subjective sensation of some foreign body in the throat, etc.

Pathogenesis. For the excess type, caused by stagnation of the liver qi, obstruction of turbid phlegm, or obstruction of lung qi due to hidden fire in the lung and stomach affected by exopathogen. For the defi-ciency type, caused by yin deficiency of the liver and kidney, or lung and stomach; resulting in malnutrition of the throat.

Indistinctive Pulse

It means that the pulse extremely soft, feeble, and barely palpable. Indistinctive pulse indicates deficiency of yin, yang, qi, and blood. It can be seen as shock, collapse, or chronic and weak syndromes.

Indolence of Limbs

Symptoms. Lassitude and relaxation of the limbs.

Pathogenesis. Usually caused by weakness of the spleen, the spleen fails to transport essence and malnutrition of the limbs.

Induced Period of Acupuncture Anesthesia

It is needed that a procedure of manual or electric stimulation to raise the pain threshold of the patient before surgical operation. The period from insertion of the needle with the occurrence of the needling response and the application of certain proper stimulation forms until the analgesic effect is produced, so that the surgical operation can be performed. The duration of the period mainly depends on the characteristics of the selected acupuncture points and stimulation forms, usually 15-30 minutes. If the acupuncture points is located on the nerve trunk or branch, the induced period may take less time, while if the acupoint is far from the area of operation, the induced period may last a little longer.

Inducing Diuresis for Treating Stranguria

A therapy to treat stranguria with prescriptions, whose actions are removing dampness to induce diuresis, and clearing away heat.

Pathogenesis. Caused by retention of damp-heat in the bladder and disturbance in qi transformation of bladder.

Indication. Frequency and urgency of micturition, burning pain in urethra, dark and turbid urine.

Inducing Diuresis with Bland Drugs

One of the methods to eliminate dampness, which is using inducing diuresis drugs to eliminate dampness through urination.
Indication. Symptoms of dampness as diarrhea, urinary incontinence.

Inducing Qi

An acupuncture point method. It refers to: 1. After the generation of the needling sensation, the needle is pressed by slow insertion and slow withdrawal. Apply the method to dredge and regulate the meridian qi to normal, relieve the pathogenic qi in case it gets deeper and restore the vital-qi, so as to cure the disease. 2. The method of making the needling sensation move along the course of meridian, also called qi-guiding method.

Inducing Resuscitation

It is a method of restoring life or consciousness after collapse or apparent death.
Therapeutic Principle. Using drugs with fragrant and pungent in nature and migratory drugs.

Inducing Resuscitation with Aromatic and Warm Drugs

It refers to the therapy of warming yang, inducing resuscitation and restoring consciousness with aromatic and warm drugs whose actions are inducing resuscitation and promoting qi circulation.
Indication. Sudden faint, lockjaw, pale face, cold limbs.

Induction Qigong

It is a maneuver in Qigong that causes the practitioner to relax the whole body, breathe evenly and smoothly, eliminate distracting thoughts to reach a tranquil state through the induction by the practitioner himself or someone else using signals such as consciousness, breath, words, sound, etc.

Indurated Mass between the Waist and Hip

It refers to the mass appearing between the waist and the hip.
Symptoms. The cellulitis brings about numbness and pain and difficulty to be subdued and ulcerated. It is hard like a stone. The skin color is normal.
Pathogenesis. Caused by the stagnancy of cold qi and blood stasis.
Therapeutic Principle. Dispelling cold, activating blood flow and removing blood stasis.

Indurated Mass of Knee

It refers to the swollen mass appearing in the knee.
Symptoms. Swelling knee, hard as a stone, in the normal skin color and difficulty to be subdued and ulcerated.
Pathogenesis. Caused by the accumulation of blood stasis due to the deep attacking of pathogenic cold into the deficiency body.
Therapeutic Principle. Dispelling bold, activating blood flow and removing blood stasis.

Inebriate Achnatherum Herb

It is the whole herb and root of Achnatherum inebrians (Hance) Keng. (Gramineae).
Effect. Detoxicating and subduing swelling.
Indication. Pyogenic infection and ulcerous disease of skin, and arthralgia.

Infantile Acute Asthma

Symptoms. Sudden attack of asthma with rapid breathing, flaring of nares, and fullness of the chest and hypochondrium.
Pathogenesis. Usually caused by excessive phlegm and heat, which invade the heart, and lung.

Therapeutic Principle. Releasing the lung to dissipate phlegm and clearing away pathogenic heat.

Infantile Blepharitis
Symptoms. One kind of ulcerative marginal blepharitis.
Pathogenesis. Caused by acquired affection of pathogenic wind in addition to immersion of canthi in turbid liquid when a newly-born infant is bathed.

Infantile Convulsion
Symptoms. Spasm, clenching, twitching, shivering, opisthotonos drawing, squinting and staring. The doctor of Chinese traditional medicine thought of the sudden attack, high-fever, annoyance and thirst as acute infantile convulsion, and considered the slow attack, low-fever and fatigue as chronic infantile convulsion.
Therapeutic Principle. Arresting convulsion and tranquilizing mind, clearing away heat, expelling wind and removing phlegm.

Infantile Convulsion due to Vomiting and Diarrhea
Symptoms. Purple face, cold extremities, opening the eyes when sleeping, and convulsion of hands and legs.
Pathogenesis. Usually caused by the splenic weakness, shortage of the body fluid and malnutrition of the muscular system.
Therapeutic Principle. Strengthening the spleen, regulating the stomach, tonifying qi and producing body fluid.

Infantile Cornea Softening
Symptoms. Dark-field blindness after birth, followed by ocular dryness, turbidity, or even erosion and impairment of the black.
Pathogenesis. Mostly caused by impairment of the spleen and stomach and hypoactivity of qi and blood that result from improper feeding of infant.

Therapeutic Principle. Invigorating the spleen, clearing away heat, and nourishing the liver to improve visual acuity.

Infantile Deaf and Mute
It is classified into two types: the congenital and the acquired.
Pathogenesis. The acquired deaf and mute are caused by the stagnancy of functional activities of qi in the meridians and collaterals and the closed orifices after febrile disease or epilepsy induced by terror.
Therapeutic Principle. Clearing away the meridians and promoting the flow of qi, also with acupuncture. Generally, the therapeutic result is better if the patient still has a little auditognosis.

Infantile Diarrhea
It has three types:
1. Diarrhea due to damp-heat.
   Symptoms. Thin or watery stool with yellow color and foul smell, fever and thirst, burning sensation of the anus, scanty and dark urine.
   Pathogenesis. Caused by attack of exogenous summer dampness, which disturbs the spleen and stomach, and leads to dysfunction of the spleen and occurrence of diarrhea.
   Therapeutic Principle. Clear heat and remove dampness.
2. Diarrhea due to improper diet.
   Symptoms. Abdominal distention and pain, pains relief after diarrhea, foul smell of the stools, eructation or vomiting.
   Pathogenesis. Improper diet: retention of the undigested food damages the intestine and stomach, which leads to indigestion and failure to distinguish water from food and to the occurrence of diarrhea.
   Therapeutic Principle. Promote digestion to remove stagnation.
3. Diarrhea due to yang-deficiency.
   Symptoms. Intermittent diarrhea or prolonged diarrhea, watery stools or stools with undigested food, diarrhea

occurring after eating, poor appetite, lassitude and fatigue.

Pathogenesis. Prolonged illness leading to deficiency of the spleen and stomach, insufficiency of kidney-yang.

Therapeutic Principle. Invigorate the spleen and warm the kidney.

Infantile Eczema

Symptoms. Commonly occurring on the head and face of the baby, sometimes extending to other parts of the body.

Pathogenesis. Mostly caused by allergic constitution; accumulation of wind, dampness, and heat in muscles and skin.

Infantile Erysipelas

Symptoms. At the beginning of the disease, the infant has a fever and is restless with crying, then the skin turns red as if it is covered with red paint. The red area is getting larger and larger. The infants under one year are susceptible to the disease.

Pathogenesis. Usually caused by fetal toxicosis or pathogenic wind-heat-toxin.

Therapeutic Principle. Clearing away heat, and detoxifying from the interior.

Infantile Headache

It is clinically divided into two types:

1. Headache due to wind cold.

   Symptoms. Aversion to cold and fever, pain in the vertex and temple.

   Pathogenesis. Caused by the derangement of qi and blood and the blockage of the meridians resulting from wind-cold attacking the collaterals of vertex.

   Therapeutic Principle. Expel wind-cold.

2. Headache due to internal heat.

   Symptoms. Dry nose, pain in the eyes radiating to the vertex and teeth, pain without definite time.

   Pathogenesis. Caused by overeating fleshy and greasy food leading to disorder of the digestive function of the spleen and stomach, which causes accumulated food to grow into fire, and the

fire flames up along the Stomach Meridian.

Therapeutic Principle. Clear heat from the Stomach Meridian.

Infantile Jaundice due to Stomach-heat

Symptoms. High fever, sudden yellow body, thirst and intention of abdomen, dark and difficult urine, and constipation.

Pathogenesis. Usually caused by Yangming stomach heat, accumulation of damp pathogens in the body.

Therapeutic Principle. Clearing away heat and promoting diuresis.

Infantile Malnutrition

Symptoms. In the early stage, yellow face and thin body, good appetite, dry or loose stool, restlessness, much sweat and grinding teeth in sleeping.

Pathogenesis. Deficiency of spleen-yang and malnutrition due to feeding improperly.

Therapeutic Principle. Regulate the spleen and stomach.

Infantile Malnutrition with Abdominal Distention

Symptoms. Patients are gradual emaciation, full abdomen with clearly-seen vessels, fever, lack of energy, shortness of breath.

Pathogenesis. The abdominal distention due to infantile malnutrition.

Therapeutic Principle. Relieving the stagnation, strengthening the spleen and clear away the heat.

Infantile Malnutrition with Ascariasis

Symptoms. Malnutrition and dysentery, atrophy of the muscles.

Pathogenesis. Caused by ascarids in abdomen and infantile malnutrition.

Therapeutic Principle. Expel the ascarids and strengthen the spleen.

Infantile Malnutrition with Cough

Symptoms. Cough due to infantile malnutrition.

Pathogenesis. Caused by impairment of the lung due to infantile malnutrition with fever.

Therapeutic Principle. Clearing away heat in lung.

Infantile Malnutrition with Dampness

Symptoms. Sore appear in the anus, or in the mouth and nose.

Pathogenesis. Long-term dysentery, gastrointestinal weakness or heat in the organs, on taking too much fat and sweet.

Therapeutic Principle. Clearing away heat and damp, expelling ascarises.

Infantile Malnutrition with Diarrhea

Symptoms. Blue-yellow face, full abdomen, loss of appetite, cold days and fever nights, mass in the abdomen.

Pathogenesis. Usually caused by dysfunction of the spleen due to immoderate eating and drinking.

Therapeutic Principle. Strengthening the spleen and regulating the stomach.

Infantile Malnutrition with Swelling

Symptoms. Cough, stuffiness in the chest, swelling of abdomen, edema of head, arms and legs.

Pathogenesis. Usually caused by obstruction of the lung-qi and dysfunction of the spleen.

Therapeutic Principle. Clearing the lung and eliminating damp, excreting water and regulating the spleen.

Infantile Malnutrition with Thirst

Symptoms. Thirst due to malnutrition, preference for drinks.

Pathogenesis. Usually caused by stomach heat, or lack of saliva.

Therapeutic Principle. Clearing away pathogenic heat, requlating the function of stomach, tonifying qi and produce saliva.

Infantile Massage

It is a specially designed massage method to prevent and treat the infantile diseases. According to the infantile physiological and pathological conditions, there are special acupuncture points and manipulations to prevent cold, fever vomiting, diarrhea, stagnancy of food, infantile malnutrition, enuresis, prolapse of rectum, convulsion, etc.

Infantile Metopism

Symptoms. Unclosing fontanel, acute distention of muscles and tendons, projected blue vessels, pale face, vomiting of sputum and saliva. If long-lasting, chronic infantile convulsion will appear.

Pathogenesis. Caused by invasion of the pathogenic wind into the brain and spinal cord, because of metopism.

Therapeutic Principle. Dissipating wind and eliminating sputum.

Infantile Mouth Swelling

Symptoms. The fleshy swelling in the infant mouth as high as fungiform.

Pathogenesis. Because of the excessive fire of the fetus or heat pathogens in the stomach.

Therapeutic Principle. Clearing away heat and detoxifying.

Infantile Myasthenia

Symptoms. Deficiency and flaccidity of the muscles, loose skin and emaciation of the infant.

Pathogenesis. Usually caused by immoderate diet, malnourishment, qi deficiency of the spleen and stomach.

Therapeutic Principle. Tonifying the spleen and stomach.

Infantile Postcibal Diarrhea

Symptoms. Diarrhea after the infant eats enough food and repeating diarrhea till there is no food in the stomach.

Pathogenesis. Caused by indigestion of food due to deficiency of the spleen and the stomach.

Therapeutic Principle. Strengthening the spleen and tonifying the stomach.

Infantile Pyo-bloody Dysentery

Symptoms. Distention and pain in the abdomen, tenesmus, dysentery with pus and blood in the stool, aversion to cold and cold limbs, etc.

Pathogenesis. Usually caused by deficiency and weakness of the spleen and stomach, and attack of cold and dampness into the body, or improper diet of cold and raw food.

Therapeutic Principle. Warming the middle-energizer and relieving dysentery.

Infantile Retardation of Walking

Symptoms. The infant cannot walk after one, even two or three years old.

Pathogenesis. Usually caused by flaccidity of muscles and bones due to insufficiency of the liver and kidney, deficiency heat of the spleen and stomach.

Therapeutic Principle. Replenishing the liver and kidney, reinforcing the spleen and nourishing the stomach, and strengthening the muscles and bones.

Infantile Tic

Symptoms. Spasm, severe pain of the abdomen, pain with bending down, shortness of breath, scream with fear, blood streaks and spots in the eyes, black stool, and alternative chillness and fever.

Pathogenesis. Caused by affection of heat, wind and fright during pregnancy.

Therapeutic Principle. Calming endopathic wind and relieving pain.

Infantile Vomiting due to Improper Diet

Symptoms. Frequent vomiting with sour mucus, yellowish juice or clear saliva, abdominal distention and eructation, anorexia, etc.

Pathogenesis. Mostly caused by improper diet, that damaged the spleen and stomach.

Therapeutic Principle. Strengthen the spleen and stomach, eliminate undigested food.

Infantile Vomiting with Diarrhea and Fever

Symptoms. Fever, vomiting, diarrhea, accompanied by abdominal fullness, failure of food intake and irritability, etc.

Pathogenesis. Mostly caused by the affection of exopathogens and improper feeding.

Therapeutic Principle. Relieve exopathogens and regulate stomach to relieve vomiting and diarrhea.

Infection on Palm

Symptoms. Have millet-like red spots at the beginning, followed by hard swelling with vesicle and small deep-rooted boils, which are numb, painful and itching. In the case of severe syndrome, the vesicle will change from bright to dark, and the swelling and pain will become acute, or even ulcerate muscles and bones.

Pathogenesis. Caused by the excessive fire-toxin of heart and pericardium Meridian and collateral.

Therapeutic Principle. Pricking the bright vesicle at the beginning, and using heat-clearing and detoxifying drugs as oral administration.

Infection with Swollen Head

Symptoms. At the very onset, fever, aversion to cold, flushed swollen face; then progression of fever, thirst with preference for drink, dysphoria, flushed swollen and enlarged face, severe sore throat, yellowish coating of red tongue, and rapid and replete pulse.

Pathogenesis. An acute epidemic disease due to seasonal wind-warm pathogens. It is characterized by flushed swollen face usually occurring in winter and spring.

Therapeutic Principle. Mainly clearing away heat and toxic substances.

Inflammation of Throat

It refers to laryngeal obstruction due to inflammation, which is a general designation of guttural swelling and pain.

Symptoms. One case: red swelling, feverish pain and dysphagia, accompanied by headache, cold and heat, etc. Another case: pharyngeal tidal red, odynophagia and subjective uncomfortable sensation of the pharynx when the patient coughs, accompanied by general yin deficiency.

Pathogenesis. Caused by invasion of wind-heat and pathogenic toxic in the throat in the former case. Caused by flaring up of deficiency five due to yin insufficiency in the letter case.

Therapeutic Principle. Dispelling wind and clearing away heat, or nourishing yin and reducing pathogenic fire.

Inflammatory Diseases of Foot

Symptoms. Swelling, itching and watering between the toes of the foot, and heat appearing on the sole.

Pathogenesis. Caused by deficiency of qi and blood, the downward flow of noxious dampness.

Therapeutic Principle. In the case of red swelling, hot pain, ulceration and pyorrhea to remove obstruction. In the case of white stretching swelling pain without ulceration, to warm and nourish yang-qi.

Influenza

It refers to serious case of cold i.e. epidemic cold.

Symptoms. High fever, aversion to cold, headache, arthralgia, listlessness and tiredness, thirst, sore throat, reddish tongue with white fur, etc.

Therapeutic Principle. Expelling exogenous pathogen and clearing away heat and toxic substances.

Inguinal Hernia

Also called qi of the small intestine, or yin-type hernia.

Symptoms. Distention and pain of the lower abdomen and scrotum. The testis enters into the abdomen when the patient is in the lying position. The testis comes down to the scrotum when the patient is in the standing position. For serious hernia, the prolapsed substance can only be put back into the abdomen with the help of the hand.

Pathogenesis. Mostly caused by sinking of qi deficiency and injury of the collaterals resulting from overwork or carrying too much weight.

Therapeutic Principle. Tonifying and elevating the spleen-qi, and alleviate pain.

Injury between Temporal and Sphenoid Bones

Symptoms. Local inflammation, cyanosis, pain, dizziness, and even unconsciousness seen in serious cases.

Cause. Usually caused by trauma.

Therapeutic Principle. In mild cases, treatment given by external application of relieving swelling ointment and immobilization with many-tailed bandage. In the serious cases with coma and unconsciousness, give first aid treatment.

Injury by Overstrain

Symptoms. Less serious cases: fatigue, short breath and disinclination to talk, poor appetite; the more serious cases: chest pain, bleeding of mouth and nose.

Pathogenesis. Overstrain or traveling long distance with heavy load lead to the injury of internal organs, qi and blood.

Therapeutic Principle. For the former, focus on recuperation, accompanied by tonifying qi and blood. For the latter, invigorating qi to accelerate hemostasis, dispersing blood stasis, take note of exercises and avoiding overload.

Injury of Blood Vessels of Lung by Heat

1. Heat of excess type.

Symptoms. Mostly acute disease, hemoptysis, fever, flushed face, reddish tongue with yellowish fur.

Pathogenesis. Stasis of exogenous pathogen changes into heat and injury of the blood vessels of the lung by heat.

2. Fever of deficiency type.

Symptoms. Mostly chronic disease, less hemoptysis, sputum mixed with blood, tidal fever in the afternoon, flushing of zygomatic region.

Pathogenesis. Deficiency of yin fluid of both the lung and the kidney, impairment of the lung by fire of deficiency type.

Injury of Coccyx

Symptoms. Local swelling pain, exacerbation of pain by pressure, bony crepitus in movement, and restriction of walking, sitting, lying and turning the body.

Cause. Usually caused by trauma and impact.

Therapeutic Principle. Manual reduction and immobilization.

Injury of Emotion

Symptoms. Mental and emotional disease, pain and stiffness of the waist and back stretch, and pallid complexion, etc.

Pathogenesis. Injury of the mind and emotion.

Therapeutic Principle. Nourishing the heart and calming mind.

Injury of Forehead

Symptoms. External wound and edema of face. If there is internal injury and blood stasis, patient will be vomiting, epistaxis, coma, pectoralgia, and anorexia.

Cause. Usually caused by trauma and impact.

Therapeutic Principle. Arresting bleeding, inducing appetite and digestion, removing blood stasis and relieving pain.

Injury of Meridians

Symptoms. In less serious cases: unsmooth passage of meridians, disharmony of qi and blood, the obstruction of blood flow, light swelling and pain in local parts. In more serious cases: rapture of the vessels, blood going away from the vessels, blood stagnated in the body or overflowing out of the body, and apparent swelling pain in the injured parts.

Pathogenesis. Injury of qi and blood in meridians caused by trauma.

Injury of Muscle and Tendon

Symptoms. Local pain, cyanosis, edema and flatulence, and even difficulty in extension and flexion of joint.

Cause. Mainly caused by trauma, twisting and contusion.

Therapeutic Principle. Promoting blood circulation to remove blood stasis, relieve rigidity of muscles and activate the meridians and collaterals, simultaneously by acupuncture and moxibustion, massage and cupping.

Insect Wax

It is the processed wax secreted from the trunk of Ericerus pela (Chavannes) Guerin, Fraxinus chinensis Roxb. Ligustrum lucidum Ait (Oleaceae).

Effect. Stopping bleeding, promoting tissue regeneration and arresting pain.

Indication. Hematuria, hemafecia, cutting wounds with bleeding, skin and external disease and chancre, etc.

Inserting the Needle as if Injecting

One of the methods of needle insertion.

Method. When inserting the needle, the doctor holds the lower part of the needle body with the thumb and index finger, and exposes a length of 0.2 cun above the tip of the needle, then inserts the needle into the point swiftly. It is suitable for perpendicular puncture.

Inserting the Needle by Twirling

One of the methods of needle insertion.

Method. Inserting the needle by twirling the needle handle when the needle fails to be inserted quickly because of the soft body of the needle, e.g. one made of gold or silver, or the skin around the selected point is so hard that the needle can be inserted swiftly; the twirling method is used.

Inserting the Needle through a Pipe

One of the methods of needle insertion.

Method. When inserting the needle, the doctor puts a small hollow pipe, which is a bit shorter than the needle, vertically on the point, places a flat-handle filiform needle in the pipe, knocks the exposed handle quickly to enable the needle tip to be punctured into the skin, and then takes away the pipe. This method can reduce the painful sensation during insertion.

Inserting the Needle under Pressure of Finger

One of the methods for inserting the needle.

Method. When inserting the needle the doctor holds the root of the needle with the thumb and index fingers of the right hand, presses straight on the acupoint with the middle or the ring finger, keeps the body of the needle closely against the finger, then inserts the needle into the point quickly, using the pressure of the thumb and index fingers. This method is suitable for the insertion of the short needle and can be manipulated only with one hand.

Inserting the Needle while Pinching the Skin

One of the methods for inserting the needle.

Method. While the skin at the point region is pinched by the thumb and the index finger of one hand, the needle held by the other hand, is inserted into the pinched skin. It is commonly used for inserting the needle in shallow and thin regions of the skin.

Inserting the Needle while Unfolding the Skin

One of the methods for inserting the needle.

Method. After unfolding and tightening the skin adjacent to the acupuncture point on both sides with the left thumb and index finger, puncture the acupuncture point with the needle held in the right hand. Applicable where the skin is flaccid and perpendicular needling is required, such as the acupoints on the abdomen.

Insomnia due to Deficiency of the Heart and Spleen

Symptoms. Difficulty in getting to sleep, dream-disturbed sleep or liability to waking, palpitations, forgetfulness, liability to sweating, pale complexion, lassitude, mass in the stomach, watery stools.

Pathogenesis. Caused by excessive contemplation, consuming the heart and spleen deficiency of qi and blood, and failure of nourishment of the heart.

Therapeutic Principle. Invigorate qi and nourish blood.

Insomnia due to Derangement of the Stomach

Symptoms. Shallow sleep, feverish sensation in the chest, fullness of the stomach, eructation, dizziness and blurred vision, vomiting and hiccups with phlegm and saliva, yellow and greasy tongue coating.

Pathogenesis. Caused by improper diet leading to disorder of the spleen and stomach, excessive accumulation of dampness, and stagnant phlegm producing heat. The phlegm-heat flares up to disturb the heart and mind.

Therapeutic Principle. Resolve phlegm, regulate the stomach and tranquilize the mind.

Insomnia due to Excessive Heat

Symptoms. Fever, mental irritability, restlessness, insomnia and rapid pulse, etc.

Pathogenesis. Caused by exogenous heat pathogen injuring the qi system and the heat impairing mind.

Therapeutic Principle. Clearing away heat and removing dysphoria.

Insomnia due to Gallbladder-fire

Symptoms. Night restlessness, hypochondrium fullness, vexation, trance, yellowish or reddish coloration of eyes, etc.

Pathogenesis. Usually caused by depressed anger, improper diet and internal hot phlegm stagnancy.

Therapeutic Principle. Clearing the gallbladder heat.

Insomnia due to Insufficiency of Gallbladder-qi

Symptoms. Vexation and insomnia, palpitation, mental derangement, etc.

Pathogenesis. Caused by timidity due to deficiency of the gallbladder, mental disorder of qi.

Therapeutic Principle. Restoring qi and warming the gallbladder.

Insomnia due to upward Disturbance of Liver-fire

Symptoms. Dizziness and headache, sleeplessness, vexation, and sometimes accompanied by hypochondriac pain, bitter taste.

Pathogenesis. Resulting from emotional upset, causing upward disturbance of liver-fire, which leads to an unsteadiness of the mind.

Therapeutic Principle. Calm and suppress liver-fire.

Insomnia due to Yin Deficiency and Hyperactivity of Fire

Symptoms. Insomnia due to vexation, or aptness to wake during sleep, feverish sensation in the palms and soles, palpitation, dry mouth and throat, dizziness tinnitus, amnesia, emission, soreness of waist, red tongue.

Pathogenesis. Due to deficiency of Kidney-yin, and failure to nourish the heart, this leads to the flaring of heart-fire, which results in mental disorder due to heat, and mental restlessness.

Therapeutic Principle. Nourish yin to reduce pathogenic fire.

Inspecting Eyes to Differentiate Injury

It is a diagnostic method to detect location and nature of injury on the basis of observing changes of collateral branch of the large meridian and the location of ecchymosis conjunctiva.

Inspection by Visual Observing

It is one of the four methods of diagnosis including observing the patient's mental state, facial expression, complexion, physical condition, skin color, all parts on the body, tongue and coating, and the changes of urine, stool and other excreta to obtain information for establishing a diagnosis. Generally, doctor uses his eyes to observe the mental state and inspection of the tongue to make a diagnosis.

Inspection of Appearance

It is one of the methods in observation. Doctors observe mentality, expression, facial complexion, etc, to learn about the prosperity or decline of vital-qi, cold and heat, deficiency and excess, etc.

Inspection of Skin Color

It is one of inspections. Doctors evaluate the patient's illness by observing the facial color and luster of the patient. The doctor should master the diagnostic significance of the five colors, combining it with shade of color, moist or withered, bright or dim, and diffusion.

Inspection of Tongue

It is one of inspections. It refers to the method of observing the changes of the texture and color of the tongue in making diagnosis of diseases. The tongue is closely related to viscera. The doctor can know the pathological changes and the prosperity and decline of viscera, qi, blood, yin, and yang from tongue picture. The different parts of the tongue correspond to various internal organs and can reflect the pathological changes respectively. The doctor must combine the theory with the observation from other symptoms to correct conclusion.

Insufficiency and Cold of Bladder

Symptoms. Light-colored urine, frequent micturition or dripping of urine, incontinence of urine and enuresis.

Pathogenesis. Commonly results from the impairment of the urinary bladder functions, or deficiency of the kidney-yang.

Therapeutic Principle. Warming and recuperating the kidney-yang.

Insufficiency of Heart-yang

Symptoms. Severe palpitation, pain of the heart, shortness of breath, spontaneous perspiration, coldness of the body and limbs, pale mouth and tongue, pale and moist fur.

Pathogenesis. Insufficiency of yang in the body, misusing the therapy of purgation and diaphoresis or overexertion.

Therapeutic Principle. Warming and recuperating the heart-yang.

Intense Heat in both Qi and Blood Systems

Symptoms. High fever, thirst, coma and delirium, eruptions, or even hematemesis and epistaxis, deep red tongue with yellow coating and soft rapid pulse.

Pathogenesis. Due to persistence of excessive pathogenic heat in qi system together with appearance of intense heat in blood system.

Therapeutic Principle. Clearing away the heat from both qi and blood systems.

Intense Stimulation

In acupuncture, select a thicker needle and the manipulation of a large range of lifting and thrusting and twirling as well as rotating. In moxibustion, select a larger moxa cone and apply moxibustion to the point for longer time or more units of moxa cones. The method is suitable for patients whose pathological condition is acute and physical condition is strong.

Interdependence between Yin and Yang

Yin and yang depend on each other for existence. They enjoy mutual support. The physiological or pathogenic relationships between zang and fu, qi and blood, function and substance are explained with the theory of interdependence between yin and yang in TCM.

Inter-follow of Mindwill and Qi

The Qigong practitioner uses his own mind activities to influence the respiration and to go with the circulation of the internal qi so as to achieve coordination of qi and breathing and the mindwill, and finally reach the unification of mindwill and qi.

Interior Cold

Symptoms. Cold and pain in the stomach and abdomen, vomiting of watery fluid, loose stools, copious clear urine, chilly, cold limbs, pale complexion.

Pathogenesis. Usually caused by insufficiency of yang-qi or cold evil directly attacks the internal organs.

Therapeutic Principle. Warming the middle-energizer and removing cold.

Interior Deficiency

Symptoms. Short breath, palpitation, listlessness, dizziness, tinnitus, poor appetite, limb fatigue, etc.

Pathogenesis. Deficiency and consumption of qi, blood, yin and yang in zang-fu organs.

Therapeutic Principle. Restoring qi and strengthening the body resistance.

Interior Excess Syndrome

It refers to the syndrome characterized by high fever, abdominal distention, constipation, etc. caused by two pathogenesis, and should be treated by varying principles separately.

1. **Pathogenesis.** Caused by exogenous pathogen, which enters the inside as heat and is accumulated in the intestine and stomach.

   Therapeutic Principle. Relaxing the bowels with demulcents.

2. **Pathogenesis.** Caused by stagnation of phlegm and blood stasis, indigestion, and parasitic infestation.

   Therapeutic Principle. Eliminating the phlegm, regulating qi to promote blood circulation, promoting digestion, relieving dyspepsia, and killing parasites, etc.

Interior Fire

It is divided into excess and deficiency type.

1. The excess type

   Symptoms. Aphtha, dysphoria, bloodshot eyes, thirst relieved by drinking, yellow phlegm, or phlegm with pus and blood.

   Therapeutic Principle. Clearing excessive in zang-fu organs.

2. The deficiency type

   Symptoms. The syndrome usually located on a certain part of the body, such as toothache, pharynx pain, dryness of the mouth and lips, hectic fever and flushing of zygomatic region.

   Therapeutic Principle. Nourishing yin to reduce fire.

Interior Mammary Abscess

It refers to the acute inflammation of the breast during pregnancy, reddish, swelling, heat, and pain. It is difficult to heal up if ulcerous.

Pathogenesis. Mostly caused by sufficient fetal-qi, and stagnation and steaming of pathogenic heat during the third trimester of pregnancy.

Interior Pathogen

It refers to the pathogen, which attacks the interior of the body.

Pathogenesis. The injury of sexual strain and emotional depression, thereafter interior pathogen brings on disease from the inside.

Interior Water

Symptoms. Edema of the face and body, dysuria and deep pulse, etc.

Therapeutic Principle. Facilitating the flow of the lung-qi and inducing diuresis.

Intermenstrual Period Metrostaxis

Symptoms. Cyclic scanty bleeding from the vagina during intermenstruum.

Pathogenesis. Mostly caused by yin asthenia, dampness-heat, or blood stasis.

Therapeutic Principle. Restoring qi, or clearing away heat, or eliminating dampness, or removing stasis according to the pathogeny.

Intermittent Fever due to Retention of Food

Symptoms. Hunger with inability to eat, distention and fullness in epigastrium, enlarged abdomen and nausea, alternate chills and fever, or acute abdominal pain.

Pathogenesis. Caused by injury of the stomach-qi due to hunger and overeating or irregular food and drink.

Intermittent Fever of Deficiency Type

Symptoms. Moderate chills and fever, fatigue, poor appetite, spontaneous sweating.

Pathogenesis. Usually caused by the vital-qi of the body is weak, or patient's prolonged intermittent fever leading to impairment of original qi.

Therapeutic Principle. Nourishing body resistance and supplementing deficiency, or supplementing and preventing simultaneously.

Intermittent High Fever

Symptoms. Fever without chills, restlessness, chest tightness and nausea, etc.

Therapeutic Principle. Expelling pathogenic factors from exterior of the body and activating yang, and clearing away heat and producing body fluid.

Intermittent Menstruation

Symptoms. Women with intermittent menstruation with a few drops of the amount of menses, usually occurring three or four times a month, accompanied by green-yellowish complexion, occasional pain in the abdomen, and alternate chills and fever, etc.

Pathogenesis. Mostly caused by visceral dysfunction due to attack of pathogenic wind and stagnation of the liver-qi.

Therapeutic Principle. Soothing the liver, regulating the circulating of qi, and tonifying blood to expel wind.

Intermittent Pulse

It refers to the slow and weak pulse with missing beats at regular intervals. The missing beats cannot return spontaneously and last for a long time. This condition is mostly found in heart diseases, being seized with terror, traumatic injuries in serious case, etc.

Intermuscular Needling

Method. Needling deep insertion into muscular striae and interspace of muscles.

Indication. Aching pain of muscles, etc.

Internal Diabetes

Symptoms. Polyuria with thick suspension in the urine, absence of thirst, asthenia, shortness of breath, impotence etc.

Pathogenesis. Caused by impaired kidney and pathogenic heat.

Therapeutic Principle. Nourishing yin and clearing away heat, tonifying the kidney and strengthening absorption.

Internal Ear (MA)

An ear point.

Location. On the 6th section of the ear.

Indication. Tinnitus, hypoacusis, auditory vertigo.

Internal Genitalia (MA)

An ear point.

Location. At the medial 1/3 of the triangular fossa.

Function. Supporting yang and replenishing vital essence, regulating menstruation by adjusting the flow of qi and blood.

Indication. Pain, irregular menstruation, leukorrhagia, essential uterine bleeding, seminal emission, premature ejaculation, prostatitis, etc.

Internal Hemorrhoids

Symptoms. Hematochezia, and prolapse of hemorrhoids, accompanied by anal discomfort.

Pathogenesis. Caused by the downward pressure on the large intestine due to the original deficiency of zang-fu organs, improper diet and dryness-heat in the interior.

Therapeutic Principle. Removing pathogenic heat from blood, replenishing yin essence and moisturizing the viscera, dispelling wind and removing dampness by diuresis. Ligature and necrotizing therapy for hemorrhoids, etc. can be applied in the external treatment.

Internal Injury

It possesses two implications: 1. It refers to pathogenic factors impairing the function of internal organs such as emotional strain, improper diet, exhaustion and intemperance in sexual life. 2. It refers to the disease caused by the pathogenic factors mentioned above, oppositting to affection by exopathogen. It also refers to injury by a strike, fall, heavy load, or other factors without breaking the skin but impairing zang-fu organs, meridians and collaterals, and qi and blood.

Internal Injury due to Overstrain

Symptoms. Fatigue, tidal fever, night sweating, feverish sensation in palms and soles, deafness and tinnitus, xerophthalmia with photophobia, numbness of the limbs, dry mouth and sore throat, etc.

Pathogenesis. Mostly caused by injury of essence and blood due to over drink, excess of sexual intercourse, and overstrain or consumptive illness.

Therapeutic Principle. Nourishing yin and clearing away heat.

Internal Nose (MA)

An ear point.

Location. On the lower half of the medial aspect of the tragus.

Function. Soothe and dredge the nasal cavity.

Indication. Rhinitis, nasosinusitis, epistaxis.

Internal Obstruction and External Exhaustion

Symptoms. Sudden dropping of high fever, and pale complexion, clammy limbs, excessive sweating, etc. It is a dangerous syndrome.

Pathogenesis. Caused by excessive pathogens and deficiency of vital qi, over perspiration and excessive excretion occasioning the abrupt loss of yin fluid during febrile disease.

Therapeutic Principle. Removing heat from the heart to restore consciousness, and giving emergency treatment to collapse.

Interrelation of Zang and Fu

Referring to the relation and influence among zang and fu organs. The coordination of zang and fu of human body represents the mutual supply and transformation relations between yin and yang, and between exterior and interior. Meridian of zang organs linking with fu and fu's meridian with zang. The coordinations of zang and fu are: heart coordinating with small intestine, lung with large intestine, liver with gallbladder, spleen with stomach, kidney with urinary bladder, pericardium with tri-energizer.

Interrogation of Chest and Abdomen

It refers to inquiring about pathological changes of chest, hypochondrium, and gastric cavity. The doctor should pay more attention to the site of pathologic change, nature of pain, whether liking or disliking cold and warm, accompanying symptoms, etc. Inquiry about chest is to comprehend the pathologic change in the heart and lung. Inquiry about hypochondrium is to comprehend the pathologic change in the liver and gallbladder. Inquiry about gastric cavity is to comprehend the pathologic change in the kidney, stomach intestine, urinary bladder, uterus, Vital and Front Middle Meridians.

Interrogation of Cold and Heat

It refers to inquiring about the fever and aversion to cold of the patient. The doctor can differentiate interior and exterior, deficiency and excess, qi and blood, yin and yang of an illness. There are four clinical cases: aversion to cold and fever, only cold without fever, only fever cold and alternate attacks of chills and fever.

Interrogation of Diet and Taste

It refers to inquiring about the changes of diet, likes and dislikes of taste including thirst and drinking water, appetite and the amount of diet, abnormal taste in mouth, etc. of the patient. Thereby the doctor can learn the function of the spleen and stomach, diagnose progress and regression of illness.

Interrogation of Ear and Eye

It refers to requiring about pathogenic changes of the ears and eyes. The doctor should pay attention to whether there is tinnitus, deafness, ear pain, and reappearance of sounds, itching and pain of the eyes. They reflect pathogenic changes of liver and kidney.

Interrogation of Head and Body

It refers to inquiring about the pains of the head and the body, because headache and pantalgia are the common symptoms. According to duration, location, and nature of pain, duration of relieving pain or pain with or without cold and heat, etc., the doctor can differentiate yin and yang, exterior and interior, cold and heat, insufficiency and excess.

Interrogation of Onset of Diseases

It refers to inquiring about the time of onset, cause, course, treatment, characteristics and changes of the main symptoms. It is of great significance to learn the law of the nature, onset, development and changes of a disease and to guide differentiation of syndromes and treatment.

Interrogation of Sleep

It refers to inquiring about the abnormal states of sleep of the patient in order to learn the circulation of defensive energy, prosperity and decline of yin and yang.

Interrogation of Sweating

It refers to inquiring about sweating. By the method doctor can differentiate pathogenic and vital contention, deficiency and excess, interior and exterior, and yin and yang of an illness.

Interrogation of Urination and Defecation

It refers to inquiring about the patient's stool and urine. By this method the doctor can know digestion function and metabolism, and differentiate cold and heat, deficiency and excess of an illness.

Intestinal Colic in Child

Symptoms. Acute abdominal pain, bending loins and cry accompanied by cold feed, blue lips, sweat on forehead, etc.

Pathogenesis. Usually caused by debility, and stagnating cold in the small intestines.

Therapeutic Principle. Warming middle-energizer to promote the flow of qi.

Intestinal Laxation due to Protracted Diarrhea

It possessed two implications:

1. It refers to the syndrome of general chronic diarrhea.

   Symptoms. Diarrhea with indigested food, dim complexion, lassitude, cold limbs, tastelessness and anorexia, etc.

   Pathogenesis. Usually caused by protracted diarrhea or erroneous administration of purgatives resulting in the deficiency of the spleen and stomach, sinking of qi of middle-energizer, the failure of consolidation and absorption.

   Therapeutic Principle. Elevating the spleen-qi, and puncturing the points of Zusanli (S 36), Neiting (S 44), and Tianshu (S 25), etc.

2. It refers to the syndrome of laxation with rectal mucosa.

   Pathogenesis. Caused by chronic diarrhea.

   Therapeutic Principle. Invigorating qi to consolidate intestine, and elevating the spleen-qi and astringing to arrest diarrhea.

Intestine Morbidity

Symptoms. Dysuria, abdominal fullness, lienteric diarrhea.

Pathogenesis. Dysfunction of the large and small intestines.

Therapeutic Principle. Inducting urine and strengthening the function of the spleen.

Intolerable Headache

Symptoms. Severe headache radiating to the brain and the top of the head, hands and feet cold, extending to elbows and knees, etc.

Pathogenesis. Caused by the invasion of pathogen into the brain.

Therapeutic Principle. Strengthening yang-qi, refreshing the brain, calming and absorbing the kidney-qi.

Intolerance of Cold due to Yang Deficiency

Symptoms. Intolerance to cold, cold hand and foot, spontaneously sweating, etc.

Pathogenesis. Caused by deficiency and weakness of yang-qi, failing to warm muscles, skin and hair.

Therapeutic Principle. Warming and exerting yang-qi.

Intoxication due to Misuse of Drugs

It refers to the poisoning effect of drug administration. It is mainly caused by misuse of poison medicines, mistaking drugs, taking the unqualified or deteriorated medicines, and taking over-dose of medicines, etc.

Intradermal Needle

A small needling instrument specially made of wire of stainless steel, embedded beneath the skin. They are divided into granular intradermal needle and intradermal needle of thumb-tack shape.

Inula Flower   ⊛ I-3

It is the capitulum of Inula britannica L. var. chinensis (Rupr.) Reg. (Compositae).

Effect. Dispelling phlegm, inducing diuresis and descending the adverse rising of qi to arrest vomiting.

Indication. Cough and asthma due to accumulation of phlegm and fluid in the lung, the feeling of stuffiness and fullness in the chest caused by retention of phlegm and fluid, eructation, vomiting, etc.

Invasion by Cold after Delivery

Symptoms. Chills with fever, headache, anhidrosis or sweating.

Pathogenesis. Generally due to a severe deficiency of qi and blood leading to the failure of superficial qi to protect the body and allowing an invasion of cold evils.

Therapeutic Principle. Strengthen the body energy and clear the pathogenic factors.

Invasion by Wind

It possesses three implications:

1. A mild case with exogenous wind evil affecting the defensive energy, which is circulating superficially in the body.

   Symptoms. Aversion to cold, stuffy and running nose, sneezing and discomfort all over, etc.

   Therapeutic Principle. Dispelling wind and relieving exterior syndrome.

2. Syndrome of exogenous febrile disease due to attack of small intestine and Bladder Meridians by wind.

   Symptoms. Aversion to wind, spontaneous perspiration, fever, etc.

   Therapeutic Principle. Regulating defense system and nutrient system.

3. Exopathic febrile disease caused by the invasion of pathogenic wind.

   Symptoms. Aversion to wind, fever, heat exhaling, discomfort all over, etc.

   Therapeutic Principle. Dispelling wind, relieving exterior syndrome and clearing away heat.

Invasion by Wind after Delivery

Symptoms. Nasal obstruction, thin nasal discharge, spontaneous perspiration, aversion to wind.

Pathogenesis. Mostly caused by invasion from wind evil due to deficiency of qi and blood after delivery.

Therapeutic Principle. Support body energy to eliminate evils.

Invasion of Blood Stasis into Spine

Symptoms. Numbness of body, or allergy, or prickly pain, or burning pain and even flaccidity.

Pathogenesis. The entry of blood stasis into spine as a result of injury of lumbar muscle and tendon.

Therapeutic Principle. Promoting blood circulation and remove blood stasis, relieving pain by regulating qi.

Invasion of Exterior Pathogen Invading Interior

It refers to a pathogenic change of the internal invasion of pathogenic factor from the exterior into the interior due to external invasion by pathogens and weakened body resistance or improper therapy.

Invasion of Hyperactive Liver-qi

Symptoms. In the case of upward drive of the hyperactive liver qi: dizziness, headache, fullness and pain of the chest and hypochondrium, flushed complexion, tinnitus, deafness, and even hematemesis. In the case of transverse drive: abdominal distention and pain, belching and regurgitation, and irregular menstruation.

Pathogenesis. A morbid state of upward or transverse invasion of the hyperactive liver-qi resulting from stagnation of the liver-qi or emotional depression and anger.

Therapeutic Principle. Calming or soothing the liver.

Invasion of Large Intestine by Heat

It refers to the acute and febrile diarrhea.

Symptoms. Abdominal pain, burning sensation of the anus, scanty dark urine.

Pathogenesis. Dysfunction of transportation due to invasion of large intestine by heat.

Therapeutic Principle. Clearing away heat and toxic material, alleviating pain and removing dampness.

Involuntary Contraction due to Cold

It refers to the contraction of meridians and collaterals, spasm of tendons and muscles, and sluggish circulation of qi and blood when body is attacked by evil cold. The symptoms are pain, anhidrosis, etc.

Irregular Menstruation due to Kidney Deficiency

Symptoms. Irregular thin and pale menses, accompanied by dim complexion, dizziness, tinnitus, lassitude loin and legs, nocturnal polyuria, etc.

Pathogenesis. Caused by exhaust and impair the essence and blood, and weakened kidney-qi due to sexual intercourse, pregnancy and labor, etc., which lead to accumulation and flooding of stagnant blood in the uterus.

Therapeutic Principle. Invigorating the kidney to regulate menstruation.

Irregular Menstruation due to Stagnation of Liver-qi

Symptoms. Irregular menstrual cycle; profuse or scanty menstrual flow; purplish and dark in color; distending pain in the breast, chest and hypochondrium, etc.

Pathogenesis. Mostly caused by dysfunction of the liver due to emotional depression and the disorder of qi leading to the disorder of blood circulation and irregularity of the uterus in storing blood.

Therapeutic Principle. Soothe the liver and regulate the circulation of qi.

Irregular Red Vein

Symptoms. Red veins, in different thickness and density, dotting the white vertically and horizontally. It is accompanied by astringent eyes, photophobia, and plenty of secretion and tears.

Pathogenesis. Usually caused by long suffering from trachoma, or long stimulation by smoke-dust and sand blown by wind, and overuse of eyes leading to stagnation of superficial venules of the white.

Therapeutic Principle. Eliminating pathogenic factors and dissipating blood stasis.

Irritable Feverish Sensation in Chest

Pathogenesis. Caused by uprising of the heart-fire, excessive heat in the lung and stomach, deficiency of yin-fluid and blood, the attack of exopathogen evil into the interior.

Irritated Epiphora with Cold Tear

Symptoms. Marked by dacryorrhea in wind, dizziness, tinnitus, soreness and weakness of the waist and knees.

Pathogenesis. Usually caused by deficiency of both the liver and kidney, insufficiency of essence and blood, invasion of external wind, malnutrition of the eye, or obstruction of lacrimal passage.

Therapeutic Principle. Tonifying the liver and kidney.

Irritated Epiphora with Warm Tear

Symptoms. Marked by dacryorrhea in wind, conjunctival congestion, xenophthalmia and ophthalmalgia photophobia, aversion to heat, a flushing face, dry pharynx.

Pathogenesis. Usually caused by invation of external wind-heat, excessive heat in the liver and lung or yin deficiency of the liver and kidney and the flaring up of deficiency fire.

Therapeutic Principle. For the external wind-heat type, expelling wind and clearing away heat; for the asthenia yin causing excessive pyrexia type, nourishing yin and calming fire.

Itching and Pain in Anus

It refers to itch and pain in the anus.

Pathogenesis. Mostly caused by damp-heat in the large intestines, and attack of exopathogenic wind or disturbance of parasites.

Itching due to Wind

It is one type of itching.

Symptoms. Severe skin pruritus, short duration of illness, paroxysm, and occurrence or deterioration by attack of wind and heat.

Pathogenesis. Mostly caused by attack of pathogenic evil wind, stagnated heat in the skin, and incoordination of qi and blood.

Therapeutic Principle. Clearing away heat, expelling wind and removing heat from the blood.

J

Jamaica False Valerin Herb

It is the whole herb or root of Stachytarpheta jamaicensis (L.) Vahl (Verbenaceae).

Effect. Enhancing diuresis, releasing blood stasis, heat and detoxicating.

Indication. Heat stranguria and gonorrhea, rheumatic arthralgia, traumatic injuries, ecchymoma and swelling pain, swollen and sore throat, and swelling and pain of carbuncle.

Japan Clover Herb

It is the whole herb of Kummerowia striata (Thunb.) Schindl. (Leguminosae).

Effect. Removing dampness, heat and detoxicating, nourishing the spleen.

Indication. Fever owing to common cold, summer vomiting and diarrhea, malaria, dysentery, hepatitis, heat stranguria and gonorrhea.

Japanese Ardisia Herb

It is the whole plant of Ardisia japonica (Hornst.) Bl. (Myrsinaceae).

Effect. Removing dampness, blood stasis, and cough to dispel phlegm, enhancing diuresis and blood circulation.

Indication. Cough with profuse phlegm, jaundice owing to damp-heat pathogen, edema, traumatic injuries, rheumatic arthralgia and abdominal pain owing to amenorrhea.

Japanese Butterbur Rhizome

It is the rhizome of Petasites japonicus (Sieb. et Zucc) F. Schmidt (Compositae).

Effect. Detoxicating, removing blood stasis, swelling and pain.

Indication. Tonsillitis, suppurative infections on the body surface, snake bite, traumatic injuries, etc.

Japanese Buttercup Herb
⊛ J-1

It is the whole herb of Ranunculus japonicus Thunb (Ranunculaceae) with root.

Effect. Removing pain, swelling, jaundice, asthma and preventing attack of malaria.

Indication. Arthroncus of knees, toothache, migraine, rheumatic arthralgia, malaria, sarcoptidosis, tinea, and stomachache, etc.

Japanese Camellia Flower

It is the flower of Camellia japonica L. (Theaceae).

Effect. Relieving heat from blood, removing blood stasis and swelling, inducing hemostasis.

Indication. Hematemesis, epistaxis, metrorrhagia, fresh-bloody stool, dysentery with bloody stool, stranguria complicated by hematuria, traumatic injuries, scald, etc.

Japanese Cayratia Herb

It is the whole herb or root of Cayratia japonica (Thunb.) Gagnep. (Vitaceae).

Effect. Removing swelling, heat and enhancing diuresis, detoxicating.

Indication. Furuncles, swellings, carbuncles, sores, parotitis, erysipelas, numbness due to pathogenic wind-dampness, jaundice, dysentery, hematuria, cloudy urine, etc.

Japanese Climbing Fern Spore

It is the ripe spore of Lygodium japonicum (Thunb.) Sw. (Lygodiaceae).

Effect. Enhancing diuresis and treating stranguria.

Indication. Stranguria owing to heat, stranguria from urolithiasis, stranguria with hematuria and stranguria marked by chyluria.

Japanese Cudweed Herb

It is the whole herb of Gnaphalium japonicum Thunb. (Compositae).

Effect. Removing exterior syndromes, clearing away heat, enhancing acuity of vision and inducing diuresis.

Indication. Common cold, cough, headache, sore throat, bloodshot eyes and dysopia, dysuria, stranguria with turbid urine, leukorrhagia, suppurative infections on the skin, such as furuncles and boils, etc.

Japanese Dock Root

It is the root of Rumex japonicus Houtt. (Polygonaceae).

Effect. Releasing heat from the blood, ceasing bleeding, killing parasites and curing tinea.

Indication. Bleeding owing to heat and blood, and scabies, chronic eczema, etc.

Japanese Eurya Twig and Leaf

It is the branch and leaf or fruit of Eurya japonica Thunb. (Theaceae).

Effect. Removing wind, dampness and swelling, and ceasing bleeding.

Japanese Felt Fern Rhizome

It is the rhizome of Pyrrosia lingua (Thunb.) Farw. (Polypodiaceae) and many other species of the same genus.

Effect. Enhancing diuresis, removing stranguria, flatulence, consumptive fever and ceasing bleeding.

Indication. Stranguria, qi distention in the chest and diaphragmatic region, hematemesis and traumatic bleeding.

Japanese Gala Rhizomengal

It is the rhizome or the whole herb of Alpinia japonica Mig. (Zingiberaceae).

Effect. Warming the middle-energizer, removing cold, wind and enhancing blood circulation.

Indication. Gastric and abdominal cold pain, arthralgia and myalgia owing to pathogenic wind-dampness, hematemesis owing to overstrain, traumatic injuries and irregular menstruation.

Japanese Hop Herb

It is the whole plant of Humulus scandens (Lour.) Merr. (Moraceae).

Effect. Removing heat, blood stasis and toxic substances, and promoting diuresis.

Indication. Stranguria, dysuria, malaria, diarrhea, dysentery, pulmonary tuberculosis, pulmonary abscess, pneumonia, pellagra, hemorrhoids, noxious carbuncles and scrofula.

Japanese Maesa Root

It is the root and leaf of Maesa japonica (Thunb.) Moritzi (Myrsinaceae).

Effect. Removing wind, epidemic toxin and swelling.

Indication. Headache owing to common cold and dizziness.

Japanese Metaplexis Herb or Root

It is the whole herb or root of Metaplexis japonica (Thunb.) Mak. (Asclepiadaceae).

Effect. Tonifying the essence and energy, stimulating milk secretion and detoxication.

Indication. Consumptive disease, internal injury resulting from overstrain, impotence, leukorrhea, hypogalactia, erysipelas and swelling carbuncles.

Japanese Pagoda Tree Bark

It is the bark or root phloem of Sophora japonica L. (Leguminosae).

Effect. Removing wind, dampness, swelling and pain.

Indication. Physical rigidity, skin numbness and hypoesthesia, aphthae resulting from febrile disease, ulcerative gingivitis, inflammation of the throat, hematochezia, cellulitis, hemorrhoid, unhealing ulcer, pruritus genitalium, scald bum, etc.

Japanese Plum Fruit

It is the fruit of prunus salicina Lindl. (Rosaceae).
Effect. Removing heat from the liver, enhancing the production of body fluid and inducing diuresis.
Indication. Hectic fever owing to consumption, diabetes and ascitic fluid.

Japanese Plum Leaf

It is the leaf of Prunus salicina Lindl. (Rosaceae).
Effect. Removing heat, arrest convulsion, and enhancing diuresis.
Indication. High-fever in children, epilepsy due to terror, edema and incised wound.

Japanese Plum Root

It is the root of Prunus salicina Lindl. (Rosaceae).
Effect. Removing heat and detoxicating.
Indication. Diabetes, stranguria, dysentery, erysipelas and toothache.

Japanese Plum Root-bark

It is the root phloem of Prunus salicina lindl. (Rosaceae).
Effect. Removing heat and enhancing the adverse flow of qi downward.
Indication. Diabetes, vexation, sensation of gas rashing reversed flow of qi, leukorrhagia and toothache

Japanese Premna Root

It is the root of Premna microphylla Turcz. (Verbenaceae).
Effect. Removing heat and detoxicating.
Indication. Malaria, traumatic injuries, toothache owing to wind fire, burn, etc.

Japanese Premna Stem or Leaf

It is the stem and leaf of Premna microphylla Turcz. (Verbenaceae).
Effect. Removing heat and swelling.
Indication. Malaria, diarrhea, carbuncles, furuncles, poisoning swellings, traumatic bleeding, etc.

Japanese Rose Flower

It is the flower of Rosa multiflora Thunb. (Rosaceae).
Effect. Removing summer-heat, adjusting the stomach and ceasing bleeding.
Indication. Hemoptysis owing to summer-heat, thirst, diarrhea, dysentery, malaria, wounds.

Japanese Rose Root

It is the root of Rosa multiflora Thunb. (Rosaceae).
Effect. Releasing heat, dampness and wind, and enhancing blood circulation and detoxicating.
Indication. Pulmonary abscess, diabetes, dysentery, arthritis, paralysis, hematemesis, epistaxis, hemafecia, frequent micturition, enuresis, irregular menstruation, traumatic injuries, furuncle.

Japanese Snakegourd Fruit

It is the fruit of Trichosanthes cucumeroides (Ser). Maxim. (Cucurbitaceae).
Effect. Removing heat, blood stasis, enhancing the production of body fluid and lactation.
Indication. Diabetes, jaundice, regurgitation of food from the stomach, amenorrhea, lack of lactation, subcutaneous swelling, etc.

Japanese Snakegourd Root

It is the root of Trichosanthes cucumeroides (Ser.) Maxim. (Cucurbitaceae).
Effect. Removing heat and blood stasis, and enhancing the production of body fluid and blood circulation.

Indication. Extreme thirst due to febrile disease, jaundice, constipation owing to accumulation of heat, dysuria, amenorrhea, masses in the abdomen, carbuncles, sores and other pyogenic skin diseases, etc.

Japanese Snakegourd Seed

It is the seed of Trichosanthes cucumeroides (Ser.) Maxim. (Cucurbitaceae).

Effect. Remove heat to cool the blood.

Indication. Hematemesis owing to the consumptive lung disease, jaundice, dysentery, hematochezia, etc.

Japanese Sophora Flower

⊛ **J-2**

It is the flower-bud of Sophora japonica L. (Leguminosae).

Effect. Releasing pathogenic heat from blood and ceasing bleeding, clearing away liver heat and lowering blood pressure.

Indication. Different bleeding, especially hematuria and hemafecia, hypertension.

Japanese Stephania Root

It is the root or stem leaf of Stephania japonica (Thunb.) Miers (Menispermaceae).

Effect. Removing heat, wind and dampness, detoxicating.

Indication. Malaria, dysentery, rheumatic arthralgia, edema, stranguria with turbid urine, swollen and sore throat, suppurative infections on the skin, etc.

Japanese St. Johns Wort

It is the whole herb of Hypericum japonicum Thunb. (Guttiferae).

Effect. Removing swelling and heat, enhancing diuresis and detoxicating.

Indication. Jaundice owing to damp-heat, dysentery, infantile convulsion, malnutrition, tonsillitis, acute appendicitis, abscess and snake bite.

Japanese Thistle Herb

It is the root and whole plant of Cirsium japonicum DC. (Compositae).

Effect. Ceasing bleeding by removing pathogenic heat from the blood and curing carbuncles by removing blood stasis, promoting diuresis, lowering blood pressure.

Indication. Hemoptysis, epistaxis, metrorrhagia, metrostaxis, hematuria, and sores, carbuncles and other pyogenic skin diseases.

Japanese Wormwood Herb

It is the whole herb of Artemisia japonica Thunb. (Compositae).

Effect. Enhancing diaphoresis, removing heat and killing parasites.

Indication. Fever owing to common cold, phthisical cough, tidal fever, infantile malnutrition with fever, malaria, aphthae, scabies, tinea and eczema.

Japanese Xylosma Bark

It is the bark of Xylosma japonicum (Walp.) A. Gray. (Flacourticeae).

Effect. Removing dampness and heat.

Indication. Jaundice, scrofula and noxious carbuncles.

Japanese Yam

It is the rhizome of Dioscorea nipponica Mak (Dioscoreaceae).

Effect. Enhancing digestion, diuresis and blood circulation, relaxing muscles, and removing phlegm, clearing away toxic materials and relieving swelling.

Indication. Rheumatic arthralgia, chronic tracheal catarrh, indigestion and subcutaneous swelling.

Jaundice

Symptoms. Yellowish body, eyes and urine.

Pathogenesis. Mostly resulting from seasonal exopathogen, improper diet, damp-heat or cold-damp blocking in the middle-energizer, leading to the bile to overflow the skin of the whole body, including yang jaundice, yin jaundice and acute jaundice, etc.

Jaundice Disease

It is one of thirty-six types of jaundice.

Symptoms. Bluish complexion round the mouth, aversion to listen, or psychosis-like acts, etc.

Therapeutic Principle. Removing the frightening and calming the mind.

Jaundice due to Accumulation of Stagnant Blood

Symptoms. Yellowish body, amnesia, mass or distention in the chest and hypochondrium, fullness and hardness in the lower abdomen, diuresis and black stool.

Pathogenesis. Owing to the combination of blood stasis and heat-evil remaining in the lower-energizer, blood stasis stagnated in the liver and gallbladder.

Therapeutic Principle. Enhancing the blood circulation, releasing blood stasis, heat and the depressed liver-qi.

Jaundice due to Blockage of Bile Excretion

Referring to jaundice owing to abevacuation of bile.

Symptoms. Yellow-greenish body and eye, fullness in the chest.

Pathogenesis. Resulting from sudden fear, bile excretion due to impairment of the gallbladder-qi.

Therapeutic Principle. Calming the mind and allaying excitement, and arresting discharge.

Jaundice due to Blood Retention

Symptoms. Yellow skin all of over body, fullness and rigidity in the lower abdomen, and mania, etc.

Pathogenesis. Retention of stagnant heat in the interior and the cholorrhagia.

Therapeutic Principle. Removing the stagnated heat by catharsis.

Jaundice due to Cold-dampness

Symptoms. Yellow-brown discoloration of the skin and sclera, anorexia, oppressed feeling in the stomach and abdominal distention, shapeless stool and oliguria.

Pathogenesis. Due to the accumulation of pathogenic cold and dampness, the deficiency of spleen-yang and the cholorrhagia.

Therapeutic Principle. Warming the middle-energizer and removing dampness.

Jaundice due to Damp-heat

Symptoms. Jaundice, fever with chills, heaviness sensation in the limbs, dark urine or difficulty in urination, etc.

Pathogenesis. Owing to the heat in the spleen and stomach with the invasion of exopathic wind-dampness, the obstruction of striae of skin, muscles and viscera and the retention of damp-heat in the interior.

Therapeutic Principle. Removing dampness and heat from both exterior and interior.

Jaundice due to Febrile Disease

Pathogenesis. Due to the exterior syndrome of febrile disease in the exterior with the excess of damp-heat in the interior which steams the liver and gallbladder, leading to the cholorrhagia.

Therapeutic Principle. Removing dampness and heat.

Jaundice due to Liver-fire

Symptoms. Yellowish sclera, dysphoria, restlessness, anger with higher voice and mania like alcohol drunk, etc.

Pathogenesis. Due to excessiveness of the liver-fire, disturbance of mind by phlegm-fire.

Therapeutic Principle. Releasing fire from the liver and phlegm, calming the mind.

Jaundice due to Sexual Intemperance

Symptoms. Yellowish skin and sclera, fever of the sole and palm, aversion to cold, dark forehead, spasmodic distention and fullness of the lower abdomen, etc.

Pathogenesis. Usually owing to the overwork or sexual intemperance.

Therapeutic Principle. Nourishing the kidney to remove stasis.

Jaundice due to Stagnation of Liver-qi

Symptoms. Sudden vomiting, fever, general aching, yellow complexion and eyes after abatement of fever, etc.

Pathogenesis. Due to emotional depression, the stagnation of the liver-qi and the failure of the liver to distribute.

Therapeutic Principle. Smoothing the liver, adjusting the circulation of qi, removing dampness by diuresis and invigorating the spleen.

Jaundice with Heart Involved

Symptoms. Dysphoria with smothery sensation, sweating, excessive thirst, desire for drinking and yellowish pigmentation of the skin without the sclera involved.

Pathogenesis. Due to the impairment of the spleen and stomach by improper diet, over-drinking and the internal accumulation of stagnated heat.

Therapeutic Principle. Enhancing the spleen, releasing dampness and the fire from the liver.

Jaundice with Thirst and Frequent Urination

Symptoms. Yellow body and eyes, thirst, frequent urination, emaciation with polyphagia and hypochondriac pain.

Pathogenesis. Due to improper diet, excessive drinking and impairment of overstrain.

Therapeutic Principle. Removing damp-heat and heat from the liver, and enhancing blood circulation.

Java Treebine Herb

It is the whole herb of Cissus javana DC. (Vitaceae).

Effect. Removing wind, exterior syndromes, swelling and blood stasis, and reuniting bone, muscle and ligament.

Indication. Urticaria, eczema, allergic dermatitis, fracture, lacerated wound of tendon and muscle and numbness owing to wind-dampness.

Javan Waterdropwort Herb

It is the whole herb of Oenanthe javanica (Bl.) DC. (Umbelliferae).

Effect. Removing heat and enhancing diuresis.

Indication. Dire thirst, jaundice, edema, stranguria, leukorrhagia, scrofula, mumps, etc.

Jaw (MA)

It is an auricular point.

Location. On the 3rd area of the ear lobe.

Indication. Toothache, functional disorder of mandibular articulation.

Jew's Ear

It is the daughter product of Auricularia auricula (L. ex. Hook.) Underw. (Auriculariaceae).

Effect. Releasing heat from the blood and ceasing bleeding.

Indication. Dysentery with bloody stool, blood stranguria, metrorrhagia and metrostaxis, hemorrhoid, etc.

Jiache (S 6)

It is a meridian acupuncture point.

Location. On the cheek, one finger breadth anterior and superior to the mandibular angle, in the depression where the masseter muscle is prominent.

Indication. Facial paralysis, swelling of cheek, toothache, trismus, aphonia, stiffness and pain in neck.

Method. Puncture perpendicularly 0.3-0.4 cun, or obliquely in the direction of Dicang (S 4) 0.7-0.9 cun. Perform moxibustion 5-10 minutes with warming moxibustion.

Jiafeng (Ex-B)

Referring to a set of four extra acupuncture points.

Location. On the back, at the superior and inferior ends of the medial border of the scapula, four points altogether, two on each side.

Indication. Pain in the scapula and rheumatalgia.

Method. Puncture obliquely toward the lateral side 1 cun. Perform moxibustion 3-5 moxa cones or 5-10 minutes with warming moxibustion.

Jiagen (Ex-LE)

It is a set of four extra acupuncture points.

Location. Four points on the medial and lateral corners of each big toe.

Indication. Hernia.

Method. Puncture perpendicularly 0.1 cun.

Jiaji (Ex-B 2)

It is a set of extra acupuncture points.

Location. On the low back, 17 points on each side, below the spinous processes from the lst thoracic to the 5th lumbar vertebrae, 0.5 cun lateral to the posterior midline.

Indication. Diseases related to the upper limbs: points from the first to the third thoracic vertebra. Diseases related to the thoracic area: points from the 1st to the 8th thoracic vertebra. Diseases related to the abdomen: points from the 6th thoracic vertebra to the 5th lumbar vertebrae. Diseases related to the lower limbs: points from the lst to the 5th lumbar vertebra.

Method. Puncture obliquely 0.3- 0.5 cun or tap with a plumb-blossom needle. Perform moxibustion 5-15 minutes.

Jiali (Ex-HN)

It is an extra acupuncture point.

Location. In the mouth, on the buccal mucosa, 1 cun lateral to the mouth angle.

Indication. Jaundice, pestilence, aphthae in children, ulceration of gums.

Method. Puncture obliquely 0.1-0.2 cun, or prick to bleeding.

Jianjing (G 21)

It is an acupuncture point.

Location. On the shoulder, at the midpoint of the line joining Dazhui (GV 14) and the acromion.

Indication. Rigidity and spasm of head and nape, pain in the shoulder, arm and back, cough, apoplexy.

Method. Puncture perpendicularly 0.5-0.8 cun and apply moxibustion to the point with 3-5 moxa cones or for 5-10 minutes.

Notice. Deep insertion is forbidden.

Jianju (Ex-UE)

It is an extra acupuncture point.

Location. On the flexor side of the forearm, 3.2 cun proximal to the crease of the wrist, between the tendons of the long palmar muscle and the radial flexor muscle of the wrist.

Indication. Sabre and bead string shaped scrofula.

Method. Puncture perpendicularly 0.5-1.0 cun. Perform moxibustion 3-5 moxa cones or 5-10 minutes with warm moxibustion.

Jianli (CV 11)

It is an acupuncture point.

Location. In the upper abdomen, 3 cun superior to the umbilicus on the anterior median line.

Indication. Stomachache, thoracic oppressed feeling, vomiting, edema, abdominal distention, and anorexia.

Method. Puncture perpendicularly 1-1.5 cun. (Do not apply it to the pregnant woman). Perform moxibustion 3-7 moxa cones or for 5-15 minutes.

Jianliao (TE 14)

It is an acupuncture point.

Location. In the shoulder region. Posteroinferior to the acromion in the depression about 1 cun posterior to Jianyu (LI 15).

Indication. Inability to lift the shoulder, hemiparalysis owing to apoplexy.

Method. Puncture perpendicularly 1-1.5 cun. Perform moxibustion 3-7 units of moxa cones or for 5-15 minutes.

Jianneishu (Ex-UE)

It is an extra acupuncture point.

Location. 1 cun straight below the midpoint of the line connecting Jianyu (LI 15) and Yunmen (L 2).

Indication. Difficulty to raise arms owing to pain in the shoulder and arm.

Method. Puncture perpendicularly 0.5-1.0 cun. Perform moxibustion 3-5 moxa cones or 5-10 minutes with warming moxibustion.

Jianneiyu (Ex-CA)

It is an extra acupuncture point.

Location. In the superior lateral part of the thoracic wall, 0.5 cun lateral to Zhongfu (L 1).

Indication. Pain in the shoulder and arm.

Method. Puncture perpendicularly 0.5-1 cun. Perform moxibustion 3-5 moxa cones or 5-10 minutes with worming moxibustion.

Jiansanzhen

It is an acupuncture point, including Jianyu (LI 15), Jianqian, 1 cun superior to the end of the anterior axillary fold, and Jianhou, 1.5 cun superior to the end of the posterior axillary fold.

Indication. Scapulohumeral periarthritis, brachial palsy or paralysis.

Method. Puncture perpendicularly 1-1.5 cun each.

Jianshi (P 5)

It is an acupuncture point.

Location. On the palmar surface of the forearm, 3 cun above the transverse crease of the wrist.

Indication. Cardiopalmus, cardialgia, pains of sternocostal part, stomachache,

malaria, madness, epilepsy, aphonia, pain of the elbow and arm, etc.

Method. Prick perpendicularly 0.5-1 cun. Perform moxibustion to the point for 5-10 minutes or 3-5 moxa cones.

Jianshu (Ex)

It is an extra acupuncture point.

Location. On the shoulder, on the midpoint of the line connecting Jianyu (LI 15) and Yunmen (L 2).

Indication. Difficulty to raise arm owing to pain in the shoulder and arm, etc.

Method. Puncture perpendicularly 0.5-1.0 cun. Perform moxibustion 3-5 moxa cones or 5-10 minutes with warming moxibustion.

Jiantou (Ex-UE)

It is an extra acupuncture point.

Location. In the process of the acromioclavicular joint, i.e. medial and superior to Jianyu (LI 15).

Indication. Tinea, toothache, aching pain in the shoulder and arm, periarthritis of shoulder.

Method. Puncture perpendicularly 0.5-1 cun. Perform moxibustion for 3-7 cones, or mile-warm moxibustion with moxa stick for 5-15 minutes.

Jianwaishu (SI 14)

It is a meridian acupuncture point belonging to the Small Intestine Meridian of Hand-taiyang.

Location. On the back, below the spinous process of the lst thoracic vertebra, 3 cun lateral to the posterior midline.

Indication. Pain and soreness in the shoulder and back, stiff neck, cold-pain in arm.

Method. Puncture obliquely 0.3-0.6 cun. Avoid deep needling for protecting the lung. Perform moxibustion 3-5 moxa cones or 5-15 minutes with warming moxibustion.

Jianyu (LI 15)

It is an acupuncture point.

Location. On the upper position of the deltoid muscle in the shoulder region, in the depression anterior and inferior to the acromion when the arm is abducted or raised.

Indication. Omalgia, aching of the elbow and arm, brachial palsy or paralysis, scapulohumeral periarthritis, etc.

Method. Puncture perpendicularly 1-2 cun. Perform moxibustion with 3-5 units of moxa cones or for 5-10 minutes.

Jianzhen (SI 9)

It is an acupuncture point.

Location. Posterior and inferior to the shoulder joint, 1 cun superior to the posterior axillary fold with the arm adduction.

Indication. Pain of shoulder, difficult to lift hand, pain in supraclavicular fossa, tinnitus, deafness, toothache, submental swelling, scrofula.

Method. Puncture perpendicularly 1-1.5 cun. Do not needle deeply toward the chest for fear of injuring the lung. Perform moxibustion to the point with 3-7 units of moxa cones or for 5-15 minutes.

Jianzhongshu (SI 15)

It is an acupuncture point.

Location. On the back, inferior and 2 cun lateral to the spinous process of the seventh cervical vertebra.

Indication. Sore shoulder, backache, rigid nape, cough, dyspnea, spitting of blood.

Method. Puncture obliquely 0.5-0.8 cun. Do not needle deeply toward the chest for fear of injuring the lung. Perform, moxibustion to the point with 3-5 units of moxa cones for 5-10 minutes.

Jianzhugu (Ex-B)

It is an extra acupuncture point also named Jianzhu.

Location. On the shoulder, on the high point of the process of the scapular acromion.

Indication. Scrofula, pain of shoulder and arm, difficult to raise and move hand.

Method. Perform moxibustion 3-7 moxa cones or 5-15 minutes with warming moxibustion.

Jiaosun (TE 20)

It is a meridian acupuncture point.

Location. On the head, above the ear apex. Just on the hair margin.

Indication. Swelling and pain in the ear; redness, swelling and pain of the eye; blurred vision, toothache, dry lips, rigidity of the neck, headache.

Method. Puncture subcutaneous 0.3-0.5 cun. Perform moxibustion 1-3 moxa cones of 3-5 minutes.

Jiaoxin (K 8)

It is a meridian acupuncture point.

Location. On the medial side of leg, 2 cun above Taixi (K 3) and 0.5 cun anterior to Fuliu (K 7), posterior to the medial border of the tibia.

Indication. Irregular menstruation, metrorrhagia, prolapse of uterus, diarrhea, constipation, painful and swollen testis.

Method. Puncture perpendicularly 0.8-1 cun. Perform moxibustion 3-5 moxa cones or 5-10 minutes.

Jibeiwuxue (Ex-B)

It is a set of five extra acupuncture points on the back.

Location. The first point, at the spinous process of the 2nd thoracic vertebra; the second point, at the sacral apex, lower end of sacrum; the third point, at the midpoint of the connection line between the two points mentioned above; plus further two points, five in total.

Indication. Disorder of head, epilepsy induced by terror, infantile convulsion, etc.

Method. Perform moxibustion to the five points 3-5 moxa cones for each point.

Jieji (Ex-B)

It is an extra acupuncture point.

Location. On the back, at the posterior midline, in the depression below the spinous process of the 12th thoracic vertebra.

Indication. Infantile dysentery, proctoptosis, epilepsy and indigestion, etc.

Method. Puncture obliquely 0.5-1 cun. Perform moxibustion 3-5 moxa cones or 5-15 minutes.

Jienue (Ex-CA)

It is an extra acupuncture point.

Location. On the chest, 4 cun directly below the nipple.

Indication. Malaria, pain in the chest and hypochondrium.

Method. Perform moxibustion 3-5 moxa cones or 5-10 minutes with warming moxibustion.

Jiexi (S 41)

It is a meridian acupuncture point.

Location. In the central depression of the crease between the instep of the foot and leg.

Indication. Edema in the face and hand, flushed face and eye, headache, dizziness, abdominal distention, constipation.

Method. Puncture perpendicularly 0.4-0.8 cun. Perform moxibustion 3-5 minutes with warming moxibustion.

Jigujiezhong (Ex-B)

It is an extra acupuncture point.

Location. On the posterior midline, at the vertebra, with the same level as nipples.

Indication. Cough.

Method. Perform moxibustion 3-5 moxa cones or 5-10 minutes with warming moxibustion.

Jijupikuaixue (Ex-B)

It is an extra acupuncture point.

Location. On the lower back, below the spinous process of the lst lumbar vertebra, 4 cun lateral to the posterior midline.

Indication. Abdominal masses, etc.

Method. Puncture perpendicularly 0.5-1 cun. Perform moxibustion 3-5 moxa

cones or 5-15 minutes with warming moxibustion.

Jimai (Liv 12)

It is an acupuncture point.

Location. On the lateral side of the pubic tubercle, 2.5 cun lateral to the anterior midline.

Indication. Lower abdominal pain, vulva pain, prolapse of uterus, hernia, irregular menstruation, pain of thigh, etc.

Method. Puncture perpendicularly 0.5-0.8 cun. Perform moxibustion to the point with 3-5 moxa cones or for 5-10 minutes.

Jimen (Sp 11)

It is a meridian acupuncture point.

Location. On the medial side of the thigh and on the line connecting Xuehai (Sp 10) and Chongmen (Sp 12), 6 cun above Xuehai.

Indication. Dysuria, enuresis, swelling and pain in the groin, eczema of scrotum.

Method. Avoid the artery. Puncture perpendicularly 0.5-1 cun. Perform moxibustion 5-10 minutes with moxa sticks.

Jingbailao (Ex-HN 15)

It is an extra acupuncture point.

Location. On the nape, 2 cun directly above Dazhui (GV 14) and 1 cun lateral to the posterior midline.

Indication. Scrofula, asthma, hemoptysis, cough, pulmonery tuberculosis, general aching after childbirth, stiff neck, etc.

Method. Puncture perpendicularly 0.3-0.6 cun. Perform moxibustion 5-10 minutes with moxa sticks.

Jingbi (Ex-HN)

It is an extra acupuncture point.

Location. On the neck, 1 cun above the point on the junction of the medial 1/3 and lateral 2/3 of clavicle, on the posterior border of the clavicula head of sternocleidomastoideus muscle.

Indication. Paralysis and numbness of upper limbs, pain in arm and shoulder, etc.

Method. Puncture perpendicularly 0.5-1 cun. Do not puncture downward deeply, to avoid injuring the lung.

Jinggu (B 64)

It is an acupuncture point.

Location. On the external side of the foot, inferior to the tuberosity of the 5th metatarsal bone, at the junction between the reddish and whitish skin.

Indication. Lumbar spasm and pain, headache, rigid nape.

Method. Puncture perpendicularly 0.3-0.5 cun. Perform moxibustion to the point with 3-5 moxa cones or 5-10 minutes with warming moxibustion.

Jingmen (G 25)

It is a meridian acupuncture point belonging to the Gallbladder Meridian of Foot-shaoyang, the Front-mu point, of the kidney, also named Qifu, Qishu.

Location. On the lateral side of the waist, 1.8 cun posterior to Zhangmen (Liv 13), below the free end of the 12th rib.

Indication. Borborygmus, diarrhea, abdominal distention, pain in the loin and hypochondriac region.

Method. Puncture obliquely 0.5-0.8 cun. Perform moxibustion 3-5 moxa cones or 5-10 minutes.

Jingming (B 1)

It is an acupuncture point.

Location. In the depression of the slightly superior border (about 0.1 cun) of the inner canthus.

Indication. Congestion swelling and pain of the eye, lacrimation due to wind, internal and external pterygium, opacity, color blindness.

Method. Ask the patient to close his eyes when pushing the eyeball gently to the lateral side and fixing it with the left hand. Puncture perpendicularly 0.5-1.0 cun along the orbital wall. It is not advisable to

twirl or lift and thrust the needle to a large extent. Press the puncture site for a while after the withdrawal of the needle to avoid bleeding. Moxibustion is forbidden.

Jingning

It is a massage point.

Location. At seam juncture between the 4th and 5th metacarpal bones.

Operation. Nipping manipulation.

Function. Resolving phlegm, releasing stagnancy and adjusting qi.

Indication. Asthma, retching and infantile malnutrition.

Jing Points

1. **Location.** At the tips of the extremities, like the mouths of springs from the meridian-qi.

   Indication. Diseases in the zang-organs characterized by fever, coma, vexation, etc, and for emergency treatment and measurement of meridians and collaterals.

2. Referring to one of the Five Shu Points.

   Location. Above the ankle and wrist, as if the flow of water, representing the circulation of qi in the meridians.

   Indication. Asthma, cough, chill and fever, sore throat, etc.

Jingqu (L 8)

It is a meridian acupuncture point.

Location. On the radial side of the palmar surface of the forearm, 1 cun above the transverse crease of the wrist, in the depression between the styloid process of the radius and radial artery.

Indication. Cough, dyspnea, sore throat, distention, fullness and pain in the chest.

Method. Puncture perpendicularly 0.2-0.3 cun, avoiding the artery. Perform moxibustion 3-5 minutes with warming moxibustion.

Jingxia

It is an acupuncture point.

Location. 3 cun above Jiexi (S 41), 1 cun to the lateral margin of the tibia.

Indication. Foot downward, paralysis of lower limb.

Method. Puncture perpendicularly 1-1.5 cun.

Jingzhong (Ex-HN)

It is an extra acupuncture point.

Location. At the midpoint of the pupil.

Indication. Cataracta, a long-time inability to see. Modern cataractopiesis with a gold or metal needle is traced from the application on this acupoint.

Jinjin (Ex-HN 12), Yuye (Ex-HN 13)

They are two extra acupuncture points.

Á?LocationÁÀOn the vein of the left and right sides of the frenulum of the tongue.

Indication. Heaviness, pain and swelling in the tongue, aphtha, inflammation of the throat, vomiting, diarrhea, jaundice, diabetes, aphthosis, glossitis, tonsillitis, and acute gastroenteritis.

Method. Prick to cause little bleeding with a triangular needle.

Jinmen (B 63)

It is a meridian acupuncture point.

Location. On the external side of the foot, directly below the anterior border of the external malleolus, in the depression lateral to cuboid bone.

Indication. Sore knee and lumbago, numbness of lower limb, swelling pain of external malleolus, tendon spasm of shank, dizziness, headache, epilepsy, infantile convulsion.

Method. Puncture perpendicularly 0.3-0.5 cun. Perform moxibustion 3-5 moxa cones or 5-10 minutes moxibustion.

Jinsuo (GV 8)

It is a meridian acupuncture point.

Location. On the back and on the posterior midline, in the space between the 9th and 10th spinous processes of the thoracic vertebrae.

Indication. Manic-depressive disorders, epilepsy induced by terror, clonic convul-

sions, stiffness of the back, stomachache, jaundice, spasm of muscles.

Method. Puncture obliquely 0.5-1 cun. Perform moxibustion 3-5 moxa cones or 5-10 minutes moxibustion.

Jinwei

1. Myasthenia, a type of flaccidity syndrome.

   Symptoms. Muscular contracture of limbs gradually leading to the disability to movement.

   Pathogenesis. Owing to the liver-heat and the deficiency of yin-fluid and blood, the withering of fasciae.

   Therapeutic Principle. Removing the heat, enriching the blood and the liver.

2. Referring to the impotence.

   Pathogenesis. Due to the excess of sexual intercourse, the deficiency of liver-yin and kidney-yin, the myasthenia of the urogenital region and impotence.

Jiquan (H 1)

It is a meridian acupuncture point.

Location. In the center of the axilla, the pulsation point of the axillary artery.

Indication. Pain in the costal region, pain in the chest or abdomen, pain in the shoulder and arm, palpitations, shortness of breath, depression and grief, retching, dry throat, excessive thirst.

Method. Puncture perpendicularly, avoiding artery, 0.2-0.5 cun. Perform moxibustion 1-3 moxa cones or 3-5 minutes moxibustion.

Jisanxue (Ex-B)

Referring to the general name for the three extra acupuncture points on the spinal column.

Location. One at the posterior midline 1 cun below Yamen (GV 15), the second is Taodao (GV 13), and the third below the spinous process of the 5th lumbar vertebra.

Indication. Convulsive disease, lumbo-dorsal neuralgia, etc.

Method. Puncture perpendicularly 0.5-1 cun. Perform moxibustion 3-5 moxa cones or 5-15 minutes with warming moxibustion.

Jiudianfeng (Ex-UE)

It is an extra acupuncture point.
Location. On the palmar side of the middle finger, slightly anterior to the midpoint at the transverse crease of the distal interphalangeal articulation.
Indication. Vitiligo.
Method. Moxibustion.

Jiulao (Ex-B)

It is an extra acupuncture point
Location. At the tip of the 3rd thoracic vertebra.
Indication. Consumptive disease with night sweat, cough with sticky sputum and blood, emaciation with sallow complexion, mental fatigue and inertia, etc. Caused by consumption.
Method. Perform moxibustion 3-7 moxa cones or 5-15 minutes with warming moxibustion.

Jiuqueshu (Ex-B)

It is an extra acupuncture point.
Location. On the posterior midline, between the spinous processes of the 4th and 5th thoracic vertebrae.
Indication. Cough, asthmatic breath, bronchitis, neurasthenia, etc.
Method. Perform moxibustion 3-7 moxa cones or 5-15 mimutes with warming moxibustion.

Jiuquzhongfu (Ex-CA)

It is an extra acupuncture point.
Location. On the middle axillary line, 3 cun below the 7th intercostal space.
Indication. Pleuritis, pain in the chest and rib, and abdominal pain, etc.
Method. Puncture obliquely 0.3-0.5 cun. Perform moxibustion 3-5 moxa cones or 5 minutes with warming moxibustion.

Jiuwei (CV 15)

It is a meridian acupuncture point.
Location. On the upper abdomen and on the anterior midline, 1 cun below the xiphisternal synchondrosis.
Indication. Cardiac pain, palpitation, epilepsy, mania, fullness and pain in the chest, cough with dyspnea, vomiting, hiccups, regurgitation, stomachache.
Method. Puncture obliquely downward 0.4-0.6 cun. It is not advisable to puncture deep. Perform moxibustion 3-5 moxa cones or 5-10 minutes with warming moxibustion.

Jiuweiguduan (Ex-CA)

It is an extra acupuncture point.
Location. At the inferior border of the tip of the xiphoid process of the sternum.
Indication. Infantile malnutrition, and indigestion.
Method. Puncture 0.3 cun. Apply moxibustion with 5-30 moxa cones.

Jiuxiao (Ex-B)

It is an extra acupuncture point.
Location. On the back. Put a rope round the nape with the rest dropped to the xiphoid process, then turn the ring backwards with the midpoint of the dropped length overlapping the Adam's apple, and the point on the vertebra touched by the end of the rope is Jiuxiao (Ex-B) point.
Indication. Asthma, cough and bronchitis, etc.
Method. Perform moxibustion: 3-7 moxa cones or 5-15 minutes with warming moxibustion.

Jiuxuebing

It is an extra acupuncture point.
Location. At the highest spot of the crest of the 3rd sacral vertebra.
Indication. Spitting blood, epistaxis, hemafecia, epistaxis, hematochezia, metrorrhagia, etc.
Method. Perform moxibustion 5-7 moxa cones or 10-15 minutes with warming moxibustion.

Jizhong (GV 6)

It is a meridian acupuncture point.

Location. At the midline of the back, in the depression below the spinous process of the 11th thoracic vertebra.

Indication. Stiffness and pain in the waist, jaundice, diarrhea, dysentery, malnutrition of children, hemorrhoid, hemafecia and scrofula prolapse of anus.

Method. Puncture obliquely 0.5-1 cun. Perform moxibustion 3-5 moxa cones or 5-10 minutes with warming moxibustion.

Jizhu

It is a massage point.

Location. On the straight line from the Dazhui (GV 14) point to Changqiang (GV 1) point on the back.

Operation. Nipping and pushing manipulations.

Function. Adjusting yin, yang, qi and blood circulation, zang-fu organs and clearing meridians and collaterals.

Indication. Diseases owing to the disorders of zang-fu, yin, yang, qi and blood flow.

Joint of Meridians

Referring to the connections among the 12 meridians. The three yin meridians of the hand and three yang meridians of the hand are connected at tip, the three yang meridians of the hand and the three yang meridians of the foot, at head and face, the three yang meridians of the foot and three yin meridians of the foot, at toe, and the three yin meridians of the foot and three yin meridians of the hand, in the abdomen and chest, the twelve meridians through these connections linking the yin and yang one another, like a ring without end.

Joint Puncture

Referring to one of the five needling techniques, for treating painful tendons around the joints.

Method. Directly puncture the muscles and ligaments around the joints of the four limbs, avoiding impairing the meridians and causing bleeding.

Indication. Muscular rheumatism and pain in the muscles and tendons.

Jueyin Cough

Symptoms. Drastic cough, with the tongue stretching out, nausea and even vomiting.

Therapeutic Principle. Removing the depressed liver and cough.

Jueyinshu (B 14)

It is a meridian acupuncture point.

Location. On the back, at 1.5 cun lateral to the spinal process between the 4th and 5th thoracic vertebrae.

Indication. Precordial pain, palpitation, depressed chest, cough, vomiting, cardio, etc.

Method. Puncture obliquely 0.3-0.5 cun. Perform moxibustion 3-7 moxa cones or 5-15 minutes moxibustion.

Jueyunxue (Ex-CA)

It is an extra acupuncture point.

Location. On the abdomen, 1-2 cun region below the umbilicus. Woman accept moxibustion this point, she can stop delivering the baby.

Jugu (LI 16)

It is a meridian acupuncture point.

Location. On the shoulder, in the excavation between the clavicular acromial extremity and the scapular spine.

Indication. Sore shoulder, back and upper limbs, difficulty in flexion and extension of the upper limbs, epilepsy due to terror, spitting blood and scrofula, goiter.

Method. Puncture perpendicularly or obliquely downwards 0.4-0.6 cun; avoiding deep puncture, for protecting the thoracic cavity, otherwise maybe leading to a pneumothorax. Perform moxibustion 3-5 moxa cones or 5-10 minutes moxibustion.

Juice Vesiculation

It refers to the method of using garlic to rub the skin to treat diseases.

Indication. Tuberculosis.

Juliao (G 29)

It is a meridian acupuncture point.

Location. On the hip at the midpoint of the line connecting the superior spinal process of the anterior ilium and the greater trochanter of thigh.

Indication. Pain and numbness in the waist and leg due to stagnation, paralysis, foot flaccidity and hernia.

Method. Puncture perpendicularlly or obliquely 1-1.5 cun. Perform moxibustion 3-5 moxa cones or 5-10 minutes moxibustion.

Juliao (S 3)

It is a meridian acupuncture point.

Location. With the eyes look forward, directly below the pupil, on the level with the inferior edge of the nasal wing.

Indication. Deviated mouth and eyes, tremor of eyelids, nebula, toothache, swelling of the lips and cheeks.

Method. Puncture subcutaneously or obliquely 0.3-0.6 cun. Perform moxibustion 3-5 moxa cones with warming moxibustion.

Juquan (Ex-HN 10)

It is an extra acupuncture point.

Location. At the midpoint of the dorsal midline of the tongue.

Indication. Stiffness of the tongue, paralysis of the tongue muscle, asthma, cough, etc.

Method. Puncture perpendicularly 0.1-0.2 cun, or prick to cause bleeding.

Juque (CV 14)

It is a meridian acupuncture point.

Location. At the upper abdomen, 6 cun above the center of the umbilicus on the anterior median line.

Indication. Chest pain, precordial pain, vexation, nausea, vomiting, cough with dyspnea, abdominal distention and sudden pain, acid regurgitation, jaundice, diarrhea and dysentery.

Method. Puncture perpendicularly 0.5-1 cun, avoiding deep insertion. Perform moxibustion 3-5 moxa cones or 5-10 minutes moxibustion.

K

Kaempferi Dutchmanspipe Root

It is the stem root of Aristolochia Kaempferi Willd. (Aristolochiaceae).

Effect. Removing pain, heat, toxic substances and enhancing blood circulation.

Indication. Dysentery, pain in the chest and abdomen and snake bite.

Kangong

It is a massage point.

Location. On the cross-line from the beginning of the eyebrow to the end.

Operation. Partial-pushing manipulation.

Function. Restoring consciousness, enhancing vision, removing wind, cold and headache.

Indication. Fever and headache owing to common cold and eye diseases.

Kansui Root

It is the root tuber of Euphorbia kansui Liou (Euphorbiaceae).

Effect. Releasing water retention, Purging heat and relaxing bowels, relieving swelling and masses.

Indication. Edema, ascites, hydrothorax, etc.

Katsumadau Galangal Seed

It is the dried ripe seed of Alpinia Katsumadai Hayata (Zingiberaceae).

Effect. Releasing dampness, warming the middle-energizer and enhancing flow of qi.

Indication. Abdominal distention and pain, vomiting and diarrhea due to accumulation of cold-dampness in the spleen and stomach.

Kidney

1. Referring to one of the five zang organs. The kidney and urinary bladder possess a relationship of exterior and interior, including three main functions: (1) Storing the essence and being the congenital foundation and source of a human growth and development; (2) Being concerned with water metabolism, for maintaining the balance and metabolism of body fluid; (3) Being in charge of the bones and producing marrow.

2. Referring to an auricular point (MA).
   Location. Below the bifurcating point, between the superior and inferior antihelix crus.
   Indication. Pyelonephritis, lumbago, tinnitus, double hearing, emission, impotence, neurasthenia, dyspnea, glaucoma, irregular menstruation.

3. Referring to another auricular point.
   Location. At the lower part of the back auricle.
   Indication. Headache, insomnia, dizziness, irregular menstruation.

Kidney Attacked by Cold

Symptoms. Cold and pain of the loin and knees, abdominal distention and loose stool, deafness.

Pathogenesis. Owing to the kidney attacked by pathogenic cold, the deficiency of the kidney-yang and the excess of pathogenic cold in the interior.

Therapeutic Principle. Warming and nourishing the kidney-yang.

Kidney Collateral

It is a meridian and collateral, one of fifteen collaterals. If the meridian suffers from pathologic changes, such syndromes as reversed flow of qi, vexation, and anuria for excess pains in spinal column for deficiency can be found.

Kidney Diarrhea

Symptoms. Long time of diarrhea, diarrhea before dawn, abdominal pain without fixed spot, pain connected with loin and back.

Pathogenesis. Mainly owing to the insufficiency of kidney-yang, deficiency-cold of the Kidney Meridian, leading to failure in storage.

Therapeutic Principle. Nourishing the kidney and invigorating the primordial qi.

Kidney Hernia

Symptoms. Pain under the umbilicus, or acute pain all around the body under the umbilicus, with frequent but clear urination.

Therapeutic Principle. Warming yang, removing cold, spasm and pain.

Kidney Impairment due to Overstrain

Symptoms. Pain in back, loin, waist and lower extremities, oligospermia and frequent urination, etc.

Pathogenesis. Great intensity of weight lifting, long sitting on damp places, excess of sexual intercourse, attack by wind during sweating, etc.

Therapeutic Principle. Nourishing kidney and removing pathogenic factors.

Kidney-leaf Mountainsorrel Herb

It is the whole herb of Oxyria digyna (L.) Hill. (Polygonaceae).

Effect. Removing heat and enhancing diuresis.

Indication. Stagnation of the liver-qi, hepatitis, scurvy, etc.

Kidney Qi

Referring to the functional activities of the kidney, such as growth, development and sexual ability, etc.

Kidney-wind

1. **Symptoms.** Hyperhidrosis and aversion to wind, inability to stand owing to rachiagia, etc.

   Pathogenesis. Attack by exopathogens, failure of the kidney in opening and closing leading to overflow of water into muscles.

2. Referring to edema syndrome due to nephropathy.

   Symptoms. Edema, anorexia.

   Pathogenesis. Owing to excessive sexual intercourse, consumption of kidney essence, insufficiency of the kidney-qi.

   Therapeutic Principle. Removing pathogenic factors and tonifying the kidney.

Kidney-yang

It refers to the functional activities of the kidney, also refers to the power for the living activities in the body. The kidney-yang is of importance for warming all the zang-fu organs in the body so as to provide them with energy.

Kidney-yin

The kidney-yin is derived from the kidney essence and serves as material base for functioning of the kidney-yang. The kidney-yin is of importance for nourishing the organs in the body.

Kind Complexion

It is a diagnostic method. The bright and moist complexion of a patient indicates inexhaustion of the vital-qi and essence of the viscera, slight and shallow pathologic changes.

Knee (MA-AH 3)

Referring to an auricular point here.

Location. On the middle portion of the superior antihelix crus.

Indication. Pain and dysfunction at the corresponding part of the body, swelling and pain of the knee joint.

Knotted-flower Phyla Herb

It is the whole herb of Phyla nodiflora (L.) Greene. (Verbenaceae).

Effect. Removing wind, heat, swelling and detoxicating.

Indication. Sore-throat, tonsillitis, suppurative infections on the body surface, dysentery of heat type, stranguriaa, ulcerative gingivitis, herpes zoster, etc.

Kongzui (L 6)

It is an acupuncture point, belonging to the Lung Meridian.

Location. On the radial side of the forearm palm, 7 cun superior to the transverse crease of the wrist, on the line joining Chize (L 5) and Taiyuan (L 9).

Indication. Headache, febrile disease without sweating, cough, dyspnea, hemoptysis, aphonia, swelling sore throat, sore shoulder, sore elbow and arm.

Method. Puncturing perpendicularly 0.5-1 cun and performing moxibustion to the point with 5-7 moxa cones or 5-15 minutes.

Korean Pine Seed

It the seed of pinus koraiensis Sieb. et Zucc. (Pinaceae).

Effect. Tonifying the body fluid, calming the endopathic wind, moistening the lung and laxation bowels.

Indication. Dizziness, dry cough, hematemesis and constipation.

Kouheliao (LI 19)

It is a meridian acupuncture point.

Location. On the upper lip, directly below the lateral border of the nostril on the level with shuigou (GV 26).

Indication. Pyogenic infection of nose, nasal polyp, epistaxis, stuffy nose, watery nasal secretion, wry mouth, lockjaw.

Method. Puncturing perpendicularly or obliquely 0.3-0.5 cun. Moxibustion is forbidden.

Kuangu (Ex-LE 1)

It is an acupuncture point, belonging to the extraodinary points.

Location. Above the knee, 1.5 cun lateral and medial to Liangqiu (S 34),2 points on one thigh.

Indication. Swelling and pain in the knees, thigh and leg, severe and migratory arthralgia.

Method. Puncture obliquely 0.5-1 cun and perform moxibustion to the point for 5-15 minutes or 3-7 moxa cones.

Kufang (S 14)

It is a meridian acupuncture point.

Location. On the chest, in the lst intercostal space, 4 cun lateral to the anterior midline.

Indication. Cough, asthma, purulent sputum mixed with blood, distending pain in the chest and hypochondrium.

Method. Puncturing obliquely 0.5-0.8 cun towards the interior. Perform moxibustion 3-5 moxa cones or 5-10 minutes with warming moxibustion.

Kunlun (B 60)

It is an acupuncture point.

Location. Posterior to the external malleolus of the foot, in the excavation between the tip of the external malleolus and tendo calcaneus.

Indication. Headache, dizziness, swelling and pain of eye, epistaxis, rigidity and spasm of neck and back, lumbosacral pain, swelling and pain of heel, malaria, vulvar swelling and pain, dystocia and retention of placenta.

Method. Puncturing perpendicularly 0.5-0.8 cun and performing moxibustion to the point with 3-5 moxa cones or 5-10 minutes.

Kusnezoff Monkshood Root
⊛ K-1

It is the root tuber of Aconitum kusnezoffii Reichb. (Ranunculaceae). Its functions and indications are the same as those of Sichuan aconite root.

Kweichow Sage Herb

It is the whole herb of Salvia cavaleriei
Levl. (Labiatae).

Effect. Releasing heat from the blood and
ceasing bleeding.

Indication. Hematemesis,   hemoptysis,
epistaxis, dysentery with bloody stool,
metrorrhagia.

L

Labor-like Pain

The sudden onset of abdominal pain in the 8th or 9th month of pregnancy before the stage of labor, which abates and departs after 3 or 4 days.

Lacerated Wound of Muscle and Tendon

It refers to complete breaking-off of tendon in a certain part due to powerful external force, such as torsion, contusion, and traction.

Symptoms. Severe dysfunction, obvious local pain, swelling, blood stasis and ecchymosis, and deformity, etc.

Therapeutic Principle. Mainly by operation.

Laceration of Muscle and Tendon

It is a lacerated injury of some parts of tendons due to powerful external force, such as torsion, contusion and traction.

Symptoms. The morphologic change varies with strength of the external force, direction of action, and severity of the injury. Such symptoms may be seen as local slight swollen, pain, partial dysfunction, etc.

Therapeutic Principle. It can be convalesced by massotherapy in combination with rest.

Laciniate Blumea Herb

The whole herb or leaf of Blumea laciniata (Roxb.) DC. (Compositae).

Effect. Expelling wind-dampness and dredging the meridians and collaterals.

Indication. Rheumatic arthralgia and traumatic injuries.

Ladybell Root

The dried root of Adenophora tetraphylla (Thunb.) Fisch. or A. stricta Miq. (Campanulaceae).

Effect. Nourishing yin, removing heat from the lung, dispelling phlegm, and replenishing qi.

Indication. Dryness cough due to the lung-heat, phthisic cough due to yin deficiency, dysphoria with smothery sensation and thirst.

Lalanggrass Rhizome

The rhizome of Imperata cylindrica (L.) Beauv. Var. Major (Nees) C.E. Hubb. (Gramineae).

Effect. Arresting bleeding, removing heat and promoting diuresis.

Indication. Epistaxis, hemoptysis, hematemesis, hematuria due to invasion of blood by pathogenic heat, stranguria, due to heat dysuria, edema, and jaundice due to pathogenic damp-heat.

Lama (Ex-B)

An extra point.

Location. On the scapular region and on the line connecting Tianzong (SI 11) and the extreme end of the posterior axillary line 1.5 cun from Tianzong (SI 11).

Indication. Laryngitis.

Method. Puncture perpendicularly 0.5-1.0 cun.

Lambsquarters Herb

The young herb of Chenopodium album L. (Chenopodiaceae).

Effect. Removing heat, eliminating dampness and destroying parasites.

Indication. Dysentery, diarrhea, eruption, insect bite, etc.

Lance Needle

An acupuncture point instrument. One of the Nine Needles. Its tip is sharp and prismatic. It is also called the three-edged needle. It is used for blood-letting by pricking and discharging pus.

Indication. Carbuncle, swelling, acute febrile disease, etc.

Langdu Root

The root of Euphorbia fischeriana Steud, Euphorbia ebracteolata. Hayata (Euphorbiaceae).

Effect. Expelling retained water, dispelling phlegm, promoting digestion and destroying parasites.

Indication. Ascites, abdominal pain due to parasitic infestation, chronic tracheal catarrh, cough, asthma, tuberculosis of lymph node, bone tuberculosis, tuberculosis of epididymis, scabies, tinea and hemorrhoid, etc.

Lankong Lily Bulb

The bulb of Lilium lankongense Franch (Liliaceae).

Effect. Clearing away heat from the lung, relieving cough, purging intense heat and tranquilization.

Indication. Tuberculosis, chronic bronchitis, hematemesis due to chronic cough, insomnia, absent-mindedness, etc.

Lanmen (Ex-CA)

Two extra points.

Location. 3 cun lateral to Qugu (CV 2).

Method. Puncture perpendicularly 0.5-1.0 cun. Perform moxibustion 3-5 moxa cones or 5-10 minutes with warming moxibustion.

Lanweixue (Ex-LE7)

One of the extra acupoints.

Location. The most painful place on pressing anterior and lateral to the small leg, about 2 cun directly below Zusanli (S 36).

Indication. Acute and chronic appendicitis, acute and chronic enteritis, flaccid paralysis of the lower limb, puffy leg, etc.

Method. Puncture perpendicularly 1-1.2 cun. Moxibustion is applicable.

Laogong (P8)

An acupuncture point on the pericardium meridian.

Location. In the palm, between the 2nd proximal to the 3rd metacarpal bone, below the tip of the middle finger when a fist is formed. Select it when the hand is in supine position.

Indication. Apoplectic coma, heart pain, aphthous ulcer, sunstroke, hematemesis, mania, epilepsy, etc.

Method. Puncture perpendicularly 0.3-0.5 cun and apply moxibustion to the point for 3-5 minutes.

Laolong

A massage point.

Location. At the part 0.1 cun behind the nail of middle finger.

Effect. Expelling wind and relieving convulsion.

Indication. Infantile convulsion, etc.

Method. Nipping manipulation is applied.

Large Accumulation of Phlegm-heat in Chest

A kind of accumulation of phlegm-heat in the chest.

Symptoms. Fullness, pain and tenderness in the chest and abdomen, thirst, dryness of the tongue, hectic fever, etc.

Pathogenesis. Usually caused by pathogenic heat in the interior and the accumulation of phlegm and fluid.

Therapeutic Principle. Relieving accumulation, eliminating retained fluid and purging away heat.

Large Collateral of Spleen

One of the fifteen collaterals, which derives from acupoint Dabao and comes out from the point at 3 cun below acupoint Yuanye (G22), and spreads in the hypochondriac region.

Large Collateral of Stomach

One of fifteen large collaterals and located in the area of heart beat below the left breast where pectoral qi converges. It is the ancestry of qi of twelve meridians. The moving condition directly reflects the changes of stomach-qi and source and stream of qi and blood.

Large Collaterals

It refers to fifteen main collaterals which consists of twelve collaterals connected with twelve meridians, the front middle meridian and the back middle meridian and an extra collateral, (Large collateral of spleen). They are more important parts and guide countless tiny collaterals all over the body. They can strengthen the link between exterior and interior of twelve meridians and play a part in linking the front, the back and the lateral.

Large Heavenly Circuit

A maneuver in Qigong. It refers to the second stage of the Iner Elixir Pellet Prowess maneuver, namely, the process of training qi to transform it into vitality. At this stage the essence qi circulates through the regular and extra meridians (except the Conception and Governor Vessels). The maneuver has the functions of integrating vitality with qi and strengthening health and prolonging life.

Large Intestinal Asthenia

Symptoms. Chronic diarrhea, dyspepsia, prolapse of rectum, etc.
Pathogenesis. Qi deficiency in the large intestine.
Therapeutic Principle. Invigorating the spleen, replenishing qi and arresting discharge.

Large Intestinal Damp-heat

Symptoms. Frequent purulent and bloody stool, abdominal pain, scanty dark urine, burning feeling on anus seen usually in enteritis and dysentery, amebic dysentery and acute colitis.

Pathogenesis. It results from the impairment of the stomach and intestine caused by irregular and unclean diet.
Therapeutic Principle. Clearing heat and drying dampness.

Large Intestinal Heat

A disease and syndrome caused by overeating pungent food and affection of heat exopathogen or the lung-heat, which invades the large intestine.
Symptoms. Dry mouth with cracked lips, abdominal pain and distention, constipation swelling and painful anus, hematochezia or bleeding from hemorrhoid, scanty dark urine, yellow and dry coating of the tongue.
Therapeutic Principle. Dissipating intestinal heat and cooling blood.

Large Intestine (MA)

An auricular point.
Location. On the medial 1/3 of the superior aspect of the helix crus, opposite to Mouth.
Indication. Diarrhea, constipation, cough, and acne.

Large Intestine Disease

Symptoms. Abdominal distention with borborygmus, pain around umbilical region, constipation or diarrhea, dysentery, hematochezia and proctoptosis, ect.
Pathogenesis. Usually caused by incursion of cold or heat, wind pathogen or retention of dampness and qi deficiency into the large intestine, which lead to the dysfunction of stool transportation and transformation.
Therapeutic Principle. It should be taken according to the specific causes, such as promoting the circulation of qi and removing stasis, loosening the bowel to relieve constipation, warming the middle-energizer to expel cold, drying dampness to stop diarrhea, etc.

Large Intestine in Charge of Transportation

It refers to the physiological function of the large intestine which is to pass its content on and finally eliminate the waste. Disturbance of its function usually gives rise to diarrhea or constipation. After water and nutrients are digested and extracted in the small intestine, the remaining part joins the large intestine. Here the residue water is further absorbed and the residue is changed into feces which are discharged out of the body via the anus.

Large Intestine Meridian

One of the twelve meridians. It starts from the radial side of the index finger, and goes up the back of the hand and runs along the lateral front border of the arm to the front border of the shoulder joint, and then goes back to the spinous process of the seventh vertebrae cervicales (Dazhui (GV14)). From this point, it goes down, from the greater supraclavicular fossa, enters into the thoracic cavity, and connects to the lung. It goes down further through the diaphragm to the large intestine. Its branches go up from the greater supraclaveicular fossa, pass through the cervical part to the cheeks, enter the lower teeth, come out from the cheeks, and intercross at Renzhong. Finally, they arrive at the wings of the nose of the opposite part (Yingxiang (LI20) and join the Stomach Meridian.

Large Leaf Curculigo Rhizome

The rhizome of Curculigo capitulata (Lour.) O. Ktze. (Amaryllidaceae).

Effect. Restoring qi, regulating menstruation, expelling wind-dampness and dissipating blood stasis.

Indication. Cough due to asthenic disease, emission, turbid urine, metrorrhagia, metrostaxis, leukorrhagia, and arthralgia due to wind-dampness and traumatic injuries.

Large-leaf Gentian Root

The root of Gentiana macrophylla Pall. G. straminea Maxim, G. crassicaulis Duthie ex Burk., or G. dahurica Fisch. (Gentianaceae).

Effect. Expelling wind-dampness, relaxing muscle and removing heat of deficiency type.

Indication. Rheumatic arthralgia, tetraplegia, tidal fever and jaundice.

Large Needle

An acupuncture instrument, one of the nine needles used in ancient times. It is a needle with a long thick body and a slightly rounded tip. In ancient times, it was used to treat edema in the joint. Later generations used it to puncture after burning it to red, which is called fire needle. People in modern times use big needles, similar to large needles, with a diameter of 0.5-1mm, and a variety of length 3 cun, 5 cun, etc. They are used in subcutaneous, transverse and muscle-tendon acupuncture to treat paralysis and muscular spasm, ect.

Large qi

This term has four meanings: 1. Qi in universe. 2. Pectoral qi in the human body. 3. The large one in vital-qi. 4. The large one in pathogenic factors.

Laryngeal Aphthae

Symptoms. Aphthae in the throat. In the early stage, the patient has the sensation of a foreign body blocking the throat, tidal red, and pain. Then purulent spots of different size appear on the surface with areola around them, followed by ulceration. In that case, the patient has hoarseness, short breath and alternate attacks of chills and fever.

Pathogenesis. Mostly caused by impairment of the lung-yin due to burning of pathogenic wind-heat, and malnutrition of the throat, or by upward attack of fire in the stomach to the throat, or by insufficiency and loss of the kidney-yin, and flaring up of deficient fire.

Therapeutic Principle. Dispelling wind, clearing away heat and detoxicating, or nourishing yin and reducing fire.

Laryngeal Carbuncule

A general designation of carbuncule including retropharyngeal abscess and peritonsillar abscess.

Symptoms. Swollen and sore throat, obstruction of sufficient phlegm and saliva, and dyspnea, often accompanied by high fever and aversion to cold.

Pathogenesis. Mostly caused by imbalance of the proper harmonic interior-exterior relationship between zang-fu organs, derangement of qi and blood, and obstruction of qi due to pathogenic wind remaining for a long time in the throat. It may result in rapid formation of carbuncle.

Therapeutic Principle. Dispelling wind, clearing away heat, removing toxic substances and promoting subsidence of swelling.

Laryngeal Gelosis

Symptoms. Gelosis in the throat that is thick and mushroom-like, sensation of foreign body and pain, bloody venules seen with top appearing purplish, outflowing of turbid discharge, aphonia due to hoarseness, emaciation, etc.

Pathogenesis. Mostly caused by latent fire in the heart and stomach, upward attack of phlegm-toxin with fire interspersed, or emotional smoldering, stagnation of qi and coagulation of blood, or yin insufficiency of the liver and kidney, and flaring up of deficient fire.

Therapeutic Principle. Removing toxic substances and pathogenic fire, soothing the liver, regulating the circulation of qi, nourishing yin and promoting the flow of primordial qi.

Laryngeal Obstruction

Symptoms. Feeling of obstruction in larynx by a pedicle foreign body.

Pathogenesis. Mainly caused by flaring-up of the heart-fire.

Therapeutic Principle. Clearing away the heart-heat and purging intense heat, relieving the depressed liver and regulating the circulation of qi, and dispersing accumulation of pathogens.

Laryngeal Ulceration

Symptoms. Red swelling, pain and ulceration in the throat.

Pathogenesis. There are two types of this symptom. The deficiency type is caused by yin deficiency of the liver and kidney, and flaring up of deficient fire to the throat. The excess type is caused by heat accumulation in the lung and stomach, and upward attack of toxic fire to the throat.

Laser Irradiation of Acupoints

A therapy carried out by illuminating the acupoints with stimulated radiation from a laser, such as helium-neon laser, hydrogen ion laser, helium-cadmium laser, etc., which are frequently used.

Notice. The doctors should wear laser-protecting glasses in the course of laser irradiation and avoid the laser beam in case of damage to the eye.

Lassitude of Limbs

Symptoms. Weakness of the hand and foot.

Pathogenesis. Usually caused by the deficiency of the spleen and stomach, and failure to nourish the limbs.

Lassitude of Loin

Symptoms. Sensation of lassitude in the loin.

Pathogenesis. Mostly caused by damp-heat, sexual strain and deficiency of the kidney.

Latent Heat in the Interior

It refers to the original latent pathogenic heat, or depression of qi generating the fire in the body.

Symptoms. Thirst, dryness in the throat, halitosis, abdominal distention and pain with tenderness, constipation, scanty and dark urine, etc.

Latent Phlegm

It is one of phlegm syndrome.

Symptoms. Cough while catching cold, abundant expectoration, asthma, etc.

Pathogenesis. Caused by retention of phlegm in the chest.

Therapeutic Principle. Eliminating dampness to reduce phlegm.

Latent-wind

Symptoms. Dizziness, vertigo flushed face, etc.

Pathogenesis. Caused by dysfunction of zang-fu organs, deficiency of yin in the lower and excess of yang in the upper.

Therapeutic Principle. Nourishing yin and suppressing hyperactive yang.

Lateral Aspect

A part of the body, referring to: 1. The aspect of dorsum of the hand, namely, extensive side, which is the part in which three yang meridians of hand and their points are distributed; 2. The anterio-lateral aspect of the lower limbs, which is the part in which the three yang meridians of foot and their points are distributed.

Lateral-position Lifting-pulling-rocking Reduction

A therapeutic method for old dislocation of hip joint. A patient takes lateral recumbent position, with the healthy limb downward and the diseased one upward. One assistant holds knee joint, flexes hip joint to 90 degrees, then lifts and pulls it forward, simultaneously extends, flexes and rocks the hip joint slowly and gently. Another assistant twines a wide cloth-belt around the thigh root and pulls reversely backward. The manipulator presses and pulls anterior-inferior iliac spine backward with one hand and pushes and presses the dislocated whirlbone forward. Repeat like this until the whirlbone slips back to acetabulum.

Lateral Puncture

An acupuncture method. Using oblique insertions and lifting the needle in order to activate the meridians and promote the circulation of qi for the treatment of muscle spasm.

Lateral Recumbent Position

The patient lies on his/her side for selection of points on the side of the body of some of the points of the upper and lower limbs.

Laver

It is the lobous material of Porphyra tenera Kjellm. (Bangiaceae).

Effect. Dispelling sputum, softening hard masses, clearing away heat and promoting diuresis.

Indication. Goiter, beriberi, edema, stranguria, etc.

Laxflower Pottsia Root

It is the root of Pottsia laxiflora (Bl.) O. Ktze. (Apocynaceae).

Effect. Activating collaterals, promoting blood circulation, removing dampness, expelling wind.

Indication. Traumatic injuries, arthralgia, carbuncles and amenorrhea.

Layer of Kidney and Liver

A large of acupuncture, referring to the deep layer of muscles corresponding to the liver and kidney, tendons and bones.

Lead

It is a kind of greyish white metal chiefly refined from the ore of Galenite.

Effect. Relieving reversed flow of qi, destroying parasites and removing toxic substances.

Indication. Accumulation of phlegm with reversed flow of qi, dyspnea, furunculosis.

Leakage of Skin Striae due to Hairs Steaming

It refers to striae of skin leaking, caused by injury of skin and hair by wind-heat.

Leaking-wind

Referring to sustaining attack by wind pathogen.

Symptoms. Profuse sweating, aversion to wind, deficiency of qi, etc.

Leatherleaf Mahonia Fruit

It is the fruit of Mahonia bealer (Fort.) Carr. M. fortunei (Lindl.) Fedde, or M. japonica (Thunb.) DC. (Berberidaceae).

Effect. Clearing away heat, dispelling dampness.

Indication. Recurring fever, osteopyrexia, diarrhea, metrorrhagia, leukorrhea and stranguria.

Leatherleaf Mahonia Stem

It is the dried stem of Mahonia bealei (Fort.) Carr. or Mahonia fortunei (Lindl.) Fedde (Berberidaceae).

Effect. Clearing away heat, relieving dampness, purging intense heat and detoxicating.

Indication. Diarrhea caused by damp-heat, jaundice, bloodshot, swollen and painful eyes, toothache due to stomach-fire, carbuncle, swelling, dysentery, etc.

Left and Right Twirling

It is an acupuncture point technique, referring to the twirling and rotating direction of needling. Generally, hold the needle in the right hand. Twirling the needle with the thumb moving forward and index finger backward, is called left rotation or outward rotation; twirling the needle with the thumb backward and index finger forward is called right rotation or inward rotation.

Leitou (Ex-CA)

A set of extra points.

Location. On both lateral borders of the sterna, on the inferior edges of the lst and 2nd rib-heads; 2 on each side, 4 points in total.

Indication. Abdominal mass, cough, asthma, pleurisy, indigestion, etc.

Method. Puncture obliquely 0.3-0.5 cun. Perform moxibustion 5-10 minutes.

Leixia (Ex-CA)

An extra point.

Location. On the chest, approximately in the 4th intercostal space, 4 cun lateral to the nipple.

Indication. Abdominal pain, pleurisy, peritonitis, etc.

Method. Perform moxibustion 5-10 minutes.

Lemongrass Herb

It is the whole plant of Cymbopogon citratus (DC.) Stapf. (Gramineae).

Effect. Dispelling wind, inducing diaphoresis, dissipating blood stasis and obstruction in the meridians.

Indication. Common cold with headache, stomachache, rheumatic arthralgia and traumatic injuries.

Leopard-spot Needling

A needling technique. Using a three-edged needle to prick meridians or collaterals here and there for bloodletting. In clinical practice, it is applied when treating diseases due to pathogenic cold, heat, blood stasis, etc.

Lepidium Seed

It is the ripe seed of Descuratinia sophia (L.) Schur. and Lepidium apetalum Willd. (Cruciferae).

Effect. Removing heat from the lung, relieving asthma, inducing diuresis and subduing swelling.

Indication. Stagnation of phlegm and fluid in the lung, asthma and cough with abundant sputum, fullness in the chest and hypochondrium, and slow urination.

Lepromatous Leprosy
Symptoms. At the beginning, white patches like tinea all over the body, with eyebrows and eyelashes dropping off and later, pitting of the nasal septum, backing of the eyes and chapped lips, corresponding to nodular leprosy.
Pathogenesis. The attacking of toxins into the lung.

Leprosy
Symptoms. At the beginning initially stubborn numbness of skin and muscle, red macula and pimple in the body and face, and then swelling and ulceration without pus. It may gradually spread over the whole body if it gets severe, with the appearance of tic of limbs, swelling of the head and the face, eyes injury, nose sunk, etc.
Pathogenesis. Pathogenic factors infiltrate bone marrow and circulate into meridians, collaterals and joints for a long duration.
Therapeutic Principle. Expelling endogenous wind to relieve toxicity,
relieving superficial syndrome by means of diaphoresis, nourishing ying and invigorating qi, tonifying and nourishing vitalqi and expelling pathogens, etc. The patient must be isolated.

Lesser galangal Rhizome
It is the rhizome of Alpinia officinarum Hance (Zingiberaceae).
Effect. Warming the spleen and stomach to arrest pain.
Indication. Gastric and abdominal cold pain, vomiting, diarrhea, etc.

Lethargy
A disease is mainly marked by tiredness and inclination to sleeping. There are three types:
1. **Symptoms.** Floating or heaviness of the body, loose stool.
Pathogenesis. Prevalence of dampness.
Therapeutic Principle. Regulating the spleen and eliminating dampness.
2. **Symptoms.** Weak limbs, drowsiness or state of drunkenness.
Pathogenesis. Spleen deficiency.
Therapeutic Principle. Replenishing qi and invigorating the spleen.
3. **Symptoms.** Bitter taste, coma and eclipsia.
Pathogenesis. Heat of the gallbladder.
Therapeutic Principle. Clearing away heat and purging the gallbladder-fire.

Letting out of Skin Rashes
This is a treatment for febrile disease caused by pathogenic factor of warmth. Applying drugs to clear away heat and letting heat out to erupt skin rashes.
Indication. Higher fever at night, delirious speech frequently, faint skin rashes.

Lettuce
It is the stem leaf of Lactuca sativa L. (Compositae).
Effect. Inducing defecation and promoting lactation.
Indication. Dysuria, hematuria and galactostasis.

Lettuce Seed
It is the seed of Lactuca sativa L. (Compositae).
Effect. Promoting lactation and diuresis.
Indication. Galactostasis, scanty urination, swelling of vulva, hemorrhoids with anal fistula and bleeding in stool.

Leukorrhagia due to Dampness and Heat of Liver Meridian
The disease is one type of the symptom complex of leukorrhagia.
Symptoms. Constant dripping of sticky and foul leukorrhagia, yellowish or white and red in color, fullness sensation in the breast and chest, dizziness, bitter taste and dry throat, dark-colored urine, etc.

Pathogenesis. Mostly caused by stagnation of the liver-qi and dampness accumulated in the spleen.

Therapeutic Principle. Clearing away heat, eliminating dampness, soothing the liver, strengthening the spleen.

Leukorrhagia due to Deficiency of the Spleen

A type of leukorrhagia.

Symptoms. White or light-yellow and thick vaginal discharge, without foul smell, yellowish complexion, poor appetite and watery stools, weakness of the limbs, etc.

Pathogenesis. Commonly caused by dysfunction of the spleen in transportation, a downward flow of accumulated dampness which impairs the front middle meridian and Belt Meridian.

Therapeutic Principle. Strengthen the spleen and replenish qi, remove dampness and stop leukorrhagia.

Leukorrhagia due to Kidney Deficiency

A disease, one type of the symptom complex of leukorrhagia.

Symptoms. Persistent leukorrhagia, soreness in the waist, cold and pain in the lower abdomen, loose stool, etc.

Pathogenesis. Impairment and deficiency of the kidney-qi as a result of sexual overindulgence, pregnancy and labor.

Therapeutic Principle. Warming yang and invigorating the kidney to arrest leukorrhagia.

Leukorrhagia due to Phlegm-dampness

It is one type of the symptom complex of leukorrhagia.

Symptoms. Thick and fishy leukorrhea, accompanied by nausea, cough, loose stool, etc.

Pathogenesis. Impairment of water metabolism caused by splenic deficiency.

Therapeutic Principle. Invigorating the spleen for eliminating dampness and phlegm to arrest leukorrhagia.

Leukorrhagia due to Splenic Hypofunction

Symptoms. Plenty of constant dripping of whitish or yellowish snivel and spit-like leukorrhagia, accompanied by yellowish complexion, mental fatigue, loose stool, etc.

Pathogenesis. Caused by retention of water in the lower part of the body due to dysfunction of the spleen in transport.

Therapeutic Principle. Strengthening the spleen and replenishing qi, and elevating the spleen-yang to eliminate dampness.

Leukorrhagia during Pregnancy

Symptoms. The obvious increase of leukorrhea after pregnancy.

Pathogenesis. Mostly caused by deficiency of the spleen, or stagnation of cold and dampness.

Therapeutic Principle. Strengthening the spleen to eliminate dampness and reinforcing original qi of the fetus.

Leukorrhea due to Noxious Dampness

A type of leukorrhea.

Symptoms. White or greenish yellow vaginal discharge with foul odor, in large quantity, occasionally with blood, itching in vagina, pain in the lower abdomen, scanty dark urine, etc.

Pathogenesis. Commonly caused by invasion of noxious dampness and other filthy pathogenic factors due to deficiency of the uterine collaterals during the menstrual period or after delivery.

Therapeutic Principle. Clear away heat and toxic material, remove dampness with expel the pathogenic factors.

Leukorrhea with Bloody Discharge

Symptoms. The constant discharge of the light colored bloody mucus from the vagina.

Pathogenesis. Mostly caused by anxiety that disturbs the heart and spleen, and pathogenic fire that causes stagnation of the liver-qi.

Therapeutic Principle. Enriching the spleen-qi, clearing away fire from the heart and liver.

Leukorrhea with Greenish Discharge

Symptoms. Constant smell, dark green mucus discharged from the vagina.

Pathogenesis. Mostly caused by weakness of uterine collaterals after delivery, affection of pathogenic damp-evil, or downward flow of damp-heat of the Liver Meridian impairing the conception vessel.

Therapeutic Principle. Regulate the function of the liver, clear heat and promote diuresis.

Leukorrhea with Yellowish Discharge

Symptoms. Constant foul smell, thick, yellowish liquid discharged from vagina. In serious cases, the liquid is like tea.

Pathogenesis. Mostly caused by excessive dampness, the change from damp stagnancy to heat, and injury to the Front Middle Meridian and the Back Middle Meridian.

Therapeutic Principle. Clearing away heat, eliminating dampness, promoting diuresis, and detoxicating.

Levant Cotton Root

It is the root or root bark of Gossypium herbaceum L. (Malvaceae).

Effect. Suppliment qi, relieving asthma and regulating menstruation.

Indication. Cough and asthma caused by debility, hernia, metrorrhagia, leukorrhea and hysteroptosis.

Liangmen (S 21)

A meridian acupuncture point.

Location. On the upper abdomen, 4 cun above the center of the umbilicus and 2 cun lateral to the anterior midline.

Indication. Stomachache, vomiting, anorexia, loose stool.

Method. Puncture perpendicularly 0.5-1.0 cun, or perform moxibustion for 10-15 min.

Liangqiu (S 34)

A meridian acupuncture point.

Location. With the knee flexed, the point is on the anterior side of the thigh and on the line connecting the anterior superior iliac spine and the superior lateral corner of the patella, 2 cun above this corner

Indication. Stomachache, swelling and pain of the knee, paralysis of the lower limbs, acute mastitis.

Method. Puncture perpendicularly 0.5-1.0 cun. Perform moxibustion for 3-5 moxa cones or 10-15 minutes.

Lianquan (CV 23)

An acupuncture point.

Location. Above the laryngeal protuberance, in the depression at the superior border of the hyoid bone.

Indication. Swelling and pain of the subglossal region, aphasia with stiffness of the tongue, sudden loss of voice, oral ulceration, cough with dyspnea and asthma, fullness and pain sensation in chest, etc.

Method. Puncture obliquely 0.5-0.8 cun towards the root of the tongue. Perform moxibustion 3-5 moxa cones or 5-10 minutes.

Liaoliao (Ex-LE)

An extra acupoint.

Location. On the medial side of the knee joint, 3 cun inferior to Yinlingquan (Sp 9).

Indication. Metrorrhagia and leukorrhagia, irregular menstruation, itch and pain in the medial side of the leg due to wind-sore.

Method. Puncture perpendicularly 0.5-1.0 cun or moxibustion is applicable.

Lichenoid Dermatitis

It refers to the localized injury with clear boundary but of different size.

Symptoms. Dry and rough skin, localized injury with clear boundary, widening and deepening of skin. It can be seen in some chronic itching dermatitis.

Pathogenesis. Mostly caused by deficiency of blood and wind-dryness.

Licorice Root

It is the root and rhizome of Glycyrrhiza uralensis Fisch. (Leguminosae).

Effect. Invigorating the spleen, replenishing qi, moistening the lung, arresting cough, relieving spasm and pain and moderating the properties of other drugs.

Indication. Short breath, asthenia, poor appetite and loose stool; carbuncles, cellulitis, furuncle and boils, food or drug poisoning, etc.

Lidui (S 45)

A meridian acupuncture point.

Location. On the lateral side of the distal segment of the 2nd toe, 0.1 cun posterior to the proximal corner of the toe-nail.

Indication. Edema of the face, dry mouth, toothache, epistaxis, distention and full sensation in the chest and abdomen, cold limbs, febrile disease, frequent dreams, etc.

Method. Puncture perpendicularly 0.1 cun, or prick to cause bleeding. Perform moxibustion 3-5 moxa cones.

Lienteric Diarrhea

Symptoms. Diarrhea, indigestion of food.

Pathogenesis. Deficiency of qi and weakness of yang in the spleen and stomach, or due to attacks of pathogenic factors such as wind, dampness, cold, and heat on the bowels and stomach.

Lieque (L7)

An acupuncture point.

Location. At the radial border of the forearm, above the styloid process of the radius, 1.5 cun above the transverse crease of the wrist.

Indication. Headache, cough, dyspnea, sore throat, dental swelling and pain, rigid neck, hematuria, stiff neck, etc.

Method. Puncture subcutaneously 0.5-0.8 cun and apply moxibustion to the point for 3-5 moxa cones or 5-10 minutes.

Life-long Sterility

1. A disease, referring to infertility for life due to suffering from diseases.
2. A term of gynecology. It refers to life-long infertility by means of medicine or operation.

Life Natural Instincts

A term in qigong, referring to the life natural instincts of the human body, also referring to the brain vitality.

Life Pass

It has two meanings: 1. It refers to looking at one of the diagnosis part for infant. Life pass can be located on the distal segment of the index finger. If the collateral of the index finger can be seen in this part, it means that the disease is very serious and dangerous. 2. A term of massage, referring to the finger-print surface of the distal segment of the index finger.

Lifting

A needling method. It refers to lifting the inserted needle gently.

Lifting and Thrusting

One of the basic needling techniques. When the needle is inserted to a given depth at the point, apply lifting and thrusting of the needle, i.e. make the needle moves from the shallow layer to the deep layer by thrusting it and from the deep layer to the shallow layer by lifting it. The lifting and thrusting can well be done repeatedly.

Lifting Drug

This drug obtained by sublimating the mixture of mercury, niter and alum each in the equal amount.

Effect. Drawing out the pus and removing the necrotic tissue.

Indication. Post-rupture of carbuncles, stagnant pus, retention of slough, and difficulty for regeneration of the tissue.

Ligation Method

A treatment refers to the method of ligaturing the affected part by using thread, the silk ligature or ordinary threads, to block qi and blood of the local part in order to produce pathogenic necrotic changes and dropping off. It is applicable to neoplastic growth and hemorrhoid, etc., but prohibited to angioma and carcinomatosis swelling.

Light Diaphoretic Prescription

A term in classifying prescriptions. It is mainly consisting of drugs cold and cool in nature. Their action is slightly facilitating flow of the lung-qi.

Light Wheat

It is the unripe caryopsis of Triticum aestivum L. (Gramineae).

Effect. Tonifying qi, removing heat and arresting sweating.

Indication. Spontaneous perspiration, night sweat and hectic fever due to yin-deficiency.

Light-yellow Sophora Root

It is the root of Sophora flavescens Ait. (Leguminosae).

Effect. Removing heat and dampness, dispelling wind, destroying parasites eliminating phlegm, relieving dyspnea, calming the mind, and inducing diuresis.

Indication. Dampheat dysentery cough and dyspnea and leukorrhea, jaundice, scabies and tinea, stranguria, scrofula, scalds, etc.

Ligou (Liv 5)

A meridian acupuncture point.

Location. On the medial side of the leg, 5 cun above the tip of the medial malleolus, on the midline of the medial surface of the tibia.

Indication. Abnormal menstruation, leukorrhea with reddish discharge, hernia, difficulty in urination, painful and swollen testis, muscular atrophy of the lower extremities, etc.

Method. Puncture subcutaneously 0.5-0.8 cun. Perform moxibustion 1-3 moxa cones or 3-5 minutes.

Lilac and Moist Tongue

A tongue condition, which refers to a corpulent, tender, and moist tongue with lilac color. It can be seen in the patient with excess of cold due to yang insufficiency.

Lilac Daphne Flower Bud

It is the flower-bud of Daphne genkwa Sieb. et Zucc. (Thymelaeaceae).

Effect. Removing retained water and fluid, dissipating phlegm, arresting cough, destroying intestinal parasites and detoxicating.

Indication. Dyspnea, cough or dyspnea edema, ascites, fluid retention in the pleural cavity, abnormal urination, etc.

Lily Bulb

It is the pulpy bulb of Lilium brownii F.E. Brown var. Viridulum Baker, and Lilium pumilum DC. (Liliaceae).

Effect. Nourishing the lung to arrest cough and clearing away heart-fire to tranquilize the mind.

Indication. Cough due to lung heat, hemoptysis, restlessness of deficiency, fright-induced palpitation, insomnia and dreaminess sleep.

Lily Bulb Flower

It is the flower of Lilium brounii F.E. Brown var. Viridulum Baker (Liliaceae).

Effect. Nourishing the lung arrests cough and removing heat from the heart and tranquilizing the mind.

Indication. Cough, dizziness, vexation, insomnia and pemphigus.

Lily Disease

A disease, one of the emotional diseases.

Symptoms. Mental disturbance and restlessness, reticence, insomnia, poor appetite, bitter taste and dark urine.

Pathogenesis. Caused by yin deficiency of the heart and lung, mental depression or convalescence after a severe illness.

Therapeutic Principle. Nourishing yin to clear away heat.

Limb Flaccidity due to Deficiency of Blood

Symptoms. Weakness of hands and feet, akinesia, flaccidity of muscles, and sallow complexion, etc.

Pathogenesis. Usually caused by postpartum or excessive loss of blood, the malnutrition of muscles due to deficiency of yin blood.

Therapeutic Principle. Nourishing yin and supplementing blood.

Lime

It is the slaked lime from Limestone.

Effect. Eliminating dampness, destroying parasites, arresting bleeding, relieving pain, etc.

Indication. Scabies, tinea, moist sores, traumatic bleeding, scalds, hemorrhoid, etc.

Limonite

It is the natural powder-like brownish iron ore mainly commposed of FeO(OH).

Effect. Astringe intestines, stop diarrhea, and astringe to arrest bleeding.

Indication. Chronic diarrhea, chronic dysentery, metrorrhagia, metrostaxis, leukorrhea and hemorrhoid.

Limosis

It is one of the main symptoms of diabetes. Usually caused by the stomach-heat.

Linear Stonecrop Herb

It is the whole herb of Sedum lineare Thunb. (Crassulaceae).

Effect. Clearing away heat, subduing swelling, relieving pain and detoxicating.

Indication. Hepatitis swollen and sore throat, subcutaneous swelling, furuncle, jaundice, cholecystitis, and dysentery.

Lineiting (Ex-LE)

An extra acupoint.

Location. On the sole of the foot, between the 2nd and the 3th metatarsal bones, opposite to Neiting (S 44).

Indication. Pain in toes, infantile convulsion, epilepsy, etc.

Method. Puncture perpendicularly 0.3-0.5 cun. Perform moxibustion 3-5 moxa cones.

Lingdao (H 4)

A meridian acupuncture point, the Jing (River) point of the Heart Meridian.

Location. On the palmar side of the forearm and on the radial side of the tendon of the ulnar flexor muscle of the wrist, 1.5 cun above the transverse crease of the wrist.

Indication. Palpitations, severe palpitations, inability to speak due to stiffness of the tongue, dizziness, etc.

Method. Puncture perpendicularly 0.3-0.4 cun. Perform moxibustion 3-7 minutes.

Lingering Diarrhea

Symptoms. Protracted and incessant diarrhea, anorexia, cold limbs, shortness of breath, emaciation, etc.

Pathogenesis. Usually caused by qi exhaustion and prostration, the impairment of the spleen and kidney and the sinking of lucid yang.

Therapeutic Principle. Inducing astringency and stopping diarrhea, and strengthening the body resistance to eliminate pathogenic factors.

Lingering of Pathogenic Factor in Precardium

It refers to the long period pathogenesis.

Symptoms. Soporose state, convulsion, dementia, difficulty in speaking, etc.

Pathogenesis. Pathogenic factor of phlegm.

Linghou (Ex-LE)

An extra point.

Location. On the lateral side of the leg, in the depression inferior to the posterior border of the small head of the fibula. Posterior to yanglingquan (G 34).

Indication. Arthritis of the knee joint, sciatica, paralysis of the lower limbs.

Method. Puncture perpendicularly 0.5-1.0 cun. Perform moxibustion 3-5 minutes.

Lingtai (GV 10)

A meridian acupuncture point.

Location. On the back and on the posterior midline, in the depression below the spinous process of the 6th thoracic vertebra.

Indication. Cough, dyspnea, stiffness of the neck, rigidity and pain of the lower back, furuncle and sore, etc.

Method. Puncture obliquely upward 0.5-1 cun and apply moxibustion on the point for 5-10 minutes.

Lingual Pustule

Symptoms. Purple bubbles on the tongue, hard and painful.

Pathogenesis. Mostly caused by the toxic fire in the Heart Meridian.

Therapeutic Principle. Clearing away heat, detoxification.

Lingxu (K 24)

A meridian acupuncture point.

Location. On the chest, in the 3rd intercostal space, 2 cun lateral to the anterior midline.

Indication. Cough, asthma, pain and distention in the chest and hypochondriac region, vomiting, acute mastitis.

Method. Puncture obliquely or subcutaneously 0.3-0.5 cun. Deep puncture is inadvisable. Perform moxibustion 3-5 minutes, or 3-5 moxa cones.

Liniaoxue

An acupuncture point.

Location. 2.5 cun below the umbilicus on the median abdominal line.

Indication. Enuresis, retention of urine, difficult urination, enteritis, dysentery, etc.

Method. Puncture perpendicularly 0.5 cun and apply moxibustion to the point for 10-15 minutes, or press the point with the fingers.

Linquan (Ex-B)

An extra point.

Location. One point is 0.5 cun above the coccyx and two points are 0.5 cun respectively lateral to it, altogether three points in a line.

Indication. Gonorrhea.

Method. Apply moxibustion with 5-10 moxa cones for each point.

Linseed

It is the dried ripe seed of Linum usitatissimum L. (Linaceae).

Effect. Moistening dryness and dispelling wind.

Indication. Constipation dry skin, cutaneous pruritus, dried and withered hair.

Lip Abscess

It is mostly caused by heat accumulation in the spleen and stomach.

Symptoms. Abscess grown on the lip with uncertain locations, assumes purple appearance with hard swelling. The patient has subjective sensation of numbness at the early stage, with pain and numbness later.

Therapeutic Principle. At the early stage, subduing swelling and resolving abscess if there is exterior syndrome of alternate attacks of chills and fever. Later the abscess grows bigger and the patient possesses interior heat, mainly removing pathogenic heat from the heart and diaphragm.

Lip Erosion

It refers to erosion in the lips and mouth.
Pathogenesis. Mainly caused by excessive heat in the stomach and dampness in the Spleen Meridian.
Therapeutic Principle. Clearing away heat to remove dampness.

Lip Pustule

Symptoms. The disease appears rather inside the lip ridge, miller-like form, purple, hard, itching, numb and painful at the beginning. It is necessary to treat it soon. In the case of the delayed treatment, it will attack the inside organs and cause vertigo and nausea.
Pathogenesis. Fire-toxin in three meridians of the spleen, stomach and heart.
Therapeutic Principle. The treatment is the same with the furuncle. Clearing away heat, removing toxic material and eliminating heat from the heart to restore the consciousness. Puncture the point weizhong but not by moxibustion.

Lip Shaking

Symptoms. Uncontrolled lip shaking, slobbering, vexation and insomnia, etc.
Pathogenesis. Blood deficiency and wind-dryness, or the hypofunction of the spleen.

Lips Turning Over

It refers to the lips rolling up.
Pathogenesis. Deficiency and weakness of the spleen and stomach, failure of insufficient blood to nourish lips.

Litchi Leaf

It is the leaf of Litchi chinensis Sonn. (Spindaceae).
Effect. Astringing dampness.
Indication. Ulcers behind ears.

Litchi Nut

It is the fruit of Litchi chinensis Sonn. (Sapindaceae)
Effect. Promoting the production of body fluid, nourishing blood, regulating flow of qi and arresting pain.
Indication. Polydipsia, stomachache, furuncle, toothache and traumatic bleeding.

Litchi Root

It is the root of Litchi chinensis Sonn. (Sapindaceae).
Indication. Stomachache of stomach-cold type, seminal emission and inflammation of the throat, etc.

Litchi Seed

It is the seed of Litchi chinensis Sonn. (Sapindaceae).
Effect. Warming the middle-energizer, promoting flow of qi and arresting pain, expelling cold and resolving masses.
Indication. Hernial pain due to cold, painful and swollen testis, stomachache, abdominal pain before menstruation, and postpartum abdominal pain, etc.

Litchi Shell

It is the shell of Litchi chinensis Sonn. (Sapindaceae).
Indication. Dysentery, metrorrhagia and eczema.

Little Ground-cherry Herb or Fruit

The whole herb or fruit of Physalis minima L. (Solanaceae).
Effect. Expelling dampness and destroying parasites.
Indication. Cough, dyspnea, jaundice, scrofula, pemphigus, damp sores, dysuria, etc.

Littleleaf Dogwood Root

It is the whole plant of Cornus paucinervis Hance. (Cornaceae).
Effect. Dissipating blood stasis, arresting pain, stopping bleeding and knitting bones.

Indication. Fracture and traumatic bleeding.

Liufeng (Ex-UE)
A group of extra points.
Location. Four points, i.e. Sifeng (Ex-E 10), on the palmer side, at the center of the proximal interphalangeal joints of the 2nd to 5th fingers, and the other two points, at the middle points of the transverse crease of the metacarpophalangeal joint and the interphalangeal joint of the thumb, 6 points on each hand, 12 points in all.
Indication. Furuncle, malnutrition and indigestion in children, etc.
Method. Puncture perpendicularly 0.1-0.2 cun, or prick to squeeze out yellowish and whitish mucus.

Liver (MA-SC 5)
An auricular point.
Location. On the lateral inferior border of the cymba concha.
Indication. Hypochondriac pain, dizziness, irregular menstruation, etc.

Liver Abscess
A disease, refers to the abscess appearing on the liver lobes.
Symptoms. Chills, fever, swelling of the liver, and evident pain on touching and tapping in the liver region.
Pathogenesis. Mostly caused by the transformation of fire due to stagnation of liver-qi, blood stasis due to stagnation of qi, which is accumulated to form abscess, or by the steaming of phlegm due to accumulated dampness.
Therapeutic Principle. In the early phase, it shows the stagnation of liver-qi and the gallbladder-heat, it is advisable to remove heat from the liver, normalize function of the gallbladder, regulate the flow of qi and alleviate mental depression. In the middle phase, it shows the formation of pus and excessive fire toxin, it is advisable to purge intense heat and detoxicate with the assistance of letting out the pus. In the final phase, it shows weakened body resistance with toxin lingering, and it is advisable to invigorate qi and enrich the blood to remove toxin.

Liver and Gallbladder are Related Interior-exteriorly
The liver is a zang organ belonging to yin, while the gallbladder is a fu organ belonging to yang. They all belong to wood in the five elements and the yin and yang interior and exterior relationship is formed by connecting the Liver Meridian with the Gallbladder Meridian. The liver and gallbladder can influence each other if diseased, showing their interior-exterior relationship.

Liver Apoplexy
Symptoms. Shaking head and twitching of eyelid, hypochondriac pain, frequent bending walk, or sitting in rigidity with inability to lower the head, etc.
Pathogenesis. Usually caused by the invasion of pathogenic wind, the blockage of body fluid and blood resulting in the impairment of the Liver Meridians.
Therapeutic Principle. Dispelling wind and nourishing the liver.

Liver Being Easily Affected by Anger
It refers to upward invasion of the hyperactive liver-qi, dysfunction of expelling and purging due to consistent anger.
Symptoms. Headache, dizziness, flushed face, reversed flow of qi, even syncope and hematemesis.

Liver-blood
The blood stored in the liver often related to the liver-yin. Clinically, the syndromes of liver-blood are usually associated with bleeding and deficiency of blood, not necessarily with manifestation of yin deficiency and yang excess.

Liver-cold

A syndrome, refers to a cold syndrome resulting from deficiency of the liver-yang and hypofunction of the liver.

Symptoms. Depression, fright, fatigue cold limbs, deep thready slow pulse.

Therapeutic Principle. Warming the liver, promoting the circulation of qi and dispelling cold.

Liver Collateral

One of the fifteen collaterals, which is derived from Ligou (Liv 5), 5 cun above the medial malleolus to the Gallbladder Meridian. The branch ascends along tibia to testis, knots at the penis.

Liver Divergent Meridian

A meridian derived from Liver Meridian, at the dorsum of the foot, ascending to the margin of the pubic region, converging with Gallbladder Meridian, and running parallel with it.

Liver Edema

A kind of edema referring to edema due to hepatopathy.

Symptoms. Abdominal distention, distending pain in hypochondrium, anorexia and lassitude, etc.

Pathogenesis. Caused by stagnation of qi or the obstruction of damp-heat and accumulation of phlegm stagnancy, etc.

Therapeutic Principle. Relieving the depressed liver and inducing diuresis, removing dampness and clearing away heat, and promoting blood circulation by removing blood stasis.

Liver Epilepsy

A kind of epilepsy.

Symptoms. Bluish complexion, shaking head, wide opening eyes and alternation of joy and anger, etc.

Pathogenesis. Usually caused by the impairment of the liver by anger or hyperactivity of yang due to yin deficiency, etc.

Therapeutic Principle. Soothing the liver to stop the wind and relieving convulsion to calm the frightening.

Liver Failure

It has two implications:

1. It refers to the critical syndromes occurring in the liver failure.

   Symptoms. Pale complexion, bluish lips, blindness with open eyes, constant sweating, etc.

   Pathogenesis. Usually caused by the impairment of essence by hemorrhage, or the impairment of vital energy by hepatic disease, etc.

   Therapeutic Principle. Astringing the liver-qi and strengthening the body resistance, and treating the prostration syndrome.

2. It refers to the prostration syndrome of apoplexy with closed eyes or staring straight.

Liver-fire

It is defined as heat syndrome or symptoms of reversed flow of the liver qi due to hyperfunction of the liver.

Symptoms. It is manifested as dizziness and distending pain in the head, flushed complexion, congested eyes, bitter taste, dry throat, irritability, distending pain in hypochondrium, constipation, dark urine, red tip and edge of the tongue, taut rapid pulse and even coma, madness and vomiting.

Pathogenesis. Caused by hyperactivity of the live-yang or accumulation of heat in the Liver Meridian due to extreme seven emotions.

Therapeutic Principle. Purging the liver of pathogenic fire.

Liver-fire Epigastralgia

The epigastralgia caused by the dominant liver-fire attacking the stomach.

Symptoms. Frequent epigastralgia with hypochondriac pain, bitter taste, etc.

Therapeutic Principle. Soothing the liver, purging away the heat, and regulating the stomach.

Liver Governing Ascending of qi

It refers to the liver's dispersing and discharging functions. When these liver functions are normal, the qi ascends and regulates the vital qi and blood. If the ascending of qi is unrestraint, the hyperactivity of the liver-yang occurs, manifested by headache, dizziness and so on.

Liver-heat Attacking Lung

A morbid condition resulting from stagnation of the liver-qi.

Symptoms. Burning pain in the chest and hypochondrium, dizziness, bloodshot eyes, paroxysmal cough, little thick yellow sputum, often accompanied by irritability, dysphoria, fever, bitter taste, red tongue with thin yellow fur.

Therapeutic Principle. Purging pathogenic fire of the liver and clearing away the lung-heat.

Liver-heat Disease

Symptoms. Abdominal pain, fever, thirst, yellow urine, mental irritability with fright, hypochondriac pain, feverish sensation of hands and feet and insomnia, etc.

Pathogenesis. Caused by the invasion of the pathogenic heat into the liver.

Therapeutic Principle. Removing heat from the liver.

Liver Impairment

It is one of seven kinds of impairments and refers to the impairment of the liver.

Symptoms. Gradual emaciation and weakness, bluish hands and feet, heavy eyes, with pain in pupils.

Pathogenesis. Caused by outburst of anger and reversed flow of qi impairing the liver.

Therapeutic Principle. Soothing the liver and regulating the circulation of qi.

Liver-jaundice

One of nine types of jaundice.

Symptoms. Yellow eyes and limbs, especially eyes, cold limbs, and incessant sweating above the waist, etc.

Pathogenesis. Caused by stagnation of the liver-qi, and accumulation of damp-heat in the body.

Therapeutic Principle. Soothing the liver and regulating the circulation of qi, and eliminating damp-heat.

Liver Malnutrition

One of five kinds of malnutrition.

Symptoms. Sallow complexion, dryness and itching of eyes, more sweating and diarrhea, etc.

Pathogenesis. Usually caused by pathogenic heat latent in the Liver Meridian.

Therapeutic Principle. Purging heat away from the liver.

Liver Meridian

One of twelve regular meridians. The meridian starts from Dadun (Liv 1) on the big toe, just behind the nail. It ascends along the dorsum of the foot to the region one cun in front of the medial malleolus, then through the inner side of the lower limb, crossing the Spleen Meridian at 8 individual cun above the medial malleolus. It continues its ascent, passing through the medial side of the knee, along the medial side of the thigh, to the pubic region, curves round the external genitalia and enters the lower abdomen to qimen (Liv 14), a point about 2 cun below the nipple. From there it runs upwards via the stomach into its pertaining organ, the liver and communicates with the gall bladder. Upward, it ascends through the diaphragm along the trachea, larynx, sinus cavity, connecting with the surrounding tissues of the eye, then emerges from the forehead, and finally meets the Back Middle Meridian.

Liver-qi

This term has three meanings: 1. It refers to the essence of the liver. 2. It refers to the functional activities of the liver, which has the function of smoothing and regulating the flow of vital-qi and blood. 3. It is a short form of stagnation of the liver-qi.

Liver-qi Attacking Stomach

A morbid state of failure of the stomach to descend.

Symptoms. Mental depression, anger, anorexia, distention in the hypochondrium, distending pain in the stomach, belching, vomiting.

Pathogenesis. Caused by stagnation of the liver-qi, dysfunction of the liver to smooth and regulate the flow of qi and blood and impairment of the stomach by the reversed flow of qi.

Therapeutic Principle. Relieving depressed liver and regulating the stomach.

Liver Related to Anger

Over-anger may lead to stagnation of the liver-qi, and upward invasion of the hyperactive liver-qi. The stagnation of the liver-qi turns into fire. The relation between anger and the pathologic changes of liver is so closed.

Liver Restricting Spleen

Symptoms. Mental depression, anger, susceptibility to sigh, distending pain in chest and hypochondrium, fullness in the stomach and abdomen, borborygmus, diarrhea, etc.

Pathogenesis. Dysfunction of the spleen and stomach resulted from restriction of the spleen and stomach by excess of the liver-qi.

Liver Serves to Regulate the Activity of Vital-qi and Blood

It refers to that the liver has the functions of dispersing and discharging qi, blood, and fluid. When these functions of the liver are normal, the circulation of qi is smooth, the relationship between qi and blood is in harmony, the conditions of meridians are normal, and zang-fu organs work normally and coordinately.

Liver Signs Favorable Prognosis of Sores

One of the methods to judge the prognosis of sores.

Symptoms. Light and vigorous body, easy mind without restlessness, red lively nails, quiet and comfortable living. These show that the vital essence of the liver has not been exhausted, and that the disease has a good prognosis.

Liver Storing and Regulating Blood

It refers to the function of liver to store blood and regulate its amount, serving as a reservoir of blood. Will expel the blood stored to satisfy the need. When the body is in the state of rest, part of the blood circulating around the body is stored in the liver. The dysfunction of the liver results not only in blood deficiency or bleeding, but also in pathological changes in malnourishment of many parts by blood.

Liver-syncope

Symptoms. It appears as epilepsy, numbness with sleepiness, vomiting when awake, dizziness and fever, etc.

Pathogenesis. Rising of cold extremities of liver-qi.

Therapeutic Principle. Regulating circulation of qi and lowering the adverse flow of qi.

Liver Taking Charge of Tendons

The liver supplies the tendons with nutrients to develop physical strength. Malnutrition of the tendons due to deficiency of the liver-blood may result in numbness of the extremities, sluggishness of joint movement, spasm of the muscles and tremors of fingers.

Liver-wind

Symptoms. Dizziness, convulsion, trembling of hands and feet, or endogenous wind.

Pathogenesis. Excess of pathogenic heat or failure of the liver-yin to control the liver-yang due to yin deficiency results in abnormal rising of the liver-yang, so uncontrollable that liver-wind is stirred.

Liver-wood

This term has two meanings: 1. It refers to the liver corresponding to wood, according to the theory of the Five Evolutive Phases. 2. It refers to a massage site.

Liver-yang

Referring to vital function of the liver. It governs ascending, smoothing and regulating the flow of vital-qi and blood.

Liver-yang (MA)1

One of the auricular acupuncture points.
Location. At the upper rim of the tuberculum helix.
Indication. Chronic hepatitis.

Liver-yang (MA)2

One of the auricular acupuncture points.
Location. At the lower rim of the tuberculum helix.
Indication. Chronic hepatitis.

Liver-yang Headache

Symptoms. Dizziness, irritability, irascibility, disturbed sleep, etc.
Pathogenesis. Up-disturbance of the liver-yang.
Therapeutic Principle. Calming the liver and suppressing yang hyperactivity of the liver.

Liver-yang Vertigo

A kind of dizziness.
Symptoms. Dizziness and headache, restless sleep, irritability, flushed face, etc.
Pathogenesis. Mainly caused by discomfort of emotions, excessive vexation, internal exhaustion of liver-yin, which lead to

liver yin failing to counterbalance yang, yang-qi of the liver rising abnormally.
Therapeutic Principle. Calming the liver and suppressing the excessive yang.

Liver-yin

It refers to the blood and yin fluid in the liver. Under normal conditions, the liver-yin and liver-yang coordinate each other to maintain relative balance. When the liver-qi is in hyperactivity and the liver-yang is excess, this condition may exhaust the liver-yin while insufficiency of the liver-yin may result in hyperactivity of the liver-yang.

Lizard

The whole body of Eremias argus Peters (Lacertidae).
Effect. Eliminating scrofula.
Indication. Tuberculosis of lymph node.

Lizard-tympanites

Symptoms. Dark sallow complexion, tongue boil, fullness sensation and lingering light pain in abdomen, stool with pus and blood, emaciation and darkish sallow complexion in the serious case.
Pathogenesis. Noxious agents produced by various parasites.
Therapeutic Principle. Detoxicating, killing parasites.

Local Point Selection

One of the point selection methods, referring to the selection of the meridian acupuncture points, extra points, or Ashi points, etc. In the pain area, e.g. Quchi (LI 11) is selected for the pain in elbow, Xiyan (Ex-LE 4&5) for knee pain, Jingming (B 1) for eye diseases, Yingxiang (LI 20) for stuffy nose, Zhongwan (CV 12) for gastric abscess, Zhongji (CV 3) for enuresis, etc.

Locating Point by Finger-cun Measurement

One of the methods for locating acupoints, referring to locating an acupoint according to the stipulated length and breadth of the patient's fingers as a unit.

Location According to Anatomical Landmarks on Body Surface

One of the methods for locating points, referring to the method of determining the position of points according to anatomical signs on the body surface.

Lochiorrhea

Symptoms. Contant dripping of profuse, and stinking lochia following childbirth, accompanied by pain in the lower abdomen and vagina, tiredness, dizziness, chest tightness, shortness of breath, and loss of appetite, etc.

Therapeutic Principle. Invigorating qi and arresting hemorrhage.

Lochiostasis

It refers to the retention of Lochia, or if any, small discharge after delivery. This disease is divided into two clinical types: 1. Qi stagnation, 2. Blood stasis.

1. **Symptoms.** Retention of lochia or lochia in small amounts, distending sensation in the chest and hypochondrium, distention and pain in the lower abdomen.

   Pathogenesis. Mostly due to emotional depression leading to the stagnation of liver qi, disorderly movement of qi followed by the obstruction of blood circulation.

   Therapeutic Principle. Relieving the depressed liver, dissipating blood stasis.

2. **Symptoms.** Very little lochia discharge with dark purplish color, palpating the abdomen with the lower abdominal pain, palpable mass at the painful site.

   Pathogenesis. Mostly due to cold pathogens and cold food intake leading to the stagnation of blood.

   Therapeutic Principle. Promoting blood circulation to remove blood stasis.

Locked Chest due to Cold

Symptoms. Fullness and tenderness of the chest, constipation, vexation, absence of feeling of thirst, and seldom fever, etc.

Pathogenesis. Erroneous cold bath for Taiyang Meridian syndrome which leads to obstruction of pathogenic heat by cold, attachment of water and cold on the lung and accumulation of cold in the chest.

Therapeutic Principle. Warming and removing cold.

Locked Knee

Symptoms. While moving the knee joints or walking in a posture at a certain angle, a sudden feeling of inability to extend and flex the knee joint accompanied by pain, as if gripped by something. Then, the gripping feeling is staggered and removed by slow extention and flexion of knee joints, and normal movement is restored.

Cause. Patients with meniscus injury, or presence of corpus liberum in knee joints.

Lockjaw

Symptoms. Trismus, inability to open mouth.

Pathogenesis. Mainly caused by internal stagnated heat and exogenous wind, phlegm and qi stagnation, and stagnated meridians and collaterals. It can be seen in such diseases as apoplexy, convulsion disease, infantile convulsion, etc.

Lockjaw in Newborn

Symptoms. Convulsion and trismus, inability to suck the breasts.

Pathogenesis. Caused by tetanus due to the umbilical cord being cut off unclean and infection of the exterior pathogens. In general, it happens four to seven days after birth.

Therapeutic Principle. Relieve convulsion and calm the wind.

Lock Throat Syndrome

Symptoms. Pain in the inside and outside of the faucial isthmus with a red swelling region as big as an egg, chocking sensation in the chest, short breath, tachypnea, dysphasia, trismus, ozostomia, constipation, fever and aversion to cold.

Pathogenesis. Mostly caused by heat in the lung and stomach, repeated attack of pathogenic wind that invades and occupies the throat.

Therapeutic Principle. Dispelling wind, clearing away heat, removing toxic substances and subduing swelling, releasing pus by pricking with a needle or knife if there is formation of pus.

Loess-cake-separated Moxibustion

A kind of cake-separated moxibustion, referring to moxibustion, which uses coarse moxa-cones and mud-cakes made of clean earth and water, one cake for each moxa-cone.

Log-like Hernia

Symptoms. Orchioscirrhus and thickness of scrotal skin without pain and itching.

Pathogenesis. Mostly caused by condensation of cold-dampness.

Therapeutic Principle. Strengthening the spleen, warming the middle-energizer, and clearing and regulating water passage.

Loin as Seat of Kidney

As the kidneys are located in both sides of the lumbar spinal column, patients with kidney disease often complain of lumbago.

Long

This term has three meanings: 1. It refers to difficulty in micturition with dripping bit by bit in a small amount. The case develops slowly and belongs to a slight dysuria. 2. An old term for stranguria. 3. It refers to hunchback, a back disease with hunchback. Others say it is lameness, with inability to to walk on foot.

Longan Aril

The ripe flesh of Euphoria longan Lour. (Sapindaceae).

Effect. Nourishing the heart and spleen and supplementing qi and blood.

Indication. Severe palpitation, insomnia, amnesia, etc.

Longan Seed

The seed of Euphoria longan Lour. (Sapindaceae).

Effect. Arresting bleeding, alleviating pain, regulating flow of qi and dispelling dampness.

Indication. Traumatic bleeding, scrofula, scabies and tinea, etc.

Longestapex Beantyberry Leaf

The leaf of Callicarpa longissima (Hemsl.) Merr. (Verbenaceae).

Effect. Expelling wind and cold, dissipating blood stasis and detoxicating.

Indication. Rheumatic arthralgia, cough due to wind-cold, abdominal pain due to accumulation of cold and traumatic injuries, etc.

Longhan (Ex-CA)

An extra point, also named Longtou.

Location. 1.5 cun directly above Jiuwei (CV 15).

Indication. Stomachache, dyspnea.

Method. Puncture subcutaneously 0.2-0.3 cun. Apply moxibustion 3-10 minutes with a moxa stick.

Long Inhalation

It refers to the deep, long and difficult inhalation of the patient. It indicates decline of kidney-yang.

Long Pepper

The immatured fruit spike of Piper longum L. (Piperaceae).

Effect. Warming the middle-energizer and alleviating pain.

Indication. Vomit and hiccups due to cold in the stomach, diarrhea and abdominal pain, etc.

Long Pulse

It refers to the pulse with large extent and prolonged stroke. A long pulse with moderate tension is a normal pulse, but a long and taut pulse indicates an excess syndrome in which both the pathogenic factor and the body resistance are strong.

Long Retention of the Needle for Cold Syndromes

One of the principles of acupuncture treatment, referring to dispelling the pathogenic cold, which can be relived by retaining the needle in the treatment of cold syndrome.

Long Snake Moxibustion

One of the moxibustion methods, also named spreading moxibustion.

Method. Peel and pound some garlic and spread it on the spinal column from acupoint Dazhui (GV 14) to Yaoshu (GV 2) about 6 mm in both thickness and width. Cover the skin with mulberry paper, then apply respectively to Dazhui (GV 14) and Yaoshu (GV 2), burning cones of moxa, as big as soybeans, until the patient has the smell of garlic both in his mouth and nose. It is used for the treatment of consumptive diseases.

Longstamen Loosestrife Herb

The whole herb of Lysimachia lobelioides Wall. (Primulaceae).

Effect. Supplementing qi, relieving cough and arresting bleeding.

Indication. Cough of deficiency syndrome, swelling pain in the breast and traumatic injuries.

Long-standing Asthma

Symptoms. Recurrent attacks of dyspnea, fullness sensation and distention in the chest, etc.

Pathogenesis. Usually caused by accumulation of wind-cold and pleural effusion in lungs leading to obstruction of air passage and upward adverse flow of the lung-qi.

Therapeutic Principle. Warming the lung to dispel cold and removing fluid retention to relieve asthma.

Long-standing Lumbago

Symptoms. Lumbago and weakness of the knees and legs, aggravated by tiredness and relieved by bed rest, and repeated attack.

Pathogenesis. Mostly caused by kidney-qi insufficiency or lingering of pathogenic factors due to kidney deficiency.

Therapeutic Principle. Tonifying the kidney, sometimes together with eliminating the pathogenic factors.

Long-stored Rice

It is the polished round-grained glutinous rice stored for many years.

Effect. Nourishing the stomach, dispelling dampness and eliminating restlessness.

Indication. Asthenia of the spleen and stomach polydipsia, diarrhea, regurgitation and fasting dysentery.

Longxuan (Ex-E)

An extra acupoint.

Location. 2 cun above the transverse crease of the radial side of the forearm, at the vein 0.5 cun above Lieque (L 7).

Indication. Pain in the forearm, deviation of mouth due to apoplexy, toothache.

Method. Moxibustion. Acupuncture is forbidden.

Looking at Nose Apex

A term in qigong, referring to the condition that the eyes look naturally at the tip of the nose in qigong practice, in such a way as to help the mind concentrate and tranquilize consciousness as well as effectively avoid going to sleep.

Looking Inwards

A term in qigong, referring to a condition that in practising qigong, looking inwards at a certain part inside the body with both eyes slightly closed and concentrate the mind thereon. It serves to get rid of distracting thoughts to reach a tranquil state.

Loose Stool

This term has two meanings:

1. The disease with watery faces as the main clinical manifestation.

   Symptoms. Watery stool, anorexia, abdominal distention and listlessness of limbs, yellow complexion, etc.

   Pathogenesis. Mucus resulting from impairment due to exopathogens, improper diet and emotional stress or from weakness of the spleen and the stomach.

   Therapeutic Principle. Eliminating pathogenic factors, promoting digestion and strengthening the spleen.

2. It refers to a symptom as mucus and grimy stool.

Loquat Leaf

The leaf of Eriobotrya japonica (Thunb.) Lindl. (Rosaceae).

Effect. Dispelling sputum, relieving cough, reinforcing the stomach.

Indication. Cough due to lung-heat, asthma vomiting due to stomach-heat, dysphoria with smothery sensation and thirst.

Loranthus Mulberry Mistletoe

It is the stem of Taxillus chinesis (DC.) Danser. (Loranthaceae) with leaf.

Effect. Removing wind-dampness, nourishing the liver and kidney,

reinforcing muscles and tendons, and preventing abortion.

Indication. Rheumatic arthralgia, aching loins and knees, vaginal bleeding during pregnancy and threatened abortion.

Losing Control of Lower by Upper Deficiency

It refers to the pathogenesis that the upper-energizer cannot control the lower-energizer due to visceral dysfunction; the patient experiences frequent micturition.

Loss of Appetite

Symptoms. Declination in diet, anorexia.

Pathogenesis. Mostly caused by the interior disturbance of excess heat, cold-phlegm and damp retention, or the deficiency of the spleen and stomach.

Loss of Blood

A general term for various kinds of bleeding, such as epistaxis, hematemesis, hemoptysis, spitting blood, hemafecia and hematuria, etc.

Loss of Vitality

It refers to a state indicating unfavourable prognosis. Lack of vitality is characterized by dull eyes, unclear speech, dull complexion, abnormal breath, thin muscles, and fecal and urinary incontinence.

Loss of yang

It has two meanings:

1. It refers to deficiency of yang;
2. It refers to disappearance of the exterior syndrome.

Lotus Rhizome

The fat rhizome of Nelumbo nucifera Gaertn. (Nymphaeaceae).

Effect. Arresting bleeding, dissipating blood stasis; invigorating the spleen, improve appetite, etc.

Indication. Hematemesis hemoptysis, stranguria due to heat, etc.

Lotus Rhizome Node

The rhizome node of Nelumbo nucifera Gaertn. (Nymphaeaceae).

Effect. Dissipating stasis and astringing to arrest bleeding.

Indication. Various kinds of bleeding such as hematemesis, hematuria, metrorrhagia, etc.

Lotus Root Starch

The starch of Nelumbo. nucifera Gaertn. (Nymphaeceae), which is processed from the fat and thick lotus rhizome.

Effect. Nourishing blood, arresting bleeding, regulating the middle-energizer and promoting appetite and digestion.

Indication. Hematemesis, cough up blood, dysentery and poor appetence.

Lotus Seed

The ripe seed of Nelumbo nucifera Gaertn. (Nymphaceaceae).

Effect. Invigorating the spleen, arresting diarrhea, tonifying the kidney to arrest spontaneous seminal emission and nourishing the heart to tranquilization.

Indication. Chronic diarrhea due to deficiency of the spleen, spontaneous seminal emission and spermatorrhea due to deficiency of the kidney, palpitation, insomnia, metrorrhagia, leukorrhagia, etc.

Lotus Seed Pot-like Hemorrhoid

The hemorrhoid like a lotuspod with seeds. It corresponds to multiple external hemorrhoids or rectal polyp.

Lou (Spiral Stria of Vulva)

It refers to deformity of the external genital organ, spinning of the spiral shell-like vulva into the vagina, which affects sexual intercourse and delivery, during which dystocia occurs if the female is pregnant.

Lougu (Sp 7)

An acupuncture point.

Location. Located at the Spleen meridian, 3 cun above Sanyinjiao (Sp 6).

Indication. Abdominal distention, borborygmus, spermatorrhea, difficulty in urination, pain and flaccidity of the lower extremities, swelling and pain of the ankles, etc.

Method. Puncture perpendicularly 1.0-1.5 cun and apply moxibustion to the point for 5-15 minutes or 3-5 moxa cones.

Louyin (Ex-LE)

An extra point.

Location. 0.5 cun below the medial malleolus on the small artery.

Indication. Metrorrhagia and metrostaxis, leukorrhea with reddish discharge.

Method. Puncture perpendicularly 0.3-0.5 cun. Apply moxibustion 3-7 moxa cones or 5-10 minutes with warming moxibustion.

Lower Abdominal Pain Related to Qi

A type of hernia caused by qi-stagnation with two implications: 1. Abdominal pain with tenesmus, which becomes worse and mild alternatively. The therapeutic principle is regulating qi and alleviating pain. 2. Bearing-down pain of the scrotum due to qi-stagnation, which connects with the kidney and abdomen. The therapeutic principle is soothing the liver-qi and regulating qi circulation.

Lower Auricle Root (MA)

An auricular point, also known as Spinal Cord 2 (MA).

Location. At the inferior edge of the junction of the earlobe and cheek.

Indication. Headache, abdominal pain, asthma.

Lower Being Excessive

This term has two meanings: 1. It refers to excessive pathogenic factors in the lower part. The patient with excessive pathogenic factors in the lower part usually dreams of falling down from the high place. 2. Diagnostic method refers to the pulse excessive in cubit pulse.

Lower Cold Keeping out Upper Heat

It refers to the disorder of yin-yang in the human body and resistance of the lower cold to the upper heat. For example, in the case of the chronic dysentery due to cold of defficiency type, patient will vomit when misusing cold drugs.

Lower Confluent Points

An acupuncture point. It is a simple designation of the lower confluent points of the six fu organs at the lower limbs, belonging to the six acupoints where the meridians of the six fu organs join with the Stomach Meridian, the Bladder Meridian and the Gallbladder Meridian at the lower limbs: The Small Intestine Meridian, at the lower limbs, with Xiajuxu (S 39), the Tri-energizer Meridian with Weiyang (B 39), the Large Intestine Meridian with Shangjuxu (B 37), the Urinary Bladder Meridian with weizhong (B 40), the Gallbladder Meridian with yanglingquan (G 34), and the Stomach Meridian with Zusanli (S 36). They are mainly employed to cure diseases of the six fu-organs.

Lower Dantian

A term in qigong, referring to one of the three Dantians. There are different opinions as to its locality. Generally, it is believed to be among the navel, Mingmen and Huiyin. It is not a certain point but a three-dimensional area where the body essence, including reproductive essence, is transformed into qi and qi is trained and emitted to the outside of the body.

Lower Disease Affecting the Upper

It refers to the pathological changes showing progress of debility from a lower viscus to an upper one in the body.

Lower-energizer

This term has two meanings: 1. It is one of the tri-energizer, refers to lower portion of the body cavity from the lower part of the stomach to two lower orifices, the external urethral meatus and the anus, housing the kidney, bladder, small and large intestines, including the liver due to its physiological relation with the kidney. Its main function is clearing fluid from turbid one and discharging urine and stool. 2. It refers to the lesions of the liver and the kidney caused by warm-pathogen in anaphase and convalescence.

Lower-energizer Resembling Drainage

It refers to the lower-energizer which works like gutters, for the kidney, urinary bladder and large intestine, with the function of transporting water, clearing fluid from turbid one and discharging urine and stool just like drainage of water from ditch.

Lubrication of Stool

Referring to a therapy for treating constipation by moisturizing the intestines with drugs of moisturizing the intestines.

Lucid Ganoderma

The whole herb of Ganoderma japonicum (Fr.) Lloyd or M. Lucidum (Leyss. ex Fr.) Karst. (Polyporaceae).
Effect. Reinforcing vital essence and energy, strengthening the bones and muscles, tranquilization.
Indication. Cough, asthma, insomnia and dyspepsia.

Lucky-nut Thevetia Seed

The kernel of Thevetia peruviana (Pers.) K.Schum. (Apocynaceae).
Effect. Reinforcing the effect on the heart.
Indication. Heart failure, paroxysmal and supra-ventricular tachycardia and paroxysmal fibrillation.

Luffa   ⊛ L-1

The fresh fruit or dried, old ripe fruit after frost of Luffa cylindrica (L.) Roem or Luffa acutangula Roxb. (Cucurbitaceae).
Effect. Removing heat, dispelling phlegm and detoxicating.
Indication. Fever, excessive thirst, cough with phlegm, dyspnea, rheumatic arthralgia, galactostasis, furuncle and subcutaneous swelling.

Luffa Fruit Bundle

The vascular bundles of the mature fruit of Luffa cylindrica (L.) Roem. (Cucurbitaceae).

Effect. Dispelling wind and removing obstruction in meridians, detoxicating and eliminating phlegm.

Indication. Rheumatic arthralgia, muscular convulsion, pain in the chest and hypochondrium, cough with phlegm, galactostasis, furuncle, etc.

Luffa Seed

The seed of Luffa cylindrica (L.) Roem or L. Acutangula Roxb (Cucurbitaceae).

Effect. Promoting diuresis and purging intense heat.

Indication. Edema on the face and body, stranguria due to the urolith fresh-bloody stool, hemorrhoid, etc.

Luffa Stem

The stem of Luffa cylindrica (L) Roem or L. Acutangula Roxb. (Cucurbitaceae).

Effect. Relaxing muscles and tendons, dissipating blood stasis, invigorating the spleen and destroying parasites.

Indication. Paralysis in the extremities, irregular menstruation, edema, etc.

Lumbago and Backache

Symptoms. Dragging pain of the lumbar region and back.

Pathogenesis. Insufficiency of the kidney-qi and invasion of pathogenic wind, cold and dampness when the body is weakened.

Lumbago due to Blood Deficiency

Symptoms. Frequent lumbago, soreness and weakness of the lumbago and knees, numbness of hand and foot, pale or sallow complexion, dizziness with blurring vision.

Pathogenesis. Usually caused by the excessive loss of blood or the impairment of the heart and spleen by excessive anxiety which results in the blood deficiency and the failure in nourishing the muscles and tendon.

Therapeutic Principle. Enriching blood mainly, clearing and activating the meridians and collaterals.

Lumbago due to Blood Stasis

Symptoms. Pain in certain part of the body, stabbing pain, mild pain during the day and serious pain at night.

Pathogenesis. Caused by blood stasis.

Therapeutic Principle. Removing blood stasis and promoting qi circulation.

Lumbago due to Cold-dampness

Symptoms. Pain, cold and heavy sensation of the lower back, difficulty in turning over in bed, the pain may be relieved by heat and aggravated by cold.

Pathogenesis. Caused by the stagnancy of cold-dampness in the meridians and collaterals resulting in the obstruction of qi and blood.

Therapeutic Principle. Dispelling cold and dampness and warming meridians and collaterals.

Lumbago due to Consumptive Disease

Symptoms. Lingering pain in the waist, frequent inability to walk or stand, emaciation, shortness of breath, pain becoming more acute while overworking.

Pathogenesis. Mostly caused by kidney deficiency, overstrain, or the obstruction of the circulation of meridian.

Therapeutic Principle. Invigorating deficiency, supplementing primordial energy and strengthening the kidney.

Lumbago due to Dampness

Symptoms. Coldness, pain and heaviness in the waist as if sitting in the water, more severe pain in wet weather or after long period of sitting.

Pathogenesis. Caused by sitting in cold and damp places for a long time, or being caught in rain and dew.

Therapeutic Principle. Invigorating the spleen and dispersing dampness.

Lumbago due to Exogenous Affection

Symptoms. Excess syndrome is common.
Pathogenesis. Invasion of external pathogen into meridians and collaterals.
Therapeutic Principle. Expelling the pathogen and removing the obstruction in collaterals.

Lumbago due to Injury

Symptoms. Pain in lumbar region, swelling, and cyanosis, in serious cases, symptoms of backache can be seen, and difficulty in movement.
Pathogenesis. Caused by trauma and fall from a high place which leads to injury of lumbar muscle and stagnation of blood and qi in meridians.
Therapeutic Principle. Promoting blood circulation to remove blood stasis, relaxing muscles and tendons and activating the flow of blood and qi in meridians and collaterals, simultaneously by aupuncture and moxibustion, massage, steaming and washing with medicinal herbs.

Lumbago due to Internal Injury

Symptoms. In general, the course of deficiency syndrome is longer.
Pathogenesis. Caused by the deficiency of the liver, spleen and kidney, or phlegm-dampness, blood stasis and internal injury.
Therapeutic Principle. Reinforcing mainly the spleen and kidney, nourishing the liver subserviently, and adding drugs to eliminate dampness and phlegm, promote blood circulation and remove blood stasis according to the symptoms.

Lumbago due to Kidney Deficiency

Symptoms. Lassitude and pain of waist, aggravated on exertion, ameliorated upon lying down, relief by pressing and kneading, and repeated attack, etc.
Pathogenesis. Mainly caused by congenital defect combining with overstrain, or debility due to long-standing illness, or excess of sexual intercourse which leads to insufficiency of essence and blood and inability to nourish muscles.
Therapeutic Principle. Warming and recuperating the kidney-yang, and nourishing the kidney-yin.

Lumbago due to Pathogenic Wind

Symptoms. Wandering pain with the sensation of drawing in the loin, or with the shoulders and feet involved, or chills and fever, etc.
Pathogenesis. Impairment of the Spleen Meridian by pathogenic wind.
Therapeutic Principle. Dispelling wind, promoting blood circulation and removing obstruction in the collaterals.

Lumbago due to Qi Stagnation

Symptoms. Lumbago accompanied by fullness and distention of the abdomen and hypochondrium. The pain is like a twinge or movable pain.
Pathogenesis. Mostly caused by stagnation of qi due to melancholy, sudden sprain and contusion as well as fall.
Therapeutic Principle. Promoting circulation of qi to relieve pain.

Lumbar Movements

One of self-massage manipulations.
Operation. Incline forward and backward and rotate with the waist as center.
Indication. Health care of the waist.

Lumbar Pain (Lumbago)

Symptoms. Pathologic pain in one or both sides of the waist, or along the spinal column.
Pathogenesis. Mostly caused by deficiency of the kidney, or affection of pathogenic cold-dampness, blood stasis, sprain and contusion. It can be divided into three types: lumbar pain due to cold and dampness, lumbar pain due to overstrain, and

lumbar pain due to deficiency of the kidney.

Lumbar Sprain with Qi Blocked

Symptoms. Unbearable lumbago without local areola and swelling, inability of pronation supination and body-turning and severe pain on moving.

Pathogenesis. Mainly caused by sprain and bruise of inappropriate motion in removing heavy things, injury of the lumbar region of lower part of thoracic vertebrae, and stagnation of meridian and collateral qi and blood.

Therapeutic Principle. Promoting the circulation of qi and activating collaterals, in combination with acupuncture and moxibustion, and massage.

Lumbodorsal Pain during Pregnancy

Pathogenesis. Mostly caused by deficiency and weakness of the kidney-qi and, in addition, affection by exopathic cold and dampness invading the lumbodorsal meridians and causing qi stagnancy and sluggish flow of blood.

Therapeutic Principle. Enriching the kidney, expelling the dampness and preventing abortion.

Lumbosacral Vertebrae (MA)

An otopoint.

Location. Divide the area from the muscle of incisure of helix to the branching spot of the upper and lower cruse of the anthelix into five equal parts, the 2nd from the top, which is the point.

Function. Strengthen the vertebra and replenish the spinal cord.

Indication. Pain in the lower back, abdominal pain, pain in the waist and lower extremities and peritonitis, etc.

Lump at Right Hypochondrium

Symptoms. Dyspnea, fever and chills, oppressed feeling in the chest, vomiting and coughing up of bloody purulent sputum. If persistent for a long time, the case can become pulmonary abscess.

Pathogenesis. Accumulation of pathogens in the lung. It refers to tachypnea, and upward adverse flow of qi.

Therapeutic Principle. Reducing the lung-qi, removing phlegm and expelling the pathogenic heat.

Lump below Left Hypochondrium

Symptoms. Mass below the left hypochondrium with pain extending to the lower abdomen, cramp due to the cold of feet, often accompanied by cough.

Pathogenesis. Stasis of the liver qi and accumulation of phlegm and blood.

Therapeutic Principle. Relieving the depressed liver and regulating the circulation of qi, dispelling phlegm and removing stagnation and softening and dispelling the lump.

Lump in Breast

A disease, referring to the chronic but not suppurative masses appearing in the breast.

Symptoms. Nodular masses in the breast which are hard, painless, movable when they are being pushed, without chills and fever, of normal skin color, as seen in cases of chronic cystic mastitis and benign tumor of breast.

Pathogenesis. Mostly caused by stagnation of qi and accumulation of phlegm due to the anxiety impairing the spleen and the stagnated anger impairing the liver.

Therapeutic Principle. Regulating qi by alleviation of mental depression, dispelling phlegm and expelling accumulation of pathogen.

Lung (MA)

An auricular point.

Location. On the medial side of the middle region of the back of the ear.

Indication. Asthma, diseases of digestive system, fever, etc.

Lung (MA-IC 1)

An auricular point.

Location. Around the central depression of the cavum concha.

Indication. Cough and dyspnea, hoarseness, cutaneous pruritus, constipation, stopping smoking.

Lung and Kidney Deficiency

This term has two meanings:

1. It refers to insufficiency of the lung-qi and the kidney-qi. The lung performs the function of respiration since it takes charge of qi, while the kidney controls and promotes inspiration since it governs reception of air.

   Symptoms. The symptoms of the insufficiency of the lung-qi and the kidney-qi are dyspnea, shortness of breath, cough with profuse sputum, spontaneous perspiration, aversion to cold, cold extremities or general edema.

   Therapeutic Principle. Warming the kidney to take in air.

2. It refers to deficiency of a lung and the kidney yin.

   Symptoms. Flushed check, hectic fever, night sweat, dry cough, hoarseness, lassitude in the loins and knees, and nocturnal emission.

   Therapeutic Principle. Nourishing yin to reduce pathogenic fire both in the lung and in the kidney.

Lung and Spleen Deficiency

Symptoms. Prolonged cough, shortness of breath, fatigue, much thin sputum, poor appetite, abdominal distention, loose stool, foot back dropsy, etc.

Pathogenesis. Prolonged asthma and cough, the lung deficiency involving the spleen, or impairment of the spleen due to diet and overstrain, and the spleen deficiency involving the lung.

Therapeutic Principle. Invigorating the spleen to benefit the lung.

Lung Apoplexy

Symptoms. Oral dryness, fullness in the chest, shortness of breath, poor vision, dizziness, etc.

Pathogenesis. Invasion of pathogenic wind into the lung meridian.

Therapeutic Principle. Expelling wind, descending the adverse flow of qi and promoting blood circulation.

Lung Carbuncle

Symptoms. Chill due to fever, cough, pain in eth chest, coughing out the fetid and spitting purulent sputum mixed with blood.

Pathogenesis. Accumulation of toxic heat due to exopathic wind and cold in the lung, and by heat accumulation and blood stasis.

Therapeutic Principle. Removing heat from the lung and dissolving phlegm, detoxicating and dispelling pus, and nourishing yin and invigorating qi in the convalescence.

Lung-cold Syndrome

Symptoms. Resemble symptoms of the consumptive lung disease. Besides, saliva is spontaneously secreted in the mouth with whitish, moist, and glossy fur, and there are manifestation of yang-deficiency and exterior-cold.

Pathogenesis. Cold in the Lung Meridian belonging to syndrome yang-deficiency.

Therapeutic Principle. Warming the lung and dispelling cold.

Lung Deficiency Syndrome

The term has two meanings: 1. The diseases resulting from insufficiency of qi, blood, yin, and yang in the lung. Its main manifestations are insufficiency of lung-qi and lung-yin deficiency. 2. It refers to lung-qi insufficiency.

Lung Disorder Caused by Lochioschesis

Symptoms. Oppressed feeling in the chest, restlessness, flushed face, severe vomiting, or even dyspnea, etc.

Pathogenesis. Postpartum lochia, retained and retrograding to disturb the lung.

Therapeutic Principle. Relieving asthma and regulating the flow of qi to remove the blood stasis.

Lung-distention

This term has two meanings:

1. **Symptoms.** Cough, dyspnea, profuse expectoration, distention, and fullness in the chest, palpitation, dark lips, edema of limbs, etc.

   Pathogenesis. Mostly caused by deficiency of lung after chronic disease or invasion of pathogenic factors, accompanied by stagnation of phlegm and blood stasis.

   Therapeutic Principle. Eliminating the pathogenic factor to ventilate the lung, descending qi to remove the phlegm, warming yang to promote diuresis.

2. It refers to the distention in the chest, marked by the dyspnea and cough of deficiency type.

Lung Dryness

Symptoms. Cough without sputum, or little thick sputum difficult to discharge, thirst, dry mouth, nose and pharynx, sore throat, hoarseness, hemoptysis, etc.

Pathogenesis. Injury of the lung by pathogenic dryness or deficiency of yin of the lung.

Therapeutic Principle. Nourishing the lung to arrest cough.

Lung Excess Syndrome

Symptoms. Asthma and cough, raucous breathing, fullness sensation and distending pain in chest, abundant expectoration, yellow and thick sputum.

Pathogenesis. Invasion of the lung by overwhelming pathogenic factors, such as wind-cold, phlegm-dampness and phlegm-heat.

Lung-fire

A morbid condition due to intense heat, either of deficiency type or of excess type.

Lung Function of Dredging Water Passages

The lung function of regulating dissemination, discharge, transportation, and elimination of body fluid. If this function is impeded, oliguria and edema may occur.

Lung-heat

Symptoms. Red cheek, cough with thick sputum, chest pain, shortness of breath, and hemoptysis in severe cases.

Pathogenesis. Heat attacks the lungs or exopathogen invades the lungs and is transmitted into heat.

Therapeutic Principle. Clearing qi and purging the lung of the pathogenic fire.

Lung Hernia

Symptoms. Falling pain and distention in lower abdomen involving the testis, dysuria, etc.

Pathogenesis. Invasion of the lung by pathogenic cold.

Therapeutic Principle. Ventilating the lung, expelling cold, dispersing accumulation of pathogen.

Lung Impairment

Symptoms. Shortness of breath, cough and hemoptysis in overwork.

Pathogenesis. Caused by fire of deficiency into the lung and the impairment of the lung yin.

Therapeutic Principle. Nourishing yin and clearing away heat, regulating the body fluid and arresting cough.

Lung in Charge of Activating qi Flow, Food Essence and Fluid

It refers to the function of disseminating the lung-qi. The lung function of activating the flow of qi, food essence, and body fluid not only disseminates the body fluid throughout the body, but also controls the opening and closing of pores of sweat ducts to regulate the elimination of sweat. If lung-qi is not dispersed, stuffiness in the chest, cough and asthma, nasal obstruction, sneezing and anhidrosis may occur.

Lung Malnutrition of Infant

Symptoms. Chills and fever, cough and asthma, running nose with watery discharge, pale complexion, dryness of the skin, etc.

Pathogenesis. Improper nursing, the impairment of the Lung Meridian by accumulated heat.

Therapeutic Principle. Dispelling the wind, clearing away the heat, and nourishing the lung.

Lung Meridian

One of the twelve meridians. It starts from gastric cavity of the middle-energizer, descends to connect with the large intestine, then returns and passes through the diaphragm along the upper opening of the stomach and reaches the lung and throat. Its course is lateral and it exits superficially at Zhongfu (L 1), and then descends along the lateral side of the arm and forearm, terminates at Shaoshang (L 11).

Lung-qi

A term refers to 1. The respiratory function of the lung; 2. The breathed air; 3. The vital essence and energy in the lung.

Lung-qi Dysfunction

It refers to the disturbance of the functional activities of the lung, especially referring to its function in maintaining normal water metabolism, giving rise to oliguria and edema together with respiratory symptoms.

Symptoms. Cough, stuffy nose, oliguria, general edema and dyspnea.

Therapeutic Principle. Promoting circulation of lung-qi or descending qi.

Lung-qi Insufficiency

Symptoms. Cough, asthma with low and weak voice, pale complexion, intolerance of wind and spontaneous perspiration.

Pathogenesis. Usually lies in impairment of the lung-qi due to prolonged cough and dyspnea, or insufficient interpromoting of the elements due to deficiency of the spleen-qi and the kidney-qi.

Therapeutic Principle. Replenishing and restoring the lung-qi.

Lung-qi Obstruction

Symptoms. Aversion to cold, running a fever, stuffy and running nose, cough in upper respiratory infection, etc.

Pathogenesis. Impediment of the functional activities of the lung, resulting from exterior attacks by exopathogen of wind-cold and from the skin closing.

Lung Relating to Melancholy

Anxiety, grief, and sorrow, which affect the lung, because over-anxiety exhausts qi successively and the lung operates the qi of the whole body.

Lung Taking Charge of Qi

One of the main functions of the lung shown in two aspects: 1. The lung takes charge of the qi of respiration. The lung is the chief organ for exchanging air between the interior and exterior of the body. The lung takes in fresh air and gives off waste gas. 2. The lung also has the function of operating and regulating the qi of the whole body.

Lung-yin

It refers to yin fluid that nourishes and moistens the lungs. It is generated from essential substances of foodstuff, moistened by the kidney-yin, and used with the lung-qi to maintain the normal function of the lungs.

Lung-yin Deficiency

Symptoms. Dry cough with a small amount of glutinous sputum, afternoon fever, and night sweat, hoarseness, red and dry tongue, etc.

Pathogenesis. Impairment of the lung-yin due to prolonged invasion of the pathogenic dryness and heat, or ascribable to accumulation of phlegm-fire.

Therapeutic Principle. Replenishing yin essence and moisturizing the viscera.

Luo Gong Sha

Symptoms. Coma due to high fever, continuously productive cough, eyeballs rotating upwards.

Pathogenesis. Mainly caused by stasis in qi and blood.

Therapeutic Principle. Removing the stasis followed by administering medicine, clearing away phlegm, descending qi.

Luo (Connecting) Points

A term for the classification of the acupoints. A point at a certain place on the meridians from which each collateral branches is called Luo (Connecting) Point.

Function. Connect the two meridians of the exterior and the interior. The Luo (Connecting) Points of the Twelve Regular Meridians are all located below the joints of the elbow and knee. Add the Luo (Connecting) Points of Governor Vessel and Conception the front middle and the back middle meridians and the large Luo (Connecting) Point of the Spleen, a total of 15 points. So it is called Fifteen Luo (Connecting) Points.

1. Lieque point (L 7)
2. Tongli point (H 5)
3. Neiguan acupuncture point point (P 6)
4. Zhizhen point (SI 7)
5. Pianli point (LI 6)
6. Waiguan acupuncture point point (G 37)
7. Gongsun point (Sp 4)
8. Dazhong point (K 14)
9. Shaoyin point (Liv 5)
10. Feiyang point (B 58)
11. Fenglong point (S 40)
12. Guangming point (G 37)
13. Jiuwei point (CV)
14. Changjiang point (GV)
15. Dabao point (Sp 21)

Luoque (B 8)

A point on the Bladder Meridian.

Location. On the head, 5.5 cun directly above the midpoint of the anterior hairline and 1.5 cun posterior to Tongtian (B 7)

Indication. Vertigo, tinnitus, stuffy nose, deviation of the mouth, mania, madness, blurred vision, swelling of the neck, goiter.

Method. Puncture subcutaneously 0.3-0.5 cun. Apply moxibustion 1-3 moxa cones or 3-5 minutes of warming moxibustion.

Lushang (Ex-B)

A set of extra points.

Location. On the caudal, one middle-finger length directly above the tip of the coccyx, the other two are half of the middle-finger length beside the first point, 3 points in total.

Indication. Hemorrhoid, hematochezia.

Method. Apply oxibustion 3-7 moxa cones or 5-10 minutes with warming moxibustion.

Luxi (TE 19)

An acupuncture point on The Triple-energizer Meridian.

Location. Posterior to the auricle root, at the junction of the upper 1/3 and lower 2/3 of the line along the helix linking Yifeng (TE 17) and Jiaosun (TE 20).

Indication. Headache, tinnitus, deafness, toothache, infantil convulsion, etc.

Method. Puncture subcutaneously 0.3-0.5 cun and apply moxibustion to the point for 3-5 minutes.

Luxu Granulation

Symptoms. Though this disease is not very painful or quite itchy, it will bleed constantly if injured by mistake. With passing of time, general debility will appear. Some of it correspond to skin carcinoma.

Pathogenesis. Mostly caused by the stagnation of damp-phlegm, qi and blood.

Therapeutic Principle. Regulating qi and blood, resolving phlegm and promoting diuresis.

Lying Postures

Postures in acupuncture, divided into supine postures, side recumbent posture and prone posture.

M

Maceration

It is a method using the finished decoction to wash or soak the affected region to make the injury of skin clean and clear away the pathogenic factors.

Indication. The opening of a sore stays unhealed, with watery pus or slough after the ulceration of sores, dermatosis, and the swelling pain of internal hemorrhoid and external hemorrhoids, etc.

Therapeutic Principle. Washing, bathing and soaking.

Macrostem Onion **M-1**

It is the bulb of Allium macrostemon Bge. (Liliaceae).

Effect. Activating the circulation of yang-qi, dispersing accumulation of pathogen, keeping the adverse qi down ward and removing stagnation of intestines.

Indication. Stuffiness sensation and pain in the chest, angina pectoris, stagnation of qi in the spleen and the stomach, diarrhea and dysentery with tenesmus, etc.

Macula

Referring to patches on the surface of skin.

Symptoms. The maculae originate from the chest and then spread out to the abdomen, back and limbs. It is red, purple, and dark in color, patch spot in shape, accompanied by fever, restlessness, thirst, even vague mind and delirium.

Pathogenesis. Heat stagnation in Yangming Meridian which affects the blood system and comes out through the muscle during epidemic febrile disease.

Therapeutic Principle. Clearing away the stomach-heat and detoxicating, and removing heat from blood and removing macula.

Macula after Vomiting and Diarrhea

Symptoms. Appearance of purple macula on the skin after vomiting and diarrhea.

Pathogenesis. Rootless fire wandering outside due to stomach deficiency.

Therapeutic Principle. Tonifying the spleen and stomach, warming the meridians and stopping bleeding.

Macula Caused by Violent Heat-pathogen

Symptoms. High fever, dysphoria, insomnia with restlessness, red and swollen head and face, swollen and sore throat, vomiting pus and blood, nausea, abdominal pain, thirst due to dryness, raving, diarrhea, etc.

Pathogenesis. Obstruction of tri-energizer, pathogens in nutrient system and defence system, burning of qi and blood.

Therapeutic Principle. Clearing away heat and toxic material, and removing heat from the blood to relieve feverish rash.

Madeiravine Bulbil

It is the bud of Boussingaultia gracilis Miers var. Pseudopasselloides Bailey (Basellaceae).

Effect. Warming and invigorating the stomach and spleen, strengthening the loins and knees, subduing swelling and eliminating blood stasis.

Indication. Pain of the waist and knees, traumatic injuries, fracture, etc.

Magnetite

It is the ore of magnetic iron.

Effect. Restrain yang, easing mental strains, improving eyesight and hearing, helping inspiration and relieving asthma.
Indication. Palpitation, insomnia, dizziness, headache, epilepsy and mania due to hyperactivity of the liver or the heart; deafness, tinnitus, blurred vision due to deficiency of the liver and kidney; short breath due to failure of the kidney in receiving air, etc.

Magnolia Bark

It is the dried trunk bark or branch bark of Magnolia officinalis Rehd. et Wils, or M. biloba (Rehd. et Wils.) Cheng (Magnoliaceae).
Effect. Activating circulation of qi, eliminating dampness, invigorating the function of the spleen, allaying asthma and removing food stagnation.
Indication. Gastric and abdominal distention with pain, vomiting and diarrhea due to dyspepsia, cough and asthma with abundant expectoration.

Magnolia Flower   ⊛ M-2

It is the flower-bud of Magnolia biondii Pamp., M. denudata Desr., M. Sprengeri Pamp. (Magnoliaceae).
Effect. Expelling wind and cold, clearing the nasal passage.
Indication. Affection by wind-cold exopathogens, headache with stuffy nose, nasal discharge due to rhinitis and nasosinusitis.

Magnolia Fruit or Seed

It is the fruit or seed of Magnolia officinalis Rehd. et Wils. or M. biloba (Rehd et Wils.) Cheng (Magnoliaceae).
Effect. Regulating flow of qi, warming the spleen and stomach, promoting digestion and removing food stagnancy.
Indication. Distention in the stomach.

Magpie

It is the meat of Pica pica sericea Gould (Anatidae).

Effect. Clearing away heat, dispelling accumulation of pathogen, treating stranguria and relieving thirst.
Indication. Stranguria due to urolithiasis, accumulation of phlegm in the chest, diabetes, epistaxis, etc.

Malaria

A infectious disease.
Symptoms. Intermittent rigor, and high fever and sweating. It often occurs in summer and autumn or in forest and mosquito breading area.
Pathogenesis. A disease caused by malarial parasites. In traditional Chinese medicine, it is thought to be caused by the attack of the body by pathogenic malaria, mountainous evil air, and wind, cold, summer heat and dampness in Shaoyang Meridian, nutrient system, and defensive system.

Malaria due to Depression

Symptoms. Chills and fever like malaria, attacking at regular time, fullness sensation in chest and hypochondrium, worsening at night, distention in the lower abdomen, loose and unsmooth stool.
Pathogenesis. Depression for a long time.
Therapeutic Principle. Removing heat from the liver and relieving the depressed liver, and nourishing blood and promoting blood circulation.

Malaria with General Debility

1. A kind of malarial disease.
   Symptoms. Lassitude, acratia, short breath, anorexia, sallow complexion, thinness, recurrence of malarial disease whenever overstrained, alternate attack of chills and fever.
   Pathogenesis. Vital-qi deficiency, internal injury caused by overstrain followed by affection of the pathogenic factor of malarial disease.
   Therapeutic Principle. Strengthen the body resistance and eliminate pathogenic factors, supplement qi and nourish blood.

2. Referring to long-standing incurable malaria, which is transmitted into three yin meridians.

Symptoms. Intermittent chill, high fever, sweating accompanied by disease related to three yin meridians.

Pathogenesis. Attack of body by pathogenic factors of malarial disease which invade the nutrient system and the defensive system.

Therapeutic Principle. Removing obstruction in meridians, promoting the circulation of qi and nourishing yin.

Malignant Boil

It is a more serious type of boils.

Symptoms. Redness, pain, and itching in the swelling locality. After rupture, it is still difficult to heal.

Pathogenesis. Wind heat involving noxious dampness.

Therapeutic Principle. Clearing away heat and detoxicating, and subduing swelling and removing stasis.

Malignant Malaria due to Heat

Symptoms. High fever with slight chills, or without cold, headache, restlessness and pain of the limbs, flushed face and redness of the eye, oppressive feeling in the chest and vomiting, constipation, burning sensation during urination even unconsciousness and delirium.

Pathogenesis. The invasion of mountainous evil air and malarial pathogens into the body with excessive yang leading to interior stagnation of noxious heat and mental disturbance.

Therapeutic Principle. Detoxicate and remove mountainous evil air, reduce heat and promote salivation accompanied by eliminating heart fire to restore consciousness.

Malnutrition due to Ascariasis

Symptoms. Weak constitution, sudden abdominal pain, vomiting watery saliva, blue-yellow face, restlessness in mind and a liking to eat strange food.

Pathogenesis. The delayed ascariasis.

Therapeutic Principle. Dispelling ascarides and replenishing deficiency.

Malnutrition due to Infantile Dyspepsia

Symptoms. Yellowish face and thin body, lack of vigour, abdominal distention, soft bone and baldness.

Pathogenesis. Stagnant milk.

Therapeutic Principle. Clear away heat, strengthen the spleen and reinforce the stomach, and stop the child from drinking the milk.

Malnutrition of Cold Type

Symptoms. Darkish complexion and swelling of the eyelids, thin body, weakness and diarrhea with thin and white foam, etc.

Pathogenesis. Deficiency of cold in the spleen and stomach with improper diet.

Therapeutic Principle. Warming the middle-energizer, invigorating the spleen and reinforce the stomach.

Malt

It is the ripe seed, which dried after germinating, of Hordeum vulgare L. (Gramineae).

Effect. Improving digestion, strengthening the stomach and lactifuge.

Indication. Dyspepsia, anorexia, epigastric and abdominal distention due to food stagnation, stopping milk secretion, etc.

Malt Extract

It is the cooked powder of polished glutinous rice or polished round-grained rice mixed with malt decocted on a gentle fire.

Effect. Invigorating the spleen and replenishing qi, moistening the lung and relieving cough.

Indication. Impairment of the spleen due to overstrain, cough due to the lung deficiency, asthenia, poor appetite, abdominal pain due to cold of deficiency type, etc.

Manchurian Rhododendron Leaf

It is the branch leaf or flower of Rhododendron micranthum Turcz. (Ericaceae).
Effect. Dispelling wind, removing obstruction in the meridians and arresting bleeding.
Indication. Bronchitis, dysentery, postpartum aching and fracture.

Mandibular Dislocation

Symptoms. Unilateral dislocation is characterized by inclination of mandible to the healthy side; bilateral dislocation, the mandible hanging forward and down, inability of closing mouth, speaking and chewing accompanied by salivation.
Pathogenesis. Deficiency of liver-yin and kidney-yin, insufficiency of blood and qi, muscular relaxation, over open of mouth of external injury.
Therapeutic Principle. Holding-elevating reduction. In the case of deficiency of liver, kidney, blood and qi: invigorating qi and enriching blood, nourishing the liver and kidney; For external injury: promoting blood circulation to remove blood stasis in combination with acupuncture and moxibustion.

Manehurian Tubergaurd

It is the fruit of Thladiantha dubia Bge. (Cucurbitaceae).
Effect. Decreasing the adverse flow of qi, dispelling dampness and dissipating stasis.
Indication. Jaundice, dysentery, regurgitation, hemoptysis with chest pain and lumbar sprain.

Mangchangxue (Ex-CA)

An extra acupuncture point.
Location. On the right side of the abdomen, on the midpoint of the line connecting the anterior superior iliac spine and the umbilicus.
Indication. Acute appendicitis, diarrhea, etc.

Method. Puncture perpendicularly 1.0-1.5 cun. Perform moxibustion with 3-5 moxa cones or for 5-10 minutes.

Manshurian Aristolochia Stem

It is the lianoid stem of Aristolochia manshuriensis Kom. (Aristolochiaceae), or Clematis armandii Franch and the same genus Clematis montana Buch.-Ham. (Ranunculaceae).
Effect. Inducing diuresis, treating stranguria, expelling heat and promoting lactation, activating the joints.
Indication. Scanty dark urine, acute urinary infection, edema canker sores due to inflamed heart-fire, vexation, amenorrhea and scanty lactation after delivery.

Mantis Egg-case

It is the egg-case of Tenodera sinensis Saussure, and Statilia maculata (Thunb.) (Mantidae).
Effect. Invigorating the kidney, supporting yang and treating spontaneous emission and reducing the frequency of urination.
Indication. Emission, impotence, enuresis, nocturia, leukorrhagia due to deficiency of the kidney-yang.

Manyflower Glorybower Root

It is the root of Clerodendron cyrtophyllum Turcz. (Verbenaceae).
Effect. Clearing away heat and detoxicating, expelling wind and dampness.
Indication. Epidemic encephalitis, common cold with high fever, headache, dysentery, jaundice, toothache, epistaxis, swollen and sore throat, etc.

Manystem Stonecrop Herb

It is the stem leaf of Sedum multicaule Wall. ex Lindl. (Crassulaceae).
Effect. Clearing away heat, detoxicating, arresting bleeding and dispelling wind-dampness.
Indication. Swollen and sore throat, epistaxis, dizziness, due to wind-heat,

arthralgia due to wind-dampness, eczema and suppurative infections on the body surface.

Mapleleaf Goosefoot Herb
It is the whole herb of Chenopodium hybridum L. (Chenopodiaceae).
Effect. Promoting blood and qi circulation, removing toxic substances and promoting subsidence of a swelling.
Indication. Irregular menstruation, metrorrhagia, metrostaxis, hemoptysis due to tuberculosis of the lung and hematuria, rheumatic arthralgia, traumatic injuries.

Margin of Tongue
It refers to the two edges of the tongue. They indicate conditions of the Liver and the Gallbladder Meridians.
Function. Diseases can be diagnosed by observing the conditions of the margin of the tongue. The blue and purple margin of the tongue with blue and purple ecchymosis is one of the manifestations of blood stasis in the Liver Meridian.

Marrow
It is one of the extraordinary organs, consisting of bone marrow and spinal cord formed by the kidney essence and foodstuff.
Function. Nourishing bone and invigorating brain.

Mary Rhododendron Leaf and Twig
A Chinese medicine. It is the flower, leaf, twig and root bark of Rhododendron mariae Hance (Ericaceae).
Effect. Relieving cough and eliminating phlegm.
Indication. Acute and chronic bronchitis.

Masaikai Caper Seed
It is the seed of Capparis pterocarpa Chun, or Capparis masaikai Levl. (Capparidaceae).

Effect. Clearing away heat, promoting the production of body fluid and quenching thirst.
Indication. Exogenous febrile diseases, thirst due to summer-heat, measles, swollen and sore throat, food retention due to improper diet, pyogenic infections, etc.

Massage
It is one of the traditional maneuvers applied to treat diseases externally.
Function. On the body points, a series of manipulations can be used to regulate functions of physiology and pathology so as to achieve effective results.

Massage along the Meridian
An auxiliary manipulation in acupuncture, referring to a procedure for promoting the needling effect.
Method. Pressing with the fingers gently on the upper or lower parts of the related acupoints along the meridians and collaterals.
Function. Promote the flow of meridian-qi and make the needling response appear more easily.

Mass by Blood Stasis
Symptoms. Pain in the abdomen, feeling the fixed lump while pressing.
Pathogenesis. Blood stasis, the stagnation of the meridians.
Therapeutic Principle. Strengthening the body resistance to eliminate pathogenic factors, and promoting blood circulation by dissipating stasis.

Mass due to Accumulation of Pathogenic Factor
Symptoms. Accumulation of pathogens in the chest, diarrhea, or mass in the hypochondrium down to the side of umbilicus with pain referring to the lower abdomen into spermatic cord.
Pathogenesis. Deficiency of the zang organ and yang, accumulation of severe pathogenic cold, and stagnation of qi and blood.

Therapeutic Principle. Warming zang-organ and expelling accumulation.

Mass due to Dryness

Symptoms. A half cup-like mass movable up and down and dragging pain in the hypochondrium, heavy sensation in the waist and back, sore feet after standing long, spontaneous perspiration, dysphoria, vomiting, dyschesia, etc.

Pathogenesis. Tiredness and anger during menstrual period in summer, leading to blood stasis and dry abdominal mass.

Therapeutic Principle. Removing blood stasis and moistening, removing obstruction and relieving pain.

Mass due to Water Retention

Symptoms. General edema, preference for drinking aversion to food, appearance of water sound by pressing on the abdomen, free mass without fixed location, etc.

Pathogenesis. Kidney deficiency, the obstruction of meridians and collaterals and the accumulation of fluid.

Therapeutic Principle. Reinforcing the kidney, strengthening the spleen and promoting flow of qi and blood circulation.

Masses of Pathologic Mucoid Substance

Symptoms. Large or small swelling masses, which heal here and set on there, and may appear anywhere.

Pathogenesis. Blockage in the meridians and collaterals due to phlegm with cold-dampness.

Therapeutic Principle. Cauterize the masses with a thin red-hot needle.

Mass in Abdomen

Symptoms. There are two types.
1. The mass is fixed in shape, painful in certain location.
2. The mass is unshaped, movable and painful without certain location.
   It is often seen in pathological changes of lower-energizer and in female cases.

Pathogenesis. Depressed emotion, injury of improper diet, injury of the liver and spleen, disharmony of zang-fu organs and stagnation of qi and blood stasis for a long time.

Therapeutic Principle. In the first case, promoting blood circulation to remove blood stasis. For the second case regulating the circulation of qi and removing stagnation.

Mass of Turbid Qi

Symptoms. Abdominal fullness and distention without pain, etc.

Pathogenesis. Purging by mistake during the exogenous febrile disease due to the failure of the unrelieved pathogen to go to the exterior resulting in the mass of turbid qi.

Therapeutic Principle. Regulating the flow of qi, dissipating mass and relieving distention and fullness.

Match-head Moxibustion

A moxibustion technique.

Method. Cauterizing the selected points rapidly with a burning match.

Indication. Epidemic parotitis, etc.

Mated Needling

A kind of needling

Method. For treating diseases of the internal organs, the acupoints on the chest and the abdomen and those on the back can be selected. Be sure to puncture these points obliquely so as not to damage the internal organs.

Measles

It is an acute eruptive infectious disease.

Symptoms. The reddish rashes appearing on the skin after having a fever 3 to 4 days.

Pathogenesis. Measles toxin affecting the meridians of the lung and the spleen, then erupting out of the skin in spring and winter.

Therapeutic Principle. Dispelling and clearing away the pathogenic germs.

Measles Complicated by Laryngitis and Aphonia

Referring to hoarseness resulting from measles and obstruction of seven orifices by heat pathogens.

Therapeutic Principle. Moistening the lung and promoting the production of the body fluid and removing heat pathogen from the throat.

Measles Complicated by Pneumonia

Symptoms. Delayed high fever, cough, short breath, rale in the throat, etc.

Pathogenesis. Debilitated young child, deficiency of the vital-qi, excessive pathogenic toxin, or repeated affection of seasonal pathogens, or invasion to the lung by measles, obstruction in the lungs.

Therapeutic Principle. Clearing away heat and toxin, ventilating the lung and dissipating the phlegm.

Measles with Dysentery

Symptoms. Measles get better, but with fever, adhesive stool with pus and blood, abdominal pain, tenesmus, vomiting with anorexia and fatigue, and purple stagnant superficial venule of the index finger.

Pathogenesis. Excessive measles toxin. The toxin is removed to the large intestine.

Therapeutic Principle. Clearing away toxin and heat, dispelling damp and relieving dysentery.

Measles with Dyspnea and Wheezing

Symptoms. Dyspnea and sound produced by the collection of sputum in the throat.

Pathogenesis. Obstruction of the lung by phlegm-fire.

Measles without Adequate Eruption to Expel Toxins

Symptoms. Measles which should appear, spots without adequate eruption or too rapid disappearance of measles.

Pathogenesis. Internal obstruction of toxins resulting from many pathogenic factors.

Therapeutic Principle. Ventilating the lung and promoting eruption with other therapy pursuant to the symptoms.

Measles with Sore Throat

Symptoms. Painful swelling in the throat and even difficulty to drink due to the measles.

Pathogenesis. Stagnation of the exterior pathogenic factors, measles without adequate eruption and toxin heat going up to the throat.

Therapeutic Principle. Eliminating the pathogens and relieving pharyngeal swelling.

Meat Mass

A kind of mass diseases.

1. It refers to accumulation with phlegm stagnancy and hard mass in the abdomen caused by preference for eating meat.

   Therapeutic Principle. Dissipating mass and removing accumulation.

2. Referring hard, cup-like mass below the navel of female, amenorrhea, emaciation.

   Therapeutic Principle. Dissipating mass and removing stagnant accumulation.

Medicated Tea

It is a solid dosage form made of coarse-powdered drugs and adhesive excipient. Patient can drink as tea after infusion with boiling water.

Medicated Wine

A dosage form. It refers to a preparation made by soaking the drugs in wine for a period of time and removing the drugs after boiling. Either oral administration or external application.

Indication. Invigorating weak body, general asthenia, rheumatic pain and traumatic injury.

Medicinal Evodia Fruit

It is the immature fruit of Evodia rutaecarpa (Juss.) Benth. E. rutaecarpa (Juss.) Benth. var. officinalis (Dode) Huang or Evodia rutaecarpa (Juss.) Benth. var bodinieri (Dode) Huang (Rutaceae).

Effect. Warming up the stomach and relieving pain, soothing the liver, lowering the adverse flow of qi and drying dampness, lowering blood pressure.

Indication. Gastric and abdominal cold pain, acid regurgitation, diarrhea due to cold deficiency, vomiting, pain caused by disturbance of lower legs due to pathogenic cold and dampness, etc.

Medicinal Evodia Root

It is the root or the root phloem of Evodia rutaecarpa (Juss.) Benth. (Rutaceae).

Effect. Promoting flow of qi, warming the middle-energizer and destroying parasites.

Indication. Gastric and abdominal cold pain, diarrhea, dysentery, lumbago, hernia, abdominal pain due to amenorrhea and oxyuriasis.

Medicinal Indionmulberry Root

It is the root of Morinda officinalis How. (Rubiaceae).

Effect. Reinforcing the vital function of the kidney especially that of the sexual organs, strengthening yang, dispelling wind and eliminating dampness.

Indication. Impotence and premature ejaculation, frequent urination, sterility due to uterine coldness, irregular menstruation, cold pain in the lower abdomen, frigidity in women, aches or lassitude in the loins and knees, etc.

Medicine Terminalia Fruit

It is the ripe fruit of Terminalia chebula Retz. (Combretaceae).

Effect. Astringing intestine to correct diarrhea, astringing the lung to stop cough, descending qi and relieving sore throat.

Indication. Chronic diarrhea, chronic dysentery, proctoptosis, asthma and cough due to lung deficiency or aphonia due to chronic cough.

Meeting Yin and Yang

A massage manipulation.

Operation. Push at Yinyang point from the two sides of the hand to the center thereof.

Function. Reducing phlegm and dissipating the accumulation thereof. Regulating the blood and qi and removing the sputum and saliva.

Indication. Accumulation of phlegm and cough with phlegm, choking sensation in the chest, etc.

Meichong (B 3)

A meridian acupuncture point.

Location. On the head, directly above Cuanzhu (B 2), 0.5 cun above the anterior hairline, on the line connecting Shenting (GV 24) and Qucha (B 4).

Indication. Epilepsy, headache, dizziness, vertigo, blurred vision, stuffy nose.

Method. Puncture subcutaneously 0.3-0.5 cun. Moxibustion is applicable.

Melancholia

Symptoms. Emotional stress, emotional vexation, distending pain in hypochondrium, or being susceptible to anger and cry, sensation of foreign body obstruction in pharyngeal portion and insomnia, etc.

Pathogenesis. Due to emotional depression accumulated after a considerable period of time.

Therapeutic Principle. For excess syndrome: soothing the liver and regulating the circulation of qi in combination with promoting circulation of blood, resolving phlegm, removing dampness by diuresis, clearing away heat and promoting digestion, etc.; For deficiency: invigorating qi, enriching blood, strengthening body resistance, etc.

Melancholia

Symptoms. Dysphoria and insomnia.

Pathogenesis. Excessive anxiety and melancholy.

Therapeutic Principle. Regulating qi by alleviation of mental depression and tranquilizing mind.

Meniere Disease

Symptoms. Sudden attack of dizziness, accompanied by tinnitus, deafness, nausea, vomiting, etc.

Pathogenesis. Fire-transmission due to stagnation of the live-qi, which goes up to disturb the orifices on the head, or by malnutrition of the aural orifice due to deficiency of the spleen and kidney, or by upward invasion of body fluid due to pathogenic cold which results from deficiency of the kidney-yang, etc.

Therapeutic Principle. Clearing away heat from the liver, or strengthening the spleen and replenishing the kidney to warm yang and decreasing dampness, etc.

Menopausal Syndrome

Symptoms. Dizziness, tinnitus, hot sensation and sweating, palpitation, insomnia, dysphoria, liability to anger, tidal fever, edema in the face and lower limbs, loose stool, menstrual disorder, emotional uneasiness, etc.

Pathogenesis. Kidney deficiency.

Therapeutic Principle. In the case with kidney-yang deficiency, warming and enriching the kidney-yang; in the one with kidney-yin deficiency, nourishing the kidney-yin; in the one with deficiency of both yin and yang, nourishing both yin and yang.

Menophania Amenorrhea

Referring to amenorrhea in the unmarried female.

Symptoms. Amenorrhea, darkish and yellowish complexion, and edema all over the body.

Pathogenesis. Girls at fourteen or fifteen wash their hands and feet or clothes in cold water just before the start of their first menstruation out of unawareness, their menstrual blood becomes coagulable because of cold, and fails to flow.

Therapeutic Principle. Inducing menstruation and promoting blood circulation.

Menorrhagia

Symptoms. Timely menstrual cycle with profuse menstrual blood discharge, or menstrual period delayed more than 7-8 days, and with more than normal blood. In the clinic, there are three types: menorrhagia due to deficiency of qi menorrhagia due to blood-heat and, menorrhagia due to blood stasis.

Therapeutic Principle. In the first case, hemostasis by invigorating qi to reinforce the vital meridian; in the second case, clearing away heat from blood to arrest bleeding; in the last case, promoting circulation to dissipating stasis and stop bleeding.

Menostasis due to Coitus in Menstrual Period

Referring to the menostasis caused by the impairment of the uterine blood vessels due to sexual activity in menstrual period.

Therapeutic Principle. Regulating qi and blood.

Menostaxis

Symptoms. Menstruation lasting more than seven days, or even half a month with basically normal menstrual cycle.

Pathogenesis. Blood stasis due to qi stagnation, or by interior heat due to yin deficiency.

Therapeutic Principle. In the former case, promoting blood circulation to remove stasis and stop bleeding, in the latter, nourishing yin and clearing heat to stop bleeding.

Menstrual Blood Color

Referring to the color of the menstrual blood. Normal menstrual blood is dark-red. Its color changes with pathological changes of the body. Pale indicates qi or blood deficiency; purplish red or crimson shows blood heat; dark-purple is caused by blood stasis; dark-black results from coagulation of cold; bright red responds to fever of deficiency type; alternating of red with yellow confirms damp-heat; mostly with leukorrhea verifies noxious dampness.

Menstrual Fever

Symptoms. Repeated fever during, before or after menstruation.

Pathogenesis. Production of interior heat due to yin deficiency of the liver and kidney, or by unbalance between yin and yang due to qi and blood deficiency.

Therapeutic Principle. Nourishing yin and clearing heat, or invigorating qi and consolidating superficial resistance, and nourishing blood to regulate the nutrient system.

Menstrual Migraine

Symptoms. Unbearable headache during, before or after menstruation.

Pathogenesis. 1. Both qi and blood deficiency especially during menstruation. 2. Stagnation of the liver-qi. 3. Blood stasis and meridian obstruction.

Therapeutic Principle. Regulating qi and blood, clearing and activating the meridians and collaterals, and in addition, nourishing yin and blood in the first case; clearing heat and purging fire in the second case; promoting blood circulation to dissipating blood stasis for the last one.

Menstruation in an Unfixed Period due to Kidney Deficiency

Symptoms. Irregular menstrual cycles with scanty, thin and light-colored menses, soreness and weakness of the waist and knees, dizziness, tinnitus.

Pathogenesis. Constitutional deficiency of kidney-qi and excess of sexual intercourse or multiparity resulting in dysfunction of the kidney in storing and impairment of the Front Middle and Vital Meridians.

Therapeutic Principle. Nourishing the kidney and regulate menses.

Mental Confusion due to Phlegm

Symptoms. Wheezing sound in the throat, oppressed feeling in chest, haziness coma in severe case.

Pathogenesis. Phlegm due to retention of dampness or from accumulation of phlegm in the heart caused by emotional depression.

Therapeutic Principle. Dispelling phlegm for resuscitation.

Mental Derangement

Symptoms. Mental aberration, delirium, alternation of grief and joy, abnormal behaviour or trance and amnesia, etc.

Pathogenesis. The internal impairment by seven emotions, the attack of the heart by phlegm-fire, or insufficiency of the heart-qi.

Mental Disturbance due to Phlegm-fire

Symptoms. Vexation, palpitation, bitter taste, insomnia, excessive dreaming with fright, amentia, restlessness, etc.

Pathogenesis. Phlegm-fire disturbing the mind.

Therapeutic Principle. Clearing away heat, expelling phlegm, and tranquilizing mind and removing restlessness.

Meridians and Collaterals

The pathways for the circulation of qi and blood throughout the human body composed of meridians and collaterals. The ones running longitudinally are termed meridians; the ones branching out of the meridians and connecting all parts of the body are termed collaterals. This system of meridians and collaterals includes: Twelve Regular Meridians, Branches of the Twelve Regular Meridians, Eight Extra Meridians, Fifteen Collaterals, Muscles along the Twelve Regular Meridians and Twelve Cutaneous Regions, etc. Among them, the Twelve Regular Meridians are the main meridians, while the Fifteen Collaterals are the main collaterals. They run in length and breadth, scattering throughout the whole body and connecting the interior and exterior, zang-fu organs and extremities, thus forming an organic integrity.

Meridian Transmission Phenomenon

It refers to the transmission of the acupuncture feeling induced during needling along the course of the meridians, or all kinds of cutaneous reaction occurring along the meridians. In some people, the phenomenon may result from moxibustion, electrification, and pressure, stimulating acupoints or in the process of practising Qi gong. The sensations may vary due to different stimuli and constitutions. Meridian transmission phenomenon is very significant for research of the essence of meridians and collaterals.

Method of Leading the Needling Sensation

An acupuncture point manipulation.

Method. Press the region inferior to the acupoint with the fingers to move the needling reaction upward; press the region superior to the acupoint with the fingers to make the needling reaction downward.

Metrorrhagia after Anger

Symptoms. Sudden flooding or dripping of menstrual blood after great anger.

Pathogenesis. Affection of the liver by anger, failure of the liver to restore blood, resulting in uncontrollable menstruation.

Therapeutic Principle. Calming the liver to dissipate stagnation and nourishing blood to stop bleeding.

Metrorrhagia and Metrostaxis

Symptoms. Sudden massive bleeding prior to or beyond the menstrual period, or incessant dripping of blood from the uterus. Including light but lingering menstrual blood during menstruation. In the process of the disease, bursting may turn into leaking and vice versa, therefore, the two cannot be separated and are often termed together as bursting-leaking.

Pathogenesis. Impairment and debility of the Vital and Front Meridians, which therefore fail to control the blood.

Metrorrhagia and Metrostaxis due to Blood-heat

Symptoms. Bleeding in dark-red color with foul smell, thick bleeding, discharge, dry mouth, restlessness and irritation.

Pathogenesis. Exogenous heat evil attacking, or eating pungent food leading to heat attacking the Vital and Front Meridians and irregular uterine bleeding.

Therapeutic Principle. Eliminate pathogenic heat from the blood to stop bleeding and regulate menstruation.

Metrorrhagia and Metrostaxis due to Blood Stasis

Symptoms. Stasis clots in uterine bleeding, abdominal pain and tenderness which is relieved by the discharge of blood clots.

Pathogenesis. Accumulation of blood stasis, dysfunction of the Vital and Front Meridians with failure to hold blood in the meridians.

Therapeutic Principle. Promoting blood circulation to remove blood stasis and arrest uterine bleeding to regulate menstruation.

Metrorrhagia and Metrostaxis due to Damp-heat

Symptoms. Uterine bleeding with dark-red color, accompanied by massive leukorrhea with white or yellowish green color and foul odor, itching and pain of the vulva.

Pathogenesis. Retention and accumulation of damp-heat in the lower-energizer resulting in impairment of the uterine collaterals.

Therapeutic Principle. Clearing away heat and decreasing diuresis.

Metrorrhagia and Metrostaxis due to Qi Deficiency

Symptoms. Metrorrhagia, or dripping of menstrual and light red menstruation, pale complexion, short breath, poor appetite.

Pathogenesis. The constitutional insufficiency of the spleen, or improper diet and impairment of the spleen-qi, deficiency of qi in the middle-energizer, inability to control blood, debility of the Vital and Front Middle Meridians.

Therapeutic Principle. Invigorating qi to strengthen its power to control blood circulation.

Metrorrhagia and Metrostaxis due to Qi Stagnation

A type of metrorrhagia and metrostaxis.

Symptoms. Metrorrhagia and metrostaxis, distention and pain in the hypochondrium, vexation, restlessness, sometimes sigh.

Pathogenesis. The stagnation of the liver-qi, fire transmitted from qi stagnation, the disorder of storing blood.

Therapeutic Principle. Stop bleeding by relieving the depressed liver and qi to arrest bleeding and regulate menstruation.

Metrorrhagia and Metrostaxis due to Yang Insufficiency

Symptoms. Metrorrhagia, or dripping blood, cold-pain in the lower abdomen, cold limbs, aversion to cold, preference for warm, loose stools.

Pathogenesis. Insufficiency of kidney-yang, dysfunction in storing essence, debility of the Vital and Front Meridians.

Therapeutic Principle. Warm and recuperate the kidney yang, astringe to arrest menstruation.

Metrorrhagia and Metrostaxis due to Yin Deficiency

Symptoms. Profuse menses or incessant dripping of blood with scarlet color, dizziness, tinnitus, dysphoria with feverish sensation in chest, insomnia, night sweat, soreness and debility of waist and knees.

Pathogenesis. Insufficiency of the kidney-yin, resulting in hyperactivity of fire of deficiency type, leading to failure to control blood.

Therapeutic Principle. Nourishing the liver and kidney, and clearing away heat to reinforce meridians.

Metrorrhagia due to Accumulation of Phlegm

Symptoms. Fullness in the stomach, abdominal pain around the navel, relief of pain after blood is discharged, fullness while blood stops.

Pathogenesis. Accumulation of phlegm and salvation in the chest, inability of clear qi to up, and blocking in meridians.

Therapeutic Principle. Regulating qi and dissipating phlegm.

Metrorrhagia due to Qi Collapse

Symptoms. Fatigue, lassitude, sleepy dyspnea and profuse bleeding with activity.

Pathogenesis. Deficiency and collapse of the spleen-qi and stomach-qi, and debility of the Vital and Front Meridians leading to blood prostration as a result of improper diet and overstrain.

Therapeutic Principle. Invigorating the spleen and qi, and recuperating depleted yang.

Metrorrhagia due to Sprain or Fall

Symptoms. Abdominal pain when pressed.

Pathogenesis. Falling from hight, or injury from sprain and contusion leading to debility of the Vital and Front Meridian to release extravasated blood.

Therapeutic Principle. Promoting blood circulation to dissipating stasis.

Metrorrhagia with Watery Diarrhea

Symptoms. Metrorrhagia with watery discharge or diarrhea once or twice a day, short of breath, lassitude, sleepy and fatigue.

Pathogenesis. Impairment of the spleen and stomach leading to failure of the spleen to keep blood in the vessels, or heart-fire invading the spleen due to irregular eating or physical fatigue.

Therapeutic Principle. Dispelling dampness or tonifying middle-energizer.

Metrostaxis with White Discharge

Referring to incessant metrostaxis accompanied by whitish discharge.

Pathogenesis. Qi deficiency of the spleen and lung.

Therapeutic Principle. Strengthening the spleen and tonifying the lung.

Mexican Tea Herb

It is the whole plant with fruiting part of Chenopodium ambrosioides L. (Chenopodiaceae).

Effect. Expelling wind, promoting the circulation of qi, killing parasites, stimulating menstrual discharge and relieving pain.

Indication. Rheumatic arthralgia, dysmenorrhea, amenorrhea, ascariasis, skin eczema and snake bite.

Mianyan (Ex-HN)

An extra acupuncture point.

Location. On the face, level with both sides of the protruding point of the wing of nose; under the junction of lateral one-quarter of the infraorbital margin and medial three-quarters of the infraorbital margin.

Indication. Deep-rooted sore on the head and face.

Method. Puncturing perpendicularly 0.2-0.3 cun.

Middle Cymba Conchae (MA)

An auricular point.

Location. In the center of the cymba conchae.

Indication. Low fever, abdominal distention, biliary ascariasis, hypoacusis, and parotitis. Acupuncture is applicable.

Middle-energizer

It is one of the tri-energizer.

Location. Between the diaphragm and umbilicus navel.

Function. Helping the spleen and stomach in decomposing and digesting food, eliminating waste products, transforming food essence, sending food essence upward and turbid substance downward. It is source of vital energy and blood.

Middle-energizer Fullness

Symptoms. Fullness and distention in the abdomen, lassitude, difficulty in walking and standing, vomiting after eating, etc.

Pathogenesis. Obstruction of the middle-energizer.

Therapeutic Principle. Relieving distention and fullness.

Middle Finger Cun

A term in acupuncture. It refers to the length of the middle segment of the middle finger, taken as the standard of measurement. It means that one cun is equivalent to the distance between the cross-striations on the radial side of the first and second dactylopodites of the patient's middle finger.

Function. Locating acupoints on the back transversely and on the limbs perpendicularly.

Middle-Qi

It refers to qi in the stomach and the spleen. The stomach-qi's physiological function is receiving, digesting and transforming water and foodstuff, ascending clarity, descending turbidity and controlling all the blood of the body. The spleen-qi's function is fixing the internal organs at their original locations and preventing prolapse of the rectum and uterus and ptosis of other internal organs.

Middle Triangular Fossa (MA)

An auricular point.

Location. At middle 1/3 of the triangular fossa.

Function. Clearing away heat to relieve asthma.

Indication. asthma.

Midget Crab-apple Fruit

It is the fruit of Malus micromalus Mak. (Rosaceae).

Effect. Promoting digestion to relieve dyspepsia and stopping diarrhea.

Indication. Diarrhea and dysentery.

Migraine

Symptoms. Headache on one side accompanied sometimes by ophthalmalgia or nausea and vomiting, etc.

Pathogenesis. Upper invasion of wind-phlegm or by hyperactivity of fire due to deficiency of blood.

Therapeutic Principle. Expelling wind and dredging obstruction in meridians, regulating the flow of qi and eliminating phlegm and invigorating both qi and blood.

Migratory Arthralgia

Symptoms. Aching of the limbs and joins with migratory pain, limitation of the joints; or aversion to wind and fever.

Pathogenesis. Attack of wind, cold, and damp evils, which block the meridians and collaterals with predominantly wind-evil.

Therapeutic Principle. Deoppilating the obstruction of the meridians and collaterals, expel pathogenic factors to relieve pain.

Mild Cold

Symptoms. Headache, stuffy nose, heavy voice, running nose, frequently sneezing without fever and aversion to wind.

Pathogenesis. Catching cold by cooling or attacked by cold.

Therapeutic Principle. Dispersing exo-pathogen, soothing, regulating and promoting the dispersing function of the lung.

Mild Heatstroke

Symptoms. Dizziness, headache, fever, lack of perspiration, vomiting, restlessness, thirst, lassitude, and sleepy.

Pathogenesis. Stagnant summer-heat and dampness in the exterior part of the body.

Therapeutic Principle. Clearing away summer-heat from the body by diaphoresis, and regulate the function of the middle-energizer to dispel dampness.

Mild Moxibustion

Referring to moxibustion therapy by warming the local place without scorching the skin.

Method. For direct moxibustion, ignite one end of a moxa stick, put the ignited end directly above the local place to warm it, 0.5-1 cun or so away from the place till red spots appear without pain. For indirect moxibustion the interposing thing and moxa cone should be properly moved according to the patient's reaction. For a child or a patient with syncope and disturbance of perception in the local place, the doctor should control the temperature of moxibustion by putting his index finger or middle finger on the place so as to avoid scalding the patient.

Indication. Stagnant pain due to wind-cold pathogens and so on.

Mild-moxibustioner

A moxibustion apparatus.

Method. Prepare a tube made of metal, with dozens of small holes in the bottom, and a smaller tube with over ten small holes in it, place argyi wool or medical powder in the smaller tube. When the moxibustion is applied, ignite it and put the tube on a certain position to make the heat go through the skin and muscle.

Function. Regulating qi and blood, warming the middle-energizer to dispel cold.

Indication. Especially suitable for women, children and those who are afraid of needles.

Mild Numbness

Referring to a numbness disease.

Symptoms. Numbness of the skin, pale tongue with white coating and floating pulse, etc.

Pathogenesis. The pathogen in the meridians and collaterals, the pathogen is still in the skin without the impairment of tendon and bone.

Therapeutic Principle. Eliminating pathogenic factor to activating meridians and collaterals, and regulating qi, and blood.

Mild Wind Syndrome

Symptoms. Sensation of worm sprawling inside muscle. It is often accompanied by other symptoms of zang-fu, qi and blood.

Pathogenesis. The interior excess of yangqi due to the obstruction of defensive energy by wind evil.

Therapeutic Principle. Inducing diaphoresis to dispel wind evil.

Miliaria

Symptoms. Groups of papular eruptions appear on the skin, red, itching, with small blisters or small pustule. Mostly found in children.

Pathogenesis. Summer-heat or dampheat.

Therapeutic Principle. Clearing away summer-heat and promoting diuresis.

Milk-food Vomiting

Symptoms. The infant vomits with signs of milk or indigested food, fullness of the abdomen. Slight fever, and damp heat, poor appetite.

Pathogenesis. Due to eating excessive milk or food, or improper diet.

Therapeutic Principle. Promoting digestion, relieving stasis, and decreasing eating and drinking.

Millet

It is the kernel of Setaria italica (L.) Beauv. (Gramineae).

Effect. Normalizing the function of the stomach and spleen, tonifying kidney, eliminating heat and detoxicating.

Indication. Fever due to deficiency of the spleen and stomach, regurgitation, vomiting, poor appitite, diabetes and diarrhea.

Millet Sprout

It is the dried germinant fruit of Setaria italica (L.) Beauv. (Gramineae).

Effect. Promoting digestion and regulating the stomach, strengthening the spleen and replenishing qi.

Indication. Dyspepsia, anorexia due to hypofunction of the spleen, etc.

Mimasclike Rosewood Leaf

It is the leaf of Dalbergia mimosoides Franch. (Leguminosae).

Effect. Relieving inflammation and removing toxic substances.

Indication. Furuncle carbuncles, subcutaneous swelling, viper bite and phlegmon.

Mingguan (Ex-CA)

An extra acupuncture point.

Location. Directly below the nipples, 4 cun above the umbilicus.

Indication. Edema, dysuria, dyspnea, abdominal distention, vomiting and nausea, incontinence of stool, persistent pain in the hypochondrium.

Method. Moxibustion is applicable.

Mingmen (GV 4)

1. An acupuncture point.

   Location. On the posterior midline of the lower back, in the depression below the spinous process of the second and the third lumbar vertebrae.

   Indication. Waist pain due to overstrain, stiffness of the spine, enuresis, frequent micturition, emission, impotence, premature ejaculation, leukorrhea with reddish discharge, repeated abortion, dizziness and tinnitus, epilepsy, terror, cold limbs.

Method. Puncture perpendicularly 0.5-1.0 cun. Perform moxibustion with 3-7 moxa cones or for 5-15 minutes.

2. It means the vital gate or gate of life, which is believed to be closely related to the kidney. Its main functions are the root of primordial qi acting as the primary motivating force for the life activities. It stores the essence of life, with close relation to the human reproduction. It is the source of yang-qi and the house of water and fire. It stores the kidney-yang.

Ministerial Fire

1. Referring to the fire (yang-qi) originating from the gate of life stored in the liver, gallbladder and the tri-energizer in cooperation with the king fire, which originates from the heart.

   Function. It can warm and nourish the zang-fu organs and promote their functional activities. The excessive ministerial fire results in diseases.

2. The part of fire controlled by the kidney that promotes the sexual potency.

Mirabilite

It is the crystal of the refined mirabilite from the sulphate minerals, which mainly contains hydrated sodium sulphate.

Effect. Clearing away heat and softening hard masses by purgation.

Indication. Constipation due to accumulation and retention of heat of excess type, sore throat, canker sores, bloodshot eyes, carbuncle and ulcers, externally for acute mastitis, etc.

Miscellaneous Qi

It refers to the various epidemic diseases except the six evils in the nature. Certain pathogen-qi of miscellaneous qi can only attack certain zang-fu organs and certain

meridians and collaterals to cause certain diseases.

Moderate Stimulation

An acupuncture point, moxibustion fashion, referring to the stimulating intensity of acupuncture and moxibustion, between strong and weak stimulation.

Moellendorf's Spikemoss Herb

It is the whole herb of Selaginella moellendorfii Hieron. (Selaginellaceae).

Effect. Removing heat from the blood bleeding, and inducing diuresis.

Indication. Hemoptysis, hemafecia, metrorrhagia, traumatic bleeding, jaundice, stranguria and infantile convulsion.

Moist and Glossy Tongue Fur

Referring to tongue coating with excessive moisture, damp and glossy, and even start of saliva drip.

Pathogenesis. Insufficient yang-qi, stagnation of water-damp, phlegm retention, and floating upward onto the surface of the tongue.

Moistening Being Basis of Complexion

It refers to a diagnostic method if complexion of the patient keeps bright and moist, it suggests exhaustion of the stomach-qi, indicating favourable prognosis. If complexion remains withered and dusky, it suggests exhaustion of the stomach-qi, indicating unfavourable prognosis.

Moisturize Dry-heat by Clearing Bowels

It is one of the therapeutic methods to treat constipation resulting from accumulation of heat obstruction of qi in fu organs impairment of body fluid.

Indication. Constipation, halitosis and lip boil, flushed complexion, scanty dark urine.

Mole Cricket

It is the dried intact insect of Gryllotalpa africana Pal. de Beauvois (Gryllotalpidae).
Effect. Inducing diuresis and relaxing the bowels.
Indication. Edema, stranguria caused by the passage of urinary stone, ascites and retention of urine, scrofula, subcutaneous swelling, malignant boils, etc.

Moleplant Seed

It is the ripe seed of Euphorbia lathyris L. (Euphorbiaceae).
Effect. Dispelling retained water and decreasing edema, eliminating blood stasis and resolving masses.
Indication. Edema, ascites, difficulty in urination and defecation, masses in the abdomen and amenorrhea.

Monkey Bezoar

It is the biliary calculus of Macaca mulatta Zimmermann (Macacaceae).
Effect. Expelling phlegm and relieving convulsion, clearing away heat and detoxication.
Indication. Asthma and cough due to accumulation of phlegm, infantile epilepsy induced by terror, etc.

Monkshood Cake

A kind of medicinal cake for moxibustion.
Preparation. Grind monkshood into powder and mix it with warm water to make small cakes of about 0.6-1 cm thick, then make several holes in the center for indirection moxibustion.

Moody State during Menstruation

Symptoms. It refers to anxiety and irritability, depression, insomnia; or even mania and restlessness during and before menstruation; commonly restoration to normal condition after the menstruation.
Pathogenesis. 1. Malnutrition of heart blood due to qi and blood insufficiency; 2. Disturbance of mental state because of fire-transmission due to liver stagnation.

Therapeutic Principle. In the first case, nourishing blood to calm the mind; in the second case, clearing away fire from the liver and relieving convulsion to tranquilize the mind.

Moonwort

It is the plant of Botrychium ternatum (Thunb.) Sw. (Botrychiaceae) with root.
Effect. Clearing away heat, calming the liver and relieving cough.
Indication. Dizziness, headache, hematemesis, epilepsy, acute conjunctivitis, sore throat, carbuncles and other pyogenic infections on the body surface.

Mor Angelica Root

It is the root of Angelica morii Hayata (Umbelliferae).
Effect. Invigorating the middle-energizer and replenishing qi.
Indication. Diarrhea due to deficiency of the spleen-yang, cough due to cold of deficiency type, snake bite etc.

Morbid Leukorrhea due to Kidney Deficiency

Symptoms. Profuse leukorrhea with whitish and watery discharge, the lower abdomen cold, soreness and pain of the waist, frequent urination especially at night, loose stools.
Pathogenesis. Constitutional insufficiency of kidney-qi or marriage at an early age, or multiparity leading to impairment of the kidney, deficiency of the primary qi and unconsolidation of the Front and the Belt Meridians.
Therapeutic Principle. Warm and recuperate the kidney-yang to consolidate and control the Front and the Belt Meridians.

Morning Convulsion

Symptoms. High fever, flushed face, superduction of the eyes, spasm of neck and limbs, etc.
Pathogenesis. Up-stirring of the liver wind by flaming of the liver-fire.

Therapeutic Principle. Nourishing the kidney and clearing away the liver-fire.

Morning Sickness due to Liver Heat

Symptoms. In the early stages of pregnancy, vomiting, dry mouth, bitter taste, fullness and distention in the stomach, mental depression, dizziness.

Pathogenesis. Stagnated heat in the Liver Meridian, leading to attack on the stomach.

Therapeutic Principle. Clearing away heat from the liver and regulate the stomach; reduce the adverse flow of stomach-qi to arrest vomiting.

Morning Sickness due to Phlegm Stagnation

Symptoms. In the early stage of pregnancy, vomiting with phlegm-salivation, feeling of oppression in the chest and loss of appetite, palpitations and short breath, lack of taste.

Pathogenesis. Dysfunction of the spleen in transportation, phlegm-dampness produced in the interior.

Therapeutic Principle. Strengthen the spleen and reduce phlegm, decrease the adverse flow of qi and regulate the stomach.

Morning Sickness due to Stomach-cold

Symptoms. In the early period of pregnancy, vomiting of watery fluid, cold extremities, aversion to cold, dull pain in the stomach and abdomen, preference for warmth and pressing etc.

Pathogenesis. Original deficiency and cold in the spleen and stomach, aggravated by reverse flowing of sufficient qi in the Vital Meridian after pregnancy, leading to stomach dysfunction.

Therapeutic Principle. Warming the stomach and relieving vomiting.

Morning Sickness due to Stomach Deficiency

Symptoms. Epigastric distention and fullness, nausea, vomiting, even instant vomiting when eating food, lassitude and sluggishness, pale tongue with whitish coating.

Pathogenesis. Constitutional deficiency of the spleen and stomach, excessive qi in the Vital Middle Meridian during pregnancy, leading to the failure of stomach-qi to descend.

Therapeutic Principle. Strengthen the spleen and stomach, regulate qi and decrease the adverse flow of stomach-qi.

Morning Sickness due to Stomach-heat

Symptoms. Vomiting, vexation, flushed complexion, thirst for cold drink, constipation, red tongue with yellowish coating.

Pathogenesis. Constitutional heat in the stomach, excessive qi in the Vital Middle Meridian during pregnancy resulting in the failure of the stomach-qi to descend.

Therapeutic Principle. Clear away heat from the stomach; decrease the adverse flow of stomach-qi to stop vomiting.

Morning Vertigo

Symptoms. Dizziness when getting up in the morning, which disappears a moment later and never occurs during the day, and so on.

Pathogenesis. Yang-deficiency or solid phlegm-stagnation.

Therapeutic Principle. Depriving dampness and dispelling sputum, and invigorating the spleen and regulating the stomach.

Motherwort Herb

It is the whole herb of Leonurus heterophyllus Sweet (Labiatae).

Effect. Invigorating blood circulation to dissipate blood stasis, relieving edema by inducing diuresis.

Indication. Irregular menstruation, distending pain in the lower abdomen, amenorrhea, postpartum abdominal pain due to blood stasis, lochiorrhea, traumatic injuries, swelling and pain, dysuria and edema.

Mountain Spicy Tree Fruit

It is the fruit of Litsea cubeba (Lour) Pers. (Lauraceae).

Effect. Warming the middle-energizer and relieving pain.

Indication. Abdominal pain, epigastric, vomiting and hiccups due to cold in the stomach, etc.

Mountain Spicy Tree Root

It is the root and rhizome of Litsea cubeba (Lour.) Pers. (Lauraceae).

Effect. Dispelling wind, removing dampness, regulating flow of qi and relieving pain.

Indication. Common cold, rheumatic arthralgia, stomachache and beriberi.

Moutan Bark

It is the root bark of Paeonia suffruticosa Andr. (Ranunculaceae).

Effect. Removing heat from blood, promoting blood circulation and eliminating blood stasis.

Indication. Eruptions, hematemesis, epistaxis, hemafecia, hectic fever with consumptive fever due to yin-deficiency, night fever; amenorrhea and menorrhagia abdominal masses, traumatic injuries, suppurative infections on the body surface, etc.

Mouth (MA-ICS)

An otopoint.

Location. On the posterior and superior border of the orifice of the external auditory meatus.

Function. Clearing heat-fire, and removing pathogenic wind.

Indication. Facial paralysis, stomatitis, cholecystitis, cholelithiasis.

Moving Landmarks

One of the anatomic marks of body surface. Referring to lacunas, pitting, wrinkles and prominences, etc, appearing at the joints, muscles, tendons, and skin.

Function. With these landmarks, the location of some acupoints can be determined.

Moxa Cone

A cone-shaped moxa is made with sharp tip and flat base for application of moxibustion. According to the needs of moxibustion, moxa cones vary in size, large, medium and small.

Moxa Cone Moxibustion

A moxibustion method.

Method. Putting a burning moxa cone on the acupuncture point of the body surface, divided further into direct moxibustion and indirect moxibustion.

Moxa Stick

It is made of mugwort. In general, it is made by adding a certain drug in to the moxa during preparation, making 20 g of pure moxa (a small amount of fragrant and dry drug powder can be added into moxa to strengthen the action) on cotton paper 9cm in length and 15cm in width, then folding the two ends of the cotton paper, and rolling it closely and sealing its openings with egg white, then drying and storing it for use.

Moxa Stick Moxibustion

Method. A specially-made moxa stick to smoke and cauterize the point, including mild moxibustion and pecking moxibustion.

Moxa Wool

The main material for moxibustion. It is processed from moxa leaves. Collect the leaves in summer while the plant is exuberant, dry and grind them, remove the stalks and impurities, making a fine, soft wool-like substance.

Moxibustion at Eight Points for Beriberi

It refers to the eight effective points for treating beriberi with moxibustion. The points are Fengshi (G 20), Futu (S 32), Dubi (S 35), Xiyan (Ex-LE 5), Zusanli (S 36), Shanglian (LI 9), Xialian (LI 8) and Xuanzhong (G 39).

Moxibustion by Steaming with Herbal Medicine

A kind of moxibustion, referring to a moxibustion method of steaming the acupoints with herbal medicinal fluid to achieve the purpose of treatment.

Moxibustion Dipper

A moxibustion apparatus, composed of two parts. The upper part is formed by a spring holder wound up with metal wire, and the lower part is made of artifical leather or asbestos pad. On either side of the pad, there is a silk ribbon for fixing the moxa holder.

Application. The moxa wool is placed inside the holder and lit for warming moxibustion.

Moxibustion for Health Protection

A moxibustion method used to keep one's general health by improving the body resistance.

Method. Commonly moxibustion points are Zusanli (S 36), Guanyuan (CV 4), Qihai (CV 6), Gaohuang (B 43), etc.

Moxibustion of Sore

Method. Use the heat and the effects of the drugs of moxibustion to dredge the meridians, to relieve stagnation and remove toxic substances.

Indication. The beginning of the skin and external diseases, including yang and yin syndromes.

Moxibustion Technique

It refers to the method by which diseases are treated by burning, fumigating or ironing with moxa wool, etc.

Moxibustion with Alum

A form of indirect moxibustion in which an herbal cake containing black alum and other drugs is used as the separation. Apply one cake to the affected part and place a moxa cone upon the cake for moxibustion.

Indication. Extended hemorrhoids and fistula.

Moxibustion with Warming Needle

A term in acupuncture.

Method. While retaining the needle in proper depth, ignite a ball of moxa wool, wrapping the handle of the needle to cause the conduction of heat into the selected point through the needle body. Usually 1-3 balls of moxa wool are burned at each moxibustion.

Function. Promoting the flow of qi and the blood circulation by warming channels.

Indication. Arthralgia aggravated by cold; numbness.

Muchuang (G 16)

An acupuncture point.

Location. On the head, 1.5 cun superior to the anterior hairline and 2.25 cun lateral to the median line of the head, 1 cun behind Toulinqi (B 15).

Indication. Headache, dizziness, redness and pain of eye, optic atrophy, facial edema, pain in outer canthus, and epilepsy due to terror.

Therapeutic Principle. Puncture subcutaneously 0.3-0.5 cun and apply moxibustion to point with 1-3 units of moxa cones or for 3-5 minutes.

Mulberry

It is the ripe spike of Morus alba L. (Moraceae).

Effect. Nourishing yin and blood, tonifying the kidney promoting production of the body fluid and moistening the bowels.

Indication. Dizziness, blurred vision, tinnitus, insomnia, premature grey hair, thirst and diabetes constipation.

Mulberry Bark

It is the bark of Morus alba L. (Moraceae).

Effect. Clearing away heat from the lung, relieving asthma, inducing diuresis and subduing swelling.

Indication. Asthma and cough due to heat in the lung, edema and dysuria.

Mulberry Leaf

It is the leaf of Morus alba L. (Moraceae).

Effect. Dispelling wind and clearing away heat, removing intensive heat from the liver and improving acuity of sight.

Indication. Dizziness, headache, sore throat, thirst, cough due to heat in the lung, hematemesis.

Mulberry Twig

It is the twig of Morus alba L. (Moraceae).

Effect. Expelling pathogenic wind, relieving obstruction in the meridians and inducing diuresis.

Indication. Rheumatic arthralgia, spasm of limbs, and edema.

Mule Calculus

It is the stone in the stomach of Equus asinus L., Equus caballus L. (Equidae).

Effect. Arresting convulsion and detoxicating, clearing away heat and dissipating phlegm.

Indication. Infantile acute convulsion, interior heat and phlegm, delirium, depressive psychosis, etc.

Multicolored Vaginal Discharge

Symptoms. Continuous mucous discharge with filthy and various colors and fetid smell from the vagina.

Pathogenesis. Downward flow of damp and heat pathogens into the lower-energizer, accumulating to form toxin, and impair the Vital Front and the Belt Meridians.

Therapeutic Principle. Strengthening the spleen to eliminate dampness, expelling pathogenic factors, clearing heat and warming yang.

Notice. For this kind of patient, be careful to see whether the genitals have a malignant tumor.

Multiple Abscesses due to Blood Stasis

Symptoms. Stretching swelling and pain normal skin color. It mostly appears in the deep parts with rich and thick muscles of the limbs and the trunk, Persistent attacks.

Pathogenesis. Swelling due to stagnation of pathogenic damp-heat from skin injury into the muscles, retention of blood stasis due to traumatic injury, multiple abscess in the meridians and collaterals due to postpartum lochiorrhea, etc.

Therapeutic Principle. In the case of muscular injury due to overstrain, regulating the nutrient and dissipating blood stasis, clearing away heat and eliminating dampness; For traumatic injury, regulating the nutrient system and dissipating blood stasis. For postpartum blood stasis, regulating the nutrient and dissipating blood stasis.

Multiple Abscess with Summer-heat and Dampness

Symptoms. White stretching swelling on the affected skin with slight fever and pain, fever with aversion to cold, and arthralgia, etc.

Pathogenesis. The suffering from the summer-heat and dampness at the beginning, and then the affection of cold.

Therapeutic Principle. Detoxicating, clearing away summer-heat and dissipating dampness.

Mumps

An acute viral infectious disease.

Symptoms. It is an acute viral infectious disease. It mostly occurs in children during the winter and spring with sudden onset, swelling and pain in the parotid region under the ear. For the mild case, swelling of the parotid region under the ear, difficulty in chewing, accompanied by aversion to cold, fever, slightly yellow tongue coating. In the severe case, redness, swelling and pain of the parotid region, difficulty in chewing, high fever and headache, irritability, thirst, constipation, scanty dark urine, sometimes accompanied by vomiting, swelling and pain of the testis, even coma and convulsion, yellow tongue coating,

Pathogenesis. Invasion by a wind-warm virus into the mouth and nose which blocks the Shaoyang Meridian and stagnates in the cheek.

Therapeutic Principle. In the mild case, dispel wind to relieve exterior syndrome and clear heat and toxins. In the severe case, clean away heat, remove toxins, and activate obstruction in meridians and collaterals to reduce edema.

Muscle Particle in Eyelid

Symptoms. Muscle particles, as tiny as grains, yellow and soft, growing in the eyelid or at the edge of the eyelid. The tears inside, and astringent pain.

Pathogenesis. Wind-heat in the Spleen Meridian.

Therapeutic Principle. Scraping to bleed and applying the drugs of removing wind from the spleen.

Muscovite

It is a kind of silicate mineral.

Effect. Improving inspiration and relieving asthma, and arresting bleeding to treat boils.

Indication. Asthma of insufficiency type, dizziness, palpitation, epilepsy, chronic dysentery, cutting wounds with bleeding, carbuncle, deep-rooted carbuncle, furuncle, etc.

Muscular Atrophy

Referring to the muscle and tendous flaccidity and numbness.

Symptoms. Numbness, and inability to raise limbs when it becomes serious.

Pathogenesis. Excessive heat of middle-energizer and spleen, failure in nourishing muscles or impairment of spleen by pathogenic dampness, dysfunction of the spleen in transport and impairment of muscles.

Therapeutic Principle. Strengthening both spleen and stomach, clearing away heat and dissipating dampness.

Muscular Contracture

Symptoms. Muscular contracture, stiffness and inability of limbs to flex and extend, etc.

Pathogenesis. Malnutrition of muscles due to the invasion of pathogenic wind-cold into muscles or the impairment of muscles by liver-fire or blood deficiency and fluid consumption.

Therapeutic Principle. Nourishing blood and liver, and relaxing muscles. In addition, expelling wind and clearing away cold, or removing heat from the liver, or nourishing yin and promoting the production of body fluid pursuant to pathogenic factors.

Musk

It is the dried secretion in the musk sac of the adult male musk deer Moschus berezovskii Flerov or M. sifanicus Przewalski or M. Moschiferus L. (Cervidae).

Effect. Inducing resuscitation and restoring consciousness, promoting blood circulation to resolve hard masses, relieving pain and expediting child delivered.

Indication. Unconsciousness and convulsion apoplexy and epilepsy precordial pain, traumatic injury, sores carbuncles masses in the abdomen, amenorrhea, etc.

Muskmelon Base

It is the base of Cucumis melo L. (Cucurbitaceae).

Effect. Causing vomiting endopathic heat-phlegm and dyspepsia internally; removing damp-heat.

Indication. Heat-phlegm, dyspepsia, and jaundice and headache due to damp-heat.

Muskroot-like Semiaquilegia Root

It is the root tuber of Semiaquilegia adoxoides (DC.) Makino (Ranunculaceae).

Effect. Clearing away heat, detoxicating, promoting the subsidence of swelling, dissipating stasis and inducing diuresis.

Indication. Sores, carbuncles, furuncle and boils, scrofula, stranguria with turbid urine, leukorrhagia, cough due to lung-deficiency, epilepsy, infantile, hemorrhoid, traumatic injuries, etc.

Mussel

It is the meat of Mytilus crassitesta Lisohke (Mytilidae) and other mussels.

Effect. Invigorating the liver and kidney, tonifying spontaneous emission and blood and treating goiter.

Indication. Dizziness, night sweat, lumbago, hematemesis, impotence, metrorrhagia, metrostaxis, leukorrhea and goiter.

Mustard Seed Moxibustion

A kind of moxibustion with herbal blister.

Method. Apply the mustard seed ground into powder to the acupoint for about 3-4 hours till blister forms in the local region.

Indication. Tuberculosis, asthma, facial hemiplegia, etc.

Muttering in Sleep

Symptoms. Talking in sleep, weak, rumble and meaningless, and stopping when awakened, but continuing muttering with eyes closed.

Therapeutic Principle. Tonifying heart-yin, clearing away heart-fire and the heat in the gallbladder, regulating the stomach function, etc.

Mutual Assistance

Drugs of similar characters and functions in certain aspects can be used together, with one as the principal and the other as subsidiary, to help increase the effects of the therapy.

Mutual Detoxication

One drug can lessen or remove the toxicity and side effects of another drug.

Muzhilihengwen (Ex-LE)

An extra acupuncture point.

Location. On the plantar side of toe, the midpoint of transverse crease of phlangeal joint.

Indication. Hernia.

Method. Puncture perpendicularly 0.2-0.3 cun. Moxibustion is applicable.

Myasthenia of Lower Limbs due to Dysentery

A disease.

Symptoms. Chills, fever, aching and weakness of feet, pain and difficulty in activities with effusion of yellow liquid from the knee joint, etc.

Pathogenesis. Insufficiency of three yang, overstrain, or affection by expathogen, or deficiency due to sexual strain after dysentery.

Therapeutic Principle. Invigorating qi, promoting blood circulation warming yang and strengthening the muscles and bones.

Myopia

Symptoms. Patient is able to see things nearby with visual clarity, but at a distance things are blurred.

Pathogenesis. Congenital disposition, insufficiency of the heart-yang, or insufficiency of the liver and kidney.

Therapeutic Principle. Nourishing the heart to promote the flow of qi, or replenishing the liver and kidney.

Myrrh

It is the resin oozed out of the tree trunk of Commiphora myrrha Engl. (Burseraceae) or other species in the same genus plants.

Effect. Promoting blood circulation, relieving pain, relieving swelling and promoting tissue regeneration.

Indication. Epigastralgia amenorrhea, dysmenorrhea, pain due to traumatic injuries, sores and ulcers and exudative skin infections.

Mysorethorn

It is the seed of Caesalpinia sepiaria Roxb. (Leguminosae).

Effect. Clearing away heat, dispelling dampness and destroying parasites.

Indication. Dysentery, diabetes, and malnutrition of children, etc.

N

Nacre

It is the pearly layer in the shell of Hyriopsis cumingii (Lea) and Cristaria plicata (Leach) (Naiadidae) or Pteria martensii (Dunker) (Pteriidae).

Effect. Calming the liver and suppress yang, removing heat from the liver and improving acuity of vision.

Indication. Dizziness, headache, tinnitus, restlessness, insomnia due to deficiency of the liver and kidney, and hyperactivity of the liver-yang; swollen and painful eyes due to heat in the liver or blurred vision due to deficiency of the liver-qi, etc.

Nail-like Boil

It refers to furuncle, which is small in size, deep-rooted, hard like nails.

Pathogenesis. Mostly caused by improper diet, with the external affection of wind and fire-toxins, or traumatic infection.

Therapeutic Principle. Clearing away heat and toxic material.

Nail-like Boil of Ten Fingers

It refers to the disease of nail-like boil appearing on the middle finger, which affects the fingers nearby.

Therapeutic Principle. Stabbing the digital root of the ending joint to squeeze the extravasated blood and use drugs internally to clear away heat and toxic material.

Nail-like Crust Skin

Symptoms. Dry, contracted, hard outer skin, which affects good muscle, swelling and pain, etc.

Pathogenesis. Loss of blood in the case of blood stasis and heat accumulation due to traumatic injury.

Therapeutic Principle. Let out the stasis and dirty things immediately. Take drugs for supplementing qi and promoting tissue regeneration, cutting off the dead muscle should be avoided.

Nail-like Scar

Symptoms. Scabs do not drop off for a long time after the healing of smallpox.

Pathogenesis. Mostly caused by exterior deficiency.

Nail-line Furuncle

Symptoms. Redness swelling, heat and pain along one side of the nail. It can spread to the other side of the nail, and even invade under the nail in the severe case.

Pathogenesis. Pathogenic poison which affects the broken skin.

Therapeutic Principle. Clearing away heat and removing toxic material, cutting and evacuating pus.

Nail-pressing

Referring to pressing the acupoint with the left thumbnail to make insertion of the needle easier. It can reduce pain while inserting and strengthen the needling sensation.

Nail-scratching

It refers to an auxiliary needling manipulation. It means scratching along the meridian with the nail of the thumb to promote the movement of stagnated pathogens, while the needle is inserted.

Nangdi (Ex-CA)

An extra acupuncture point.

Location. On the midpoint of the posterior crossed crease of the scrotum in male.

Indication. Hernia, scrotal eczema, testitis, etc.

Nanyinfeng (Ex-CA)

An extra acupuncture point.

Location. Right in the centre of the juncture of the root of the penis and the scrotum.

Indication. Jaundice, testitis, insanity, etc.

Naohu (GV17)

A meridian acupuncture point.

Location. On the head, 2.5 cun directly above the midpoint of the posterior hairline, 1.5 cun above Fengfu (GV 16), in the depression on the upper border of the external occipital protuberance.

Indication. Headache, vertigo, hoarseness of voice, stiffness of the neck, epilepsy, etc.

Method. Puncture horizontally along the skin 0.5-0.8 cun. Apply moxibustion 3-5 minutes.

Naohui (TE 13)

A meridian acupuncture point.

Location. On the lateral side of the upper arm and on the line connecting the tip of the olecranon and Jianliao (TE 14), 3 cun below Jianliao (TE 14), and on the posteroinferior border of the deltoid muscle.

Indication. Swelling pain in the shoulder, scapular area and arm, goiter, scrofula, eye disorders, etc.

Method. Puncture perpendicularly 0.8-1.2 cun. Perform moxibustion 3-7 moxa cones or 5-15 minutes.

Naokong (G 19)

A meridian acupuncture point.

Location. On the head and on the level of the upper border of the external occipital protuberance or Naohu (GV 17), 2.25 cun lateral to the midline of the head, 1.5 cun directly above Fengchi(G 20).

Indication. Headache, dizziness, tinnitus, pain and stiffness of the neck and nape, epilepsy, palpitation due to fright, etc.

Method. Puncture horizontally 0.3-0.5 cun. Moxibustion is applicable.

Naoshu (SI 10)

A meridian acupuncture point.

Location. On the shoulder, above the posterior and of the axillary fold, in the depression below the lower border of the scapular spine.

Indication. Aching and swelling in the shoulder, inability to ride of the arm, rigidity on the neck and nape.

Method. Puncture perpendicularly or obliquely 1.0-1.5 cun. Moxibustion is applicable.

Notice. Deep puncture toward the chest is forbidden, for fear of damaging the lung. Perform moxibustion 3-7 moxa cones or 5-15 minutes.

Nape Carbuncle

Symptoms. At the beginning Fengfu (GV 16) Point as millet-like shape, burning, swelling, and pain. The pain can be felt even in the head, shoulder and neck. Gradually it will enlarge like a plate, reddish, and easy to ulcerate.

Pathogenesis. Stagnation of wind-heat, stagnancy of qi and blood due to earlier accumulated heat, and wind-evil in the exterior.

Therapeutic Principle. Clearing away heat and toxic material or operation.

Nardostachys Root

It is the rhizome and root of Nardostachys chinensis Batal and N. jatamansi DC. (Valerianaceae).

Effect. Promoting the circulation of qi, relieving pain, clearing liver and activating the spleen-energy.

Indication. Chest distress, abdominal distention, anorexia and epigastralgia.

Nasal Acupuncture

An acupuncture point therapy by needling particular points on the nose, but this therapy is not extensively used in clinic.

Nasal Bacterium

Symptoms. Prolonged and constant running of bloody and watery discharge that is filthy and fishy, or by turbid and purulent nasal discharge with blood interspersed.

Pathogenesis. Accumulation of phlegm and turbid discharge, stagnation of qi and blood, and stagnation of fire-toxin.

Therapeutic Principle. Removing phlegm dispersing pathogenic accumulation, promoting the circulation of qi and blood, softening and resolving hard lumps, purging intense heat and detoxicating.

Nasal Disability to Smell

1. **Symptoms.** Nasal obstruction, red swelling of the nasal meatus.

   Pathogenesis. Obstruction of sufficient wind-heat and pathogenic toxin.

2. **Symptoms.** Pale swelling and distention of the nasal meatus.

   Pathogenesis. Deficiency of the lung and spleen qi.

3. **Symptoms.** Swelling and distending, dark reddish meatus.

   Pathogenesis. Stagnation of pathogenic factors in meridians and collaterals, and coagulation of qi and blood.

4. **Symptoms.** Substantial masses blocking in the nose.

   Pathogenesis. Upward attack and coagulation of pathogenic dampness.

Nasal Discharge

It is mucus secreted by the nasal membrane and has the function to moisten the nasal cavity. It is also the lung fluid.

Nasal Dryness

Symptoms. Dryness in the nose, atrophy of sarcolemma, and large nasal cavity, etc.

Pathogenesis. Insufficiency and deficiency of the lung, and malnutrition of the nose.

Therapeutic Principle. Nourish yin to moisten dryness, invigorate the spleen, replenish qi, enrich the blood and moisten the dryness.

Nasal Furunculosis

Symptoms. Local redness, swelling and pain around the furuncle that is small, deep-rooted, hard and nail-like with yellowish and whitish purulent spots on top.

Pathogenesis. Impairment of skin by digging of the nose and pulling-out of the vibrissa nasal hair, and outward attack of wind-heat and pathogenic toxin, or overeating of food rich fatty and pungent in taste, and stagnation of pathogenic fire-toxin.

Therapeutic Principle. Dispelling wind, clearing away heat, detoxicating and subduing swelling.

Nasal Polyp

Symptoms. It refers to lump in the nasal cavity, grape-like, glossy, soft and movable, which blocks the nasal cavity and results in impeded respiration.

Pathogenesis. Stagnation of wind dampness and heat in the Lung Meridian.

Therapeutic Principle. Removing heat from the lung to relieve the dispersing function of the lung-qi, purging dampness and resolving lump.

Nasal Sore

Symptoms. Red swelling of skin, erosion, scab, burning itching, prolonged disunion and repeated attacks in the vicinity of the anterior naris.

Pathogenesis. Damp-heat accumulation in the Lung Meridian, invasion of evil factors, disorder of the spleen and stomach.

Therapeutic Principle. Clearing away heat, detoxicating and removing dampness.

Natant Salvinia Herb

It is the whole plant of Salvinia Natans (L.) All. (Salviniaceae).

Effect. Clearing away heat, detoxicating, promoting blood circulation, relieving pain, dispersing dampness and detumescence.

Indication. Fever due to asthenia of the viscera, general edema, furuncle, eczema, burns, etc.

Natural Indigo

It is the pigment in the leaf of Baphicacanthus cusia Bremek. (Acanthaceae), Polygonum tinctorium Ait. (Polygonaceae), or Isatis tinctoria L. (Cruciferae).

Effect. Clearing away heat, detoxicating, cooling the blood and diminishing swelling.

Indication. Seasonal febrile disease, high fever in children, hematemesis, epistaxis, subcutaneous swelling, snake and insect bite, oral ulcer, mumps, and skin infections.

Nausea

It refers to desire for vomiting due to adverse rising of the stomach-qi.

Pathogenesis. Stagnation of cold, heat, dampness, phlegm and food, or pathological changes in other viscera, leading to disorder of the stomach qi.

Nearby Bleeding

Symptoms. Passing the fresh blood before defecation.

Pathogenesis. Accumulation of damp-heat in the large intestine burning yin collaterals.

Therapeutic Principle. Clearing away heat and promoting diuresis, and improving blood circulation to remove blood stasis.

Nearby-needle Puncture

Method. Insert a needle perpendicularly into the affected parts, and then another needle obliquely toward the first needle at a nearby point.

Indication. Lingering arthralgia-syndrome with obvious and fixed tenderness.

Nearby Neural Segment Point Selection

One of the methods of point selection, referring to selecting acupoints located at the same or neighboring spinal neural segment. In clinical treatment and acupuncture anesthesia and the trouble or the location of the operation are controlled by the same or proximal segement of the spinal cord. For example, point selection on the upper limbs for disease or operations of the chest, on the lower limbs for disease or operations of the abdomen. Local point selection or nearby point selection both belong to this method.

Nearby Point Selection

One of the point selection methods, which means the selection of relevant points near the diseased area for acupuncture. The range is larger than that of local point selection, e.g. select taiyang (Ex-HN 5) for ophthalmopathy; Waiguan (TE 5) for pain in the wrist; Yinshi (S 33) and yanglingquan (G 34) for pain in the knee joint, etc.

Nearly Prostrate due to Asthma

Symptoms. Breathing with whoop, raising shoulders and covering abdomen.

Pathogenesis. The exhaustion and damage of the renal yin fluid due to heat pathogen in summer.

Near-sighted Disease

Symptoms. Blurred vision, hypopsia. Eye pain insomnia, forgetfulness, etc.

Cause. Reading, writing or short-distance work in dim light or with incorrect posture, or overtime. In addition, it can also be caused by congenital deficiency, or yin deficiency of the liver and kidney.

Therapeutic Principle. Nourishing the liver and kidney, replenishing qi to improve eyesight.

Nebula-encroaching upon Eye

Symptoms. There are small grey and white alveoli around the boundary of the black, confluent into patches for the serious case, photophobia, pricking pain with tear, and repeated attack.

Pathogenesis. Excessive heat in the liver and lung or deficient yin inducing vigorous fire.

Therapeutic Principle. Clearing away heat and purging fire or nourishing yin and clearing away heat.

Neck (MA-AH 10)

An auricular point.

Location. On the border of cavum conchae, anterior to Cervical Vertebrae (MA-AH 8).

Indication. Stiff neck, swelling and pain of neck.

Neck Rigidity

It refers to the muscular rigidity, tension and pain of the nape.

Pathogenesis. Invasion of the Taiyang Meridian by pathogenic wind, cold and dampness, or the attack of summer-heat, the exhaustion of the body fluid and the malnutrition of muscles or caused by sprain and contusion, prolonged sitting and the improper position of the head during sleeping.

Necrotic Mass of Breast

It refers to ulcer or necrotic mass of the breast with unbearable pain, lasting a long time with no sign of recovery.

Necrotizing Therapy for Hemorrhoids

It refers to the therapy of using erosive drugs to apply on the surface of the hemorrhoids or to insert into the hemorrhoids to let the hemorrhoids wither, necrose, and drop off.

Needle-embedding

One of the acupuncture therapies. To embed a subcutaneous needle in intradermal or hypodermic of an acupuncture point.

Method. Grip the cutaneous needle with a pair of tweezers, place the tip of the needle directly on the selected acupoint, then insert the needle slowly 0.3-0.8 cun. Fix the needle with adhesive plaster. The duration of retaining needle depends on the specific conditions.

Needle-holding Hand

An acupuncture point term. Both hands work together when inserting the filiform needle. Usually one hand, the right hand, controls the needle and inserts the needle rapidly through the skin into the body, so as to apply various proper manipulation techniques, such as lifting, thrusting, twirling, or rotating. So this hand is called needle-holding hand.

Needle Lifting

A form of needling manipulation, referring to the method of lifting or withdrawing the needle while the reducing method is applied.

Needle-like Finger Pressing

Methods to use fingers rather than needles, such as pressing, fingernail pressing or poking, etc.

Needle-steadying Technique

It refers to a method of inserting the needle into the acupuncture point. Hold the needle handle with the thumb, index, and middle fingers of one hand while the other hand helps by pressing the skin at the same time, making the tip of the needle get swiftly through the skin and further into the tissue. This method is primarily employed by using a needle of 1.5 cun long.

Needle-test of Pre-acupuncture-anesthesia

A term in acupuncture. Before the operation, an acupuncture trial should be made to determine the patient's tolerance of acupuncture. On the basis of the patient's endurance, the needling technique is clearly known.

Needle Transmission

A term of acupuncture.

1. It refers to the acupuncture therapy applied and employed.
2. It refers to manipulations after the insertion of the needle which twirling-rotating and lifting-thrusting techniques are used to induce, keep, and promote needle sensation. The continuous or intermittent needle transmission is done according to the pathological condition.

Needle-withdrawing

A term for a needling technique. It refers to the method of withdrawing the needle from the acupoint, when the needling has finished. To withdraw the needle quickly or slowly depends on the patient's condition and the requirements of the different methods of reinforcing and reducing. In general, fast withdrawing is to remove pathogenic factors, while slow withdrawing is to reinforce the body resistance. Too powerful and casual withdrawal of the needle should be avoided.

Needling Contraindication

It refers to immediate needling, inapplicable to patients during the time of fright, indignation, fatigue, overeating, hunger, thirst, intercourse, intoxication, expedition, depression, etc. In addition, it is not advisable to puncture such specific points as those very close to the principal viscera, organs, or tissues, or under certain conditions, such as pregnancy. Modern clinic practice proves non-absoluteness for the contraindication. Nevertheless, it is necessary to manipulate with caution.

Needling Method

1. It refers to the acupuncture therapy employed.

2. The general term for the puncturing and manipulating methods of various needling instruments.

Needling Methods of Midnight-noon Ebb-flow

It refers to adjunct acupuncture point selection according to time, i.e. calculating the excessive and deficient time of the flowing and ebbing of qi and blood by the designated days and hours. The flow of qi and blood changes with the time. The points open with the excess of qi and blood, and close with deficiency.

Needling Reduction

It involves the coordination of fixation and application of steel needles to penetrate the skin to restoration the fracture and dislocation, which are hard to be reduced by manual reduction.

Needling Response

1. It refers to the patient's sensation of soreness, distention, pressure, numbness, etc. in the local or comparatively large area;
2. The response of the operator's fingers that the needle is sinking, as if slightly sucked.

Needling Treating Five Pathogenic Factors

It is a needling theory, which refers to different needling techniques for treating different diseases. Five pathogenic factors refer to the pathogens of carbuncle, excess, faintness, heat, and cold. For the five pathogenic factors there are five needling principles, and use of five different needle instruments.

Negundo Chastetree Fruit

It is the fruit of Vitex negundo L. Var. Cannabifolia (Sieb. et Zucc.) Hand-Mazz. (Verbenaceae).

Effect. Dispelling pathogenic wind and eliminating phlegm downward qi and relieving pain.

Indication. Cough with asthma, heat-stroke, stomach-ache, and leukorrhagia, etc.

Negundo Chastetree Leaf

It is the leaf of Vitex negundo L. var. cannabifolia (Sieb. et Zucc.) Hand. -Mazz. (Verbenaceae).

Effect. Expelling pathogenic wind from the body surface, invigorating qi and promoting the function of spleen and stomach, destroying parasites and relieving pain.

Indication. Common cold, bronchitis, stomachache, abdominal pain due to eruptive disease, vomiting, diarrhea, dysentery, rheumatalgia, etc.

Neiguan (P 6)

A meridian acupuncture point.

Location. On the palmar side of the forearm, 2 cun above the transverse crease of the wrist, between the tendons of the long palmar muscle and radial flexor muscle of the wrist.

Indication. Palpitation, cardialgia, thoracic and hypochondriac pain, vomiting, stomachache, faintness, convulsive pain of the elbow and arm, etc.

Method. Puncture perpendicularly 0.5-0.8 cun. Apply moxibustion 3-5 moxa cones or 5-10 minutes.

Neihuaiian (Ex-LE 8)

Location. On the medial aspect of the foot, at the tip of the medial malleolus.

Indication. Toothache, sore throat, spasm of the medial side of the leg.

Method. Prick to cause litte bleeding. Apply moxibustion to the point with 5-7 moxa cones

Neihuaiqianxia (Ex-LE)

An extra acupuncture point.

Location. One-finger width anterior to the midpoint of the inferior border of the medial malleolus.

Indication. Regurgitation and vomiting.

Neijingming (Ex-HN)

An extra acupuncture point.

Location. On the lacrimal caruncle of the inner canthus.

Indication. Red eyes with swelling and pain, blurred vision, optic atrophy, etc.

Method. Puncture perpendicularly in the medial side of the orbit 0.5-1.0 cun, with no twirling, lifting or thrusting of the needle. Moxibustion is forbidden.

Neitaichong (Ex-LE)

An extra acupuncture point.

Location. On the dorsum of foot, at the medial side of the tendon of the long extensor muscle of the great toe, parallel with Taichong (Liv 3).

Indication. Hernia, insomnia, difficult breathing.

Method. Puncture perpendicularly 0.1 cun. Apply moxibustion 3 minutes.

Neiting (S 44)

A meridian acupuncture point.

Location. On the dorsal of the foot, at the margin of the web between the 2nd and 3rd toes.

Indication. Toothache, sore throat, deviation of the mouth, epistaxis, diarrhea, dysentery, pain and swelling of the dorsum of foot, febrile diseases.

Method. Puncture obliquely 0.1 cun. Apply moxibustion 3-5 moxa cones, or 5-10 minutes.

Neixiyan (Ex-LE 4)

An extra acupuncture point

Location. In the depression medial to the patellar ligament with the knee fixed.

Indication. Gonarthrosis with peripheral soft tissue inflammation, beriberi.

Method. Puncture obliquely 0.5-0.7 cun from the anterior of the medial side to the posterior of the lateral side, at a 45 degree angle with frontal section. Moxibustion is applicable.

Neiyangchi (Ex-UE)

An extra acupuncture point.

Location. 1 cun above Daling (P 7) which is on the crease of the wrist.

Indication. Stomatitis, sore throat, tinea unguium, infantile convulsion, etc.

Method. Puncture perpendicularly 0.5-0.8 cun. Moxibustion is applicable.

Neiyingxiang (Ex-HN 9)

An extra acupuncture point.

Location. In the nostril, at the junction between the mucosa of the ala cartilage of the nose and the nasal concla. Opposite to Shangyingxiang (Ex-HN 8)

Indication. Sudden pain of the eyes, nasal obstruction, sore throat, headache, febrile disease, sunstroke, vertigo etc.

Method. Prick with a three-edged needle to cause bleeding.

Neizhiyin (Ex-LE)

An extra acupuncture point.

Location. On the medial side of the small toe, about 0.1 cun lateral to the corner of the toe nail.

Indication. Infantile spasm, syncope, etc.

Method. Prick needling to cause bleeding.

Neonatal anuria

It means that the newborn infant does not urinate after two days of the birth.

Pathogenesis. Unless physiologic deformity, it is caused by neonate heat accumulated in the urinary bladder, or congenital defect of the urinary bladder and qi stagnated in the urinary bladder.

Therapeutic Principle. Clearing away heat and diuresis, tonifying qi and diuresis.

Neonatal Jaundice

It refers to the jaundice of newborn infant.

Pathogenesis. Affection of damp-heat or stagnation of cold-damp of the pregnant mother, transferred to the fetus.

Therapeutic Principle. Clearing away heat, removing damp, strengthening and warming the spleen, and reducing jaundice, etc.

Neurodermatitis due to Blood Deficiency and Wind-dryness

One type of neurodermatitis.

Symptoms. In addition to the general symptoms, prolonged course of disease, dryness and thickness of local skin with white bits coming off, looking like the skin of a cattle collar.

Pathogenesis. Prolonged illness without cure, insufficiency of the nutrient blood meridians and collaterals loose nourishment of blood.

Therapeutic Principle. Enrich the blood and moisten the dryness.

Neurodermatitis due to Heat-transformation of Wind-damp Pathogen

One type of neurodermatitis.

Symptoms. Besides the general symptoms of neurodermatitis, accompanied by erythra, ulceration, wet and blood crust.

Pathogenesis. Stagnation of wind, damp and heat pathogens in the superficial muscle skin and meridians.

Therapeutic Principle. Dispel wind, clear heat and promote diuresis.

Nieru (Ex-HN)

An extra acupuncture point.

Location. On the midpoint of the line connecting the lateral end of the eyebrow and the corner of the outer canthus.

Indication. Epidemic febrile disease, headache, vertigo, eye diseases and facial paralysis, etc.

Method. Puncture subcutaneously 0.3-0.5 cun.

Night Blindness after Measles

Symptoms. Dry eyes, nyctalopia and cloudiness of cornea.

Pathogenesis. Injuring yin due to measles virus, deficiency of the blood in the liver and poor moistening of the eyes.

Therapeutic Principle. Replenishing yin for improving visual acuity.

Night Fever

Symptoms. Mostly low fever, or accompanied by vexation and restless sleep, etc.
Pathogenesis. Indigestion, deficiency of blood or yin, accumulation of evils in the yin meridians, etc.

Nightmare

Symptoms. Patient's crying in fear due to frightening dream or sudden waking-up with the sensation of a heavy load on the body, which makes him unable to move.
Pathogenesis. Excessive heart-fire.
Therapeutic Principle. Nourishing the heart to calm the mind and clearing away the heart-fire.

Nightshade-leaf Ironweed Herb

It is the leaf, root, or whole herb of Vernonia solanifolia Benth. (Compositae).
Effect. Expelling wind-dampness and arresting itching.
Indication. Postpartum arthralgia caused by wind-dampness, itching of skin, etc.

Night Sweat

Symptoms. Hectic fever, flushing of zygomatic region and dry throat, etc.
Pathogenesis. Disorder of the defensive qi, deficiency of yin and presence of internal heat.
Therapeutic Principle. Nourishing yin and removing fire.

Nine Kinds of Accumulation

A category of diseases in TCM. It refers to nine kinds of accumulation: indigestion, alcoholic dyspepsia, qi stagnation, saliva accumulation, hypochondriac nodes, accumulation of phlegm, fluid accumulation, extravasated blood retention and retention of meat.

Nine Kinds of Jaundice

A category of diseases in TCM. It refers to nine kinds of jaundice: the jaundice of the stomach, heart, kidney, intestine, chyluria, tongue, marrow, muscle, and liver.

Nine Needles

A category of ancient needles. Nine different needles, namely, shear, round-point, spoon, lance, stiletto, round sharp filiform, long and big needle are involved. They are different from each other in shape, size, and function.

Nine Needling

A term in acupuncture, referring to curing different diseases by means of nine different ancient needling techniques.

Nine Orifices

It refers to seven orifices, two eyes, two ears, two nostrils, and the mouth, together with the urethra, including the vagina, and the anus.

Nine Orifices Bleeding

1. It refers to bleeding from the mouth, ear, and nose at the same time.
2. It refers to nine orifices bleeding simultaneously.

Nine Pains

It refers to the nine kinds of pain symptom complex of the females: pain due to the vaginal injury, pain in the vagina due to strangury, ardor urine, pain due to cold, abdominal pain during menstruation, pain due to qi extention, worm-like biting pain in the vagina due to sweating, hypochondriac pain and lumbocrural pain.
Therapeutic Principle. Activating the meridians by removing stasis, and stopping pain according to the differentiation of syndromes and detection of the causes.

Nine-six Reinforcing-reducing

A reinforcing-reducing method of acupuncture, in ancient times 9 is taken as a yang number and 6 as a yin number. In later years, 9 and 6 are respectively taken as a basic number for reinforcing and reducing method. It means the numbers serve as a standard of times for twirling lifting and thrusting the needle.

Nipping Manipulation

A massage manipulation.
Operation. Nail-press the point.
Function. Causing resuscitation and dispelling convulsion.
Indication. Syncope, apoplexy, etc.

Nipple Cracks

Symptoms. The skin and muscle of nipple and the mammary areola cracks, excretes lipid and water, yellow crusts, dry and cracked pains. All these symptoms are more serious in lactation. It is mostly found in breast-feeding women.
Pathogenesis. The combination of the liver-fire with damp-heat in yangming meridian.
Therapeutic Principle. Clearing away the liver-fire and eliminating dampness and heat.

Nocturnal Cough

Symptoms. Constant cough only at night, relief at dawn, bitter taste and dryness throat, hypochondriac pain etc.
Pathogenesis. Deficiency of the kidney-yin, hyperactivity of fire due to yin deficiency, impairment of the lung by the fire of deficiency type.
Therapeutic Principle. Nourishing yin to reduce pathogenic fire and nourishing the lung to arrest cough.

Nocturnal Emission

Symptoms. Emission due to dreaming accompanied by premature ejaculation, dizziness, irritability and insomnia, soreness of the waist and tinnitus, etc.
Pathogenesis. Seeking sexual pleasure, over-anxiety or excessive heart-fire.
Therapeutic Principle. Clear heart-fire, nourish yin and stop nocturnal emission.

Nodular Varicosity

It refers to a mass-like pathogenic change formed by the crisscross of varicose vein of the body surface, mostly appearing in the lower limbs. The tumor is soft or hard with nodes, twined with blue veins, which are even exposed like earthworms in the more severe case.
Pathogenesis. Stagnation of blood in the lower body, the crisscross and the twining of choroid due to long periods of work by standing, shouldering a heavy load or pregnancy, etc.
Therapeutic Principle. Promoting blood circulation to remove blood stasis, relaxing muscles and tendons to dissolve lumps. Banding up with an elastic bandage is applicable in the external treatment.

Nodules of Breast

Symptoms. Nodular masses in the breast resembling a plum or an egg, painless and movable, without change in colour of the skin, fever, disappearance or enlargement along with joy or anger.
Pathogenesis. Anxiety impairing the spleen and anger impairing the liver leading to the stagnation of qi and phlegm or by deficiency of the liver and kidney which leads to lack of nourishment of meridians and collaterals of breast.

Nodules of Breast due to Stagnation of Liver-qi

Symptoms. Nodular masses in the breast, which are painless, without change in skin color, unmovable, accompanied by dizziness, distending pain in the lower abdomen. The flow of menses is not smooth, etc.
Pathogenesis. Depression of liver-qi stagnation of qi and blood, leading to the obstruction of the mammary collaterals.
Therapeutic Principle. Soothe the liver and regulate the circulation of qi.

Noma

Symptoms. At the early stage, formation of hard nodes in the gum and cheek with reddish, swelling and painful, which become ulcerous and then emit bloody and watery purplish black discharge with an unbearably stinking smell. This acute morbid condition progresses rapidly and is often found in infants.

Pathogenesis. Insufficiency and deficiency of vital qi, and existence of residual toxin after recovery from illness, plus repeated affection by exopathogenic factors which accumulate to attack upward to the gum.

Therapeutic Principle. Removing toxic material and clearing away heat to eliminate ulcer.

Non-endo-exopathogenic Factors

It mainly refers to such factors causing diseases: improper diet, fatigue, trauma, sexual indulgence, bites by insects and beasts, and drowning.

Non-scarring Moxibustion

It generally refers to mild, warm feeling to the patient, with no festers or scars left on the skin.

Method. Place a small moxa cone on the point, ignite it until the local skin feels pain, without burning the skin and then remove it for another one until the skin becomes flush.

Non-swallow of Gargling Water

Symptoms. Dry throat and mouth cavity, patient should only use water to gargle the mouth cavity without swallowing it.

Pathogenesis. Invasion of the blood systems by pathogenic heat and blood stasis.

Normal Breathing

It refers to normal, calm breathing. The doctor should first quieten his own respiration, concentrate his attention, and when he has normal breathing, take the patient's pulse.

Normal Person

It refers to healthy person with qi and blood in order. It is one of the diagnostic methods; the doctor compares the normal respiration and pulse condition of healthy persons with those of unhealthy ones.

Normal Sense of Mouth

It refers to no sense of bitter, dryness, or thirst in the mouth; able to talk freely, with good taste for food.

Nose as Orifice to Lung

The nasal functions of breathing and smelling are mainly dependent on the free movement of the lung-qi, and unobstructed respiration. Invasion of the lung by exopathogen impair the purifying and descending functions of the lung and brings about nasal pathogenic changes such as nasal obstruction, water nasal discharge, hyposmia, dryness of nasal cavity, etc.

Nose-flaring and Chest-sticking-out

It refers to severe difficulty in breathing, accompanied by the fanning of the nasal wing and the chest sticking out far.

Nose-inhaling and Mouth-exhaling Method

It refers to the respiration method. It is suitable for those with chest distress or blocked respiration.

Notoginseng

It is the root of panax notoginseng (Burk.) F. H. Chen (Araliaceae).

Effect. Arresting bleeding, reducing swelling, eliminating blood stasis and relieving swelling and pain by promoting blood circulation.

Indication. Various kinds of internal and external bleedings, traumatic injuries with blood stasis, swelling and pain and angina pectoris.

Notopterygium Root

It is the rhizome and root of Notopterygium incisum Ting, ex H. T.

Chang or N. forbesii Boiss. or N. forbesii Boiss. (Umbelliferae).

Effect. Dispelling cold to relieve exterior syndrome, expelling wind, removing dampness and relieving pain.

Indication. Aversion to cold, fever, headache and general pain due to affection by exopathogenic wind-cold; arthralgia caused by wind-cold-dampness, etc.

Nourishing Diarrhea

Symptoms. Diarrhea, excessive thirst and vomiting, little diet and borborygmus, lassitude of limbs and sleepiness etc.

Pathogenesis. Deficiency of the spleen and stomach, and stagnation of food.

Therapeutic Principle. Invigorating the spleen and replenishing qi, promoting digestion and removing stagnation food and arresting diarrhea.

Nourishing Yin and Suppressing Excessive yang

It is a therapy to treat hyperactivity of the liver yang.

Indication. Distending pain in the head, dizziness, tinnitus flushed face, restlessness, irritability insomnia, dreaminess, etc.

Noxious Dampness

1. It is formed by stagnation of dampness.
2. A cause of the disease in TCM. It may cause hematochezia when it occurs in the intestine or cause ulcer, pus, and putrid fluid of the shank when it invades the muscles and skin of the lower limbs.

Noxious Dryness

It refers to a syndrome of fire-toxin due to pathogenic dryness.

Symptoms. Red eyes with swelling and pain, conjunctival blepharitis and sore throat.

Therapeutic Principle. Clearing away heat and purging fire, removing toxin.

Noxious Heat

It refers to the toxicant due to accumulation of pathogenic heat. It is the main cause of carbuncle and sore, etc.

Noxious Heat in Blood System

1. It is mostly seen in epidemic febrile disease.

   Symptoms. High fever, hematemesis, epistaxis, hematochezia, dense dark red spots on skin, or coma etc.
2. It generally refers to some acute surgical pyogenic infection.

Numbness and Unconsciousness

It refers to the sensory disturbance of the skin, with numbness of the limbs or even no feeling of pain and itch.

Pathogenesis. Deficiency of qi and blood, or the stagnation of qi and blood, the accumulation of cold-dampness and sputum in the meridians and collaterals.

Numbness due to Insufficiency of Blood

Symptoms. Numbness in the hypochondrium, shoulder and back.

Pathogenesis. Malnutrition of the diaphragm region due to blood insufficiency of the nutrient and superficial defensive system.

Therapeutic Principle. Nourishing qi and blood.

Numbness of Feet

It refers to uneasiness and numbness of the feet.

Pathogenesis. Invasion of collaterals by wind-dampness, or deficiency of qi with damp phlegm, and obstruction of blood stasis.

Numbness of Finger

It refers to a symptom of ill sensation of numbness of fingers.

Pathogenesis. Stagnation of qi and blood, and obstruction of qi in meridians.

Numbness of Skin

It refers to the numbness of skin without pain, itching, cold and heat. It usually occurs at the ends of extremities.

Pathogenesis. Invasion of exopathogen into the skin and the stagnancy of qi and blood circulation.

Numb Tongue

Symptoms. Numbness of the tongue, anorexia, bitter taste and vexation and abundant phlegm, etc.

Pathogenesis. Depression of seven emotions, phlegm-transmission due to heart-fire, stagnation of phlegm in meridians and collaterals, or deficiency of blood.

Therapeutic Principle. Regulating qi, clearing away heat from the heart, nourishing blood to activate meridians.

Nutgalls

It is the gall of Cynips gallaetinctoriae Olivier (Apidae), the gall parasitized on the twig of Quercus infectoria Olivier (Fagaceae).

Effect. Reinforcing the kidney, controlling nocturnal emission, astringing the lung and arresting blood.

Indication. Chronic diarrhea, hemafecia; emission, cough, hemoptysis, toothache, traumatic bleeding, and slow-healing etc.

Nutgrass Galingale Rhizome

It is the rhizome of Cyperus rotundus L. (Cyperaceae).

Effect. Soothing the liver, regulating flow of qi to relieve pain, regulating menstruation and preventing miscarriage.

Indication. Distending pain in the hypochondrium due to the stagnation of the liver-qi, chest and abdominal distention with pain, irregular menstruation, amenorrhea, dysmenorrhea and distending pain in the breasts, abortion.

Nutmeg

It is the ripe seed of Myristica fragrans Houtt. (Myristicaceae).

Effect. Warming the spleen and stomach, promoting flow of qi, astringing the bowels and arresting diarrhea.

Indication. Chronic diarrhea, abdominal distention and pain, loss of appetite and vomiting.

Nutrient Being Stored in Spleen

It refers to the function of storing nutrients and blood in the spleen.

Nutrient system-qi

It refers to the essential substance or energy circulating in the meridians and blood vessels and nourishes all the organs and tissues. It comes from food essence transformed and transported by the spleen and stomach. It originates from the middle-energizer.

Nuxi (Ex-LE)

An extra acupuncture point.

Location. On the heel and in the center of the calcaneus.

Indication. Vomiting, diarrhea, spasm, osteomyelitis of the maxillary bone, gingival infection, palpitation, mental disorders, etc.

Method. Puncturing perpendicularly 0.2-0.3 cun. Moxibustion is applicable.

Nuxvomica Seed

It is the ripe seed of Strychnos nux-vomica L. or Spierriana A. W. Hill (Loganiaceae).

Effect. Clearing and activating the meridians and collaterals, resolving masses, subduing swelling and relieving pain.

Indication. Rheumatic arthralgia, spasm, numbness, sequela of infantile paralysis, and traumatic injuries with pain.

Oblique Insertion
It refers to puncturing at an angle of 30-60 degrees with the skin of the point. It is applicable to acupoint on the chest, hypochondrium, and upper back where the muscle is thin and with important internal organs near by. Oblique insertion can avoid damaging internal organs. It must also make a needling sensation.

Obliqueness and Exhaustion
A term of pulse conditions in TCM. Obliqueness refers to no pulse in one hand; exhaustion means that there are no pulses in two hands.

Oblongleaf Kadsura Stem or Root
It is the stem or root of Kadsura oblongifolia Merr. (Megnoliaceae).
Effect. Dispelling wind, removing dampness, regulating the intestine and stomach, promoting flow of qi and stopping pain.
Indication. Common cold, rheumatic arthralgia, diarrhea, vomiting.

Observation of Physical Condition and Behavior
It refers to a method of observing the patient's physical condition and behavior to establish diagnosis of a disease. The physique, development, and nutrition are helpful to detect excess and deficiency of qi and blood, ebb and flow of the pathogenic factor and of the bodily resistance, etc.

Obstinate Cold Syndrome
Symptoms. Pale complexion, aversion to cold, cold limbs, vomiting clear salivation, abdominal pain, loose stools with indigested food, frequent clear urine, impotence, soreness and lassitude in the lumbus and knees with cold sensation, etc.
Pathogenesis. Shortage of genuine yang and prolonged pathogenic cold in the body.
Therapeutic Principle. Warming yang and dispelling cold.

Obstructed Cough
Symptoms. Cough with shortness of breath, strong fishy taste in throat, coughing with black blood, etc.
Pathogenesis. Blood stasis in the lung, dysfunction of the lung-qi and obstruction of the air passage.
Therapeutic Principle. Promoting blood circulation and flow of qi, and facilitating the flow of the lung qi to relieve cough.

Obstruction and Rejection
Symptoms. Vomiting, abdominal pain, abdominal distention and constipation.
Pathogenesis. Improper diet, over-exertion, stagnation of pathogenic cold, heat stagnation, accumulation of blood stasis, internal accumulation of costive, or gathering of roundworms, etc.
Therapeutic Principle. Relaxing the bowels, promoting circulation of qi to stop pain, promoting blood circulation and eliminating retained fluid or treatment by operation.

Obstruction of Kidney Meridian
Symptoms. Lumbago, emission, spasm of lower extremities with inability to stand upright.

Pathogenesis. Rheumatism involving the bone for years, combined with affection by pathogenic, or impairment of bones by over-fatigue, or impairment of the kidney through excess of sexual intercourse.

Therapeutic Principle. Tonifying the kidney and expelling pathogenic factors.

Obstruction of Liver-qi

Symptoms. Thirst, frequent urination, hypochondriac pain, abdominal distention, etc.

Pathogenesis. Long-lasting muscular rheumatism with the attack of external pathogen or due to anger impairing the liver, the stagnation of the liver-qi.

Therapeutic Principle. Soothing the liver and removing the pathogenic factor.

Obstruction of Lung due to Phlegm Dampness

Symptoms. Cough, expectoration of white and thick sputum which is easily expectorated, or asthma, stuffiness in the chest, vomiting and nausea.

Pathogenesis. Obstruction of phlegm dampness, dysfunction of clarifying and sending down the lung-qi.

Therapeutic Principle. Ventilating the lung and dispersing phlegm, or alleviating asthma and cough.

Obstruction of Qi in the Chest due to Blood Stasis

Symptoms. Stabbing pain in the chest, radiating to shoulder and back, purple lips and tongue.

Pathogenesis. Long-term depression, resulting in stagnation of blood, blockage of the collaterals leading to obstruction of yang-qi in the chest.

Therapeutic Principle. Removing blood stasis, arresting pain by removing obstruction in the meridians and collaterals.

Obstruction of Qi in the Chest due to Cold of Insufficiency Type

Symptoms. Chest pain radiating to the back, palpitation, oppressed feeling in the chest and shortness of breath, aversion to chill, cold limbs.

Pathogenesis. Insufficiency of chest-yang, or invasion of yin-cold evil when the body is deficient, leading to the stasis of cold and qi.

Therapeutic Principle. Strengthen yang to disperse cold.

Obstruction of Qi in the Chest due to Phlegm Turbidity

Symptoms. Distention and pain in the chest, short breath, cough, expectoration of whitish sputum.

Pathogenesis. Obstruction of qi in chest, resulting from stagnation of phlegm-dampness.

Therapeutic Principle. Promote the flow of yang and resolve turbidity.

Obtuseleaf Erycibe Stem

It is the old root or stem of Erycibe obtusifolia Benth. (Convolvulaceae).

Effect. Relieving exterior syndrome, inducting diaphoresis, removing wind-dampness, expelling the pain, subduing swelling, inducing miosis.

Indication. Rheumatic arthralgia, hemiplegia, swelling and pain due to traumatic injuries, primary glaucoma.

Obvious Emaciation and Muscular Atrophy

It refers to deficiency of spleen-qi, resulting in excessive emaciation, so exposing the bones of the shoulders, arms, buttock, thigh and tibia. It can be found in patient with late chronic consumptive disease, etc.

Occiput (MA)

An auricular point.

Location. At the posterior superior corner of the lateral aspect of the antitragus.

Function. Tranquilizing the mind, stopping pain and eliminating pathogenic wind.

Indication. Dizziness, headache, insomnia, bronchial asthma, etc.

Occlusion of Summer-heat

It refers to internal summer-heat and external occlusion of wind-cold.

Symptoms. Headache, fever, aversion to chill, thirst, muscular contracture, gastric fullness and anhidrosis, etc.

Therapeutic Principle. Dispelling cold to relieve exterior syndrome, removing summer-heat and eliminating hygrosis.

Occurrence of Cold Syndrome in Case of Extreme Heat

A pathogenesis. According to the theory of transformation between yin and yang, yang-heat syndrome may show symptoms of pseudo-heat under certain conditions, commonly resulting from exhaustion of the vital-qi.

Symptoms. Cold in the limbs, profuse sweating, very weak pulse.

Occurrence of Wind Syndrome in Case of Extreme Heat

It refers to a morbid condition occurring in a febrile disease.

Symptoms. High fever with coma, muscular rigidity, convulsion or opisthotonos. Mostly seen in infantile convulsion due to high fever, epidemic meningitis, encephalitis B, toxic dysentery, and septicemia.

Pathogenesis. Malnutrition of muscles and tendons due to impairment of ying-blood and the Liver Meridian by excess pathogenic heat.

Ocular Perforated Injury

It refers to ocular trauma with perforating injury to the eyeball.

Symptoms. Acute ophthalmic pain, photophobia, lacrimation, severe vision weakness, etc.

Pathogenesis. Eyeball rupture due to stab with something sharp, or rapid collision with tiny foreign substance, then the invasion of pathogenic toxin to impair qi, blood, meridians and collaterals.

Therapeutic Principle. Taking therapeutic measures based on depth and location of the injury, surveying foreign substances and degree of the pathogenic toxin interspersed.

Odoriferous Rosewood

It is the heart-wood in the root of Dalbergia odorifera T. Chen (Leguminosae).

Effect. Promoting blood circulation to remove blood stasis and stopping bleeding to arrest pain.

Indication. Pain in the hypochondrium due to the stagnation of qi and blood stasis, traumatic injuries and traumatic bleeding, vomiting, abdominal pain, coronary heart disease, etc.

Offensive Odour in Hiccups

It refers to spoiled odour of undigested food in hiccups.

Pathogenesis. Deficiency and weakness of the spleen and stomach, unfavourable digestion and stagnation of qi.

Oil Rape Seed

It is the seed of Brassica campestris L. (Cruciferae).

Effect. Promoting blood circulation, relieving the stagnation of qi, diminishing swelling and dissolving mass.

Indication. Abdominal pain due to stagnation of blood after childbirth, dysentery with bloody stool, pyogenic infections and hemorrhoids complicated by anal fistula.

Oiltea Camellia Seed

It is the seed of Camellia oleifera Abel. (Theaceae).

Effect. Promoting flow of qi and dispelling the stagnation of qi.

Indication. Abdominal pain due to stagnation of qi.

Ointment

A dosage form. It refers to a half-solid form of preparation made by mixing appropriate matrix and drugs, and applying it easily to the skin and mucosa, and acting on the affected local region.

Old Trauma

Any injuries, failing to recover after more than two weeks, whether treated or not, all belong to old trauma.

Symptoms. Clinical symptom is no more obvious than the acute ones and probably without clear history of external injury, but it has close relations with seven emotions, six evils and tiredness, which are usually the important reasons for exacerbation of a disease.

Therapeutic Principle. Promoting blood circulation and relaxing muscles and tendons.

Oligospermia

Symptoms. Less sperm, or even one or two drops in sexual intercourse.

Pathogenesis. Congenital deficiency, or excess sexual intercourse, mind overstrain, improper diet, etc. resulting in consumption of essence.

Therapeutic Principle. Nourishing the kidney and replenishing the vital essence.

Omalgia

Symptoms. Aching pain in the diseased shoulder, more serious at night and restriction of movement.

Pathogenesis. Bodily weakness of the aged, deficiency of liver-yin and kidney-yin, deficiency of both qi and blood, failure in nourishing muscles and tendons, simultaneously overwork and injury, and attack by cold and dampness, which lead to failure of blood to nourish muscles and tendons, stagnation of damp and turbid in meridians and shoulder joint.

Therapeutic Principle. Manipulation of massage.

Omei Mountain Bamboo Leaf

It is the tender leaf of Sinocalamus affinis (Rendle) McClure (Gramineae).

Effect. Clearing away the heart-fire and arresting excessive thirst.

Indication. Strangury due to pathogenic heat, hematuria, dizziness, constipation, dark micturition with pain, etc.

Omoto Nipponlily Root and Rhizome

It is the root and rhizome of Rohdea japonica Roth. (Liliaceae).

Effect. Exerting a tonic effect on the heart to induce diuresis, clearing away heat, detoxicating and stopping bleeding.

Indication. Heart failure, swelling and sore throat, diphtheria, edema, hemoptysis, furuncle, erysipelas, snakebite, burns and scalds, etc.

Omphalia

It is the dried sclerotium of Omphalia lapidescens Schroet. (Polyporaceae).

Effect. Killing parasites.

Indication. Taeniasis, ancylostomiasis and ascariasis.

Onion

It is the bulb of Allium cepa L. (Liliaceae).

Effect. Removing toxic materials.

Indication. Wound, ulcer and Trichomonas vaginalis.

Opening Tianmen

A massage manipulation.

Operation. Push straight and upward from the Zanzhu (B 2) point.

Function. Dispersing wind and expelling exogenous pathogen, inducing resuscitation and restoring consciousness, and tranquilizing the mind.

Indication. Exopathic affection, fever, headache, infantile convulsion, etc.

Ophicalcite

It is a marble containing ore of green serpentine.

Effect. Stopping bleeding and removing blood stasis.

Indication. Internal hemorrhage, such as hemoptysis, hematemesis with blood stasis. Powdered drug is used externally as hemostatic for incised wounds. Internal hemorrhage, such as hemoptysis, hematemesis with blood stasis.

Opisthotonos

Symptoms. Arching up backwards of the waist and back.

Pathogenesis. Accumulation of pathogenic factors in meridians, or impairment of body fluid by excessive heat or insufficiency of yin-blood, failure in nourishing muscles and tendons, contracture and spasm.

Oppressive Feeling and Vertigo after Delivery

Symptoms. Vertigo and blurred vision, depression and stuffiness, poor appetite with vomiting, constipation, sweating in the head without sweating in the body.

Pathogenesis. Lost profuse blood after delivery, deficiency of surface qi, excessive sweating, invasion of pathogenic cold in the deficiency, vital-qi cannot dispel the pathogens, and rushes up adversely.

Therapeutic Principle. Strengthening the resistance of the body to eliminate the pathogenic factors and regulating yin and yang.

Optic Atrophy

The affected eye has a fine outward appearance and periphery, but its visual acuity gradually declines to blindness.

Pathogenesis. Insufficiency of the liver and kidney, or deficiency of both the heart and spleen, insufficiency of vital essence, blood and body fluid, or traumatic ocular and cephalic injury, tumor oppression and obstruction of meridians due to blood stasis.

Therapeutic Principle. The excess type and the deficiency type should be distinguished from each other first. For the defi-

ciency type, nourish the liver and kidney and invigorate the heart and spleen; for the excess type, soothe the liver, regulate the flow of qi and promote the circulation of blood for elimination of stasis. Acupuncture therapy is applicable.

Oral Aphtha

It refers to yellowish or greyish-whitish ulcer spots in different size, dotting the mucous membrane of the mouth.

Pathogenesis. Accumulation of heat or fire in the spleen and stomach, or yin deficiency of the body, or febrile diseases that injure yin.

Therapeutic Principle. For the accumulation of heat in the spleen and stomach, clearing the stomach and purging intense heat. For fire caused by yin deficiency, nourishing yin and extinguishing fire.

Oral Aphtha during Menstruation

It refers to repeated attack of the oral mucosa and tongue before or during menstruation, with complete recovery following menstruation.

Pathogenesis. Fumigating and steaming of the stomach heat or hyperactivity of fire due to yin deficiency.

Therapeutic Principle. Clearing away the stomach-heat or nourishing yin to reduce pathogenic fire.

Ordos Wormwood Herb

It is the stem leaf and flower-bud of Artemisia ordosica Krasch. (Compositae).

Effect. Expelling wind and dampness, drawing the pus out and removing toxic substances.

Indication. Rheumatic arthritis, common cold, sore throat, sores, furuncle, carbuncles and swelling, etc.

Organ Cold

1. **Symptoms.** Cold limbs, slight blue lips and face, no appetite, abdominal pain, borborygmus, diarrhea like water, cry at

night, etc. Mostly seen in the infant less than l00 days old.

Pathogenesis. Affection of cold during delivery or giving the infant a cold bath, or navel invaded by cold.

Therapeutic Principle. Warming the middle-energizer to disperse cold.

2. It refers to the cold syndrome of the internal organs due to yang-deficiency of the organs.

Symptoms. Fullness and distention of the abdomen with cold pain, being susceptible to heat and aversion to cold.

Oriental Buckthorn Root

It is the root or root bark of Rhamnus crenata Sieb. et Zucc. (Rhamnaceae).

Effect. Clearing away heat, removing dampness, destroying intestinal worms and detoxicating.

Indication. Scabies, tinea, furuncle, leprosy, ascariasis, etc.

Oriental Cockroach

It is the whole worm of Blatta orientalis L. (Blattidae).

Effect. Removing blood stasis, subduing swelling and detoxicating.

Indication. Masses in the abdomen, malnutrition in children, boils and furuncles, tonsillitis, subcutaneous swelling, snake bite, etc.

Oriental Variegated Coralbean Bark

It is the dried bark of Erythrina variegata L. var. orientalis (L.) Merr. (Leguminosae).

Effect. Expelling wind and dampness, clearing the meridians and collaterals, removing blood stasis to relieve pain.

Indication. Pain from rheumatism, spasm of limbs and neurodermatitis and chronic eczema.

Oriental Water plantain Rhizome

It is the tuber of Alisma orientalis (Sam.) Juzep. (Alismataceae).

Effect. Promoting urination and excreting dampness, purging heat.

Indication. Edema, dysuria, diarrhea, strangury with turbid urine, leukorrhagia, etc.

Oriental Wormwood

It is the young plant or flowering tops of Artemisia capillaris Thunb. or A. scoparia Waldst et Kitaib. (Compositae).

Effect. Clearing away heat and removing dampness, treating jaundice.

Indication. Hepatitis with jaundice, exudative sores with yellowish liquid.

Oroxylum Seed

It is the seed of Oroxylum indicum (L.) Vent. (Bignoniaceae).

Effect. Moistening the lung, regulating the liver and normalizing the function of the stomach, and promoting tissue regeneration.

Indication. Cough, throat inflammation, hoarseness, stomachache due to emotional depression and the hyperactive liver-qi, protracted sores and unhealing of ulcer, etc.

Orpiment

It is the ore of sulfide mineral Orpiment (As_2S_3).

Effect. Eliminating dampness, destroying parasites and detoxication.

Indication. Scabies, tinea, malignant boil, snake bite, sting, cough with asthma due to cold-phlegm, abdominal pain due to parasites, etc.

Orthodox Abdominal Respiration

It is one of the breathing methods commonly adopted in Qigong practice. It refers to the method of respiration in the dilated abdomen while inhaling and contracting the abdomen while exhaling. The method is suitable for weak, aged people.

Osteoarthrosis

Symptoms. Arthralgia, inability to raise the heavy limbs, and joint deformity.

Pathogenesis. Internal invasion of pathogenic wind, cold dampness accumulated in bones which fight against visceral qi and the bones.

Therapeutic Principle. Tonifying the kidney to eliminate the evils factors.

Osteoarticular Tuberculosis

Symptoms. Hectic fever and night sweat, lower afternoon fever, articular swelling and pain, and sinus occuring after the ulceration.

Pathogenesis. Invasion of certain joint by tuberculin due to congenital defect, postpartum, and general debility, etc.

Therapeutic Principle. Oral administration and external application of medicinal herbs or by operation to remove focus, according to patients' condition.

Otorrhagia

Symptoms. Bleeding from ear or appearance of bruising, without pain or swelling, emission and dysphoria, otalgia, insomnia and bitter taste, red tongue, etc.

Pathogenesis. Deficiency of the kidney, or accumulation of heat in the liver and gallbladder, or excessive drinking.

Therapeutic Principle. Nourishing yin, clearing heat, purging the liver of pathogenic fire, arresting bleeding, etc.

Oval Leaf Aspidistra Rhizome

It is the rhizome of Aspidistra typica Baill. (Liliaceae).

Effect. Promoting blood circulation, removing blood stasis, knitting bones, stopping pain, clearing away heat and detoxicating.

Indication. Dysentery, malaria, rheumatic arthralgia, lumbocrural pain due to the kidney deficiency, traumatic sprain, fracture, snake bite, etc.

Ovate Catalpa Fruit

It is the ripe fruit of Catalpa ovata G. Don. (Bignoniaceae).

Effect. Inducing diuresis and diminishing swelling.

Indication. Edema.

Ovate Catalpa Root Bark

It is the root bark or root phloem of Catalpa ovata G. Don (Bignoniaceae).

Effect. Clearing away heat, removing toxic materials and destroying parasites.

Indication. Fever due to exogenous febrile disease, jaundice, regurgitation, skin pruritus and scabies.

Ovate Leaf Holly Bark

It is the bark or root bark of Ilex rotunda Thunb. (Aquifoliaceae).

Effect. Clearing away heat and detoxication, improving diuresis and stopping pain.

Indication. Common cold, fever, tonsillitis, swollen and sore throat, acute and chronic hepatitis, gastric ulcer, duodenal ulcer, rheumatic arthritis, traumatic injuries and scalds and burns.

Overabundance of Amniotic Fluid

It refers to edema in the pregnant woman and abdominal distention after 5th or 6th months pregnancy.

Symptoms. Overall edema, abnormal expansion of the abdomen, oppressed chest, short of breath and serious dyspnea, unable to lie down.

Pathogenesis. Dysfunction of the spleen in transportation due to qi deficiency, retention and accumulation of water within the uterus and then diffusion all over the body.

Therapeutic Principle. Invigorating the spleen and promoting diuresis.

Overacting of Five Emotions

A cause of disease. The activity of the five emotions, anger, joy, anxiety, melancholy and fear, is based on the essence and energy of the five zang-organs as their material. Excessive five emotions may disturb the normal flow of qi and blood of the internal organs, or cause the functional disorder and morbid conditions.

Oyster Shell

It is the shell of Ostrea gigas Thunb. and O. talienwhanensis Crosse or O. rivularis Gould (Ostreidae).

Effect. Calming the liver and subduing hyperactivity of the liver-yang, softening and resolving hard lumps and inducing astringency, when calcined.

Indication. Irritability, palpitation, insomnia, dreaminess, dizziness, deafness, tinnitus sweating due to debility, scrofula, seminal emission, leukorrhagia, etc. In addition, it can also be used in case of gastrorrhoea.

P

Paddy-field Dermatitis

Symptoms. It usually appears in the region of hand forks, at the beginning, swelling, white putrefaction, wrinkles, followed by erosion, running water, itching and pain due to friction.

Pathogenesis. The external soaking of dampness and local friction.

Therapeutic Principle. Washing it with alum water. In the case of ulceration, it is advisable to apply Powder of Indigo Naturalis.

Pain due to Pathogenic Wind in Collaterals

Symptoms. Headache, pain of muscles and bones in the neck, shoulder, back, waist and leg, etc.

Pathogenesis. Insufficiency of vital qi and blood, with the attack of pathogenic wind in the collaterals.

Therapeutic Principle. Expelling pathogenic wind and cold, removing obstruction in the meridians and, invigorating qi and blood.

Pain due to Qi Disorder

Symptoms. Fullness and pain in the chest, pricking pain in the abdomen and hypochondrium, lumbago with hernia and mass, etc.

Pathogenesis. Emotional stress, obstruction of turbid phlegm, improper diet, overtiredness, etc.

Therapeutic Principle. Promoting the flow of qi to relieve stagnation.

Painful Swelling on Body

It refers to the whole body surface swelling blocks that have not ulcerated. It is classified into yang and yin syndromes.

Symptoms. In the yang syndrome, red swelling, pain, body fever and headache. In the yin syndrome, the skin color of the swollen part is normal, slight pain without heat, without the whole body symptoms, but with the low fever in the afternoon and night sweat, etc. after pyogenesis.

Therapeutic Principle. For the yang syndrome, clearing away heat and detoxicating, removing blood stasis and removing dampness by diuresis. For the yin syndrome, expelling pathogenic cold from meridians, removing obstruction in the meridians and resolving phlegm.

Painful Swelling on Maxillofacial Region

Symptoms. At the beginning, the appearance of a swelling like a red bean. Gradually it increases to a few, burning, red, swelling, and painful. After ulceration, yellow water flows out. It mostly appears in the mandible positions of the face.

Pathogenesis. The stagnation of wind-heat in the Stomach Meridian to attack upward.

Therapeutic Principle. Dispelling wind and clearing away heat.

Pain-test of Pre-acupuncture-anesthesia

It refers to the test of pain-endurance before operation, based on the test results, regulating the point prescription, and also predicting the effect of acupuncture anesthesia. At present, dolorimetres are applied to testing pain.

Paleaceous Knotweed Rhizome

It is the rhizome of Polygonum paleaceum Wall. (Polygonaceae).

Effect. Dissipating blood stasis and arresting bleeding, depressing upward reverse flow of qi and relieving pain.

Indication. Chronic gastritis, gastric ulcer, duodenal ulcer, dyspepsia, irregular menstruation, general edema and traumatic injury, snake bite, etc.

Pallas Pit Viper

It is the whole body without internal organ of Agkistrodon halys (Pallas) (Crotalidae).

Effect. Expelling pathogenic wind and counteracting toxic substances.

Indication. Leprosy, pellagra, hemorrhoid, etc.

Palmate Girardinia Herb

It is the whole herb or root of Girardinia palmata (Forsk.) Gaud. (Urticaceae).

Effect. Expelling pathogenic wind, expelling pathogenic factors from exterior the body, promoting flow of qi, eliminating phlegm, and removing fire and detoxicating.

Indication. Cough due to common cold, chest distress, abundant sputum, skin pruritus, noxious carbuncles, etc.

Palmer Pustule

Symptoms. It appears at Laogong (P 8) on the palm, high swelling of the palm and the dorsum of hand, acute pain, accompanied by fever, headache.

Pathogenesis. Traumatic infection, excessive fire-toxin.

Therapeutic Principle. Clearing away heat and toxins. In the case of pus, it is appropriate to cut in order to drain the pus.

Palm-leaf Raspberry Fruit

It is the immature fruit of Rubus chingii Hu. (Rosaceae).

Effect. Tonifying the kidney to arrest spontaneous emission, improving eyesight and reducing urination.

Indication. Emission, spermatorrhea, enuresis, frequent urination due to impairment of the kidney-qi; consumptive disease, blurred vision.

Palm-pressing Manipulation

A massage manipulation.

Operation. Press acupoint or the affected region of the body surface with one palm or both palms, or palms overlapped together.

Function. Relaxing muscles and tendons, warming middle-energizer to dispel cold.

Indication. Stomachache, headache, aching pain and numbness of extremities, etc.

Palm-rubbing Manipulation

A massage manipulation.

Operation. Keep the palm on the affected part, with the wrist joint as the center, and rotate the palm rhythmically along with the forearm.

Function. Regulating middle-energizer and qi, promoting digestion and removing stagnated food, and promoting the peristalsis of the stomach and intestines.

Indication. Gastric and abdominal pain, food stagnancy, fullness of abdomen, stasis of qi, injury of the chest and hypochondria, etc.

Palpating Manipulation

A massage manipulation.

Operation. Rub the two palms together until the palms feel hot and then immediately put one palm on the affected part, so that the heat permeates the subcutaneous tissues. The manipulation is only used on the epigastrium and repeated many times until the local part feels warm.

Function. Dispelling cold and dredging collaterals.

Indication. Gastric and abdominal pain, diarrhea, dysmenorrhea, etc.

Palpebral Edema of Newborn

Symptoms. Swelling eyes that cannot be opened, red face and dry lips, etc.

Pathogenesis. The heat stagnated in the spleen.
Therapeutic Principle. Clearing the spleen and dispelling the heat.

Palpitation due to Blood Deficiency

Symptoms. Palpitation and restlessness, dizziness and blurring of vision, shortness of breath.
Pathogenesis. Insufficiency of heart-blood and the heart failing to be nourished.
Therapeutic Principle. Strengthening qi and nourishing blood, tonifying heart to calm the mind.

Palpitation due to Blood Stasis

Symptoms. Progressive palpitations for many years, shortness of breath during physical activity, or paroxysmal chest pain, sallow complexion, dark purple lips and tongue. In severe cases, cold body and limbs, inability to lie flat due to cough and dyspnea, edema, feeble pulse.
Pathogenesis. Stagnation of qi and blood stasis and failure to nourish the heart.
Therapeutic Principle. Promoting blood circulation to strengthen functions of the heart.

Palpitation due to Fluid Retention

Symptoms. The palpitation accompanied by the feeling of stuffiness and fullness in the chest, dizziness and nausea, scanty urine, etc.
Pathogenesis. The fluid retention in the interior and the attack of the heart by retained fluid.
Therapeutic Principle. Activating yang and removing fluid retention from the interior.

Palpitation due to Fright during Convalescence

Symptoms. Fatigue and weakness, palpitation due to fright, inclination due to being frightened, dreaminess and insomnia, etc.
Pathogenesis. Blood deficiency and failure to nourish the meridians of the heart and liver during the convalescence.
Therapeutic Principle. Nourishing the heart to calm the mind and warming the gallbladder to tranquilize the mind.

Palpitation due to Phlegm-fire

Symptoms. Palpitations appear and fade at frequent intervals, irritability, restlessness, oppressing feeling in the chest, dizziness, insomnia and dreamy sleep, cough with pituitary sputum, dark urine, yellow greasy tongue coating.
Pathogenesis. Impairment of the spleen resulting from improper diet, and the formation of phlegm due to excessive dampness, which stagnates and produces heat, and phlegm-fire which disturbs the inside of the body.
Therapeutic Principle. Purging intense heat, dispelling phlegm, and arresting convulsion.

Palpitation due to Qi Deficiency

Symptoms. Uncontrollable palpitations, panic, short breath, polyhidrosis of the palm center, sleeplessness which can be eased by the patient lying in a peaceful position, thin and white tongue coating.
Pathogenesis. Yang-qi deficiency, the heart lacking warmth and nourishment.
Therapeutic Principle. Supplementing qi and tranquilizing the mind.

Pancreas-Gallbladder (MA-SC 6)

Location. An auricular meridian acupuncture point between the two points of Liver (MA-SC 5) and Kidney (MA).
Indication. Cholecystitis, cholelithiasis, ascariasis of biliary tract, herpes zoster, otitis media, pancreatitis and migraine.

Pangguangshu (B 28)

A meridian acupuncture point.

Location. On the sacrum and on the level of the 2nd posterior sacral foramen, 1.5 cun lateral to the meridian sacral crest.

Indication. Abdominal pain, diarrhea, constipation, pain and stiffness and pain of the lower back, swelling and pain of the vulva, and stranguria with turbid urine, scanty dark urine, seminal emission, enuresis.

Method. Puncture perpendicularly or obliquely 0.8-1.0 cun. Perform moxibustion 3-5 moxa cones or 5-10 minutes with warming moxibustion.

Paniculate Fameflower Root

It is the root of Talinum paniculatum (Jaca.) Gaertn (Portulacaceae).

Effect. Strengthening the spleen, tonifying the lungs, relieving cough and regulating menstruation, promoting the body fluid and lactation.

Indication. Diarrhea, cough with blood-stained sputum, dizziness, tidal fever, night sweat, lack of lactation, irregular menstruation, leukorrhea, emission etc.

Paniculate Swallowwort Root

It is the root and rhizome of Cynanchum paniculatum (Bge.) Kitag. (Asclepiadaceae).

Effect. Dispelling wind, relieving pain and itching, smoothing and activating the meridian, relieving cough and dyspnea, clearing away toxic material and relieving swelling.

Indication. Rheumatic arthralgia, lumbago, abdominal pain, toothache, traumatic injury, eczema, rubella, neurodermatitis and snake bite.

Papaya Fruit

It is the fruit of Carica papaya L. (Caricaceae).

Effect. Invigorating qi and promoting the function of the spleen and stomach, dissipating blood stasis and relieving heat stagnation.

Indication. Stomachache, dysentery and difficulty in urination and defecation, arthralgia due to wind, etc.

Papermulberry Bark

It is the bark phloem of Broussonetia papyrifera (L.) Vent. (Moraceae).

Effect. Promoting diuresis and arresting bleeding.

Indication. Edema with ascites, cough, dysentery with bloody stool, metrorrhagia, etc.

Papermulberry Fruit

It is the fruit of Broussonetia papyrifera (L.) Vent. (Moraceae).

Effect. Nourishing the kidney, removing heat from the liver and improving eyesight.

Indication. Consumptive disease, blurred vision, opacity, edema, etc.

Papermulberry Root

It is the tender root or root of Broussonetia papyrifera (L.) Vent. (Moraceae).

Effect. Clearing away heat, removing heat from the blood, promoting diuresis and eliminating blood stasis.

Indication. Cough with hematemesis, edema, metrorrhagia, traumatic injuries, etc.

Paralysis

It refers to the failure of limbs.

Symptoms. Limbs fail to move.

Pathogenesis. Deficiency of the liver and the kidney, insufficiency of qi and blood, or the invasion of evil-wind into meridians and collaterals.

Therapeutic Principle. Promoting blood circulation to remove obstruction in meridians, and nourishing muscles and tendons. Besides, there should be the comprehensive treatment with acupuncture, moxibustion and massage.

Paralytic Strabismus

Symptoms. Sudden strabismus with limited rotation of the eyeball, ambiopia, sometimes accompanied by nausea, vomiting, etc.

Pathogenesis. Pathogenic wind affects the meridian, or wind-phlegm blocks the meridian.

Therapeutic Principle. Dispelling pathogenic wind, removing phlegm, promoting blood circulation and remove obstruction in the meridians, with application of acupuncture and moxibustion.

Parasite stasis

Symptoms. Abdominal pain appearing and fading at frequent intervals, noisy gastric cavity, or even vomiting ascaris, etc.

Pathogenesis. The deficiency of qi in middle-energizer and eating food stained with parasite eggs by mistake.

Therapeutic Principle. Invigorating the spleen and reinforcing the stomach, and killing intestinal parasites.

Paronychia

Symptoms. It appears on the back of the finger, right after the root of the nail, like half a red date, fat and swelling.

Pathogenesis. Traumatic infection or the stagnation of fire in the zang and fu organs.

Therapeutic Principle. Clearing away heat and toxic material, subduing swelling and alleviating pain.

Paroxysmal Diarrhea

Symptoms. Abdominal distention, borborygmus at night, diarrhea at dawn, anorexia, fatigue and weakness.

Pathogenesis. Spleen deficiency and excessive dampness.

Therapeutic Principle. Invigorating the spleen and eliminating dampness.

Parting-pushing Manipulation

A massage manipulation.

Operation. Pushing from the center of the point separately to both sides with both hands using slight force and moderate speed.

Pathogenesis of Meridians and Collaterals

A term that refers to morbid changes resulting from direct or indirect affection of pathogenic factors on the meridians and collaterals. The main manifestations are excessive or deficient qi and blood along the meridians and collaterals, disorder, stagnation and obstruction of qi and blood and even exhaustion of them in severe cases.

Pathogenic Action

It refers to six climatic conditions, as pathogenic factors: wind, cold, summer-heat, dampness, dryness and fire, invading human body, and leading to disease occurrence, when insufficiency of vital-qi of the human body and low resistance to disease.

Pathogenic and Vital Contention

It refers to the conflicts between the ability to resist diseases and pathogenic factors. The result of the conflict determines not only the deficiency and excess of the disease, but also the occurring development and the final result of the disease.

Pathogenic Damp-heat Syndrome

It refers to the pathogenic factor that exists in four seasons, mostly in the long summer. It can cause the damp-warm syndrome, slow onset of the disease, less change, easy damage to spleen and stomach, stagnated and inhibited functional activities of qi, and finally long course of disease. It is difficult to cure and easy to recur.

Pathogenic Dryness

It is one of the six atmospheric pathogenic factors easily impairing yin. Patient can have the symptoms such as dry cough, chest pain, dryness in the mouth, nose, and the skin.

Pathogenic Dyspnea

Symptoms. Dyspnea, tachypnea, blockage sensation in the throat or desire for vomiting, or fever, and deep-sited pulse, etc.

Pathogenesis. The invasion of the lung by pathogenic cold, the obstruction of the air passage and accumulation of the lung qi.

Therapeutic Principle. Warming the lung, dispelling cold and relieving dyspnea.

Pathogenic Factor Lingering in Tri-energizer

1. It refers to the syndrome due to damp-heat pathogen lingering in the tri-energizer and qi system.

   Symptoms. Cough with chest distress, abdominal distention, loose stool, difficult urination, etc.

2. It generally refers to the pathologic changes of metabolic disturbance of water and body fluid due to dysfunction in the tri-energizer.

   Symptoms. Fullness in the chest and hypochondrium, oppressed feeling in chest, contracture in the lower abdomen, abnormal urination, etc.

Pathogenic Heat Accumulated in Blood System

Symptoms. Feverish body is aggravated at night, local stabbing pain, dark red tongue, etc.

Pathogenesis. Usually due to the impairment of yin by blood-heat, the stagnation of blood circulation; or blood stasis retention, then becoming pathogenic heat.

Therapeutic Principle. Removing pathogenic heat from blood and removing blood stasis.

Pathogenic Position

It refers to the body part where pathogens invade. The different invaded sites are due to the different nature of pathogens. For example, it is easy for wind pathogens to invade the upper part of human body,

damp pathogens to invade the lower part of human body. It is easy for cold pathogens to damage yang-qi, heat pathogens, to damage yin-body fluid.

Pathogenic Wind due to Spleen Deficiency

Symptoms. Physical lassitude coma, inability to talk, slight convulsion of the hand and foot, cold sensation over the limbs, etc.

Pathogenesis. Mostly caused by internal wind resulting from damage to the spleen due to vomiting and diarrhea or misuse of drugs of cold nature or by spleen deficiency.

Therapeutic Principle. Warming and nourishing the spleen and stomach to expel wind.

Patrinia Herb

It is the whole herb of Patrinia scabiosaefolia Fisch. ex Link. or P. villosa Juss. (Valerianaceae) with root.

Effect. Dissipating pathogenic heat from the blood, detoxicating, treating boils, evacuating pus, eliminating blood stasis and relieving pain, tranquilizing.

Indication. Acute appendicitis, pulmonary abscess, boils due to toxic heat, bloodshot swollen and painful eyes, vexation, insomnia, insanity, dysentery, leukorrhea with reddish discharge, etc.

Patting Manipulation

A massage manipulation.

Operation. Pat the affected body surface gently and rhythmically, with one or both palms and the metacarpophalangeal joints slightly flexed.

Function. Relaxing muscles and tendons and promoting the blood circulation, often performed at the beginning and the end of massotherapy.

Indication. Aching pain due to wind and dampness, local dysarthrosis and muscular spasm.

Pea

It is the seed of Pisum sativum L. (Leguminosae).

Effect. Regulating the middle-energizer, keeping the adverse qi downward, inducing diuresis and clearing away toxic materials.

Indication. Cholera cramp, beriberi, subcutaneous swelling, etc.

Peach Kernel

It is the kernel of Prunus perica (L.) Batsch, or Prunus davidianna (Carr.) Franch. (Rosaceae).

Effect. Promoting blood circulation to remove blood stasis, moistening the bowels to relieve constipation.

Indication. Constipation due to dryness of the intestines, dysmenorrhea, amenorrhea due to blood stasis, postpartum abdominal pain due to retention of blood stasis, masses in the abdomen, traumatic injuries and.

Peanut

It is the seed of Arachis hypogaea L. (Leguminosae).

Effect. Moistening the lung and stomach.

Indication. Dry cough, regurgitation, lack of lactation, and beriberi.

Pearl

It is the lustrous concretion found in the double-shell animal of Pteria mareensii (Dunker) (Pteriidae) and Hyriopsis cumingii (Lea) (Naiadidae).

Effect. Calming the mind and relieving palpitation, clearing away liver fire, astringing ulcers and promoting tissue regeneration.

Indication. Palpitation, epilepsy, infantile convulsion; red eyes with painful swelling, slow-healing sores and ulcers.

Pearl-like Node

Symptoms. A node in ear lobe and slight itching pain.

Pathogenesis. Mostly caused by invasion of pathogenic wind due to blood heat and accumulation of heat-toxin.

Therapeutic Principle. Removing heat from blood to eliminate wind and removing toxic substances to dissolve lumps.

Pecking Manipulation

A massage manipulation.

Operation. Slight flexing of all the fingers of both hands to form a claw-like shape and rub the certain region with the tips of two hands fingers up and down alternately, briskly and rhythmically as if chicken pecking grains.

Function. Alleviating pain and tranquilizing the mind.

Indication. Headache and insomnia.

Pectoral Qi

1. It is a combination of the food energy with the fresh air inhaled, stored in the chest. Pectoral qi promotes the respiratory movement through the respiratory tracts and, therefore, has something to do with speaking, voice, and respiration.
2. It relates the circulation of blood, which is associated with the temperature and acivities of limbs, visual and auditory ability, and heartbeat and rhythm.

Peking Euphorbia Root

It is the root of Euphorbia pekinensis Rupr. (Euphorbiaceae).

Effect. Promoting diuresis to reduce edema, subduing swelling and resolving masses, purging heat and relaxing the bowels.

Indication. Edema, ascites, hydrothorax boils and pyogenic infections.

Penetrating Needling

A needling technique.

Method. Puncture two or more adjoining points in one insertion of the needle. Straight penetration can be applied to the corresponding points on the medial and lateral or anterior and posterior of the four limbs. Oblique or subcutaneous penetration can be applied to neighbouring points on the superior and inferior parts.

Penis Carcinoma

It refers to the carcinoma of the glans penis.

Pathogenesis. Mostly caused by the deficiency of liver-yin and kidney-yin, and the attacking of fire of deficiency type, leading to the blockage in meridians and collaterals and the accumulation of pathogens in the penis.

Therapeutic Principle. In the early phase, dispersing stagnated liver qi, solving phlegm to remove accumulation of pathogen. In the middle phase, clearing away heat and eliminating dampness, purging intense heat and detoxicating. In the final phase, invigorating qi and blood, regulating the stomach and spleen.

Penis Sore

Symptoms. Sore on the penis, red skin with foul damp water, very itchy and painful.

Pathogenesis. Caused by the movement of the dampness and heat of the Liver Meridian due to dirty sexual intercourse.

Therapeutic Principle. Spread catechu over the affected part, releasing heat and toxic material from blood.

Penis Tuberculosis

Symptoms. Cavernosa with cord-like or plaque-type subcutaneous induration which can be felt in the dorsum penis. The penis is painful during erection, low fever, red skin weakness of limbs.

Pathogenesis. Caused by deficiency of the kidney and liver qi the stagnation of internal turbid phlegm due to the impair transportation and transformation of the stomach and the spleen.

Therapeutic Principle. Strengthening the spleen and stomach, resolving phlegm and masses, or nourishing yin to reduce pathogenic fire.

Penitis

Symptoms. Pain and itching, or swelling on the penis, persistent erections, or impotence with white, sticky discharge, etc.

Pathogenesis. Caused by the damp-heat of the Liver Meridian and the kidney impairment due to sexual strain.

Therapeutic Principle. Eliminating dampness and heat.

Pennywort Lawn Herb

It is the whole herb of Hydrocotyle sibthorpioides Lam. (Umbelliferae).

Effect. Clearing away heat, inducing diuresis, subduing swelling and detoxicating.

Indication. Hepatitis with jaundice, dysentery, stranguria, urinary tract infection, opacity, pertussis, swollen throat, carbuncles, cellulitis, furuncles, ecchymoma due to traumatic injuries, etc.

Pepper Fruit

It is the dried fruit of Piper nigrum L. (Piperaceae).

Effect. Warming the middle-energizer to relieve pain.

Indication. Cold in the stomach, gastric abscess and abdominal pain, vomiting, diarrhea, etc.

Peppertree Pricklyash Peel

It is the ripe seed of Zanthoxylum bungeanum Maxim., or Z. schinifolium Sieb. et Zucc. (Rutaceae).

Effect. Promoting diuresis and relieving asthma.

Indication. Edema and ascites, phlegmatic cough, etc.

Perforated Tuberculous Cervical Lymphonodes

It refers to the scrofula on the neck part.

Symptoms. Swelling and pain clustered scrofula, with some healed and some ulcerating. After ulceration, pus flows out without stopping.

Therapeutic Principle. Detoxicating and resolving masses, removing the necrotic tissue and promoting granulation.

Perianal Abscess

Symptoms. In the acute phase, red, swelling, heat and pain, etc. in the local part. After ulceration, they may all form anal fistula.

Pathogenesis. Caused by downward flow of damp-heat.

Therapeutic Principle. For excess syndrome, removing heat from the blood and toxic substances; for deficiency syndrome, replenishing the vital essence, removing heat and eliminating dampness.

Periappendicular Abscess

Symptoms. Metastatic pain in the right lower abdomen, nausea, vomiting, tenderness, tight abdominal skin, tenderness of lanweixue point (appendicealgia), accompanied by fever, headache.

Pathogenesis. Mostly caused by stasis of qi and blood, transformation of damp-heat in the interior, stagnation of turbid qi due to improper diet, melancholy and anxiety, walking in a hurry.

Therapeutic Principle. Promoting abdominal circulation and purging heat, promoting circulation of qi and removing blood stasis, clearing away toxins.

Pericardium Meridian of Hand-jueyin

It is one of the twelve regular meridians, which starts from the chest and pertains to the pericardium. It passes through the diaphragm and in turn, joins the upper-, middle- and lower-energizer. The thoracic branch exits superficially at Tianchi (P 1) near the nipple, and descends along the midline of anterior side of the arm to Zhongchong (P 9) at the midpoint of tip of the middle finger. The other branch is derived from the palm, goes along the fourth finger to the end of the ulnar side of the finger, and joins the Tri-energizer Meridian of Hand-shaoyang.

Perilla Stem

It is the stem of Perilla frutescens (L.) Britt. or the plant of the same genus (Labiatae).

Effect. Alleviating depression to regulate qi, and preventing abortion.

Indication. Stagnation of qi in the chest and abdomen, hypochondrium, distending pain in the abdomen, threatened abortion etc.

Periotic Furuncle

Symptoms. Burning heat, itching, blister, erosion, exudate of turbid discharge, scab, around the ear etc.

Pathogenesis. Caused by upward steaming of damp-heat, or erosion of pus discharge from the purulent ear.

Therapeutic Principle. Clearing away heat and promoting diuresis.

Peristrophe Herb

It is the whole plant of Peristrophe japonica (Thunb.) Brem. (Acanthaceae).

Effect. Expelling pathogenic wind and removing heat, resolving phlegm and removing toxic material.

Indication. Cough due to pathogenic wind-heat, infantile convulsion, swollen and sore throat, pyogenic infections due to abscess and acute mastitis.

Periumbilical Colic and Testalgia due to Invasion of Cold

Symptoms. Colic pain of testicle and lower abdomen, even radiating to the chest and hypochondrium, contraction of penis, cold scrotum, chills, cold limbs, pale complexion.

Pathogenesis. Stagnation of qi and blood resulting from cold-dampness attacking the Front Middle Meridian and the Liver Meridian, and the pathogenic factors accumulating in the lower abdomen, testicle and scrotum, etc.

Therapeutic Principle. Expel pathogenic cold and dampness and dredge the meridians.

Pernicious Vomiting due to Liver-heat

Symptoms. Vomiting of bitter water, dizziness, in the severe case, even immediate vomiting after eating food.

Pathogenesis. Mostly caused by original irritability and restlessness, and deficiency of yin and blood because of collection of blood to nourish the fetus after pregnancy.

Therapeutic Principle. Clearing away heat from the liver, regulating the stomach function, and lowering the adverse flow of qi to relieve vomiting.

Perpendicular Needling

It refers to insertion whereby the needle enters at an angle of about 90 degrees between the needle and the skin surface of the point.

Persian Lilac Flower-bud

It is the flower-bud of Syringa persica L. (Oleaceae).

Effect. Warming middle energizer to expel cold, decreasing flatulence and arresting vomiting.

Indication. Hiccups due to stomach-cold, vomiting, hyperemia of gastric mucosa, etc.

Persimmon Calyx

It is the persistent calyx of Diospyros kaki L. f. (Ebenaceae).

Effect. Descending the abnormally ascending flow of qi and arresting vomiting.

Indication. Hiccups due to failure of descending stomach-qi.

Persimmon Fruit

It is the fruit of Diospyros kaki L. f. (Ebenaceae).

Effect. Clearing away heat, moistening the lung and relieving thirst.

Indication. Cough, hematemesis and oral ulcer.

Persimmon Root

It is the root or root bark of Doispyros kaki L. f. (Ebenaceae).

Effect. Removing pathogenic heat from blood and stopping bleeding.

Indication. Metrorrhagia, dysentery with bloody stool and hemorrhoid.

Persistent Epistaxis

It refers to the constant bleeding from the nose.

Symptoms. Pale complexion, giddiness and dizziness.

Pathogenesis. Deficiency of the spleen-qi.

Therapeutic Principle. Invigorating qi and accelerating hemostasis and stopping bleeding.

Persistent Erection

Symptoms. Persistent penile erection, inability to ejaculate, or spermatorrhea.

Pathogenesis. Usually caused by the excessive fire-toxin in the interior, or overtaking aphrodisiac, or excessive sexual intercourse causing the yin deficiency of the liver and kidney and floating-up of asthenic yang.

Therapeutic Principle. Nourishing yin and purging fire.

Persisting Edema

Symptoms. General edema, abdominal distention, prolonged disease frequent attack, etc.

Pathogenesis. Usually caused by the deficiency of the spleen and kidney resulting in the disorder of uncontrolled water.

Therapeutic Principle. Strengthening the spleen, reinforcing the kidney and removing dampness to relieve edema.

Perspiration due to Spleen Deficiency

Symptoms. Sweating, lassitude and asthenia, anorexia and abdominal distention, etc.

Pathogenesis. Mostly caused by the spleen deficiency and the failure of the spleen to guide the body fluid.

Therapeutic Principle. Invigorating the spleen and replenishing qi.

Perspiration of Hands and Feet

Symptoms. Constant dampness and perspiration of the hands and feet.
Pathogenesis. Mostly due to the damp-evaporation of the spleen and stomach. For feverish sensation in palm and sole due to the deficiency of yin-fluid and blood; for cold hands and feet, it is ascribable to deficiency of middle-energizer yang.

Perspiration Over Precordial Region due to Blood Deficiency

Symptoms. Sweating just over the chest, but not on other parts; the more anxiety, the more sweating.
Pathogenesis. Impairment of heart blood because of excessive anxiety.
Therapeutic Principle. Nourishing the heart blood.

Pertussis

It is a respiratory infectious disease commonly seen in children under the age of 5.
Symptoms. Paroxysmal continuous cough followed by special inspiratory roaring, or cock-crowing echo, and expectoration with foam.
Pathogenesis. Usually caused by prevalent epidemic toxin invading the lung and leading to stagnation of phlegm and qi, and impairment of purifying and descending function of the lung.
Therapeutic Principle. Ventilating the lung and resolving phlegm, purging the lung of pathogenic fire and expelling phlegm, and moistening the lung and nourishing yin, etc.

Pestilence

It refers to acute infectious disease caused by affection by epidemic pathogens. There are two types.

1. Epidemic disease with pathogens of the exterior or interior.
   Symptoms. High fever, aversion to cold, headache and pantalgia, etc.
   Therapeutic Principle. Expelling heat from exterior and removing heat from the interior.
2. Epidemic pathogens of summer-heat accumulated in the stomach.
   Symptoms. High fever with vexation, abdominalgia with diarrhea, splitting headache, coma, epistaxis, eruption, etc.
   Therapeutic Principle. Clearing away pestilence and eliminating toxic material.

Pestilence with Pimple

Symptoms. Reddening and swelling all over the body like tumors.
Pathogenesis. Seasonal noxious agent.
Therapeutic Principle. Clearing away heat and purging fire for removing toxin and subduing swelling.

Pestilence with Red Liquid Vomit

Symptoms. Projection of the chest and the hypochondrium, and liquid vomit like blood.
Pathogenesis. Attacked by seasonal noxious agent.
Therapeutic Principle. Clearing away heat and toxic materials, removing pathogenic heat from blood and resolving phlegm.

Petal Formed Meadourue Root

It is the root of Thalictrum petaloideum L. (Ranunculaceae).
Effect. Clearing away heat and toxic materials.
Indication. Red-white dysentery, carbuncle and swelling, skin and external diseases, acute eczema, etc.

Petaloid Tooth

It refers to the blood petals on tooth and gum. It can be divided into yang-blood type and yin-blood type. In case of yang-blood type, the color of the petals is violet or like dry lacquer. It is occurrence of blood due to domination of heat in the stomach. It belongs to excess type. In case of yin-blood type, the color of the petals is yellow, like soy sauce, it is due to consumption of the kidney-yin by heat and flaring-up of fire of deficiency type and it belongs to deficiency type.

Phallocrypsis

Symptoms. Contracted penis and testis, or accompanied by sensation contracture of the lower abdomen, etc.

Pathogenesis. Usually caused by invasion of Jueyin Meridian by cold, or extreme loss of yang-qi due to severe vomiting and diarrhea, or invasion of Jueyin Meridian by heat accumulated in Yangming Meridian, or heat in the liver or gallbladder.

Therapeutic Principle. Warming Jueyin Meridian and dispelling cold, recuperating depleted yang to rescue the patient from collapse, removing heat from the liver and gallbladder, etc.

Pharbitis Seed

It is the ripe seed of Pharbitis nil (L.) Choisy or P. Purpurea (L.) Voigt (Convolvulaceae).

Effect. Promoting diuresis to reduce edema, eliminating stagnancy to purge the bowels and destroying parasites.

Indication. Edema and abdominal distention, constipation, and abdominal pain due to ascariasis and taeniasis.

Pharyngeal Dryness

Pathogenesis. Caused by consumption of body fluid due to excessive heat in lung and stomach, or yin deficiency.

Therapeutic Principle. For the patient with insufficient yin and body fluid, replenishing vital essence to tonify the kidney. For the patient with impairment of body fluid due to excessive fire in the lung and stomach, clearing away fire, nourishing yin and relieving sore-throat.

Pharynx-larynx (MA-T 3)

An auricular point.

Location. At the upper half of the medial aspect of the tragus.

Effect. Removing intense heat from the pharynx and larynx, relieving sore throat.

Indication. Hoarseness, acute and chronic pharyngitis and tonsillitis, etc.

Philippine Flemingia Root

It is the root of Flemingia philippinensis Merr. et Rofle (Leguminosae).

Effect. Expelling wind and eliminating dampness by diuresis, subduing blood stasis and detoxicating.

Indication. Rheumatic arthralgia, chronic nephritis, lumbar muscle strain traumatic injuries and furuncle.

Phlegm Accumulation

Symptoms. Dizziness with blurred vision, fullness and dull pain in the chest, mass in the abdomen, difficulty in coughing up phlegm, etc.

Pathogenesis. Mainly due to deficiency of the lung and spleen qi, pathogenic phlegm stagnated in the chest, and stagnation of qi circulation.

Therapeutic Principle. Clearing up stagnation in the chest to expel the phlegm.

Phlegm Apoplexy

A kind of apoplectic stroke.

Symptoms. Sudden vertigo, coma, stiffness of the tongue, inability to raise limbs, etc.

Pathogenesis. Usually caused by domination of phlegm and damp-heat brought about by wind.

Therapeutic Principle. Resolving phlegm and expelling wind.

Phlegm Caused by Retention of Food

Symptoms. Fullness in chest and stomach, eructation and acid regurgitation, nausea, severe pain in the stomach.

Pathogenesis. Mainly caused by indigestion of food, blood stasis, and phlegm caused by retention of food.
Therapeutic Principle. Promoting digestion, resolving phlegm and removing blood stasis.

Phlegm Cough

It refers to cough due to excessive phlegm.
Symptoms. Cough and profuse sputum, with cough stopping when phlegm is dispelled, feeling of fullness and oppression in the chest and stomach, etc.
Therapeutic Principle. Eliminating phlegm and stopping cough.

Phlegm Damp Affecting the Lung

Symptoms. Cough with abundant expectoration white thick sputum which is easily expectorated, complicated stuffiness in the chest, nausea and vomiting, poor appetite, heaviness sensation in the limbs, loose stool, etc.
Pathogenesis. Phlegm stagnation which causes impairment of the normal function of clarifying and sending down the lung qi, or exopathogens such as wind-cold and cold dampness, and spleen deficiency resulting in accumulation of water and dampness which is transformed into phlegm dampness, thus affecting the lung.
Therapeutic Principle. Invigorating the spleen, reducing phlegm and removing dampness by diuresis.

Phlegm-dampness Lumbago

Symptoms. Heaviness in the waist involving the spine and back, cold pain, aversion to cold and preference for warmth. It is accompanied by diarrhea, or swelling in the waist, which is soft and painless when pressed, normal color of the skin, etc.
Pathogenesis. Caused by attack of the spleen wetness, which leads to dysfunction of spleen in transportation and transformation.
Therapeutic Principle. Removing phlegm and eliminating dampness.

Phlegm due to Qi Deficiency

It refers to the syndrome of phlegm caused by deficiency of qi.
Symptoms. Palpitations, short breath, emaciation with yellowish complexion, vomiting of clear watery fluid and phlegm-like saliva, etc.
Therapeutic Principle. Invigorating the spleen and replenishing qi.

Phlegm-dyspnea

Symptoms. Dyspnea and adverse flow of qi, abundant expectoration, fullness and distress of the chest, whitish sputum, etc.
Pathogenesis. Mostly caused by phlegm and excessive fluid retention in the lung, blockage of the qi circulation and abnormal adverse flow of the lung-qi.
Therapeutic Principle. Keeping the inspired qi going downward, dispelling phlegm and relieving dyspnea.

Phlegm-fire

Symptoms. Similar to asthma, fever accompanied by restlessness, pain in the chest, dry mouth and lips, difficulty to cough out phlegm, etc.
Pathogenesis. Caused by the combination of fire and phlegm, which is accumulating in the lung, resulting from exogenous evil, internal injury by improper diet, etc.
Therapeutic Principle. Clearing away heat and dispersing phlegm.

Phlegm-like Abscess of Auricle

Symptoms. Swelling in the auricle part with no unusual change on the skin surface. Phlegm-like abscess grown on the scaphoid fossa.
Pathogenesis. Mostly caused by stagnation of turbid phlegm that results from interior phlegm-dampness due to splenic deficiency, and exterior invasion of pathogenic wind-cold with the phlegm-dampness.
Therapeutic Principle. Eliminating the phlegm-like pus to resolve the abscess, and dispelling wind to dredge the meridian. At the early stage, suspended

moxibustion with moxa-sticks can be applied to the local part.

Phlegm-stagnation

Symptoms. Dyspnea or cough, choking sensation in the chest, obstruction in pharynx, etc.

Pathogenesis. Caused by stagnation of pathogenic phlegm and qi.

Therapeutic Principle. Removing phlegm and alleviating mental depression.

Phlegm Syndrome due to Cold

1. It refers to the chronic phlegm syndrome complicated by asthma and cough due to pathogenic cold.

   Symptoms. Whitish, clear and thin phlegm, aversion to cold and cold limbs, etc.

   Therapeutic Principle. Warming the lung and reducing phlegm.

2. It refers to the syndrome due to the struggle of yang deficiency and cold-dampness.

   Symptoms. Soreness and weakness of the legs and knees, rigidity and pain in the back and loin, cold limbs and joints with numbness, etc.

   Therapeutic Principle. Promoting the flow of qi by warming the meridians to dispel the cold-dampness.

3. It refers to the syndrome of phlegm accumulation in the kidney.

   Symptoms. Dark complexion, stranguria, cold lower limbs, panic and discharge of profuse, thin and black-spotted phlegm, etc.

   Therapeutic Principle. Invigorating the spleen, warming the kidney and resolving phlegm.

Phlegm Syndrome due to Wind

1. It is a relapse of a old phlegm syndrome, caused by wind pathogen or wind and heat pathogen.

2. It refers to phlegm retention in the Liver Meridian.

Symptoms. Pale complexion, dizziness, headache, distending pain in hypochondriac region, constipation, irritability, pale phlegm with abundant droplet.

Therapeutic Principle. Expelling wind and resolving phlegm.

Phlegm syndrome of Deficiency Type

It refers to the phlegm syndrome caused by the deficiency of primordial qi.

Symptoms. Weakness, hoarseness and shortness of breath, nausea, vomiting and diarrhea, etc.

Therapeutic Principle. Invigorating the spleen and reinforcing the kidney.

Phlyctenular Conjuctivitis

Symptoms. One or more than two bubble-like granules surrounded with blood filaments on the surface of the white of the eye. Often repeatedly attacks people of weak constitution. Uncomfortable, dull and astringent, fully recovered after diabrosis, with no sign left.

Pathogenesis. Mostly caused by dryness-heat in the Lung Meridian, or insufficiency of the lung-yin, and local stagnation of qi and blood stasis.

Therapeutic Principle. Purging heat from the lung, promoting the circulation of qi and resolving the granule.

Phoenix Tree Leaf

It is the leaf of Firmiana simplex (L.) W. F. Wight. (Sterculiaceae).

Effect. Expelling wind dampness, clearing away heat and removing noxious material.

Indication. Headache, acute mastitis, ulcerative carbuncle, hemorrhoids, traumatic bleeding and hypertension.

Phthisical Cough

It refers to the chronic cough caused by exopathogen or consumption of five zang organ by over fatigue or sexual intemperance, etc.

Pianli (LI 6)

A meridian acupuncture point.

Location. On the redial side of the dorsal surface of the forearm on the line connecting Yangxi (LI 5) and Quchi (LI 11), 3 cun above the crease of the wrist.

Indication. Epistaxis, redness of the eyes, deafness, tinnitus, deviation of the mouth and eye, sore throat, edema, pain in the shoulder, arm, elbow and wrist.

Method. Puncture obliquely 0.3-0.5 cun. Apply moxibustion 3-5 moxa cones or 5-10 minutes with warming moxibustion.

Picking Therapy

It refers to the method by which the practitioner picks out the white fibrous substances or squeezes some liquid from the point or special erythra so as to treat disease. Frequently, erythra or points are located and selected on the back. Pick 1-2 dots of erythra each time. The point concerned can be selected according to the of the disease condition.

Notice. Pay attention to sterilization, and dressing of the local surface with sterilized gauze after pricking.

Pig Blood

Effect. Replenishing blood, stopping bleeding and normalizing the functioning of the large intestine.

Indication. Phlegm accumulating vertigo abdominal fullness, gastric discomfort with acid regurgitation.

Pigen (Ex-B 4)

An extra acupuncture point.

Location. On the lower back, below the spinous process of the 1st lumbar vertebra, 3.5 cun lateral to the posterior midline.

Indication. Abdominal mass, lower back pain, stomachache, hepatomegaly and splenomegaly, hepatitis, gastritis, enteritis, nephroptosis, etc.

Method. Puncture obliquely 0.5-0.7 cun. Apply moxibustion 5-7 moxa cones or 5-10 minutes with warming moxibustion.

Pig Spinal Marrow

It is the spinal cord or marrow of Sus scrofa domestica Brisson (Surdae).

Effect. Invigorating yin and tonifying marrow.

Indication. Hectic fever due to yin-deficiency, diabetes, and pyocutaneous diseases.

Pig Trotter

Effect. Enriching the blood, promoting lactation and treating cutaneous infection.

Indication. Lack of the lactation, subcutaneous swelling deep-rooted carbuncles and boils.

Pill

It is a solid globule, coated or uncoated, made from fine powder drugs with suitable excipient such as honey, water, rice paste, flour paste, wine, vinegar, drug juice, etc. The pill is characterized by being absorbed slowly, thus prolonging the therapeutic effect, being small in size, and convenient to be taken and stored.

Pillb Driedug

It is the dried intact body of Armadillidium vulgare (Latreille) (Armadillidiinae).

Effect. Dissipating blood stasis, promoting diuresis, detoxicating and relieving pain.

Indication. Chronic malaria, amenorrhea, abdominal masses, dysuria, infantile convulsion, toothache, various kinds of sores, etc.

Pilose Asiabell Root

It is the root of Codonopsis pilosula (Franch.) Nannf. (Campanulaceae).

Effect. Invigorating the spleen and replenishing qi, promoting the production of body fluid and nourishing the blood.

Indication. Short breath, thirst, sallow complexion, dizziness, and palpitation, etc.

Pilose Gerbera Herb

It is the whole herb of Gerbera piloselloides Cass. (Compositae).

Effect. Dispersing the wind, ventilating the lung, arresting cough, inducing diuresis and diaphoresis, promoting the flow of the lung-qi and blood circulation, removing toxic material, reducing swelling.

Indication. Cough due to invasion by wind, asthma, edema, abdominal distention, dysuria, infantile anorexia of milk and food, amenorrhea, traumatic injuries, carbuncles, boils, furuncle, etc.

Pinching Spine Manipulation

A massage manipulation for children.

Operation. The child is in pronation on the knee of the mother or on the bed. The doctor flexes the two indices to 90 degrees, pinches the skin and muscles in the lumbar vertebrae of the child from the Changqiang (GV 1) point upwards, and then press-pinches downwards with two thumbs alternately and push-pinches upwards along the spine to the Dazhui (GV 14) point constantly with the thumb and the index finger cooperating together. During pinching the spine, pinch it for three times and lift the skin of the back spine one time. Repeat the movements 6 times.

Function. Regulating yin and yang, clearing and regulating the meridians and collaterals, promoting the circulation of qi and blood, and improving functions of zang-fu organs.

Indication. Anorexia, digestive disorders diarrhea, and infantile malnutrition, etc.

Pinellia Tuber

It the dried stem tuber of Pinellia ternata (Thunb.) Breit. (Araceae).

Effect. Depriving the evil wetness and eliminating phlegm, disintegrating and resolving masses, and lowering the adverse flow of qi to stop vomiting.

Indication. Cough with profuse thin phlegm, nausea, vomiting and food regurgitation from the stomach, fullness in the stomach and abdomen, globus hystericus, scrofula, etc.

Pink Blood

Symptoms. Cough with pink phlegm, short breath, palpitation, lassitude, etc. The disease persists uncured and recurs easily after strain.

Pathogenesis. Usually caused by the impairment of the lung collaterals and hemorrhage due to qi deficiency.

Therapeutic Principle. Hemostasis by invigorating qi.

Pink Plumepoppy Herb

It is the whole herb of Macleaya cordata (Willd.) R. Br. (Papaveraceae) with root.

Effect. Subduing swelling, detoxicating and destroying parasites.

Indication. Suppurative infections on the body surface, tonsillitis, otitis media, trichomonal vaginitis, scalds, etc.

Pink Reineckea Herb

It is the whole herb of Reineckea carnea Kunth (Liliaceae) with root.

Effect. Clearing away heat from the lung, relieving cough, arresting bleeding and removing toxic substances.

Indication. Cough due to the lung-heat, hematemesis, epistaxis, hemafecia, traumatic injuries, conjunctival congestion and malnutrition, boils and pyogenic infections.

Pipa (Ex-CA)

An extra acupuncture point.

Location. On the anterior border of the lateral side of the clavicle in the depression of the superior border of the coracoid process.

Indication. Pain in the shoulder, failure to raise the upper limbs.

Method. Puncture perpendicularly 0.3-0.5 cun. Apply moxibustion 5 moxa cones or 5-10 minutes with warming moxibustion.

Pipewort Flower

It is the whole plant or inflorescence of Eriocaulon buergerianum Koern. and E. sieboldtianum Sieb. et Zucc. (Eriocaulaceae).

Effect. Dispelling the wind and expelling the heat, improving visual acuity and removing nebula.

Indication. Conjunctival congestion eyes with swelling pain, headache due to heat of the Liver Meridian, photophobia, headache, toothache, nebula formation etc.

Pishu (B 20)

An acupoint.

Location. 1.5 cun lateral to the Jizhong (GV 6), lower border of the spinous process of the 11th thoracic vertebra in the back.

Indication. Hypochondriac and back pain, abdominal distention, jaundice, vomiting, diarrhea, dysentery, bloody stools, edema, etc.

Method. Puncture obliquely 0.5-0.8 cun and apply moxibustion to the point for 10-20 minutes or 5-10 moxa cones.

Pityriasis Simplex

Symptoms. Whitish spots on the face with obvious round-shaped or elliptical-shaped borderline with small amount of grey-white sugar-like scale on the surface. It is usually found in children.

Pathogenesis. Caused by dirty diet accumulation and production of parasitosis in the interior, pathogens of parasites shown on facial skin due to stagnation of qi.

Therapeutic Principle. Take antiscolic orally and use Tincture of Pseudolarix externally.

Placenta of Hominid

It is the human placenta.

Effect. Tonifying kidney and vital essence, enriching blood and supplementing qi, invigorating the lung to relieve cough.

Indication. Impotence, emission, soreness of waist, dizziness, tinnitus, emaciation, hectic fever due to consumption, hypogalactia, asthma, etc.

Planning Treatment according to Diagnosis

It refers to the course of applying theory, method, prescription, and medicine clinically. Diagnosis means that the patient's symptom and signs are analyzed and summarized by such basic theory of TCM including the cause, nature and location of the disease and the patient's physical condition, etc.

Plantain Seed

It is the ripe seed of Plantago asiatica L. or Plantago depressa Wild. (Plantaginaceae).

Effect. Clearing away heat, inducing diuresis to treat morbid urination, arresting diarrhea, clearing away heat from the liver to improve the acuity of vision eliminating sputum and relieving cough.

Indication. Cough with profuse sputum due to the heat in the lung, edema, dysuria, stranguria, diarrhea due to summer-heat and dampness, bloodshot eyes, blurred vision.

Platycodon Root

It is the root of Platycodon grandiflorum (Jacq.) DC. (Campanulaceae).

Effect. Facilitating the flow of the lung-qi, resolving phlegm and relieving cough.

Indication. Cough with profuse phlegm, unsmooth expectoration, sore throat, hoarseness and pulmonary abscess, full and oppressed feelings in the chest and diaphragmatic region.

Pleural Effusion

Symptoms. Distention and fullness in the hypochondriac region, and pain on both sides during coughing and spitting saliva, even when turning over and respiring; or accompanied by retching, short breath, etc.

Pathogenesis. Mostly caused by fluid retention in the hypochondrium.

Therapeutic Principle. Eliminating fluid retention.

Pohu (B 42)

A meridian acupuncture point.

Location. On the back, below the spinous process of the 3rd thoracic vertebra, 3 cun lateral to Shenzhu (GV 12).

Indication. Pulmonary tuberculosis, cough, dyspnea, stiffness of neck, pain in the shoulder and back.

Method. Puncture obliquely 0.5-0.8 cun. Apply moxibustion 3-5 moxa cones or 5-10 minutes with warming moxibustion.

Pohuashan Mountain Moumtainash Fruit

It is the fruit, stem, and stem bark of Sorbus pohuashanensis (Hance) Hedl. (Rosaceae).

Effect. Relieving cough, dispelling phlegm, invigorating the spleen and promoting diuresis.

Indication. Chronic bronchitis, pulmonary tuberculosis and edema.

Point Aspirator

An instrument for aspirating and cupping. It is composed of a rubber ball with a valve and a special glass cup with a pipe-mouth at the bottom; they are connected by a rubber pipe.

Operation. Putting the glass cup around the chosen acupoint, then pressing the rubber ball to pump out the air in the glass cup and form a negative pressure inside the cup (about 240 mmHg).

Point Selection in Accordance with Differentiation of Syndrome

One of the point-selecting principles. Selecting the points based on the analyses on the relationship between manifestations of a disease and zang-fu organs, meridians and collaterals.

Point Selection on Disparate Meridians

A kind of point selection, contrary to point selection on the affected meridian. It refers to selecting points on other meridians, which are related to the affected meridian including interior-exterior related meridians and same-name meridians.

Point Selection on the Mated Meridian

It is one of the methods of point selection. According to the external-internal relationship between the meridians, select the point of on the meridian, which is externally-internally related to another meridian. Select an acupoint in another meridian, which is exteriorly or interiorly related to the main meridian according to the exterior-interior relationship between the meridians.

Point-ultrasonic Stimulation Therapy

It refers to the therapy of radiating the selected point with a beam of ultrasonic waves, emitted from a sound-emitting head which can penetrate into the selected point. The amount of stimulation can be controlled in accordance with the distance between the sound-emitting head and the point, and the regulation of the sound strength and the time it takes to work on the point.

Poisonous Buttercup Herb

It is the whole herb of Ranunculus sceleratus L. (Ranunculaceae).

Effect. Clearing away heat, detoxicating, dispelling pathogenic wind and dampness.

Indication. Rheumatic arthralgia, sore, carbuncles, furuncles, boils, scrofula, subcutaneous nodes, malaria and snake bite.

Poisonous Herbs Expelling Pathogen

The therapeutic application of poisonous drugs to eliminate the pathogenic factors.

For instance, scorpion and centipede are used to treat upstirring of the liver and clonic convulsion because they can relieve convulsion.

Polished Glutinous Rice

It is the whole herb of Memorialis hirta (Bl.) Wedd. (Urticaleae).
Effect. Clearing away heat and detoxicating, reducing swelling invigorating the spleen and arresting bleeding.
Indication. Dysentery, leukorrhea, infantile malnutrition, hematemesis, acute mastitis, traumatic bleeding, furuncle, carbuncle, scrofula, etc.

Polished Round-grained Rice

It is the kernel of Oryza sativa L. (Gramineae).
Effect. Tonifying the spleen for supplementing qi, invigorating the spleen and stomach, relieving restlessness and thirst, and arresting diarrhea and treating dysentery.
Indication. Diarrhea, dysentery, etc.

Poloborry Root

It is the root of Phytolacca acinosa Roxb. (Phytolaccaceae).
Effect. Promoting diuresis to reduce edema, subduing swelling and dissolving lumps, eliminating phlegm to alleviate cough, inducing defecation.
Indication. Edema with ascites, constipation, dysuria, subcutaneous swelling, etc.

Polymyositis and Dermatomyositis

1. **Symptoms.** Extreme pain of muscle, sweating, flaccidity of limbs, numbness of skin, and coma, etc.
   Therapeutic Principle. Expelling cold and wetness.
2. It refers to the stagnation of spleen-qi. It is developed from rheumatism of muscle.
   Symptoms. Lassitude of limbs, stuffiness, fullness and dull pain in the abdomen and stomach, seasonal purgation of stool, poor appetite, yellowish face, swollen feet, etc.
   Therapeutic Principle. Invigorating the spleen and eliminating wetness.

Polyorexia Involving Middle-energizer

1. **Symptoms.** Polyorexia with less drinking of water and scanty dark urine.
   Pathogenesis. Mainly caused by excess of stomach-fire in the middle-energizer and over-decomposition of food.
2. **Symptoms.** Frequent urination without feeling thirsty.
   Therapeutic Principle. Clearing away stomach-heat and purging fire, nourishing yin and promoting the production of body fluid.

Polyphagia and Marasmus

Symptoms. Polyphagia and hunger, weak constitution, frequent micturition and dry stool, etc.
Pathogenesis. Caused by the yin impairment by excessive heat of Yangming Meridian.
Therapeutic Principle. Clearing away the stomach-heat and purging intense fire, replenishing yin essence and moistening the viscera.

Pomegranate Leaf

It is the leaf of Punica granatum L. (Punicaceae).
Effect. Detoxicating and treating wounds.
Indication. Traumatic injuries, for external application.

Pomegranate Rind

It is the peel of Punica granatum L. (Punicaeae).
Effect. Astringing the intestines, relieving diarrhea, destroying parasites, inducing astringency and arresting bleeding.
Indication. Chronic diarrhea and dysentery, hemafecia, proctoptosis; abdominal pain due to parasitic malnutrition, metrorrhagia, metrostaxis and foul leukorrhea, ascariasis, filariasis, ect.

Pomegranate Root

It is the root bark of Punica granatum L. (Punicaceae).

Effect. Killing parasites, astringing the intestines and arresting leukorrhagia.

Indication. Ascariasis, cestodiasis, chronic diarrhea and dysentery, and leukorrhea with reddish discharge.

Poor Appetite

It refers to feeling hungry yet without appetite.

Pathogenesis. Deficiency of the spleen and stomach, leading to the impairment of the transporting function.

Poppy Capsule

It is the ripe capsule of Papaver somniferum L. (Papaveraceae).

Effect. Arresting persistent cough, relieving dysentery with astringents, and alleviating pain.

Indication. Chronic cough, chronic diarrhea and dysentery, pain in the chest or abdomen, emission or spermatorrhea, etc.

Pork

It is the meat of Sus scrofa domestica Brisson (Surdae).

Effect. Moisturizing dryness by nourishing yin.

Indication. Consumption of body fluid due to febrile disease, emaciation, irritating dry cough and constipation.

Pork Gall

Effect. Clearing away heat from the lung, eliminating sputum, removing heat and toxins.

Indication. Cough of heat type, profuse sputum, pertussis, asthma, bloodshot, swollen and painful eyes, inflammation of the throat, jaundice, diarrhea, boils, sore, swellings and ulcers.

Pork Liver

Effect. Invigorating the liver, tonifying the blood and improving acuity of vision.

Indication. Sallow and dull complexion due to blood deficiency, night blindness, conjunctival congestion, edema.

Pork Pancreas

Effect. Tonifying the lung, reinforcing the spleen and moistening dryness.

Indication. Cough and hemoptysis due to deficiency of the lung, dyspnea, dysentery, alactation and cracked skin of the hands.

Pork Spleen

Effect. Strengthening the spleen and stomach and promoting digestion.

Indication. Anorexia and indigestion.

Pork Tripe

Effect. Tonifying consumption and strengthening the spleen and stomach.

Indication. Fragility, diarrhea, dysentery, diabetes, frequent urination and infantile malnutrition.

Positive Exogenous Febrile Disease

It refers to the disorder due to affection of cold pathogen in winter.

Symptoms. Fever with cold aversion, headache, pain of the nape, rigidity of lumbar vertebra, general pain of the body.

Therapeutic Principle. Relieving the exterior syndrome with drugs pungent in flavor and warm in property.

Postpartum Abdominal Pain

Symptoms. Hard abdomen with pain and retention of lochia.

Pathogenesis. Accumulation of putrid blood in the lower abdomen due to invasion of wind-cold into deficient viscera, leading to stagnation of qi and blood.

Therapeutic Principle. Expelling pathogenic cold from the meridian and promoting blood circulation to remove blood stasis.

Postpartum Cold Feeling

Symptoms. The woman feels cold in many regions of the body after delivery, which lasts for a long time with no sign of recovery.

Pathogenesis. Postpartum deficiency of qi and blood.

Therapeutic Principle. Supplementing qi and nourishing blood.

Postpartum Constipation

Symptoms. Normal diet, difficult bowel movements, or no bowel movements for several days, or painful and difficult defecation with dry stool, sallow complexion, dry skin.

Pathogenesis. Loss of blood, impairment of body fluids, and the inability of yin fluid to moisten the intestines.

Therapeutic Principle. Nourishing blood and moistening dryness. Acupuncture is applicable.

Notice. Administration with caution for drugs of purgation.

Postpartum Convulsion

Symptoms. A sudden stiff neck, convulsions of the four limbs, even opisthotonos and lockjaw appearing after delivery.

Pathogenesis. Heavy loss of yin-blood, lack of nourishment of tendons, wind-evil attack resulting in the stir of liver-wind, or over sweating, leading to the impairment of blood and body fluids and extreme deficiency, resulting in the stir of internal wind. It is classified into invasion of wind type and internal wind type due to extreme deficiency.

Therapeutic Principle. In the case of wind invasion, with fever and chills, headache, stiff neck, dispersing the depressed liver-qi and dispelling wind; inducing resuscitation and restoring consciousness. In the case of internal wind, with pale or sallow complexion, heavy eyes, unconsciousness, nourishing yin and calming the endopathic wind.

Postpartum Deafness

Symptoms. Sudden deafness, dizziness, lassitude and debility in the loins and knees.

Pathogenesis. Caused by impairment of qi and blood, deficiency of kidney qi, and inability of essence qi to reach the ears.

Therapeutic Principle. Tonifying the kidney qi.

Postpartum Diarrhea

Pathogenesis. It can be classified into improper diet type and the type of injury of yin by pathogenic heat. Generally caused by improper diet after delivery, which injures the spleen and the stomach, leading to food remaining inside the body; or to postpartum qi and blood deficiency accompanied by the injury of yin due to heat evil; or to postpartum lochioschesis, affecting the large intestine.

Therapeutic Principle. In the case of improper diet, with abdominal pain and distention, tenesmus, removing stagnancy and purging obstruction of the fu organs. In the case of the injury of yin by pathogenic heat, with pus and blood, accompanied by fever and abdominal pain, tenesmus, fatigue, insomnia due to deficiency vexation, dry lips and thirst, nourishing blood and eliminating damp and heat.

Postpartum Edema

Symptoms. Gradual spread of edema, first to the limbs, then to the whole body, oliguria, fatigue, fullness in the epigastrium.

Pathogenesis. Generally caused by yang deficiency of the spleen and kidney after delivery, which leads to failure to transfer body fluids, resulting in the retention of body fluids in superficial muscles and skin and the limbs.

Therapeutic Principle. Invigorating the spleen and warming the kidney; promoting diuresis by restoring yang.

Postpartum Eye Pain

Symptoms. Impaired eyesight due to eye pain, photophobia, xerophthalmia, weakness of the eyelid, orbital pain and pain at the point of taiyang.

Pathogenesis. Caused by great loss of blood in delivery.

Therapeutic Principle. Enriching blood, nourishing nutrient system.

Postpartum Frequency of Urination

It can be classified into cold of deficiency type and heat deficiency type. Generally due to cold evil invading the urinary bladder, resulting from failure of asthenic superficial qi to protect the body, and causing the urinary bladder to fail to control urination; or, due to the shift of heat into the urinary bladder resulting from puerperal deficiency of kidney qi.

1. **Symptoms.** In the case of cold of deficiency: postpartum frequent urination with whitish urine, listlessness, intolerance of cold and cold limbs.

   Therapeutic Principle. Warming and strengthening the lower-energizer.

2. **Symptoms.** In the case of heat deficiency, postpartum frequent urination with difficulty and pain, distention of the lower abdomen with a dropping feeling, bitter taste.

   Therapeutic Principle. Removing heat and regulating the function of the urinary bladder.

Postpartum Haemorrhagia

Symptoms. Sudden excessive bleeding from the vagina or incessant menorrhea after delivery.

Pathogenesis. Mostly caused by early sexual intercourse in the puerperium, injury to the uterine collaterals during delivery, or retention of placenta.

Therapeutic Principle. Supplementing qi to arrest prostration.

Postpartum Hematochezia

It refers to stool with blood from the anus.

Pathogenesis. Caused by postpartum consumption yin due to excessive loss of blood, interior heat-syndrome by yin deficiency, and injury of the intestine blood vessels by heat.

Therapeutic Principle. Nourishing blood and clearing away heat.

Postpartum Hematuria

It refers to urination with blood.

Pathogenesis. Caused by puerperal deficiency of blood and qi leading to the weakening of the reserving function of the kidney, or by pathogenic heat invading and burning the bladder.

Therapeutic Principle. In the former case, invigorating qi and nourishing blood to strengthen the spleen. In the latter case, removing heat from blood and regulating collaterals.

Postpartum Hypochondriac Pain

It refers to one or both sides of the hypochondriac pain after delivery.

Pathogenesis. Generally due to the stagnation of qi and blood stasis, or puerperal severe blood loss.

Therapeutic Principle. Dissipating blood stasis by promoting blood circulation and alleviating pain by regulating the flow of qi.

Postpartum Insomnia

Symptoms. Presence insomnia, vexation, sweating, reddish complexion and thirst.

Pathogenesis. Exhaustion of qi and blood and failure of yin to keep yang well after delivery.

Therapeutic Principle. Supplementing qi, nourishing blood and tranquilizing the mind.

Postpartum Night Sweat

It refers to the parturient's night sweating during sleep, yet without sweating when awake.

Pathogenesis. Mostly caused by consumption of qi and blood during labor, leading to blood deficiency and yin insufficiency.

Therapeutic Principle. Regulating the flow of qi, replenishing blood and arresting sweating.

Postpartum Pain of Limbs

It refers to aching pain, numbness, and heavy sensation in the limbs of the parturient after childbirth.

Pathogenesis. Mostly caused by muscular malnutrition to the extremities due to blood deficiency, wind-cold and kidney deficiency.

Therapeutic Principle. In the case of blood deficiency, nourishing blood and replenishing qi, and promoting the flow of qi by warming the meridian; in the case of wind-cold, nourishing blood, expelling wind and clearing away cold to relieve pain; in the case of kidney deficiency, reinforcing the kidney and nourishing blood to strengthen the muscles and bones.

Postpartum Paralysis

Symptoms. Hemiplegia, numbness and spasm of the limbs of the parturient.

Pathogenesis. Generally caused by severe blood loss during delivery, resulting in deficiency of the meridians.

Therapeutic Principle. Invigorating qi and nourishing blood.

Postpartum Prolapse of Genital Structure

Symptoms. Hysteroptosis or the prolapse of the vaginal wall.

Pathogenesis. Generally due to the patient originally manifesting cold due to deficiency, and overstrain during delivery, leading to the sinking of qi.

Postpartum Retention of Lochia

It refers to retention of blood and putrid fluid in the uterus after presentation of the placenta, or small discharge of lochia with pain in the lower abdomen.

Pathogenesis. Mostly caused by qi stagnation or blood stasis due to cold.

Therapeutic Principle. Promoting the circulation of qi to remove stasis, or warming the meridians to expel cold and remove stasis.

Postpartum Retention of Urine

It refers to the retention of urine with hypogastric distention and pain, and restless after delivery.

Pathogenesis. Generally due to the weakness and over-consumption of qi resulting from overstrain during delivery; or excessive loss of blood leading to qi deficiency of the spleen and lung, failure to clear and regulate water passage on transfer of the urine into the bladder; or, the injury of the kidney leading to deficiency of the kidney yang, failure to dispel dampness and promote diuresis; or, to the stagnation of liver qi and the disorder of qi caused by postpartum depressed emotions, leading to disturbance in ascending and descending the clear turbid qi, and the dysfunction of the urinary bladder. The disease is clinically divided into two types: deficiency and excess.

Therapeutic Principle. In the case of deficiency, with hypogastric distention, fullness and pain, listlessness, and inertia of speech, warming the kidney, invigorating genuine qi, and promoting diuresis. In the case of excess, with hypogastric distention and pain, mental depression, distention and pain in both sides of the hypochondriac region, regulating and promoting the flow of qi, and inducing diuresis.

Postpartum Syndrome due to Wind, Cold, Deficiency, and Overstrain

Symptoms. Aversion to cold, poor appetite, diarrhea with indigested food, cold and pain in the lower abdomen, amenorrhea, etc.

Pathogenesis. Invasion of wind-cold into the body, or internal injury due to overstrain, deficiency of blood and qi.

Therapeutic Principle. Reinforcing blood and qi, warming the kidney and strengthening yang.

Postpartum Typhoid

Symptoms. Fever with aversion to cold, headache without sweat or spontaneous sweating.

Pathogenesis. Caused by pathogenic cold invading the texture and interspace of muscles resulting from qi and blood deficiency and dysfunction of the superficial defense.

Therapeutic Principle. Restoring qi, strengthening the body resistance and eliminating pathogenic factors.

Postpartum Vulva Pain

It refers to pain in the parturient woman's pudendum.

Pathogenesis. Mostly caused by infection of pathogenic factors due to birth injury, or invasion of wind into the vaginal orifice.

Therapeutic Principle. Promoting blood circulation and dispelling wind to stop pain.

Pounding Manipulation

Operation. Tap the point on the patient's body with the operator middle section or the tip of the middle finger.

Function. Relieving convulsion and tranquilizing the mind.

Indication. Night cry, infantile convulsion, dark urine with dysuria, and fever, etc.

Powder

It refers to a dosage form of drugs. There are two types, the powder for oral administration and the powder for external application. The powder is easily prepared, and convenient to use and carry, is easily absorbed, economical in administration, and liable to keep effective.

Precordial Pain due to Attack of Pestilent Factors

Symptoms. Sudden precordial stabbing pain with severe stuffiness in the chest.

Pathogenesis. Qi deficiency of viscera, psychasthenia, attack of the viscera and the heart collaterals by pathogenic and pestiferous factors.

Therapeutic Principle. Take fragrant drugs dissolving the turbid, removing obstruction in the meridians to relieve pain.

Precordial Pain due to Cold

Symptoms. Sudden precordial pain involving the back and shoulder, or lingering heart pain with cold limbs, faint breath, profuse cold sweat, loose stool, incontinence of feces and urine.

Pathogenesis. Attack of pathogenic cold or the insufficiency of the heart-yang.

Therapeutic Principle. Warming the kidney, strengthening yang-qi to dispel cold and relieve pain.

Precordial Pain due to Liver Disease

Symptoms. Precordial pain which spreads to the hypochondrium, etc.

Pathogenesis. Liver disease with the pathogen factor rising to the precordium.

Therapeutic Principle. Promoting blood circulation and removing the stagnation.

Precordial Pain due to Lung Disease

Symptoms. Tight pain in the region over the heart, cough with sputum, etc.

Pathogenesis. Attack of the heart by pathogenic factor due to lung disease.

Therapeutic Principle. Releasing lung to relieve asthma, regulating the flow of qi and promoting blood circulation to remove obstruction.

Precordial Pain due to Metrorrhagia

Symptoms. Sudden severe pain of the heart region, pale complexion and sweating, palpitation and shortness of breath and asthenia, etc.

Pathogenesis. Sudden shortage of blood due to metrorrhagia and abortion and the failure of blood to nourish heart vessels.

Therapeutic Principle. Replenishing qi, promoting the production of blood and regulating collaterals to stop pain.

Precordial Pain during Pregnancy

Symptoms. In the mild case, precordial pain appearing and fading at frequent intervals; in the serious case, pain all over chest and back with excessive fetal movement.

Pathogenesis. Combination of retention of phlegm and fluid with wind-cold, which leads to the obstruction of the chest-yang.

Therapeutic Principle. Expelling pathogenic factors to alleviate the pain, and checking the upward adverse flow of the lung or stomach-qi to prevent abortion.

Precordial Pain of Excess Type

Symptoms. Sudden cardiac pain, fullness and distention in the chest, inability to take food, constipation.

Pathogenesis. Taking food after great anger.

Therapeutic Principle. Regulating the flow of qi to dissipate stagnation.

Precordial Pain of Kidney Type

Symptoms. Pain over chest and back, irritability and sleeplessness, lassitude in loins and legs, dizziness and tinnitus, etc.

Pathogenesis. Upward rising of yin-fire, flaring-up of monarch fire.

Therapeutic Principle. Nourishing yin and tonifying the kidney, nourishing the heart to tranquilize the mind.

Precordial Pain with Feeling of Suspension

Symptoms. Precordial pain with suspending feeling, fullness and stuffiness in the chest, irritability etc.

Pathogenesis. Excessive fluid and internal pathogenic cold, reversed flow of qi or the failure of yang-qi forced by pathogenic factors to disperse, and heat due to stasis.

Therapeutic Principle. Warming yang for dispelling cold, and regulating the flow of qi to dissipate blood stasis and alleviate pain.

Pregnancy Aphthous Stomatitis

It refers to erosion of mucous membrane in the oral cavity and pain of the pregnant woman.

Pathogenesis. Blood collection to nourish the fetus, heat in the blood system, and flaring-up of the heart-fire.

Premature Ejaculation

Symptoms. Prospermia in coitus or even before coitus, easy erection of the penis, fever, night sweat, vexation, dry mouth, etc.

Pathogenesis. Deficiency of the kidney-yin and flaming of the fire from the gate of life.

Therapeutic Principle. Nourishing yin to reduce pathogenic fire.

Prepared Aconite Root

It is the product processed from the lateral roots of Aconitum carmichaeli Debx. (Ranunculaceae).

Effect. Restoring the vital function of the heart, dispelling cold, reinforcing the kidney and spleen.

Indication. Collapse and shock, spontaneous cold sweat, aversion to cold, cold limbs, aches in the loins and knees, gastric and abdominal cold pain, loose stool; edema, dysuria, arthralgia due to wind-cold dampness.

Prepared Rehmannia Root

It is the prepared root of Rehmannia glutinosa (Goertn.) Libosch. (Scrophulariaceae).

Effect. Nourishing blood to produce essence, tonifying yin and moisturizing dryness, invigorating the liver and kidney.

Indication. Sallow complexion due to blood deficiency, dizziness, palpitation, insomnia, irregular menstruation, metrorrhagia and metrostaxis, tidal fever, night sweat, seminal emission, and diabetes due to deficiency of the kidney-yin; tinnitus, deafness, premature grey hair, etc.

Prepared Soybean

It is the dried seed, which is fermented by steaming, of Glycine max (L.) Merr. (Leguminosae).

Effect. Expelling the exterior evils from the body surface, removing restlessness and soothing depressed liver.

Indication. Exterior syndromes due to affection by wind-cold exopathogens, exterior syndromes due to affection by wind-heat exopathogens, vexation, insomnia, etc.

Presenile Amenorrhea

Symptoms. Early menopause before climacteric.

Pathogenesis. Early decline of sexual function due to impairment of the kidney qi.

Therapeutic Principle. Invigorating the kidney and spleen, and nourishing blood and yin.

Pressing for Diagnosis

It refers to one of the diagnostic methods by palpating the patient's body surface such as muscle and skin, hand and feet, chest and abdomen, neck, meridians and acupoints, etc. to get a diagnostic impression of the disease.

Pressing Jingming (B 1)

A massage manipulation. One of self-massage manipulations.

Operation. Press Jingming point located in the depression, 0.1 cun above the internal canthus with the whorled surface of the thumb and index of either hand. First press downwards and then squeeze upwards. Repeat the movements for many times to cause soreness and feeling of distention.

Function. It is suitable for health care of eyes.

Pressing-kneading Jianyu (LI 15)

A massage manipulation. It is one of self-massage manipulations.

Operation. Press-knead the front depression of the end of shoulder constantly with the whorled surface of the middle finger to cause soreness and distention feeling.

Function. It is suitable for health care of the upper limbs and shoulders.

Pressing-kneading Sibai (S 2)

A massage manipulation. One of self-massage manipulations.

Operation. Press-knead the part 1 cun below the eyes constantly until soreness and distention appear.

Function. It is suitable for health care of eyes.

Pressing Manipulation

A massage manipulation.

1. **Operation.** Press the acupoint or the affected region using heavy force, often with the elbow.

   Function. Regulating qi and promoting blood circulation, relaxing muscles and tendons, and relieving pain.

   Indication. Stiffness of the lumbar muscle, persistent pain of the waist and legs.

2. **Operation.** Press the body surface with the finger, palm or knuckle.

   Function. Relaxing muscles, clearing occlusion, promoting the blood circulation and relieving pain.

   Indication. Pain of the epigastrium, headache, aching pain and numbness of extremities, etc.

Pressing String and Foulaging-rubbing

It is one of massage manipulations for children.

Operation. Foulage-rub the hypochondrium of the child with both palms up and down for many times.

Function. Regulating qi and eliminating sputum.

Indication. Cough, asthma and accumulation of sputum.

Pressing Yaoshu (GV 2)

A massage manipulation.
Operation. Press the Yaoshu (GV 2) point with the fingertip.
Function. Clearing the meridians and activating the collaterals.
Indication. Pain in the loins, paralysis of the lower limbs.

Pressure Method

A term in acupuncture. It refers to an auxiliary method of acupuncture. Before inserting the needle, press the surrounding region of the point with the thumbnail of the left hand. This auxiliary method may relieve pain from needling and help the patient in getting needling sensation.

Pricking Method

A needling method, referring to swift and superficial insertion followed by the immediate withdrawal of the needle. Usually used for blood-letting puncture.

Primary Pigmentary Degeneration of Retina

Symptoms. Night blindness and gradual narrowness of visual field which will eventually result in ablepsia.
Pathogenesis. Congenital deficiencies, insufficiency and deficiency of the liver and kidney, failure of vital essence and blood to nourish the eyes.
Therapeutic Principle. Nourishing the liver, replenishing the kidney, invigorating the spleen and promoting the flow of qi.

Prince's-feather Flower ⊛ P-1

It is the inflorescence of Polygonum orientale L. (Polygonaceae).
Effect. Dissipating blood stasis, removing food stagnancy and relieving pain.
Indication. Pain due to disorder of qi in the heart and stomach and dysentery.

Prince's-feather Herb

It is the whole plant of Polygonum orientale L. (Polygonaceae).
Effect. Expelling wind and eliminating dampness.
Indication. Rheumatic arthralgia, hernia, beriberi and sore.

Proctoptosis due to Protracted Dysentery

It refers to the syndrome of prolapse of rectum due to protracted dysentery.
Pathogenesis. Prolonged dysentery and insufficiency of splenogastric qi.
Therapeutic Principle. Invigorating the spleen and replenishing qi.

Profuse Diarrhea

Symptoms. Uncontrollable watery diarrhea, skinny physique, pale complexion, lassitude and asthenia, etc.
Pathogenesis. Deficiency of spleen with over-abundance of dampness.
Therapeutic Principle. Reinforcing the spleen and removing dampness by diuresis.

Prolapsed Hemorrhoid

It refers to the magic flower shape of the hemorrhoid.
Symptoms. Turning inside out of the anus, in the form of a magic flower, dark purple color of the flesh, pain and bleeding.
Pathogenesis. Hemorrhoid and the additional affection of pathogenic heat, the stagnation of qi and blood.
Therapeutic Principle. Removing pathogenic heat from the blood and toxic material from the body.

Prolapse of Rectum of Deficiency Type

Symptoms. Slow onset in the initial phase, distending with feeling of prolapse of anus on defecation, slight prolapse of the lower end of the rectum which may return automatically after defecation, but with the time passing, no return by itself unless it is pushed back; accompanied by sallow complexion, lassitude, listlessness, dizziness, palpitation.

Pathogenesis. Protracted diarrhea and dysentery, multiparity, constitutional insufficiency, collapse of the qi in the middle-energizer resulting in failure of control.

Therapeutic Principle. Supplement qi to make it rise.

Prolapse of Rectum of Excess Type

Symptoms. Mostly seen in acute dysentery and inflammatory hemorrhoids, distending and prolapse feeling of the anus, frequent and urgent sensation of defecation, over-exerting in defecation leading to prolapse of the rectum, accompanied by local redness and swelling, hot sensation, pain and itch.

Pathogenesis. Constipation, hemorrhoids, damp-heat accumulated in the rectum and over-exerting in defecation resulting in impairment of restraint.

Therapeutic Principle. Remove pathogenic damp-heat.

Prolonged Dysentery of Deficiency Type

Symptoms. Persistent uncontrolled dysentery, lassitude of the limbs, indigestion, pain across the abdomen, the frequent desire for defecating, etc.

Pathogenesis. Weakness and the collapse of the spleen-qi, the failure of intestines to astringe.

Therapeutic Principle. Regulating, reinforcing and inducing astringency.

Prone Needling

An acupuncture term.

Method. Withdraw the needle to the subcutaneous level, make it oblique as if it were lying down, for puncturing horizontal or retaining the needle.

Prostatitis

Symptoms. Putrid sperm emitted, mucous turbid discharge during ejaculation, light urine.

Pathogenesis. Excess of alcoholic drinking and sexual intercourse, fire hyperactivity due to insufficiency of the kidney.

Therapeutic Principle. Promoting blood circulation, nourishing yin, eliminating dampness and purging turbid urine.

Prostration due to Sexual Strain

Symptoms. Shortness of breath and fatigue, anorexia, excessive lingering diarrhea, long and thin urine, emission, spermatorrhea, etc.

Pathogenesis. Caused by discharging semen involuntarily too frequently.

Therapeutic Principle. Tonifying the kidney to arrest spontaneous emission.

Protrusion of Tongue

It refers to protruding tongue, which is unable to contract. There are three different types: heat of excess type, deficiency of yin type, and cold of deficiency type.

Symptoms. For above three types, the symptoms are characterized by deep red and swollen tongue with much saliva, dry and fissured tongue, and cold limbs, involuntary drooling and light tongue respectively.

Pathogenesis. Heat of excess type is ascribable to flaring heart-fire; deficiency of yin being in the late stage of febrile disease, impairment of yin and existence of heat; cold of deficiency type to deficiency of yang-qi in the middle-energizer, the spleen and stomach.

Therapeutic Principle. Clearing away the heart-fire, replenishing the vital essence and removing heat, as well as warming and invigorating middle-energizer yang are suitable methods for these three types respectively.

Protuberance of Abdomen

Symptoms. Sudden fullness and distention in abdomen with arm protuberance in the stomach and intestines, and pain in the epigastrium.

Pathogenesis. Improper diet, impairment of regulation of cold and warm, and dysfunction of intestines and stomach.

Therapeutic Principle. Regulating the circulation of qi, relieving distention and expelling stagnation.

Pruritic Dermatosis

Symptoms. Itching eruptions all over the body, itching of the skin with water flowing out when they are torn by scratching, dysphoria with thirst.

Pathogenesis. Mostly caused by the retention of damp-heat in the liver and the spleen, and attack of wind on the skin and muscle.

Therapeutic Principle. Nourishing the blood to expel wind, and detoxicating.

Pruritus Cutis

It refers to one of skin disease, which is itching severely with scratch marks, blood crusts, pachyderma, etc. after being scratched.

Symptoms. Paroxysmal itching which is even serious at night. It usually causes lesions as scratch marks, blood crusts, chromatosis, and leather-transformation due to scratching.

Pathogenesis. Stagnation of damp-heat in the skin which has not been dispelled and removed, or by forming of wind and transformation of dryness, the loss of nourishment of the skin due to blood-heat, blood deficiency and hyperactivity of the liver.

Therapeutic Principle. Clearing away heat, eliminating dampness and expelling the wind, or removing heat from blood, moistening, nourishing the blood and calming the liver.

Pruritus Vulvae

Symptoms. Intolerable pruritus in the vulva of vagina, even with pain in severe cases, vexation, insomnia, restlessness, fullness in the stomach, sticky mouth with bitter taste, dark urine, leukorrhea with yellowish, thick and foul discharge.

Pathogenesis. Excess of dampness due to insufficiency of the spleen, depression of the liver generating pathogenic fire, or dirty vulva, long-time sitting on damp place, and invasion of germs to the vulva.

Therapeutic Principle. Clear heat and promote diuresis in combination with relieving the depressed liver.

Pseudopterygium

Symptoms. Membrane-like or band-like adhesion between the white and black eyeball.

Cause. Traumatic injury of eye or nebula grown at the periphery of the black.

Therapeutic Principle. No need for therapy if the region is tiny enough. Operation advisable if it covers a relatively large area.

Pseudostellaria Root

It is the root ruber of Pseudostellaria heterophylla (Mig.) Pax ex Pax et Hoffm. (Caryophyllaceae).

Effect. Replenishing qi and promoting the production of body fluid.

Indication. Poor appetite due to deficiency of the spleen, lassitude and asthenia, palpitation, spontaneous sweating, cough due to lung-deficiency, thirst due to deficiency of body fluid, loose bowels, etc.

Pterygium

Symptoms. Encroachment of pterygium to the cornea, in the mild case, the affected eye is uncomfortable with astringent itching; in the serious case, the pterygium covers the pupil and affects visual acuity.

Pathogenesis. Obstruction of wind-heat in the Heart Meridian and Lung Meridian due to its sufficiency, qi stagnation and blood stasis.

Therapeutic Principle. Dispersing wind, clearing away heat, nourishing yin, reducing pathogenic fire, removing obstruction in the meridians and dissipating blood stasis. It is also advisable to use the surgical method.

Ptosis of Eyelid

Symptoms. The upper eyelid is unable to lift by itself to cover partially or wholly the pupil. There are the congenital ptosis and acquired ptosis.

Pathogenesis. Congenital deficiencies, insufficiency of the spleen yang which results in inability to control the eyelid, or deficiency of the liver and insufficiency of blood, invasion of the eyelid by wind, or traumatic injury.

Therapeutic Principle. Warming the spleen and nourishing the kidney for the congenital ptosis; nourishing the spleen and stomach to promote the flow of qi and dispelling wind to dredge the meridian for the acquired one. Acupuncture therapy is also applicable.

Puberuious Glochidion Leaf

It is the branch leaf of Glochidion puberum (L.) Hutch. (Euphorbiaceae).

Effect. Clearing away heat to promote diuresis and detoxicating to reduce swelling.

Indication. Dysentery, jaundice, stranguria with turbid urine, leukorrhagia, common cold, swollen and sore throat, ulcerative carbuncles, furuncles, etc.

Puberulous Glochidion Root

It is the root of Glochidion puberum (L.) Hutch. (Euphorbiaceae).

Effect. Clearing away heat to relieve diuresis and promoting blood circulation, detoxication.

Indication. Dysentery, malaria, jaundice, gonorrhea, cough due to overstrain, rheumatic arthralgia, metrorrhagia, metrostaxis, sore throat, toothache, subcutaneous swelling, traumatic injuries, etc.

Pubescent Angelica Root

It is the root of Angelica pubescens Maxim. F. biserrata Shan et Yuan (Umbelliferae).

Effect. Expelling pathogenic wind and dampness, relieving pain and expelling cold and promoting sweating to expel the exogenous evils from the body surface.

Indication. Arthralgia due to wind-dampness, especially arthralgia in the lower part of the body, superficial syndrome of affection by exopathogenic wind-cold with damp-evil, common cold, toothache.

Pucan (B 61)

A meridian acupuncture point.

Location. On the lateral side of the foot, in the depression posterior and inferior to the external malleolus, 1.5 cun directly below Kunlun (B 60).

Indication. Weakness and flaccidity of the lower limbs, pain in the heel, epilepsy, fainting spell, lumbago, beriberi, swelling of the knee.

Method. Puncture perpendicularly 0.3-0.5 cun, and apply moxibustion to the point for 5-10 minutes or 3-5 units of moxa cones.

Pudendum Hernia

Symptoms. Swelling scrotum without itching or painful sensation, numbness and sensation of heaviness, falling, distention and pain.

Pathogenesis. Sitting for a long time on damp earth, resulting in cold-dampness passing down.

Therapeutic Principle. Expelling dampness, regulating the circulation of qi, and removing the stagnation.

Pueraria Flower

It is the flower-bud of Pueraria lobata (Willd.) Ohwi. (Leguminosae).

Effect. Relieving acute alcoholism and activating the spleen.

Indication. Dizziness, headache due to excessive drinking, dysphoria with thirst, fullness in the chest, anorexia, vomiting, acid regurgitation, etc.

Pueraria Root

It is the root of Pueraria lobata (Willd.) Ohwi. (Leguminosae).

Effect. Removing evil factors from the superficies and muscles, invigorating the spleen-yang, promoting the skin eruptions, clearing away heat and promoting the production of body fluid to quench thirst.

Indication. Fever due to exopathy, headache, anhidrosis, stiffness and pain in the neck and back; measles at the early stage, inadequate eruption of measles; diarrhea due to pathogenic damp-heat or deficiency of the spleen, dysphoria with smothery sensation, diabetes, etc.

Pu'er Tea Leaf

It is the leaf of Camellia slinensis O. Ktze. var. assamica Kitamura (Theaceae).

Effect. Promoting meat digestion, eliminating wind phlegm, clearing away heat, removing toxic substances, promoting production of the body fluid to quench thirst.

Indication. Abdominal pain due to eruptive disease, dysentery, etc.

Puff-ball

It is the dried sporophore of Calvatia gigantea (Batsch ex Pers.) Lloyd, C. Lilacina (Mont. et Berk.) Lloyd and Lasiosphara fenzlii Reich. (Lycoperdaceae).

Effect. Clearing away lung heat, relieving sore throat, removing toxic substances and arresting bleeding.

Indication. Cough due to the lung-heat, aphonia, swollen and sore throat, hematemesis, epistaxis, traumatic bleeding, etc.

Puffiness of Eyelid

Symptoms. Swelling, feeble and ball-like eyelid, without suppuration and pain response when pressed, normal skin color.

Pathogenesis. Deficiency of the spleen and lung, or by yang deficiency of the spleen and kidney.

Therapeutic Principle. Invigorating the spleen, replenishing the kidney and promoting the flow of qi.

Pulmonary Cellulitis

Symptoms. Cough with bloody and purulent sputum, stuffiness in the chest, bitter taste in the mouth, melena, etc.

Pathogenesis. Impairment of the meridians and collaterals of the lung and stomach by excessive alcohol.

Therapeutic Principle. Purifying the lung, purging the stomach-fire and removing heat from blood to stop bleeding.

Pulmonary Shock due to Postpartum Putrid Blood

Symptoms. Cough with dyspnea, and blackish color around areas of the mouth and nose.

Pathogenesis. Extravasated blood entering the Lung Meridian.

Therapeutic Principle. Improving the function of the lung, and removing stasis to promote blood circulation.

Pulmonary Tuberculosis

An infectious and chronic prostrating disease.

Symptoms. In the beginning, slight cough, poor appetite, fatigue, sputum mixed with blood. Long term cases manifested by severe cough, afternoon fever, night sweating, dry mouth with a desire to drink a lot, hemoptysis, insomnia, oppressive and painful feeling in the chest, spermatic emission, amenorrhea etc.

Pathogenesis. Deficient vital-qi of the body, decline in resistance and the infection of tubercular bacillus.

Therapeutic Principle. Tonifying the lung and strengthening the spleen.

Pulsatilla Root   ⊛ P-2

It is the root of Pulsatilla chinensis (Bge.) Reg. (Ranunculaceae).

Effect. Clearing away heat, detoxicating and removing heat from the blood to stop diarrhea.

Indication. Dysentery due to damp-heat, fever due to diarrhea caused by toxic heat, abdominal pain, dysentery with pus and blood in the stool, tenesmus.

Pulse Condition

It refers to conditions of the arterial pulse including frequency, rhythm, rate, volume, force, tension, etc. According to the differentiation mentioned above, pulse can be divided into two types: normal and abnormal. The abnormal pulse is important evidence for the physician's diagnosis.

Pulse Feeling and Palpation

It is one of the four diagnostic methods. It consists of pulse feeling and palpation. The palpation is to touch, feel, press a certain part of the body to diagnose diseases combined with inspection, auscultation and olfaction, and interrogation.

Pummelo Peel

It is the external layer of pericarp of Citrus grandis (L.) Osbeck, or C. grandis Tomentosa (Rutaceae).

Effect. Regulating flow of qi to relieve depression, eliminating dampness to remove phlegm.

Indication. Cough, asthma, profuse sputum, dyspepsia and eructation.

Pumpkin Flower

It is the flower of Cucurbita moschata Duch. (Cucurbitaceae).

Effect. Eliminating damp-heat and subduing pyogenic infections.

Indication. Jaundice, dysentery, cough, and superficial infections.

Pumpkin Fruit ⊛ P-3

It is the fruit of Cucurbita moschata Duch. (Cucurbitaceae).

Effect. Tonifying the spleen for restoring qi, relieving inflammation and alleviating pain.

Pumpkin Root

It is the root of Cucurbita moschata Duch. (Cucurbitaceae).

Effect. clearing away heat, expelling dampness and promoting lactation.

Indication. Stranguria, jaundice, dysentery and galactostasis.

Pumpkin Seed

It is the seed of Cucurbita moschata Duch. (Cucurbitaceae).

Effect. Destroying parasites.

Indication. Cestodiasis and ascariasis.

Pumpkin Vine

It is the stem of Cucurbita moschata Duch. (Cucurbitaceae).

Effect. Clearing away heat from the lung, adjusting the stomach qi and removing obstruction in the meridians.

Indication. Slight fever due to pulmonary tuberculosis, stomachache, irregular menstruation and scalds.

Punctate Ardisia Root

It is the root or the whole herb of Ardisia punctata Lindl. (Myrsinaceae).

Effect. Promoting blood circulation to remove blood stasis, regulating menstruation, and eliminating wind-dampness.

Indication. Amenorrhea, dysmenorrhea, rheumatic arthralgia and traumatic injuries.

Punctate Keratitis

It is an oculopathy, referring to many tiny star-like nebula growing in the black.

Symptoms. Astringency, pain, photophobia, lacrimation and blepharal redness and swelling of the affected eye, the star-like nebula of slightly yellowish or greyish-white.

Pathogenesis. Mostly due to internal sufficiency of the liver fire and outward affection of pathogenic wind, or due to yin deficiency of the liver and kidney and flaring up of deficiency fire.

Therapeutic Principle. Removing wind, heat, nourishing yin and reducing the pathogenic fire.

Puncture Cauterization

It is one of the exterior therapeutic methods.

Method. Heat a three-edged needle over fire to red-hot on the 1.5 cm-long tip, dip it in sesame oil then prick the still hot needle 0.15-0.4 cm into the laryngeal tumor or tonsil, according to the size of tumor or tonsil, retain the needle for 1-2 seconds or withdraw it right away.

Puncture the point opposite to the Affected Side

A needling technique. It refers to cross-puncture: Prick the right side when there is illness on the left, and vice versa.

Puncturevine Caltrop Fruit

⊛ P-4

It is the fruit of Tribulus terrestris L. (Zygophyllaceae).

Effect. Calming and soothing the liver yang, dispelling pathogenic wind to alleviate itching and pain and improving eyesight.

Indication. Dizziness and headache due to hyperactivity of the liver-yang; costalgia and galactostasis due to the stagnation of the liver-qi; bloodshot eyes and lacrimation; rubella and pruritus, etc.

Pungent Flavor

Pungent flavor has the dispersing actions from superficies of the body and promoting the circulation of qi and blood. It can be used to treat affection by exopathogens, stagnation of vital energy, blood stasis, etc.

Purgation Helpful to Treat Occlusion

Cases of occlusion of excess type may be cured by drugs with purgative action, e.g.

the drugs with the action of purging intense heat and relieving constipation can be used to treat abdominal distention and pain, constipation, etc.

Purgation to Treat Interior Diseases

Effect. Relaxing the bowels, cleaning away heat and removing excessive fluid.

Indication. High fever, restlessness, abdominal distention and pain, constipation, difficulty in micturition.

Notice. Stop immediately once the therapeutic effect is achieved and should never be overdosed.

Purple-flower Holly Leaf

It is the leaf of Ilex chinensis Sims. (Aquifoliaceae).

Effect. Clearing away heat, detoxicating, removing heat from the blood and promoting tissue regeneration.

Indication. Burns and scalds, ulcer of lower limbs, eczema, carbuncles, sores, furuncles and swellings, traumatic bleeding, etc.

Purple Indian Dropseed Herb

It is the whole herb of Sporobolus indicus (L.) R. Br. var. Purpureosuffusus (Ohwi) Koyama (Gramineae).

Effect. Clearing away heat, coding blood, eliminating pathogenic heat, detoxicating and inducing diuresis.

Indication. Epidemic encephalitis, high fever with coma due to encephalitis B, infective hepatitis, dysentery, stranguria due to heat, hematuria, etc.

Purple Lips

1. Purplish red or purplish dim lip belongs to pyretic syndrome, usually appearing as excessive heat in blood system or blood stasis.

2. Purplish blue belongs to cold, usually appearing as stagnation of cold pathogen or retention and obstruction of blood in the heart.

Purple Perilla Leaf

It is the leaf of Perilla frutescens (L.) Britt var. crispal (Thunb.) Decne. (Labiatae).

Effect. Inducting sweating to disperse cold, promoting flow of qi to alleviate stagnation in the middle-energizer, and detoxicating ichthyotoxicon and crab venom.

Indication. Common cold of wind-cold type, especially with symptoms of stagnation of qi due to oppressed feeling in the chest, stagnation of qi in the spleen and stomach, chest tightness, vomiting, and abdominal pain, vomiting and diarrhea due to eating fish and crabs, etc.

Purple Tongue

The dark purple tongue with prickles, like red bayberry, indicates interior excess of noxious heat; purple, dim and dry tongue, like the color of pig liver, indicates yin exhaustion of the liver and kidney, usually seen in serious and critical condition; purple, dim and moist tongue is a sign of blood stagnation in the interior; light purple, purplish blue and smooth tongue indicates syndrome due to excessive pathogenic cold.

Purplish Rashes

Symptoms. Serious distending pain all over the body with black maculae, and darkish complexion.

Pathogenesis. Accumulation of rash toxin in viscera, and stagnation of qi and blood.

Therapeutic Principle. Pricking the points of Quchi (LI 11), Weizhong (B 40) to cause blood from veins with three-edged needles at first, then inducing vomiting.

Purslane Herb

It is the whole herb of Portulaca oleracea L. (Portulacaceae).

Effect. Clearing away heat and detoxicating, removing pathogenic heat from blood to stop bleeding, expelling dampness and alleviating itching.

Indication. Damp-heat dysentery, dysentery with purulent and bloody stool, leukorrhea with reddish discharge, carbuncles and furuncles due to fire-toxin, erysipelas, heat stranguria, stranguria complicated by hematuria, etc.

Pushing from Mingguan into Hukou

A massage manipulation.

Operation. Push from Mingguan, the palmar side of the distal segment of index finger, into Hukou, the area between the thumb and the index finger, with the whole surface of the thumb, and then nipknead Hukou with the tip of the thumb.

Function. Lowering the adverse flow of qi and generating blood, strengthening the spleen and promoting digestion.

Indication. Deficiency-weakness of the spleen and stomach, disharmony between blood and qi.

Pushing Manipulation

A massage manipulation.

Operation. Push and squeeze straight on the certain part in one direction with the finger, palm or elbow.

Function. Clearing the meridians and collaterals, regulating qi, removing stasis of blood, etc.

Indication. Muscular tension, spasm and local pain.

Pushing-pressing Manipulation with Thumb

A massage manipulation.

Operation. Press the point on the patient's body surface with the tip of the thumb.

Function. Resuscitation, promoting the blood circulation to relieve pain and regulating functions of zang-fu.

Indication. Spasm and pain of the epigastrium, painful the waist and legs, etc.

Pyogenic Infection of Back of Hand

Symptoms. At the beginning it is like awn, gradually it feels painful. In severe case, much swelling, red color, flourishing, burning heat and quick ulceration, or stretching swelling, hardness, absence of red color, heat, and slow ulceration.

Pathogenesis. Stagnation of wind-fire and damp-heat in the three yang meridians.

Therapeutic Principle. Relieving superficies syndrome by means of diaphoresis, and detoxicating.

Pyretic Stroke

One kind of apoplectic stroke.

Symptoms. Sudden coma, unconsciousness, reddish face, excessive thirst, paralysis, constipation, etc.

Pathogenesis. Mostly caused by failure of the power of qi to be in charge of blood circulation, sufficiency of the heart-fire, or insufficiency of the kidney-yang, and upward flow of deficient fire, resulting in mental disturbance.

Therapeutic Principle. Eliminate heart-fire impeded orifice to restore consciousness, or nourishing yin to reduce pathogenic fire.

Pyrexia Malaria

1. It refers to malaria with high fever.

   Symptoms. High fever with mild chills, hypohidrosis, headache, arthralgia, thirst with preference to drink, constipation and turbid urine, etc.

   Pathogenesis. Latent heat and further attacking by pathogenic malaria.

   Therapeutic Principle. Nourishing yin, promoting the production of the body fluid, clearing away heat, and expelling pathogenic factors from muscles and skin.

2. It refers to renal malaria.

   Symptoms. Muscle emaciation, carbuncle of the nape, restlessness and fever, relieved fever followed by aversion to cold, etc.

   Pathogenesis. Latent heat and further attacking by summer-heat.

   Therapeutic Principle. Nourishing the kidney and yin.

Pyrite

It is the mineral ore containing ferric sulfide of natural pyrite.

Effect. Removing blood stasis, to relieve pain, promoting reunion of fractured bone and curing wounds.

Indication. Traumatic injuries, fracture and swelling pain due to blood stasis.

Pyrolusite

It is the ore of Pyrolusite, which is the mineral of oxide.

Effect. Removing blood stasis, relieving pain, subduing swelling and promoting regeneration of the tissue.

Indication. Traumatic injuries, cutting wounds, superficial infections etc.

Pyrrosia Leaf   ✿ P-5

It is the leaf of Pyrrosia sheareri (Bak.) Ching. and P. petiolosa (Christ) Ching, or P. lingua (Thunb.) Farw. (Polypodiaceae).

Effect. Inducing diuresis, relieving urinary stranguria, clearing away lung heat, relieving cough and cooling blood to stop bleeding.

Indication. Heat stranguria, stranguria caused by the passage of urinary stone, stranguria complicated by hematuria, edema, metrorrhagia, metrostaxis, hemoptysis and epistaxis. Recently also used for acute and chronic dysentery and leukopenia.

Q

Qi

There are three meanings:

1. Qi in its physiological sense is referred to as the vital energy or basic element comprising the human body and maintaining its life activities, such as qi of the food, i.e., food energy, qi of respiration, i.e. the breathed air.

2. Since qi is invisible and its existence in the human body can only be perceived through its resulting activities of organs and tissues, it is more often referred to as physiological functions of viscera, such as the qi of zang-fu organs, i.e., the functional activities of zang-fu organs.

3. Qi can be used in pathogenic sense. In this case, it means pathogenic element or pathogenic factors.

Qi and Blood Deficiency

It refers to the syndrome that blood deficiency and qi deficiency exist simultaneously.

Symptoms. Pallid countenance or chlorosis, short breath, disinclination to talk, fatigue, vertigo, weak body, palpitation, insomnia, and numbness of extremities.

Therapeutic Principle. Replenishing qi and enriching blood.

Qi and Blood Deficiency in Heart and Spleen

Symptoms. Palpitation, dizziness, anorexia, dream-disturbed sleep, loose stool, fatigue and weakness, sallow face, stool with blood, subcutaneous hemorrhage, usually seen in neurosis or anemia.

Therapeutic Principle. Tonifying the heart and spleen.

Qianding (GV 21)

An acupuncture point.

Location. On the head, 3.5 cun directly above the midpoint of the anterior hairline and 1.5 cun anterior to Baihui (GV 20).

Indication. Epilepsy, vertigo, dizziness, pain in the vertex, rhinorrhea with turbid discharge, redness, swelling and pain of the eyes, infantile convulsion.

Method. Puncturing subcutaneously backward 0.5-0.8 cun, and applying moxibustion to the point with 3-5 units of moxa cones or for 5-10 minutes.

Qi and Yin Deficiency

It refers to the symptoms due to exhaustion of yin liquids and yang qi existing simultaneously. And it is common in the course of febrile disease and some chronic consumptive diseases.

Therapeutic Principle. Supplementing qi and nourishing yin.

Qianfaji Point (Ex-HN)

An extra point.

Location. 3 cun directly above Taiyang (Ex-HN 5), on the hairline.

Indication. Deep rooted sore at the face.

Method. Puncture subcutaneously 0.3-0.5 cun. Apply moxibustion 1-3 moxa cones or 5-10 minutes with warming moxibustion.

Qiangjian (GV 18)

An acupuncture point.

Location. On the midline of the head, 4 cun within the posterior hairline, i.e. 3 cun posterior to Baihui(GV 20).

Indication. Headache, dizziness, stiffness and pain of the neck and nape, manic-depressive disorder, epilepsy, dysphoria, insomnia, thirst.

Method. Puncturing 0.5-0.8 cun horizontally along the skin and applying moxibustion to the point for 5-10 minutes.

Qiangu (SI 2)

An acupuncture point.

Location. On the ulnar side of the hand, at the junction between the reddish and whitish skin at the end of the metacarpophalangeal transverse crease, anterior to the fifth metacarpophalangeal joint of the little finger with the fist slightly clenched.

Indication. Febrile disease without sweating, headache, tinnitus, deafness, swollen neck, sore throat, cought with fullness sensation in chest, palmar fever, pain and inability of fingers to clench, agalactia after delivery, brachialgia, contracture of the elbow.

Method. Puncturing perpendicularly 0.3-0.5 cun and applying moxibustion to the point 3-5 moxa cones or for 5-10 minutes.

Qiangyin Point

An acupuncture point belonging to the extraordinary points.

Location. Lateral to the laryngeal protuberance posterior and superior to Renying (S 9).

Indication. Muteness, and aphasia.

Method. Puncturing obliquely 1.0-1.5 cun towards the root of tongue.

Qianshencong (Ex-HN)

An extra acupuncture point, one of shencong.

Location. On the head, 4 cun above the midpoint of the anterior hairline, 1 cun anterior to Baihui (GV 20).

Indication. Apoplexy, headache, dizziness, epilepsy.

Method. Puncturing horizontally 0.3-0.5 cun along the skin and applying moxibustion: 1-3 moxa cones or 3-5 minutes with warming moxibustion.

Qianzheng (Ex-HN)

An extra acupuncture point.

Location. 0.5 cun anterior to the ear lobe, on the level of the midpoint of the ear lobe.

Indication. Facial paralysis, parotitis, ulcer in the oral cavity.

Method. Puncturing obliquely or subcutaneously 0.5-1 cun and applying moxibustion.

Qi as Commander of Blood

Qi serves as the dynamic force of blood flow, drives the blood circulating within the vessels, and promotes blood regeneration. Qi in motion renders blood circulating normally, and qi stagnation usually leads to blood stasis. When qi is sufficient, the ability to make blood is strong, whereas if qi is deficient, the blood is insufficient. The insufficiency of the spleen-qi and the excess of qi and fire bring about bleeding.

Qi as Mechanism of Guiding Body Fluid

It refers to qi having the function of regulating and controlling the excretion of body fluid. The balance of the metabolism of body fluid can be kept only by qi functional activity.

Qichong (S 30)

1. An acupuncture point.

    Location. Slightly superior to the groin, 5 cun below the umbilicus, 2 cun lateral to the anterior midline.

    Indication. Abdomen pain, hernia, irregular menstruation, morbid leukorrhea, impotence and stranguria, swelling of the vulva.

    Method. Puncturing perpendicularly 0.5-1 cun and applying moxibustion to the point with 3-5 units of moxa cones or for 5-10 minutes.

2. It is one of the extraordinary points, also called Qitang.

    Location. On the median line of the neck, at the middle on the connecting line between the thyroid notch and the notch of the presternum superior to the neck.

Indication. Cough, asthma.

Method. Puncturing perpendicularly 0.2-0.3 cun and applying moxibustion to the point with 3-7 units of moxa cones or for 5-15 minutes.

Qi Closed in Laterals

Symptoms. Pain and heavy feeling in the body, and less free movement.

Pathogenesis. Collateral branch of the large meridian is obstructed in the body, where blood stasis and stagnation of qi will occur.

Qi Deficiency

1. It refers generally to denoting the decline and weakness of the visceral vital energy.

   Symptoms. Shortness of breath, weak voice, lassitude, mental fatigue, dizziness with blurred vision, and spontaneous perspiration.

   Pathogenesis. Constitutional deficiency due to long suffering from illness, overfatigue, senile weakness, etc.

   Therapeutic Principle. Replenishing qi.

2. Particularly denoting hypofunction of the lung.

Qi Deficiency Causing Blood Stasis

It is a morbid state of slow flow and even stasis of the blood.

Symptoms. Stabbing pain fixed in location together with listlessness, lassitude, shortness of breath, etc.

Pathogenesis. Qi deficiency, which makes the function of propelling and warming blood disturbed.

Qi Deficiency Causing Cold-syndrome

It refers to the yin cold resulting from yang-qi deficiency, which fails to warm and nourish zang-fu organs; therefore, hypofunction and hypometabolism of these organs occur.

Symptoms. Aversion to cold, cold extremities, tiredness, pale face and tongue, clear urine, loose stool.

Qi Deficiency in Heart and Lung

Symptoms. Prolongation cough, shortness of breath, palpitation pale face, or even cyanotic lips, pale tongue and thready, weak pulse.

Pathogenesis. Deficiency of the lung-qi, which leads to insufficiency of the heart-qi or vice versa.

Therapeutic Principle. Invigorating lung-qi.

Qi Deficiency in Middle-energizer

Symptoms. Dull yellow complexion, abdominal distention after meals, dizziness, shortness of breath, fatigue, stomachache relieved by pressing, pale lips, thick tongue fur and weak pulse.

Pathogenesis. Hypofunction of the spleen and stomach.

Therapeutic Principle. Invigorating the spleen and replenishing qi.

Qi Deficiency of Spleen and Lung

Symptoms. Prolonged cough, shortness of breath, dyspnea, abundant expectoration, thin and white sputum, poor appetite, abdominal distention, fatigue, pale complexion, or edema of face and feet.

Pathogenesis. Prolonged illness and cough with dyspnea, or spleen impairment resulting from improper diet and overstrain. In turn, the spleen fails to transport essence of life to the lung.

Therapeutic Principle. Invigorating the spleen and benefiting the lung.

Qi Disorder

It refers to dysfunction of the internal organs at large, especially functional derangement in ascending and descending of qi.

Symptoms. Hiccups, stuffiness feeling in the chest, abdominal distention, and diarrhea.

Qi Downward

It refers to the pathological changes or failure of keeping the body fluid flowing normally due to the exhaustion of qi.

Symptoms. Distention and fullness, spermatorrhoea, enuresis, urinary and fecal incontinence, etc.

Qiduan (Ex-LE 12)

An extra point.

Location. Ten points at the tips of the 10 toes of both feet, 0.1 cun from the free margin of each toe nail.

Indication. Beriberi, paralysis and numbness of the toes, pain and swelling of the dorsum, and also first aid for apoplexy.

Method. Puncturing perpendicularly 0.1-0.2 cun or prick to cause little bleeding with a triangular needle and applying moxibustion with 1-3 moxa cones or 3-5 minutes with warming moxibustion.

Qi due to Pathogenic Cold

Symptoms. Shortness of breath, cold pain in the epigastrium and abdomen, aversion to cold and arthralgia, etc.

Pathogenesis. Qi of collaterals of viscera struggling with pathogenic cold.

Therapeutic Principle. Warming yang and dispelling cold.

Qi Dysphagia

Symptoms. Obstruction in swallowing, fullness sensation or pain in epigastrium, belching, or vomiting, etc.

Pathogenesis. Disorder of qi which is obstructed in the epigastric region.

Therapeutic Principle. Relieving stagnation and checking upward adverse flow of the lung-qi and stomach-qi, and resolving phlegm and removing obstruction in epigastric region.

Qi Exhaustion

Symptoms. In the case of deficiency type: shortness of breath that worsens at night, lacking in strength, withered skin and hair; in the case of excess type: dyspnea, fullness sensation in the chest, tendency to anger, dry mouth and throat, spitting blood, feverish sensation, profuse sweating, etc.

Pathogenesis. Insufficiency of the visceral qi and invasion by pathogenic factors or severe bleeding.

Therapeutic Principle. For the deficiency type: replenishing qi; for the last type: soothing the liver and regulating the flow of qi.

Qi Exhaustion due to Over-fatigue

It refers to exhaustion of vital essence and energy of the body due to overexertion, including physical and mental overwork, and excess of sexual intercourse.

Symptoms. Tiredness, lassitude, etc.

Qi Exhaustion Resulting from Hemorrhea

Referring to the collapse resulting from qi exhaustion due to hemorrhea.

Symptoms. Pale complexion, cold limbs, profuse sweating, thready and barely perceptible pulse, as seen in the hemorrhagic shock.

Therapeutic Principle. Hemostasis by invigorating qi, or recuperating depleted yang to stop bleeding.

Qi failure to Transform Body Fluid

Symptoms. Light red and dry tongue.

Pathogenesis. Deficiency of both the heart and spleen, and insufficiency of qi and blood, or at the late stage of epidemic febrile disease, deficiency of qi, blood and failure of body fluid to nourish the tongue.

Qi Function of Promoting Metabolism and Transformation

It refers to the metabolism of essence, qi, blood and body fluid and the transformations occurring between them, e.g. ingested food is changed into food essence, and food essence, in turn, transformed into qi, blood, and body fluid, the process of which is, in practice, the process of substances metabolising in the body, and the process of substances and energy transformation. In a narrow sense, it means the functional activities of the tri-energizer.

Qi Goiter

It refers to the soft masses in the sick area, which may subdue or enlarge with joy or anger.

Pathogenesis. Emotion depression or natural environment and climate or geographical factors.

Therapeutic Principle. Soothing the liver and regulating the circulation of qi, and regulating qi by alleviation of mental depression and promoting the subsidence of swelling.

Qigong

It refers to a method of physical and mental self-exercise. It is mainly by keeping a proper posture, adjusting breathing and concentrating the mind and uniting vital essence and energy and mentality as a whole for physical training, health preservation, and prevention and treatment of diseases.

Effect. Regulating and strengthening the functions of the various parts of the human body, inducing and developing the internal potential, preventing and curing diseases, protecting and strengthening health, supplementing Qigong intelligence and prolonging life.

It can be divided into dynamic and static Qigong according to the dynamic and static postures in its practice.

Qihai (CV 6)

An acupuncture point.

Location. On the lower abdomen on the anterior midline, 1.5 cun below the center of the umbilicus.

Indication. Abdominal pain around the navel, edema and tympanites, distention and fullness in the stomach and abdomen, constipation, diarrhea, enuresis, emission, impotence, hernia, irregular menstruation, metrorrhagia and metrostaxis, prolapse of uterus, lochiorrhea after delivery, myasthenia of limbs.

Method. Puncturing perpendicularly 0.5-1.0 cun, and applying moxibustion to the point with 3-7 unit of moxa cones or for 15-30 minutes.

Notice. Use with caution in pregnant women.

Qihaishu (B 24)

An acupuncture point.

Location. 1.5 cun lateral and inferior to the spinous process of the third thoracic vertebra.

Indication. Lumbago, immovable legs and knee, dysmenorrhea, irregular menstruation, metrorrhagia, metrostaxis, numbness and pain of lower limbs.

Method. Puncturing perpendicularly 0.5-1 cun and applying moxibustion to the point with 3-7 units of moxa cones or for 5-15 minutes.

Qihu (S 13)

An acupuncture point.

Location. On the chest, below the midpoint of the lower border of the clavicle, 4 cun lateral to the anterior midline.

Indication. Asthma, cough, distention and fullness and pain in the chest and hypochondrium, hematemesis, hiccups, back and hypochondrium.

Method. Puncturing perpendicularly 0.2-0.4 cun. Deep insertion is contraindicated. And applying moxibustion 3-5 moxa cones or 5-10 minutes with warming moxibustion.

Qi-lifting Method

A needling technique.

Method. First swiftly lifting and slowly thrusting the needle 6 times and gaining qi, the needling sensation, then twirling the needle slightly and lifting it gently to strengthen the needling sensation.

Indication. Regional numbness and cold feeling.

Qimai (TE 18)

An acupuncture point.

Location. In the head, in the center of the mastoid process behind the ear, between Yifeng (TE 17) and Jiaosun (TE 20), at the junction of the upper and middle third of the line along the helix.

Indication. Headache, deafness, blurred vision, infantile epilepsy due to fright, clonic convulsion, vomiting, etc.

Method. Puncturing 0.3-0.5 cun horizontally along the skin and applying moxibustion to the point for 3-5 minutes or 1-3 units of moxa cones.

Qimen (Ex-CA)

1. A term in TCM, referring to pores of a sweat duct, which is the opening of discharging yang-qi of the body.
2. An extra point.

   Location. On the lower abdomen, 3 cun lateral to Guanyuan (CV 4).

   Indication. Metrorrhagia, metrostaxis, prolapse of uterus, stranguria, anuresis, hernia, orchitis.

   Method. Puncturing perpendicularly 1.0-1.5 cun, applying moxibustion with 3-5 moxa cones or for 5-15 minutes.

   Notice. In the case of a pregnant woman, it is prohibited.

Qimen (Liv 14)

An acupuncture point.

Location. On the chest, directly below the nipple, in the 6th intercostal space, 4 cun lateral to the anterior midline.

Indication. Pain, distention and fullness in the chest and hypochondriac region, vomiting, cough, sensation of gas rushing, invasion of heat in the blood chamber due to febrile disease.

Method. Puncturing obliquely 0.5-0.8 cun and applying moxibustion to the point with 3-7 units of moxa cones or for 5-15 minutes.

Qi-moving Method

A needling technique.

Method. First inserting the needle 0.7 cun, then performing quick thrust and slow lift of the needle 9 times. Inserting the needle 1 cun deep after the needling reaction has been obtained, lifting the needle slightly and then inserting it to the original place. Performing all this repeatedly so as to relieve the stagnation of qi and resolve masses.

Qi Needle

1. A type of needle, referring to a filiform needle, contrary to a fire needle.
2. An acupuncture therapy, the method of injecting sterilized air or oxygen into an acupuncture point with an injector.

   Indication. Acute of chronic soft tissue injury and stiffness, etc.

Qinglengyuan (TE 11)

An acupuncture point.

Location. On the dorsum of the forearm, 2 cun to the tip of the elbow with the elbow flexed (olecranon).

Indication. Headache, yellowish eye, pain of elbow, arm and shoulder.

Method. Puncturing perpendicularly 0.8-1.2 cun and applying moxibustion 3-7 moxa cones or for 5-15 minutes.

Qingling (H 2)

An acupuncture point.

Location. On the internal side of the arm, on the connecting line between Jiquan (H 1) and Shaohai (H 3), 3 cun superior to the cubital transverse crease, in the anterior groove of the humeral biceps muscle.

Indication. Headache, yellowish eye, hypochondriac pain, scrofula, redness, swelling and pain of shoulder and back.

Method. Puncturing perpendicularly 0.5-1 cun and applying moxibustion with 3-7 units of moxa cones or for 5-10 minutes.

Qing Mass

Symptoms. Mass formation in the right hypochondrium near the back, involving the area from the shoulder blade to the leg, contracture of the waist, edema in the feet, yellowish complexion and eyes, difficult excretion of stool and urine, amenorrhea or metrorrhagia, which affects child-bearing.

Pathogenesis. Accumulation and combination of turbid blood and pathogenic wind-dampness after postpartum female with careless nutrient ingestion.

Therapeutic Principle. Expelling wind to clear away dampness and promoting blood circulation to remove stasis.

Qi of Vital Meridian Ascending Adversely

Symptoms. Qi rushing from the lower abdomen to the chest and throat accompanied by cold limbs, dysuria, or burning cheeks, dizziness and dim eyesight.

Pathogenesis. Recurrent fluid retention, hypofunction of the kidney-yang and qi of the vital meridian ascending adversely with the excessive fluid.

Therapeutic Principle. Lowering the adverse flow of qi.

Qi Pathway

1. It refers to the pathway where qi of the meridian and collateral passes, whose range is beyond the major meridians. There are four such pathways: the pathway of qi in the chest, the pathway of qi in the abdomen, the pathway of qi in the head and the pathway of qi in the nape.

Qi-phase Syndrome

It refers to the syndrome of dysfunction of qi due to the invasion of pathogenic factors to the Yangming Meridian or the lung, gallbladder, spleen, stomach or large intestine.

Symptoms. High fever without chills, dire thirst, flushed face, scanty urine, constipation, ect.

Qi Promoting Circulation of Body Fluid

It refers to the fact that the transportation and distribution of the body fluid and the excretion of sweat and urine to keep physiological balance of the metabolism of body fluid depend on the movement of ascending, descending, flowing-in, and flowing-out of qi.

Qi-promoting due to Cooperation of Respiration

It refers to the method by which the transmission of needling sensation is controlled in cooperation with the patient's respiration. If the patient's diseased part is located below the acupuncture point, it is advisable to thrust the needle, when the patient is exhaling, in order to promote the downward flow of qi; when the patient is inhaling, to promote the upward flow of qi, lifting the needle is applicable to the sick with the diseased part located above the acupuncture point.

Qi Promoting Formation of Body Fluid

It refers to the fact that the body fluid comes from water and food, which is formed in the process of digestion in the stomach and transformation of the spleen. When the qi of the stomach and spleen is sufficient, the body fluid is abundant. When qi is deficient, the functions of the spleen and stomach are affected, and body fluid is insufficient.

Qi-promoting Method

A needling manipulation, referring to all kinds of manipulation promoting needling sensation to be spread and transmitted, mainly including qi-promoting by lifting and thrusting, qi-promoting by exhaling and inhaling, qi-promoting by twirling and rotating, etc. This method can also be named the qi-regulating method.

Qi Restrained

It refers to restraining qi inside and obstruction of functional activities of qi.

Symptoms. Dyspnea due to cold in the chest, abdominal distention, etc.

Pathogenesis. Cold invading exterior and stuffing up of the barrier of the skin.

Qishangxiawufen Points (Ex-CA)

Location. On the abdomen, 0.5 cun above and below the umbilicus.

Indication. Infantile fontanel sinking, enteritis, dysentery, edema, pain due to hernia, borborygmus, abdominal distention and tympanites, gynecological diseases, etc.

Method. Puncturing perpendicularly 0.5-1 cun and applying moxibustion.

Qishe (S 11)

An acupuncture point.

Location. On the neck, at the superior border of the interior end of the clavicle, between the sternal tip of the sternocleidomastoid muscle and the clavicular tip.

Indication. Swelling and pain of throat, cough with dyspnea, dysphagia, rigidity and pain of neck, goiter, scrofula, swollen shoulder etc.

Method. Puncturing perpendicularly 0.3-0.5 cun and applying moxibustion to the point with 3-5 moxa cones or for 5-10 minutes.

Qi Sinking of Tri-energizer

Symptoms. Anorexia, loose stools, abdominal distention after eating, short breath, lassitude, prolapse of the anus, frequent urination, prolapse of the uterus, etc.

Pathogenesis. Improper diet and overstrain or prolonged illness resulting in insufficiency of the spleen yang, sinking of the spleen qi and its inability to sending food essence upward.

Therapeutic Principle. Reinforce the middle-energizer and promote qi circulation and elevate the spleen yang.

Qi Stagnation

It refers to the obstruction of qi in zang-fu organs and meridians.

Symptoms. Feeling of distention in the chest, emotional depression and pain in the hypochondrium, irritability and irascibility, anorexia, and menstrual disorders in woman.

Pathogenesis. Emotional depression, or the block of phlegm, dampness, retention of food, blood stasis, weak body and qi deficiency. The symptoms vary in different zang-fu organs and different meridians and collaterals.

Therapeutic Principle. Mainly soothing the liver and promoting qi circulation to alleviate mental depression.

Qi Stagnation due to Anger

Symptoms. Distending pain in the chest and abdomen, irregular breathing after anger, etc.

Therapeutic Principle. 1. In the case of injury to the liver by violent rage and alternate attack of distention and pain, removing stagnation and relaxing qi. 2. In the case of fire produced by depression and anger, even accompanied by dysphoria with smothery sensation, vomiting blood, epistaxis, etc., relaxing the liver, clearing away heat and removing heat from blood.

Qi Stranguria

Symptoms. Fullness and weighing down in the lower abdomen, astringent and painful micturition, etc.

Pathogenesis. Deficiency of the spleen and kidney, and heat accumulation in the urinary bladder.

Therapeutic Principle. Invigorating the spleen and replenishing qi, inducing diuresis.

Qi Tumefaction

It refers to the edema caused by the stagnation of qi.

Symptoms. Thick skin and pale complexion, lean limbs, hypochondriac distention, and fullness swelling, rising immediately after removing the pressed hand, etc.

Therapeutic Principle. Relieving the edema by regulating the circulation of qi, and eliminating dampness to relieve the fullness.

Qiuhou(Ex-HN 7)

An extra acupuncture point.

Location. At the crossing point of the lateral one-quarter and medial three-quarters of the lower border of the orbit.

Indication. Optic atrophy, optic neuritis, glaucoma, myopia, vitreous opacity, internal strabismus.

Method. In acupuncture, ask the patient to look up and gently stabilize the eye ball with the concerned fingers and puncturing perpendicularly 0.3-0.5 cun with the needle point towards the interior superior of optic foramen and with the lift-thrust but without rotation procedures. After withdrawal of the needle, press the puncture site gently for 2-3 minutes to avoid bleeding.

Qiuxu (G 40)

An acupuncture point.

Location. Anterior and inferior to the external malleolus, in the excavation on the exterior side of the long extensor tendon of the toe.

Indication. Fullness sensation in chest, flaccidity and numbness of lower limb, rigidity and pain of nape, spasm of sore foot, beriberi and nebula.

Method. Puncturing perpendicularly 0.5-0.8 cun and applying moxibustion to the point 1-3 moxa cones or for 5-10 minutes.

Qixue (K 13)

An acupuncture point.

Location. In the lower abdomen, 3 cun below the centre of the umbilicus and 0.5 cun lateral to the anterior median line.

Indication. Irregular menstruation, sterility, flatulence, diarrhea, dysentery, backache and impotence.

Method. Puncturing perpendicularly 1-1.5 cun and applying moxibustion to the point with 3-5 units of moxa cones or for 5-10 minutes.

Qizhongsibian (Ex-CA)

Extra acupuncture points.

Location. On the abdomen, at the centre of umbilicus and 1 cun superior, inferior and lateral to the umbilicus.

Indication. Chronic enteritis, all kinds of infantile spasm, abdominal pain, gastric spasm, edema, pain due to hernia, indigestion, etc.

Method. Puncturing perpendicularly 0.5-1 cun and applying moxibustion 5-7 moxa cones or 5-15 minutes with warming moxibustion.

Qizhuma (Ex-B)

Extra acupuncture point.

Location. On the back, about 1 cun lateral to the 10th thoracic vertebra.

Indication. Nameless swelling and poison, acute appendicitis, toothache, tumor, jaundice due to wind pathogen, obstinate module and scrofula, carbuncle, cellulitis, furuncle and sore on the lower part of the limbs.

Method. Apply moxibustion 3-7 moxa cones or 5-15 minutes with warming moxibustion.

Quail

It is the meat or whole body of Coturnix coturnix japonica Temminck et Schlegel (Phasianidae).

Effect. Tonifying and benefiting the five viscera, reinforcing the middle-energizer, promoting flow of qi, strengthening the muscles and tendons, removing mass-heat and promoting diuresis.

Indication. Diarrhea, dysentery, infantile malnutrition, damp arthralgia syndrome, etc.

Quanjianxue (Ex-UE)

An extra acupuncture point.
Location. On the dorsum of the hand, at the high point of the small head of the third metacarpal bone, fixing the point when a fist is made.
Indication. Congestive eyes, ocular pain, vitiligo, wart.
Method. Apply moxibustion 3-5 moxa cones.

Quanliao (SI 18)

An acupuncture point.
Location. On the face, directly below the outer canthus, in the depression of the lower border of the zygoma.
Indication. Deviated mouth and eyes, tremor of eyelids, swelling of the cheek, toothache, swollen lips, etc.
Method. Puncturing perpendicularly 0.3-0.5 cun obliquely 0.5-1.0 cun. Moxibustion is forbidden.

Quanmen (Ex-CA)

An extra acupuncture point.
Location. In the inferior border of pubic symphysis, superior to the anterior commissure of labia.
Indication. Sterility, leukorrhea with reddish discharge.
Method. Apply moxibustion 1-3 moxa cones or 5-10 minutes with warming moxibustion.

Quanyin (Ex-CA)

An extra acupuncture point.
Location. On the lower abdomen, 3 cun lateral to the point Qugu (CV 2) on the upper border of the pubic symphysis.
Indication. Swelling with bearing-down pain of one testis, orchitis.
Method. Puncturing perpendicularly 0.3-1.0 cun and applying moxibustion with 3-5 moxa cones or 5-10 minutes.

Quartan Malaria

It is a type of malaria, which attacks every two days.
Pathogenesis. Intrinsic deficiency of renal qi, the failure of superficial qi to protect the body against diseases, and the latency of malaria pathogenic factor in three-yin.
Therapeutic Principle. Strengthening the body resistance to consolidate constitution simultaneously with eliminating pathogenic factors.

Qubin (G 7)

An acupuncture point.
Location. On the head, at the crossing point between the vertical line of the anterior auricular temple at the posterior border of the hairline and the horizontal line of the auricular tip, at the level of Jiaosun (TE 20).
Indication. Migraine, swelling chin and cheek, lockjaw, sudden aphonia, vomiting, toothache, facial hemiparalysis, rigidity and spasm of neck.
Method. Puncturing subcutaneously 0.3-0.5 cun and applying moxibustion to the point with 1-3 units of moxa cones or for 3-5 minutes.

Qucha (B 4)

An acupuncture point.
Location. On the head, 0.5 cun directly above the midpoint of the anterior hairline and 1.5 cun lateral to Shenting (GV 24), at the junction of the medial and middle 1/3 of the line connecting Shenting (GV 24) and Touwei (S 8).
Indication. Headache, dizziness, stuffy nose, epistaxis, pyogenic infection of nose.
Method. Puncture subcutaneously 0.3-0.5 cun. Moxibustion is forbidden.

Quchi (Ex-LE)

An extra acupuncture point.
Location. On the medial side of dorsum of foot, anterior and inferior to the medial malleolus, in the depression between the tendons of the long extensor muscle of the great toe and the anterior tibial muscle.

Indication. Pain in the sides of lower abdomen, emission, hernia.

Method. Puncture perpendicularly 0.3-0.5 cun and apply moxibustion with 3-5 moxa cones or for 5-15 minutes.

Quchi (LI 11)

An acupuncture point.

Location. With the elbow flexed to form a right angle, at the lateral end of the cubital crease, at the midpoint of the line connecting Chize (L 5) and the external humeral epicondyle.

Indication. Febrile disease, sore throat, swelling and pain of the arm, irregular menstruation, scrofula, sore, erysipelas, abdominal pain with vomiting and diarrhea, dysentery, hypertension, vexation and fullness in the chest, clonic convulsion, depressive psychosis, malarial disease.

Method. Puncture perpendicularly 0.8-1.2 cun and apply moxibustion to the point with 3-5 units of moxa cones or for 5-10 minutes.

Quepen (S 12)

An acupuncture point.

Location. At the centre of the supraclavicular fossa, 4 cun lateral to the anterior midline.

Indication. Cough, asthma, swelling and pain of throat, pain in the supraclavicular fossa, scrofula, numbness of upper limb.

Method. Puncturing perpendicularly 0.2-0.4 cun and applying moxibustion to the point with 3-5 units of moxa cones or for 5-10 minutes.

Notice. Deep needling is forbidden.

Qugu (CV 2)

An acupuncture point.

Location. In the lower abdomen, at the middle of the superior border of the pubic symphysis on the anterior median line.

Indication. Distending pain of lower abdomen, dribbling urination, seminal emission, impotence, irregular menstruation, leukorrhea with reddish discharge, and enuresis.

Method. Puncturing perpendicularly 1-1.5 cun, and applying moxibustion to the point with 3-7 units of moxa cones or for 10-20 minutes.

Notice. Pay cautious attention when applying it to a pregnant woman.

Quick Cupping

Method. Apply the cup on the affected area and remove it at once. Do the same thing many times over the same area until the skin becomes hyperemic red.

Indication. Local skin numbness and miopragia of deficiency type.

Quisqualis Fruit

It is the fruit of Quisqualis indica L. (Combretaceae).

Effect. Poisoning and expelling parasites in the intestines and removing stagnation of food.

Indication. Ascariasis, abdominal pain due to parasitic infestation and infantile indigestion with food retention.

Ququan (Liv 8)

An acupuncture point.

Location. On the medial side of the knee, at the medial end of the popliteal crease when the knee is flexed, posterior to the medial epicondyle of the tibia, in the depression of the anterior border of the insertions of the semi-menbranous and semi-tendinous muscles.

Indication. Irregular menstruation, leukorrhea, prolapse of uterus, enuresis postpartum abdominal pain, emission, impotence, hernia, dysentery, headache, dizziness, manic-depressive disorders, swelling and pain of the front of the knee, flaccidity and numbness of the lower limbs.

Method. Puncturing perpendicularly 1.0-1.5 cun and applying moxibustion to the point with 3-5 units of moxa cones or for 5-10 minutes.

Quyuan (SI 13)

An acupuncture point.

Location. On the scapula, at the medial end of the suprascapula fossa, at the midpoint of the line connecting Naoshu (SI 10) and the spinous process of the 2nd thoracic vertebra.

Indication. Muscular contracture and pain of the scapula.

Method. Puncturing perpendicularly 0.3-0.5 cun. Oblique needling in the direction of the superior part of greater supraclavicular fossa should be avoided for fear of injuring the lung. Apply moxibustion 3-7 moxa cones or 5-15 minutes with warming moxibustion.

Quze (P 3)

An acupuncture point.

Location. On the transverse cubital crease, at the ulnar border of the tendon of the brachial biceps.

Indication. Cardialgia, palpitation, vexation due to febrile disease, fullness sensation in chest, cough with dyspnea, stomachache, vomiting, dry mouth, and spasm of cubital and brachial tendons.

Method. Puncturing perpendicularly 0.5-0.8 cun or prick the point to cause little bleeding, and applying moxibustion to the point for 3-5 minutes.

R

Rachialgia

Symptoms. Rachialgia, nape stiffness, even lumbago with the broken sensation and pulling sensation of the nape, or constant rachialgia caused by excess of sexual intercourse, lingering spinal pain.

Pathogenesis. The Bladder Meridian is attacked by pathogen, and the Back Middle Meridian is invaded by wind-cold.

Therapeutic Principle. Expelling wind, clearing away cold and resolving dampness in the former case, tonifying the kidney and replenishing essence and strengthening Back Middle Meridian in the latter case.

Radde Anemone Rhizome

The dried rhizome of Anemone raddeana Reg. (Ranunculaceae).

Effect. Expelling wind-dampness and eliminating subcutaneous swelling.

Indication. Arthralgia syndrome due to wind-damp, joint pain, and ulceration of carbuncle and swelling.

Radish Root

The fresh root of Raphanus sativus L. (Cruciferae).

Effect. Subduing food stagnancy, dispersing phlegm-heat, keeping the adverse qi flowing downward, relieving depression and detoxicating.

Indication. Dyspeptic abdominal distention, cough with aphonia and hematemesis.

Radish Seed

The seed of Raphanus Sativus L. (Cruciferae).

Effect. Promoting digestion to remove food retention, lowering the adverse flow of qi and resolving phlegm.

Indication. Distention and pain in the stomach, eructation with fetid odour and acid regurgitation due to retention of indigested food, constipation, retention of excessive phlegm and saliva, cough and dyspnea, etc.

Ragimiller Seed

The seed of Eleusine coracana (L.) Gaerth. (Gramineae).

Effect. Reinforcing the middle-energizer and promoting qi circulation and strengthening function of intestine and stomach.

Indication. Dyspepsia.

Ramie Root

The root, stem, and leaf of Boehmeria nivea (L.) Gaud. (Urticaceae).

Effect. Cooling heat from blood, relieving bleeding, clearing away heat, inducing diuresis and detoxicating, preventing abortion.

Indication. Hematuria hemoptysis, hematemesis, metrorrhagia and metrostaxis, threatened abortion, excessive fetal movement, traumatic injuries, etc.

Rangu (K 2)

A meridian acupuncture point.

Location. On the medial border of the foot, below the tuberosity of the navicular bone, and at the junction of the red and white skin.

Indication. Irregular menstruation, prolapse of uterus, pruritus vulvae, cloudy urine, emission, impotence, difficulty in urination, diarrhea, distending pain in the chest and hypochondrium, hemoptysis, neonatal tetanus in children, lockjaw, diabetes, jaundice, flaccidity and numbness of the lower limbs, pain in the dorsum of the foot.

Method. Puncture 0.5-1.0 cun perpendicularly. Moxibustion is applicable.

Ranhou (Ex-LE)

An extra acupuncture point.

Location. On the foot, 0.4 cun posterior to Rangu (KI 2).

Indication. Dyspepsia.

Method. Puncture 0.3-0.5 cun perpendicularly. Moxibustion is applicable.

Rash Lesions after Measles

Symptoms. Small rashes on the patent's skin, like scabies with itching, annoyance with poor appetite, restless sleep at night.

Pathogenesis. Usually caused by the rest measles toxin in the blood and repeated affection by wind pathogens and its stagnancy in the skin.

Therapeutic Principle. Tonifying the blood, calming the wind and relieving itching.

Raving Consciousness

Referring to one type of abnormal mentality.

Symptoms. Coma and delirium, restlessness and ravings.

Pathogenesis. Usually caused by blood stagnancy in lower-energizer and disturbance of heart by evil heat accumulating.

Realgar

The crystal mineral of Realgar, which is composed of arsenic disulfide (As_2S_2).

Effect. Detoxicating, destroying parasites, alleviating itching, eliminating dampness and relieving cough and asthma and relieving convulsion.

Indication. Boils, tinea, noxious insect, snake bite, abdominalgia caused by parasitic infestations, asthma, etc.

Recessive Fever

Symptoms. Dull fever without obvious symptom, usually found in patients with more damp-warm pathogen than heat pathogen.

Pathogenesis. Caused by fever due to accumulation of dampness and vaporizing of heat.

Rectal Polyp

Referring to the vegetation in the rectum.

Symptoms. Polyp growing in the anus in different sizes. They will project out of the anus in stool and needing to be pushed back with the fingers after stool. Fresh blood and mucus are usually dejected with feces painlessly. It is mostly found in children.

Pathogenesis. Blockage in the meridians and collaterals, the blood stasis and the stagnation of turbid qi due to the downward pressure of damp-heat.

Therapeutic Principle. Apply a ligation therapy or treat with an operation.

Rectum (MA-H 2)

An auricular point.

Location. On the end of the helix approximate to the superior tragus notch.

Indication. Constipation, diarrhea, prolapse of the rectum, internal and external hemorrhoids.

Recurrent Dysentery

Referring to the protracted dysentery, attack frequently.

Symptoms. Fatigue and weakness, anorexia, emaciation and cold limbs, etc.

Pathogenesis. Caused by long-time dysentery without proper treatment, resulting in the weakness of body resistance, the pathogenic factors inside of the body, and dysfunction of the stomach and intestine in transportation.

Therapeutic Principle. Warming the middle-energizer and clearing the bowels at the onset, together with regulating qi and resolving stagnation, strengthening the spleen and stomach, invigorating qi and blood, and warming the kidney for the patient with kidney deficiency in relieving period.

Red Bean

The dried ripe seed of Phaseolus calcaratus Roxb. or P. angularis Wight (Leguminosae).

Effect. Inducing urination, subduing swelling, detoxicating and promoting pus discharge.

Indication. Edematous swelling, distention and fullness of the abdomen, general edema caused by beriberi, pathopyretic ulcer and jaundice due to damp-heat pathogen.

Red Collaterals at Back of Ear

Symptoms. The ear feels warm, red collaterals can be seen at the back of auricle, and the root of ear is comparatively cold. It is one of the indications of symptoms of measles.

Reddened Tongue

The tongue condition is an indicator for diagnosis of a disease. The reddened tongue indicates heat syndrome.

Red Furuncle

Symptoms. Small red spots all over the body, sometimes mild, sometimes severe.

Pathogenesis. Mostly caused by wind-heat invasion of the lung, wind-heat is stagnated in the muscle and skin, or by the attacking of hear-fire into the lung to consume blood.

Therapeutic Principle. Dispelling wind and removing heat from the blood.

Red Helloysite

It is a mineral, hydrated aluminium silicate, which belongs to monoclinic system.

Effect. Stopping diarrhea with astringents, relieving bleeding; astringing and promoting regeneration of the tissue externally.

Indication. Chronic dysentery and diarrhea, hemafecia, proctoptosis, metror-

rhagia, metrostaxis, ulcer resistance, traumatic bleeding, etc.

Red-knees Fruit

The fruit of Polygonum hydropiper L. (Polygonaceae).

Effect. Warming the middle-energizer to promote diuresis, dissipating blood stasis and resolving masses.

Indication. Vomiting, diarrhea, abdominal masses, edema superficial infection, scrofula, etc.

Redleaf Litse Fruit

The fruit of Litsea rubescens Lecomte (Lauraceae).

Effect. Expelling cold and dampness, and eliminating undigested food.

Indication. Gastroenteritis, abdominal distention and pain due to cold in the stomach, retention of food, etc.

Redleaf Litse Root

The root of Litsea rubuscens Lecomte (Lauraceae).

Effect. Dispelling wind and expelling cold.

Indication. Headache due to common cold, arthralgia due to pathogenic wind-dampness, traumatic injuries, etc.

Red Lips

A disease, usually seen in children.

Symptoms. Mouth and lips are deep red in color and accompanied by restlessness, thirst and drink.

Pathogenesis. Caused by heat in spleen and stomach.

Redness, Swelling and Pain of the Eye

Symptoms. Redness of the eyes, aversion to light, lacrimation, dryness difficult to open, one eye is affected on the onset, and gradually both eyes.

Pathogenesis. Mostly caused by the affection of exopathic wind-heat leading to the stagnation of meridian qi and failure to expel stagnant fire; or by excessive fire in the liver and gallbladder, disturbing the upper along the meridians, leading to the blockage of the meridians and blood stasis and the stagnation.

Therapeutic Principle. Clear wind-heat, relieve swelling and pain.

Red Nose

Referring to a symptom that the infant's nose is red. It is caused by heat in the spleen and stomach, transferring to the nose along the Stomach Meridian.

Red Ochre

The ore of Hematite (trigonal system), mainly contains ferric oxide (Fe_2O_3).

Effect. Calming liver to stop endogenous wind, descending the adverse flow of qi, cooling the blood and aresting bleeding.

Indication. Headache and dizziness, due to hyperactive liver-yang; dyspnea, vomiting, and hematemesis and metrostaxis caused by blood-heat, etc.

Red Peony Root

The root of Paeonia veitchii Lynch. and P. Obovata Maxim. or P. lactiflora Pall. (Ranunculaceae).

Effect. Clearing pathogenic heat from blood, dissipating blood stasis and arresting pian, promoting visual acuity.

Indication. Epidemic febrile disease, macules, hematemesis, eruptions, amenorrhea, menorrhagia, subcutaneous swelling, conjunctivitis, traumatic injuries, etc.

Red Phoenix Encountering the Source

Referring to a needling technique.

Method. Insert the needle to the deep layer, lift it to the superficial tissue after acquiring qi insert the needle into the middle layer. Manipulate it by lifting it left and right. Twirl the fingers and spread the needle repeatedly as if a red phoenix were spreading her wings.

Function. Promoting the circulation of meridian-qi.

Red Psychotria Leaf and Twig

The tender twigs and leaf of Psychotria rubra (Lour.) Poir. (Rubiaceae).

Effect. Clearing away heat, detoxicating, dispelling wind and expelling dampness.

Indication. Tonsillitis, diphtheria, rheumatic arthralgia, skin and external diseases, pyogenic infections, and traumatic injuries.

Redroot Grom well Root

The Root of Lithospermum erythrorhizon Sieb. et. Zucc. and Macrotomia euchroma (Royle.) Pauls. (Boraginaceae).

Effect. Cooling blood, detoxicating promoting blood circulation and promoting the eruption of measles, moisturizing dryness to relax the bowels.

Indication. Eruptions, measles, jaundice, epistaxis, hematemesis, skin infection, eczema, burns, scalds, etc.

Red Sage Root

It is the root and rhizome of Salvia miltiorrhiza Bge. (Labiatae).

Effect. Invigorating blood circulation, removing blood stasis and tranquilizing the disturbed mind by nourishing blood.

Indication. Irregular menstruation, amenorrhea caused by stagnation of blood, epigastric and abdominal pain, masses in the abdomen, pain of limbs carbuncles and other pyogenic skin infections, high fever, delirium, restlessness, insomnia, palpitation, etc.

Red Sha

Symptoms. Red dots can be seen in skin like measles.

Pathogenesis. Usually caused by stagnation of sha toxin in the exterior of skin.

Therapeutic Principle. Relieving exterior syndrome, dissipating stagnation, detoxicating, dispelling Sha toxin by tempering-scrapping method. Abstain from hot drinks.

Red Smooth Tongue without Fur

Symptoms. Bright red tongue with smooth surface without fur.

Pathogenesis. Caused by fire of yin-deficiency to burn tongue, exhaustion of the stomach-qi and stomach-yin, and failure to produce fur.

Red Tongue Surrounded with white Fur

This kind of tongue picture indicates exhaustion and impairment of qi and fluid; white fur of tongue side is ascribable to pathogen in Shaoyang Meridian.

Red Tongue with White Fur

This kind of tongue picture indicates retention of damp-evil in diaphragm, latent pathogenic heat of nutrient system failing to penetrate out. It can usually be seen in damp-heat pestilence.

Reduced Menstruation due to Obesity

Symptoms. Scanty, thin and pale menstrual blood, or interspersion with leukorrhea.

Pathogenesis. Caused by qi deficiency due to obesity, disturbance of the spleen by pathogenic dampness, failure of food essence to change into blood, and stagnation of phlegm-dampness in the meridians.

Therapeutic Principle. Invigorate the spleen, remove dampness, nourish blood and promote menstruation.

Reed Flower

The flower of Phragmites communis Trin. (Gramineae)

Effect. Arresting bleeding and detoxicating.

Indication. Epistaxis, metrorrhagia, metrostaxis, vomiting and diarrhea.

Reedlike Sweetcane Root

The root of Saccharum arundinaceum Retz. (Gramineae).

Effect. Causing resuscitation, inducing diuresis, removing blood and activating meridians.

Indication. Jaundice, dysentery, constipation, traumatic injuries, arthralgia and myalgia, edema, etc.

Regulation of Yin and Yang

A principle of treatment of diseases. In traditional Chinese medicine, the fundamental pathogenesis of diseases is the imbalance of yin and yang due to the excess and deficiency of yin or of yang. Therefore, yin and yang should be regulated to restore the relative balance between them. If yin or yang is excessive or deficient, the method of removing the excess or invigorating the deficiency should be used.

Regulating Stomach and Qi

It refers to a therapeutic method administered for the qi stagnation in the stomach and failure of the stomach qi to descend, caused by stagnation of qi, phlegm, food and dampness, which marked as fullness in the stomach and abdominal distention, hiccups, eructation, acid regurgitation, nausea and vomiting.

Regulating Upward Adverse flow with Lowering Drugs

It refers to the use of drugs with the function of lowering to treat the syndrome caused by the adverse flow of qi pathogen.

Regurgitation of Food from the Stomach

Symptoms. Obvious pain in the upper abdomen, vomiting right after eating, exhaustion, dim complexion.

Pathogenesis. Commonly due to the insufficiency of spleen-yang and the decline of vital fire, the failure to receive and digest food.

Therapeutic Principle. Warm the spleen and stomach, regulate the stomach and check upward adverse flow of the stomach-qi.

Rehmannia Dried Root ✵ R-1

The root of Rehmannia glutinosa (Gaerth.) Libosch (Scrophulariaceae).

Effect. Clearing away heat, cooling the blood, arresting bleeding, nourishing yin and promoting the production of the body fluid.

Indication. Get fretful due to heat syndrome, fever with thirst due to pathological heat, hematemesis, epistaxis, hematuria, metrorrhagia, diabetes and constipation, etc.

Reinforcing and Reducing by Opening and Closing

Referring to a needling technique of acupuncture. After withdrawal of the inserted needle, massaging the hole to obliterate is "Reinforcing". While the inserted needle is being withdrawn, enlarging the hole by shaking the needle, but not being massaged, is "Reducing".

Reinforcing Yang with Drugs Pungent in Flavor and Sweet in Taste

It refers to a therapeutic method administered to patients with yang-deficiency and cold excess.

Symptoms. Pale faces, aversion to cold, cold limbs, clear urine, loose stool.

Relapse of Disease due to Intemperance in Sexual Intercourse

Referring to one type of relapse of disease due to overstrain.

Symptoms. Heaviness in the head, dim eyesight, lumbago, back pain, etc.

Pathogenesis. Failure of recuperation at the initial stage of recovery from a serious disease, excessive sexual intercourse resulting in impairment and loss of kidney essence.

Therapeutic Principle. Nourishing yin and the kidney.

Relapse of Disease due to Overstrain

Referring to recurrence of disease due to impairment of vital qi by overwork, or emotional disturbances, improper diet and sexual intemperance during the convalescence period.

Relative Excessiveness of Yin or Yang

It refers to the invasion of exopathogens into the body, leading to imbalance between yin and yang, i.e. pathologic changes from an excess of either yin or yang. The invasion of yang pathogens into the body brings about the pathological changes of yang excess featured with heat, while that of yin pathogens into the body results in the pathological changes of yin excess featured with cold.

Relieving Exterior Syndrome

Referring to a treatment by sweating the patient to release pathogenic qi of the muscle from the body together with sweat. It is applied to the exterior syndromes of wind-cold and wind-heat.

Relieving Exterior Syndrome of Sore

Referring to a method of using the drugs for inducing diaphoresis to relieve exterior syndrome for removing toxic substances outside the body along with sweat in order to dispel sores.

Relieving Obstruction in Qi and Blood Circulation and Activating Yang

It refers to a therapeutic method of dispersing stasis in the chest and promoting qi and blood circulation.

Indication. Pain and oppressed feeling in chest, shoulder and medial arm, shortness of breath, etc.

Remnant Heat during Convalescence

Symptoms. Paraphasia and listlessness, or the alternate attacks of chill and fever similar to malaria, red cheeks and dysphoria with smothery sensation, etc.

Pathogenesis. Caused by imcomplete diaphoresis and the heat remaining in the pericardium.

Therapeutic Principle. Removing the heat of deficiency type, supplementing qi and promoting the production of body fluid.

Removing Heat from Qi System with Drugs of Pungent Flavor and Cool Nature

It refers to a therapeutic method administered for epidemic febrile disease resulting from affection by exopathogen.

Symptoms. High fever, flushed face, not afraid of cold, but aversion to heat, profuse sweating, thirst, dark urine, red tongue with yellowish fur, etc.

Renal Cough

Symptoms. Cough, momentary deafness while coughing, lumbago and back pain, etc.

Pathogenesis. Mainly caused by the affection of cold due to deficiency of the kidney.

Therapeutic Principle. Tonifying the kidney and eliminating pathogenic factors.

Renying (S 9)

A meridian acupuncture point.

Location. On the neck, 1.5 cun lateral to the Adam apple, and on the anterior border of the sternocleidomastoid muscle where the pulsation of the common carotid artery is palpable.

Indication. Full sensation in the chest, dyspnea, swelling and pain of the throat, headache, hypertension, scrofula, goiter, vomiting, cholera morbus, dyspepsia.

Method. Puncture perpendicularly 0.2-0.4 cun.

Notice. Avoid the artery. Moxibustion is forbidden.

Repeated Abortion

Symptoms. More than three natural abortions of the pregnant woman.

Pathogenesis. Mostly caused by qi deficiency and blood insufficiency, leading to malnutrition of the fetus, or liability to abortion due to kidney deficiency, or blood heat harming the fetus.

Therapeutic Principle. Enriching qi and nourishing blood, invigorating the kidney or clearing heat and nourishing yin to prevent abortion respectively according to the concrete case.

Response to Finger

This term has two meanings.

1. It is a method of differentiating the presence of the pus of sores. It refers to the restoration of the swelling lump when the doctor relieves his finger, pressed in a sore.
2. It generally refers to the pulse felt under the finger when taking the pulse.

Restlessness of Yang Type

It refers to disturbance of hands and feet due to excessive heat.

Symptoms. Extreme thirst and desire for drinking, irritability, difficulty in defecation and urination, etc.

Therapeutic Principle. Clearing away heat to relieve restlessness, removing cardiopyrexia to tranquilize the mind.

Restoration of Yang

It refers to the recurrence of yang qi in a patient suffering the disease of yin cold. When the patient's hands and feet become warmer, which denotes the recurrence of yang qi and decline of yin cold, the condition shows relief of the disease.

Restoring Yang and Expelling Pathogenic Factors in Superficies

A treatment of administering drugs to invigorate yang together with diaphoretic to yang deficiency and affection by exopathogen.

Indication. Aversion to cold, high fever, anhidrosis, headache, etc.

Resupinate Woodbetony Herb
The stem leaf or root of Pedicularis resupinata L. (Scrophulariaceae).
Effect. Dispelling wind, expelling dampness, inducing diuresis.
Indication. Arthralgia caused by wind-dampness, leukorrhagia, dysuria, lithangiuria, scabies, etc.

Resurrection Lily Rhizome
The dried rhizome of Kaempferia galanga L. (Zingiberaceae).
Effect. Invigorating the circulation of qi, warming the middle-energizer, promoting digestion and relieving pain.
Indication. Fullness and distention in the chest, abdominal cold-pain, and mass of indigested food.

Retained Heat due to Blockage of Dampness
The heat stasis due to blockage of damp pathogen.
Symptoms. High fever in the afternoon which does not subside after perspiration, tired mentality, heaviness in the head, distention of the abdomen, anorexia, dark urine, etc.

Retardation in Hair-growing
Symptoms. The infant has no hair after birth, and the hair does not grow for a long time, or is loose and easily falls out, and yellow-withered with no lustre.
Pathogenesis. Caused by congenital deficiency and inability of yin blood to go up.
Therapeutic Principle. Tonifying blood and producing vital essence.

Retching
Symptoms. Vomiting with sound but no vomitus.
Pathogenesis. Usually due to gastric asthenia, or invasion of the stomach by pathogenic heat or cold, and disorder of the stomach-qi.

Retention of Dampness in Qi System
It refers to a pathogenesis, with corresponding symptoms of mild feverish body, pressure over the head, heavy sensation of the body, distress in the chest, poor appetite, abdominal distention.

Reversed Flow of Qi due to Retching
It refers to the symptom of retching without vomiting, which may be caused by the stomach-heat, stomach-cold, insufficiency of the stomach-qi, damage of the stomach-yin, etc.

Rhodiola Root
The whole plant of Rhodiola sacra (Prain ex Hamet) Fu (Crassulaceae).
Effect. Promoting blood circulation, relieving bleeding, removing heat from the lung and stopping cough.
Indication. Hemoptysis, cough caused by the lung-heat, gonorrhea and leukorrhea.

Rhubarb
The root and rhizome of Rheum palmatum L. or Rheum tanguticum Maxim. ex Balf. or R. officinale Baill. (Polygonaceae).
Effect. Relieving constipation, clearing away heat eliminating stagnated food and blood stasis, detoxicating, purging fire, promoting blood circulation, normalizing the functioning of the gallbladder and curing jaundice.
Indication. Constipation, hematemesis and epistaxis due to invasion of blood by heat, sore throat, gum swelling burns, boils, sores, scalds, acute jaundice, acute appendicitis, stranguria and other diseases caused by blood stasis.

Rice Fermented with Red Yeast
The rice fermented with red yeast of Monascus purpureus Went (Monascaceae), which live on the polished round grained rice.

Effect. Promoting blood circulation, to remove blood stasis and invigorating the function of the spleen to promote digestion.

Indication. Abdominal pain caused by blood stasis, flatulence due to dyspepsia, dysentery with blood and mucus, postpartum lochiorrhea, and traumatic injuries.

Rice Mass

Symptoms. Fixed mass in the abdomen, preference for eating raw rice, vomiting with water, etc.

Pathogenesis. Usually caused by deficiency of the spleen and stomach qi, indigestion together with the accumulation of phlegm.

Therapeutic Principle. Reinforcing the spleen to promote digestion.

Ricepaper Pith

The marrow in the stem of Tetrapanax papyriferus (Hook.) K. Koch (Araliaceae).

Effect. Inducing diuresis and removing dampness, clearing away heat and activating collaterals to promote lactation.

Indication. Hydrops dysuria, dribbling and painful micturition and postpartum alactation.

Rice Straw

The stem leaf of Oryza sativa L. (Gramineae).

Effect. Alleviating depression to regulate qi, and subduing stagnancy of food.

Indication. Dysphagia, regurgitation, dyspepsia, diarrhea, abdominal pain, diabetes, jaundice, hemorrhoid, burns, scalds, etc.

River Snail

The whole body of Cipangopaludina chinensis (Gray) (Viviparidae), or the animal in the same genus.

Effect. Clearing away heat and promoting diuresis.

Indication. Dysuria caused by accumulation of heat, jaundice, edema, diabetes, hemorrhoid, hemafecia, congested swollen eyes with pain, boils, swollen furuncle, etc.

Rivier Giantarum Rhizome

The rhizome of Amorphophallus rivieri Durieu (Araceae).

Effect. Eliminating phlegm to remove mass, dissipating blood stasis and relieving swelling.

Indication. Cough with sputum, retention of food, amenorrhea, traumatic injuries, subcutaneous swelling, furuncle, erysipelas and scalds.

Riyue (G 24)

An acupuncture point.

Location. In the upper abdomen, directly below the nipple, in the seventh intercostal space, 4 cun lateral to the anterior median line.

Indication. Hypochondriac pain, stomachache, vomiting, jaundice.

Method. Puncture obliquely 0.3-0.5 cun and apply moxibustion to the point for 5-10 minutes.

Rosacea

Symptoms. Reddish or purple-black apex nasi, even spreading to the wings of the nose, with skin thickening, apex of the nose enlarging.

Pathogenesis. Caused by the fumigation of lung due to the damp-heat of spleen and stomach.

Therapeutic Principle. Removing pathogenic heat from blood, and dispersing accumulation of pathogen.

Rose   ✿ R-2

It is the flower bud of Rosa rugosa Thunb. (Rosaceae).

Effect. Activating circulation of qi, relieving the depressed liver, regulating blood circulation and dissipating blood stasis.

Indication. Hypochondriac pain, gastric and abdominal distended pain, irregular menstruation, distended pain of breast before menstruation and traumatic injuries.

Rose Mallow Root or Herb

It is the root or whole herb of Urena lobata L. (Malvaceae).

Effect. Promoting circulation of qi and blood dispelling pathogenic wind, inducing diuresis, clearing away heat and detoxicating.

Indication. Fever due to exopathy, rheumatic arthralgia, stomachache, dysentery, edema, stranguria, leukorrhea, hematemesis, subcutaneous swelling, traumatic bleeding and snake bite.

Rosepink Zephyrlily Herb

It is the whole herb of Zephyranthes grandiflora Lindl. (Amaryllidaceae).

Effect. Clearing away heat, detoxicating, activating blood circulation and cooling the blood.

Indication. Traumatic injuries, bleeding due to wound hematemesis, epistaxis, metrorrhagia, snake bite etc.

Rotary Vertigo

Symptoms. Sudden attack, giddiness and whirling accompanied by nausea, vomiting and oppressed feeling in the chest.

Pathogenesis. Usually caused by the obstruction of phlegm in the middle of the gastric cavity, the failure of turbid yin to descend down and the disorder of qi activity.

Therapeutic Principle. Removing dampness to reduce phlegm and strengthening the spleen and stomach.

Roughhair Fig Root

The root or root bark of Ficus simplicissima Lour var. hirta (Vahl.) Migo (Moraceae).

Effect. Invigorating spleen, dispelling wind-dampness, strengthening the muscles and bones, dissipating blood stasis and subduing swelling.

Indication. Rheumatic arthralgia, general edema, pulmonary overstrain, traumatic injuries, amenorrhea, leukorrhagia, hypogalactia, etc.

Roughly Peripheral Pupil

Referring to the morbid state in which the pupil, with a rough periphery, is no longer round, and its iris is withering up due to malnutrition.

Pathogenesis. Mostly caused by failure to treat miosis.

Therapeutic Principle. Nourishing the liver, replenishing the kidney, clearing away heat and improving visual acuity.

Round Cardamom Seed

The dried ripe seed of Amomum kravanh Pirre ex Gagnep. (Zingiberaceae).

Effect. Resolving dampness from the middle energizer, promoting flow of qi, removing mass, promoting appetite, and arresting vomiting.

Indication. Chest oppression, distention and fullness of the chest and abdomen, retained food, stagnation of qi, and vomiting due to cold in the stomach.

Round-nebula Cataract

Symptoms. Chronic oculopathy of opacity of lens and slow hypopsia, which gradually leads to blindness.

Pathogenesis. Mostly caused by insufficiency of the liver and kidney, damp abundance due to splenic asthenia and upward disturbance of the liver-heat.

Therapeutic Principle. At early stage, mainly in nourishing the liver, replenishing the kidney, invigorating the spleen and promoting the flow of qi. Operative therapy is applicable, if the lens regularly takes the form of greyish-white turbidity and evidently blocks the pupil.

Round-Sharp Needle

A needling apparatus. The middle part of the needle is a slightly large, round and its tip is sharp and slightly thick, 5 cm in length.

Indication. Carbuncle and swelling on the body surface, arthralgia-syndrome.

Method. Deep puncturing.

Routine Treatment

A principle of treatment. The disease is treated according to methods and drugs opposite to its nature and the pathogenesis, e.g. drugs of hot nature are used to treat cold syndromes, while drugs of cold nature are used to treat heat syndromes.

Royal Jelly

It is the secretion from the posterior duct of the throat of a honey bee (Apis cerana Fabr., A. melifera L.) (Apidae) at the initial stage of growth and the melifera substances are made from the nectar.
Effect. Strengthening the constitution, tonifying the liver and reinforcing the spleen.
Indication. Weakness during convalescence, infantile malnutrition, general debility in advanced age, infective hepatitis, hypertension, rheumatic arthritis, duodenal ulcer, bronchial asthma, diabetes, irregular menstruation, etc.

Rubella due to Exopathogen

A type of rubella.
Symptoms. Bright red itching marks on skin, sudden onset, fever, thirst, cough, sore and pain in the limbs.
Pathogenesis. Mostly due to poor function of the skin and muscles and wind pathogen invading the body and accumulating in the skin.
Therapeutic Principle. Dispel wind and regulate the nutrients.

Rubella due to Menstruation

Symptoms. General itching, latent rubella, or rash and urticaria during, before or after menstruation.
Pathogenesis. Mostly caused by blood deficiency and repeated attack of pathogenic wind and heat.
Therapeutic Principle. Nourishing blood and clearing heat, and expelling wind.

Rubella due to Stomach-heat

Symptoms. Bright red itching marks appear on the skin suddenly with uneven density; stomachache and abdominal pain, loss of appetite, constipation, or diarrhea.
Pathogenesis. Mostly caused by the accumulation of heat in the stomach resulting in the retention of the heat in the skin portion of the body.
Therapeutic Principle. Clear heat to regulate the nutrient system.

Rugen (S 18)

An acupuncture point.
Location. Directly below the nipple, 4 cun to the anterior median line, at the root of the breast, in the fifth intercostal space.
Indication. Cough, dyspnea, pectoralgia, hiccups, acute mastitis, postpartum insufficient lactation, etc.
Method. Puncture obliquely 0.3-0.5 cun and apply moxibustion to the point for 5-10 minutes.

Runcinate Knotweed Herb

The whole herb of Polygonum runcinatum Buch.-Ham. (Polygonaceae).
Effect. Clearing away heat, detoxicating, activating blood circulation and eliminating swelling.
Indication. Dysentery, leukorrhagia, headache, metrorrhagia and metrostaxis, amenorrhea, mammary abscess, furuncle, carbuncle and traumatic injuries, etc.

Rush   ⊛ R-3

The dried stem pulp of Juncus effusus L. (Juncaceae).
Effect. Febrifuge, inducing diuresis, treating stranguria, clearing away heart-fire and eliminating restlessness.
Indication. Urinary infection, dribbling and painful micturition, restlessness caused by heart-heat, morbid night crying of babies, epilepsy and sore-throat.

Rushang (Ex-CA)

An extra acupuncture point.

Location. On the chest, 1 cun directly above the nipple.

Indication. Pain of breast, lack of lactation, intercostal neuralgia, etc.

Method. Apply moxibustion 3-5 moxa cones or 5-10 minutes with warming moxibustion.

Russian Boschniakia Herb

The whole herb of Boschniakia rossica Fedtsch. et Fleror (Orobanchaceae).

Effect. Tonifying the kidney, strengthening yang, nourishing essence and blood, moistening the bowels, catharsis and arresting bleeding.

Indication. Impotence inability of pregnancy, cold pain in the loins and knees, tiredness of the muscles and bones, and constipation in the aged.

Russian Fenugreek Herb

The whole herb of Trigonella ruthenica L. (Leguminosae).

Effect. Clearing away heat, subduing inflammation and stopping bleeding.

Indication. Cough caused by lung-heat and dysentery characterized by bloody stool.

Ruxia (Ex-CA)

An extra acupuncture point.

Location. On the chest, 1 cun below the nipple.

Indication. Abdominal distention and pain, pain in the chest and hypochondrium, swollen breast and lack of lactation, chronic cough, regurgitation, vomiting epigastralgia, amenorrhea.

Method. Apply moxibustion 3-5 moxa cones or 5-10 minutes with warming moxibustion.

Ruzhong (S 17)

A meridian acupuncture point.

Location. At the center of the nipple.

It is not used for acupuncture or moxibustion, but only serves as the locative mark for the points on the chest and abdomen.

S

Safflower ⊗ S-1

It is the dried flower of Carthamus tinctorius L. (Compositae).

Effect. Promoting blood circulation, dissipating blood stasis and normalizing menstruation, letting out skin eruptions.

Indication. Dysmenorrhea, postpartum abdominal pain due to retention of blood stasis and masses in the abdomen, pain and ecchymoma caused by traumatic injuries, arthralgia, stagnation of blood due to accumulation of heat, etc.

Safflower Fruit ⊗ S-2

It is the fruit of Carthamus tinctorius L. (Compositae).

Effect. Promoting blood circulation and detoxicating.

Indication. Small pox eruption, gynecopathy due to blood stasis and dysmenorrhea.

Sago Weed

It is the seed of Cycas revoluta Thunb. (Cycadaceae).

Effect. Activating meridians, promoting digestion, arresting bleeding, cough and dispelling phlegm.

Indication. Abundant expectoration, cough and wound.

Salt Interposed Moxibustion

It is a type of indirect moxibustion.

Indication. Collapse syndrome of apoplexy, abdominal distention, vomiting, diarrhea, dysuria, etc.

Method. Fill the umbilicus with salt and place a large moxa cone on the top of the salt and ignite the moxa cone. When the patient feels a little burning pain, the moxa cone will be replaced by another.

Salty Flavor

It refers to a kind of traditional Chinese medicine with salty and cold properties.

Effect. Softening and resolving hard masses and relieving constipation by purgation.

Indication. Scrofula, goiter, masses in the abdomen, and constipation due to accumulation of heat, etc.

Sampson St. John's Wort Herb

It is the whole herb of Hypericum sampsonii Hance (Hypericaceae).

Effect. Promoting blood circulation, arresting bleeding and detoxicating.

Indication. Vomit the blood, irregular menstruation, traumatic injuries, and carbuncles, furuncle and boils, etc.

Sanchi (Ex-UE)

3 extra acupuncture points.

Location. On the radial aspect and near the elbow, located at Quchi (LI 11), 1 cun above and below Quchi, a total of three points.

Indication. Febrile disease, rhinitis, pain in the elbow and arm, impeded movement of the upper limb.

Method. Puncturing 1-1.5 cun. Moxibustion is applicable.

Sandalwood

It is the dried heartwood of Santalum album L. (Santalaceae).

Effect. Regulating flow of qi and middle-energizer, promoting function of stomach, dispersing cold and relieving pain.

Indication. Pain in the chest and abdomen due to cold obstruction and qi stasis, stomachache due to cold, regurgitation and vomiting, etc.

Sanjian (LI 3)

A point on the Large Intestine Meridian.

Location. On the radial side of the second metacarpal bone, in the excavation posterior to the small head of the metacarpal bone. Select it by slightly forming a fist.

Indication. Fever, abdominal distention and borborygmus, ophthalmalgia, toothache, pain in the eye, swelling sore throat.

Method. Puncturing perpendicularly 0.5-0.8 cun and applying moxibustion to the point with 3 units of moxa cones or for 5-10 minutes.

Sanjiao (MA)

An auricular point.

Location. At the base of the concha auriculae, superior to the intertragicus notch.

Indication. Constipation, general edema, abdominal distention, and obesity.

Sanjiaoshu (B 22)

An acupuncture point.

Location. 1.5 cun lateral to the lower border of the spinous process of the first lumbar vertebra.

Indication. Abdominal distention, vomiting, diarrhea, dysentery, edema, pain and stiffness of the lower back.

Method. Puncturing perpendicularly 0.5-1 cun and applying moxibustion to the point with 5-7 units of moxa cones or for 10-15 minutes with warming moxibustion.

Sanshang (Ex-UE)

A collective term for Laoshang, Zhongshang and Shaoshang. They are extra acupuncture points.

Location. Laoshang is on the ulnar side of the thumb, 0.1 cun from the corner of the nail. Zhongshang is on the dorsal median of the thumb, 0.1 cun from the root of the nail. Shaoshang is on the radial side of the thumb, 0.1 cun from the corner of the nail.

Indication. Coma, high fever, influenza, acute tonsillitis and mumps, etc.

Method. Pricking to cause bleeding.

Sanxiao (Ex-HN)

An extra acupuncture point.

Location. On the face below Yingxiang (LI 20), at the midpoint of the nasolabial groove.

Indication. Nasal obstruction, facial paralysis and furuncle, etc.

Method. Puncturing subcutaneously 0.3-0.5 cun.

Sanyangluo (TE 8)

A meridian acupuncture point.

Location. On the dorsal side of the forearm, 4 cun above Yangchi (TE 4) and between the radius and ulna.

Indication. Sudden loss of voice, deafness, pain in the hand and arm, dental caries and toothache.

Method. Puncturing perpendicularly 0.5-1.0 cun. Apply moxibustion 3-5 units of moxa cones or 5-10 minutes.

Sanyinjiao (Sp 6)

An acupuncture point.

Location. 3 cun directly above to the tip of the medial ankle, in the excavation of the posterior margin of the medial side of the tibia.

Indication. Abdominal distention, diarrhea, irregular menstruation, morbid leukorrhea, prolapse of uterus, sterility, dystocia, seminal emission, impotence, enuresis, hernia, insomnia, etc.

Method. Puncturing perpendicularly 1-1.5 cun and applying moxibustion to the point with 3-7 units of moxa cones or for 5-15 minutes.

Notice. The method is forbidden in pregnant women.

Sarcandra Herb

It is the branch and leaf of Sarcandra glabra (Thunb.) Nakai (Chloranthaceae).

Effect. Clearing away heat, detoxicating, expelling wind and eliminating dampness, promoting blood circulation and relieving pain.

Indication. Epidemic influenza, pneumonia, acute appendicitis, acute gastroenteritis, dysentery, rheumatic arthralgia, traumatic injuries, snake-bite and cancer.

Sargassum

It is the whole thalluses of Sargassum pallidum (Turn.) C. Ag., and S. fusiforme (Harv.) Setch (Sargassaceae).
Effect. Dispelling phlegm, softening hard lumps and promoting diuresis to reduce edema, lowering blood pressure.
Indication. Goiter and scrofula hypertension.

Sargentglory vine Stem

It is the vine stem of Sargentodoxa cuneata Rehd. et Wils (Lardizabalaceae).
Effect. Clearing away heat and toxic materials, activating blood circulation and relieving pain.
Indication. Acute appendicitis, dysmenorrhea, irregular menstruation, rheumatic arthralgia, traumatic injuries, etc.

Saucer-like Mass

One of the eight masses.
Symptoms. Severe pain in the lower abdomen with a saucer-like mass which is partly touchable, pain in the waist, back and vagina, menostasia, sterility, dark yellowish complexion, etc.
Therapeutic Principle. Regulating the flow of qi to dissipate stasis.

Scabies

Symptoms. Itching, as if penetrating the bones, without feeling of pain when the affected part is being scratched.
Pathogenesis. Mostly caused by the damp-heat in the Liver Meridian.
Therapeutic Principle. Eliminating dampness and heat to destroy parasites.

Scabrous Mosla Herb

It is the whole herb of Sedum sarmentosum Bge. (Crassulaceae).

Effect. Clearing away heat, eliminating swelling and detoxicating.
Indication. Sore throat, burns, scalds and bite by insect and snake.

Scale

It refers to the fallen pieces of the callosity layer during the period of having dermatosis.
Pathogenesis. When it appears in the case of an acute febrile disease, the most probable reason is that the lingering heat has not been cleared away. When it appears in the case of a chronic disease, it is caused by the growing of wind and dryness due to deficiency of blood, and the loss of nourishment of the skin.

Scale Body

Symptoms. The infantile squamous and dry skin, like snake skin.
Pathogenesis. Usually caused by the weak qi and blood, and the under-nourished skin.
Therapeutic Principle. Enriching and activating the blood.

Scalp Acupuncture Therapy

A therapy for treating diseases by needling specific stimulation areas of the scalp.
Indication. Apoplectic sequela, numbness, vertigo, tinnitus, aphasia, etc.
Method. Subcutaneously insert the needle while twisting it slowly to a proper depth, stop inserting the needle, and don't lift and thrust the needle, then twirl the needle rapidly and greatly. After the needling sensation is obtained, twirl the needle continuously for 3-4 minutes, then retain the needle for 10-20 minutes, during which time twirl the needle 1-2 times.

Scandent Schefflera Root

It is the root or stem with leaf of Schefflera arboricola Hayata (Araliaceae).
Effect. Expelling wind, eliminating dampness, promoting blood circulation and removing blood stasis, astringlng bowel and relieving pain, relieving asthma.

Indication. Acute enteritis, rheumatic arthralgia, joint pain, nerve pain, stomachache, fracture and traumatic bleeding.

Scanty Menstruation due to Blood-cold

Symptoms. Scanty menstruation with pale or dark menses, thin discharge accompanied by intolerance to cold, cold pain over the lower abdomen with a desire for warmth.

Pathogenesis. Usually caused by yang-deficiency with formation of yin-cold in the body, deficiency in the function of transmitting qi and generating blood.

Therapeutic Principle. Warming the meridians and nourishing the blood. Acupuncture and moxibustion are applicable.

Scanty Menstruation due to Blood Deficiency

Symptoms. Scanty menstruation, or little discharge for only one or two days, pink and thin menses, sallow complexion, dizziness, palpitation, hollow pain in the lower abdomen.

Pathogenesis. Mostly caused by general weakness of the body, prolonged illness and bleeding leading to yin damage, or impairment of the spleen and stomach, insufficiency of the source for production and transformation leading to blood deficiency.

Therapeutic Principle. Enrich the blood, replenish qi and invigorate the spleen. Acupuncture is applicable.

Scanty Menstruation due to Blood Stasis

Symptoms. Little discharge in menstruation period, dark menstruation with blood clots, pricking pain in the lower abdomen and tenderness, which is relieved by the discharge of blood clots.

Pathogenesis. Mostly caused by the accumulation of cold and the stagnation of qi, the retention of blood stasis, leading to the blockage of blood circulation into the Front and Vital Meridians.

Therapeutic Principle. Promote blood circulation to remove blood stasis. Acupuncture is applicable.

Scanty Menstruation due to Emaciation

Symptoms. In late stage of a menstruation period, little discharge with scanty and pale blood, greyish complexion, dizziness, palpitation, lassitude due to qi insufficiency.

Pathogenesis. Caused by emaciated figure, qi deficiency and blood insufficiency.

Therapeutic Principle. Nourishing both qi and blood.

Scanty Menstruation due to Kidney Deficiency

Symptoms. Thin, pink and scanty menses, dizziness, tinnitus, soreness and weakness of the waist and knees.

Pathogenesis. Congenital deficiency, premature marriage, multiparity, or excessive sexual intercourse, resulting in impairment of kidney-qi and insufficiency of essence and blood, leading to deficiency of qi and blood in the Front and Vital Meridians and Uterine Collaterals.

Therapeutic Principle. Tonifying the kidney and nourishing blood. Acupuncture is applicable.

Scanty Menstruation due to Phlegm-dampness

Symptoms. Scant, light colored and thin menses with profuse leukorrhea, pale complexion, dizziness and palpitation, mild edema of the lower limbs, etc.

Pathogenesis. Obesity, or a rich fatty diet which produces phlegm-dampness in the interior obstructing the meridians, leading to stasis of blood in the Front and Vital Meridians.

Therapeutic Principle. Strengthening the spleen, eliminating dampness and resolving phlegm. Acupuncture is applicable.

Scarlet Fever

Symptoms. Swollen, painful and erosive throat, and scarlet spots on the skin.

Pathogenesis. Attack by virulent heat pathogen. The disease usually occurs in spring and winter, and is very infectious.

Therapeutic Principle. Clearing away heat and expelling poison.

Schisandra Fruit

It is the ripe fruit of Schisandra chinensis (Turcz.) Baill. or S. sphenanthera Rehd. et Wils. (Magnoliaceae).

Effect. Astringing the lung, nourishing the kidney, arresting diarrhea and nourishing the heart tranquilizing the mind.

Indication. Chronic cough and asthma of deficiency type, thirst, spontaneous and night sweat, seminal emission, enuresis, chronic diarrhea, palpitation, insomnia, etc.

Schizonepeta Herb

It is the whole herb of Schizonepeta tenuifolia Brig. (Labiatae) with inflorescence or the flowerspike.

Effect. Dispelling pathogenic heat, relieving exterior evil syndromes from the body surface and arresting bleeding, soothing throat.

Indication. Common cold of wind cold type, german measles, pruritus, incomplete eruption, epistaxis, hemafecia, metrorrhagia and metrostaxis.

Sciatic Nerve (MA-AH 6)

An auricular point.

Location. At the middle 1/3 of the inferior antihelix crus.

Indication. Sciatica.

Science of Acupuncture and Moxibustion

One branch of traditional Chinese medicine, composed of basic part and clinical part, with the former mainly dealing with the meridians, collaterals and acupoints, etc. and the latter acupuncture techniques, moxibustion techniques and therapies, etc.

Science of Chinese Massage

It is a medical science dealing with the manipulation of massage, basic function, and therapy for massage to be used to treat various diseases and symptoms.

Scorpion   ❀ S-3

It is the whole body of Buthus martensii Karsch (Buthidae).

Effect. Expelling endogenous wind to relieve convulsion, clearing away toxins, resolving hard masses and activating the collaterals to relieve pain.

Indication. Acute and chronic infantile convulsion, apoplexy, tetanus, sores, intractable headache or migraine, rheumatic arthralgia, etc.

Scraping

An auxiliary acupuncture manipulation. Referring to manipulation by scraping the needle handle with the fingernail after the needle is inserted to a certain depth.

Function. Strengthening the needling sensation or conducting and spreading the needling sensation.

Scraping Manipulation

A massage manipulation.

Operation. Push fast on the body surface with the radial side of the thumb or the whorled surfaces of the index and middle fingers, or with the border of a spoon or the rim of a coin, which have been dipped with water. Give a heavier force to the orbits than in pushing manipulation.

Function. Dispersing exterior syndrome and soothing the chest.

Indication. Stuffiness in the chest, dizziness, pathogenic summer-heat, etc.

Scraping Orbits

One of self-massage manipulations.

Operation. With the both index fingers of left and right hands flexed like a brow and the inside surface of the second joints of the two fingers kept close to the orbit, scrape the orbits from the inside to the outside, first the upper, then the lower. Repeat the movements until soreness and distention appear.

Function. Improving vision.

Indication. Health care of eyes.

Scraping Tianzhu

A massage manipulation.

Operation. Scrape the Tianzhu (B 10) downward with the edge of a spoon or a small wine cup dipped in water.

Function. Lowering the adverse flow of qi to relieve vomiting and expelling wind and removing cold.

Indication. Fever due to exopathic affections, sore throat and swelling, etc.

Scratching Manipulation

A massage manipulation.

Operation. Scratch a certain part or point with the finger-tips, with five fingers kept together and flexed like a claw.

Function. Relaxing muscles and tendons, and activating collaterals.

Indication. Injury of muscles and tendons.

Scrofula due to Phlegm Accumulation

Symptoms. At the beginning, it is like plums all over the body; with passing of time it will become slightly red, even broken and ulcerated. After ulceration, it is easy to heal.

Pathogenesis. Dysfunction of the spleen in transport, accumulate of cold and warm, capricious moods.

Therapeutic Principle. Promoting the circulation of qi and eliminating phlegm for resuscitation.

Scrofula due to Stagnation of Liver-qi

Symptoms. In the initial stage, it is a chronic infectious disease appearing on the neck and the back of the ear. One to several swollen lymph nodes, which are hard, movable when pushed, without pain. Later, the lymph nodes become more enlarged, dark red skin, intense pain. After diabrosis, a thin purulent fluid is discharged. The syndrome is accompanied by mental depression, distending pain in the chest and hypochondrium, fullness in the stomach.

Pathogenesis. Depression of liver-qi.

Therapeutic Principle. Soothing the liver and regulating the circulation of qi. Acupuncture is applicable.

Scrofula due to Wind-heat Pathogen

Symptoms. Besides general symptoms of scrofula, fever, headache, aching pain in joints.

Pathogenesis. The invasion of pathogenic wind, heat and fire.

Therapeutic Principle. Expelling wind and clearing away heat.

Scrofula due to Yin Deficiency

Symptoms. In addition to the general symptoms of scrofula, hectic fever, night sweat, cough, insomnia, dizziness, mental fatigue are also observed.

Pathogenesis. Yin deficiency of the lung and the kidney, interior scorching fire of deficiency type.

Therapeutic Principle. Nourishing yin to reduce pathogenic fire. Acupuncture is applicable.

Scrotal Abscess

Symptoms. Red swelling and hot, painful scrotum, even with brightness and tightness of the skin of the scrotum, and the formation of pus with passing of time. Fever with chills, thirst, and preference for cold drinks.

Pathogenesis. The downward flow of damp-heat of the liver and the kidney, or by the toxin due to the internal infusing of pathogenic dampness.

Therapeutic Principle. Clearing away heat and promoting diuresis. Nourishing yin and removing dampness.

Scrotal Eczema

Symptoms. At the initial stage, dryness and itching in the scrotum which may be relieved by hot water, or even worse, the occurrence of a reddish millet-like rash with fatty liquid when scratched, or burning pain. It takes a long time to be cured.

Pathogenesis. Mainly due to downward flow of damp-heat in the Liver Meridian and attack of pathogenic wind.

Therapeutic Principle. Removing heat from the liver and removing dampness by diuresis.

Scrubbing Chest

One of self-massage of manipulations.

Operation. With the right or left palm rubbing the chest using heavy force until heating. Injuring the skin should be avoided.

Function. Soothing the chest and regulating qi.

Indication. Stuffiness and blockage in the chest.

Scrubbing Dorsum of Hand

One of self-massage manipulations.

Operation. Rub the palms and dorsum of the hands against each other, from slowly to fast until heating.

Function. Self health care.

Scrubbing Elbow

One of self-massage manipulations.

Operation. Rubbing the elbow joint with the palm until periphery is heating.

Indication. Health care of the upper limbs.

Scrubbing Face

One of the health care maneuvers.

Operation. Rub the palms of both hands until warming, then rub with the palms from the forehead via the sides of the nose to the mandible. Rub reversely upwards from the mandible to the forehead. Repeat it 36 times.

Function. Promoting the blood circulation and the nervous activities of the face.

Besides, with persistent practice it will be beneficial to the beautification of the face.

Scrubbing Lower Abdomen

One of self-massage manipulations.

Operation. Keep the hypothenars of two hands close to the lower abdomen, near the Tianshu (S 25) point, and scrub up and down until heating.

Function. Strengthening the stomach.

Indication. Anorexia and distention of the epigasterium.

Scrubbing Manipulation

Operation. Rub and scrub the specified region to and fro along a straight line with the major thenar, palmar root or minor thenar on the palm. The frequency should be 100-120 times per minute.

Function. Warming the meridians and clearing the collaterals, promoting qi and blood circulation, dispelling swelling and relieving pain, strengthening the spleen and regulating the stomach, etc.

Indication. Consumptive disease of the internal organs and dysfunction of qi and blood.

Scrubbing Shoulder

One of self-massage manipulations.

Operation. Keep the palm center close to the surface of the shoulder and rub up and down until heating.

Indication. Health care of the upper limbs.

Scrubbing Waist

One of the self-massage manipulations.

Operation. Rub the hands until warming, then scrub both the lower back and the waist alternately with the two hands.

Function. Relax the muscles and tendons to promote the blood circulation, warm and recuperate the kidney-yang.

Indication. Pain in the waist and back, and diseases of the lung or the kidney.

Scrubbing Yongquan (K1)

It is a manipulation to hold toes with one hand, rub and massage the acupoint Yongquan (K1) with the other hand until the point grows warm.

Function. Regulating the heart function, lowering the blood pressure, nourishing the primordial qi of the kidney, strengthening the pedal force, dispelling dampness.

Scythian Lamb Rhizome

It is the rhizome of Cibotium barometz (L.) J. Sm. (Dicksoniaceae).

Effect. Tonifying the liver and kidney, strengthening muscles and bones and reliving rheumatism.

Indication. Pain and stiffness of the lower back, lassitude of the legs and loins, incontinence of urine, leukorrhagia, etc.

Sea-cucumber

It is the whole body of Stichopus japonicus Selenka (Stichopodidae).

Effect. Tonifying the kidney to arrest spontaneous emission and nourishing blood to moisten vital essence.

Indication. Consumption disease caused by deficiency of both essence and blood, impotence, nocturnal emission and constipation.

Searching for Primary Cause of Disease in Treatment

It refers to a therapeutic principle. For example, abdominal pain may be a result of many factors; therefore, it should be treated not only with analgesia, but also with the proper therapy by differentiating syndromes and searching for its cause on the clinical manifestations, and according to its cause.

Seasonal Cold due to Wind-cold

Symptoms. Serious aversion to cold, slight fever without sweat, headache, aching pain of limbs and joints, stuffy nose with nasal discharge.

Pathogenesis. Invasion of seasonal pathogenic wind-cold into the body.

Therapeutic Principle. Dispersing wind and cold.

Seasonal Disease

It refers to frequently encountered seasonal disease.

Pathogenesis. Six evils at all seasons, such as wind-warm syndrome in spring, summer fever, diarrhea, and dysentery in summer, autumn-dryness disease, malaria, and damp-warm syndrome in autumn, winter-warm syndrome, and exogenous febrile disease in winter.

Seasonal Epidemic Cold

Symptoms. Headache, pantalgia, alternation of cold and fever, absence of sweating, vomiting and without thirst, etc.

Pathogenesis. The sudden attack of cold which occurs in spring and summer.

Therapeutic Principle. Relieving the exterior with the warm pungent.

Seasonal Noxious Agent

It refers to painful swelling in the neck, cheek, and jaw.

Symptoms. Fever, aversion to cold, sore throat, swelling all over cheek and jaw, bright red coloration and pain after one or two days. It is similar to epidemic parotitis in Western medicine.

Pathogenesis. Epidemic seasonal noxious agents which invades the three yang meridians.

Therapeutic Principle. Dispelling pathogens, clearing away heat, removing toxic substances and promoting subsidence of swelling.

Sea-tangle

It is the whole plant of Laminaria japonica Aresch. (Zosteraceae).

Effect. Softening hard masses, dispelling phlegm, eliminating diuresis and expelling the pathogenic heat.

Indication. Goiter, subcutaneous nodules, hernia, mass in the abdomen, orchitis, edema and beriberi.

Seborrheic Dermatitis

Symptoms. At the beginning, edema of the face, or reddish face, itching. If the wind is severe, the skin will be dry with the rising of white skin scraps now and then, etc.

Pathogenesis. Usual blood dryness, overeating pungent and rich diet, accumulation of damp-heat in the stomach, external affection of pathogenic wind.

Therapeutic Principle. Dispelling wind and removing heat from the blood for the severe wind; clearing away heat and promoting diuresis for the severe dampness.

Selecting Points on the Affected Meridian

One of the principles of acupuncture treatment. A syndrome not obviously caused by deficiency or excess, should be treated with points according to the affected meridian instead of being treated by means of reinforcing or reducing.

Selection of Points according to Muscle Groups

It refers to selecting the point on the muscle or muscle group where the disease lies.

Indication. Often used for myoplegia and muscular atrophy, etc., for example, Futu (S 32) for paralysis of musculus rectus femoris, and Zusanli (S 36) for paralysis of musculus tibialis anterior, etc.

Selection of Points according to the Distribution of Nerves

It refers to selecting points pursuant to the distribution of nerves. In most of the cases Jiaji (Ex-B2) points related to the spinal nerves, and the points distributed on the neuro-plexus or nerve-trunk are selected, for example, select Neiguan (P 6) at the nervus medianus and Quchi (LI 11) at the nervus radialis to treat numbness of fingers; select Yanglingquan (G 34) at the nervus peroneus, ect.

Selection of Points on Connected Meridians

A method of selecting acupoints, among the twelve regular meridians, the meridians of the hand and foot with the same name are connected. Based on this relationship, the diseases of one meridian can be treated with the points on the connected hand or foot meridian.

Self-inferior Disease

Symptoms. Mass in the abdomen with anorexia, fear, preference for hiding in a dark place, avoidance in encountering people, etc.

Pathogenesis. Deficiency of blood.

Therapeutic Principle. Nourishing blood and the heart, and tranquilizing emotion and mind.

Self-massage

Operation. Simple manipulations to massage the certain points on the body surface with one's own hands.

Effect. Strengthening constitution and care health, relieving some symptoms and treating some diseases.

Senile Metrorrhagia

It refers to metrorrhagia before or after menopause.

Pathogenesis. Hyperactivity of ministerial fire with the result of inability to absorb and store blood due to insufficiency of yin essence at the initial stage of exhaustion of the kidney-qi and menopause.

Therapeutic Principle. Soothing the liver, strengthening the spleen and tonifying the kidney.

Senna Leaf S-4

It is the leaflet of Cassia angustifolia Vahl and C. acutifolia Del. (Leguminosae).

Effect. Dissipating stagnancy, clearing away heat, stopping blood.

Indication. Constipation due to accumulation of heat, ulcer with bleeding.

Sensation of Gas Rushing

Symptoms. Paroxysmal rushing of gas through the chest directly to the throat from the lower abdomen, gripping pain in the abdomen, choking sensation in the chest, dizziness and giddiness, palpitation and susceptibility, etc.

Pathogenesis. Rushing-up of pathogenic cold accumulated in the kidney, or flaming-up of the liver fire.

Therapeutic Principle. Promoting flow of qi and lowering the adverse flow of qi.

Sensitive Plant Herb

It is the whole herb of Mimosa pudica L. (Leguminosae).

Effect. Clearing away heat, tranquilizing the mind, aiding digestion and detoxicating.

Indication. Enteritis, gastritis, insomnia, infantile indigestion with food retention, bloodshot, deep abscess, etc.

Sensitive Plant-like Senna Herb

It is the whole herb of Cassia mimosoides L. (Leguminosae).

Effect. Clearing heat from the liver, inducing diuresis, dissipating away stasis to activate blood circulation and food stagnancy.

Indication. Jaundice due to damp-heat pathogen, vomiting and diarrhea due to summer-heat, edema, pyretic stranguria, constipation, infantile dyspepsia and boils, subcutaneous swelling.

Sensitive Plant Root

It is the root of Mimosa pudica L. (Leguminosae).

Effect. Relieving cough, dispelling sputum, eliminating diuresis, removing obstruction in the meridians, regulating the stomach and relieving stagnancy of indigested food.

Indication. Chronic bronchitis, pain due to pathogenic wind-dampness, chronic gastritis and infantile indigestion with food retention.

Sessile Alternanthera Herb

It is the whole plant of Alternanthera sessilis (L.) DC (Amaranthaceae) with root.

Effect. Clearing away heat to cool blood, inducing diuresis and detoxicating, subcutaneous swelling.

Indication. Cough with hematemesis, dysentery, stranguria, carbuncles and other suppurative infections on the body surface and eczema.

Sessile Lobelia Herb

It is the root or the whole herb of Lobelia sessilifolia Lamb. (Campanulaceae) with root.

Effect. Dispelling phlegm, reliving cough, clearing away heat and detoxicating.

Indication. Bronchitis, boils and pyogenic infections, snake bite, etc.

Seven Emotions

It refers to the seven emotional activities, namely joy, anger, melancholy, anxiety, grief, fear, and terror, meaning the response of the mind to the environmental stimuli. They are considered to be pathogenic factors resulting in functional derangement of qi, blood, and zang-fu organs, if in excess.

Seven-lobed Yam

It is the dried rhizome of Dioscorea hypoglauca palib., or D. septemloba Thunb. (Dioscoreaceae).

Effect. Clearing pathogenic dampness and dispelling wind-dampness.

Indication. Stranguria complicated by chyluria, rheumatic arthralgia, lumbago, gonalgia and dysuria.

Seven Ominous Signs

1. It refers to one of the methods of predicting prognosis of the skin and external diseases. Showing a poor prognosis, namely, (1) poor heart: unconsciousness, vexation, dryness of the tongue, purple dark sores, and dysphasia; (2) poor liver: stiff body, difficulty in look-

ing squarely at, blood and water flowing out of sore and timely palpitation due to fright; (3) poor spleen: thin physique sunken sore with stinking pus, poor appetite, and vomiting when the patient is taking drugs; (4) poor lung: withered skin, aphasia due to excessive phlegm, dyspnea, and flaring of nares; (5) poor kidney: timely thirsty, darkish complexion, dry throat, and internal condense of scrotum; (6) poor zang-fu organs: general edema of the body, vomiting and hiccups, borborygmus and diarrhea, and general mouth ulcer; (7) deficiency of qi and blood: dark sunken sore, timely flowing of dirty water, sweating with cold limbs, sleepiness, and speaking in low sounds.

2. It refers to one of the methods of prediction the prognosis of smallpox.

Seven Orifices

It refers to two ears, two eyes, two nostrils and mouth for hearing, seeing, breathing and eating. If the five viscera organs work abnormally, the seven orifices are obstructive.

Seven Points for Apoplexy

Seven experienced points used to treat apoplexy. They are Baihui (GV 20), Erqianfaji, Jianjing (G 21), Fengshi (G 31), Zusanli (S 36), Xuanzhong (G 39) and Quchi (LI 11).

Indication. Apoplexy, aphasia, hemiplegia.

Method. Apply moxibustion on the 7 points at the same time.

Severe Angina Pectoris

Symptoms. Pain in the heart as if being cut by knife, stiffness and pain in the chest and hypochondrium, vomiting clear fluid, poor appetite, extremely cold hand and foot, etc.

Pathogenesis. The pathogen of epidemic disease affecting the heart.

Therapeutic Principle. Eliminating pathogens, smoothing the meridians and relieving pain.

Severe Inflammatory Edema of Eyelid

Symptoms. Severe swelling of the eyelid, the eye tightly close, and redness of its local skin often accompanied by blood filaments in the white, hot tears and photophobia.

Pathogenesis. Mostly caused by stagnation of the liver-fire and the spleen-dampness in the eyelid, or by heat of the excess type in the Heart Meridian and toxic heat in the blood system.

Therapeutic Principle. Clearing away heat, eliminating diuresis, removing pathogenic heat from blood and detoxicating.

Sexual Strain

Symptoms. Lassitude in loin and legs, dizziness, tinnitus, listlessness, sexual hypoesthesia, spermatorrhea, seminal emission and impotence.

Pathogenesis. Excess sexual intercourse, deficiency of the kidney essence.

Shaking off Dust

One of the needling techniques.

Pathogenesis. Diseases caused by adverse rising of qi leading to distention and fullness in the chest, shaking shoulders when breathing, or dyspnea, inability to lie flat and fear of dust and smoke.

Therapeutic Principle. Decreasing the adverse flow of qi, dredging the meridians and collaterals, which can achieve a remarkable and quick effect like shaking off dust by selecting some points, such as Tianrong (SI 17), Lianquan (CV 23).

Shaking Manipulation

Operation. Hold the distal end of the patient's upper or lower limb with both hands and shake up and down in a narrow range with a heavy force continuously.

Function. Regulating qi and blood, relaxing muscles and tendons, and collaterals.

It is often used as the end manipulation of treatment.

Shangexue (Ex-HN)

An extra acupuncture point.

Location. In the mouth, at the inferior aspect of the palate raphe, at the midpoint of the superior border of the gum.

Indication. Jaundice, etc.

Method. Puncturing obliquely 0.1-0.2 cun or prick to cause bleeding.

Shangguan (G 3)

A meridian acupuncture point.

Location. Anterior to the ear, directly above Xiaguan (S 7), in the depression above the upper border of the zygomatic arch.

Indication. Headache, tinnitus, deafness, facial paralysis, facial pain, toothache, epilepsy and clonic convulsion.

Method. Puncturing perpendicularly 0.5-0.8 cun. Apply moxibustion 2-5 minutes with warming moxibustion.

Shangjuxu (S 37)

An acupuncture point.

Location. 6 cun directly inferior to Dubi (S 35), or 3 cun below Zusanli (S 36).

Indication. Abdominal pain, diarrhea, dysentery, constipation, acute appendicitis, flaccidity and numbness of lower limb, and beriberi.

Method. Puncturing perpendicularly 1-2 cun and applying moxibustion to the point with 3-7 units of moxa cones or for 5-15 minutes.

Shanglian (LI 9)

Location. 3 cun below Quchi (LI 11) on the connecting line between Yangxi (LI 5) and Quchi at the lateral anterior margin of the forearm.

Indication. Headache, dizziness, brachialgia, hemiparalysis, borborygmus, abdominal pain and dysuria.

Method. Puncturing perpendicularly 0.5-1 cun and applying moxibustion to the point with 3-5 units of moxa cones or for 5-10 minutes.

Shangliao (B 31)

An acupuncture point.

Location. In the first posterior sacral foramen of the sacral region.

Indication. Lumbago, dysuria, irregular menstruation, morbid leukorrhea, impotence and seminal emission.

Method. Puncturing perpendicularly 1-1.5 cun and applying moxibustion to the point with 3-7 units of moxa cones or for 5-15 minutes.

Shangma

A massage point.

Location. The back depression of the metacarpophalangeal joints of the ring and little fingers on the dorsum of the hand.

Operation. Kneading manipulation is mostly applied.

Function. Nourishing yin, tonifying the kidney, promoting the circulation of qi, dispelling the obstruction, and eliminating diuresis for treating stranguria.

Indication. Fever due to deficiency and cough with dyspnea, stranguria, abdominal pain, etc.

Shangqiu (Sp 5)

A meridian acupuncture point.

Location. In the depression, anterior and inferior to the medial malleolus, at the midpoint of the line connecting the tuberosity of the navicular bone and the tip of the medial malleolus.

Indication. Abdominal distention, diarrhea, constipation, dyspepsia, pain in the root of the tongue, jaundice, lassitude and drowsiness, manic-depressive psychosis, susceptive of sighs, cough, epilepsy in children, hemorrhoids.

Method. Puncturing perpendicularly 0.3-0.5 cun. Applying moxibustion 1-3 units of moxa cones or 5-10 minute with warming moxibustion.

Shangqu (K 17)

A meridian acupuncture point.

Location. On the upper abdomen, 2 cun above the center of the umbilicus, and 0.5 cun lateral to the anterior midline.

Indication. Abdominal pain, diarrhea, constipation, and abdominal mass.

Method. Puncturing perpendicularly 0.5-0.8 cun. Applying moxibustion 5-7 units of moxa cones or 10-15 minutes moxibustion.

Shangwan (CV 13)

An acupuncture point.

Location. Middle of the abdomen and 5 cun above the umbilicus.

Indication. Stomachache, abdominal distention, nausea, vomiting and epilepsy.

Method. Puncturing perpendicularly 1-2 cun. Moxibustion is applicable.

Shangxing (GV 23)

An acupuncture point.

Location. 1.0 cun inside the front hairline on the cephalic median line.

Indication. Headache, ophthalmalgia, epistaxis, psychosis, malaria and febrile disease.

Method. Puncturing subcutaneously 0.5-1 cun and applying moxibustion to the point with 3-5 units of moxa cones or for 5-10 minutes.

Shangyang (LI 1)

An acupuncture point.

Location. 0.1 cun lateral to the corner of the nail on the radial side of the index finger.

Indication. Coma due to apoplexy, febrile disease without sweating, deafness, swelling sore throat, malaria and numbness of finger.

Method. Puncturing obliquely 0.1 cun, or prick the point to cause bleeding with a three-edged needle. Applying moxibustion to the point with 1-3 units of moxa cones or for 5-10 minutes.

Shangyingxiang (Ex-HN 8)

An acupuncture point.

Location. On the sunken spot under the nasal bone and the upper end of the nasolabial groove.

Indication. Headache, allergic rhinitis, hypertrophic rhinitis, atrophic rhinitis, nasal obstruction, or thick nasal discharge.

Method. Puncture obliquely upward 0.5-1 cun along the skin.

Shangyinli (Ex-HN)

An extra acupuncture point.

Location. In the mouth, at the middle of labial frenum, opposite exteriorly to Shuigou (GV 26).

Indication. Jaundice, etc.

Method. Puncturing perpendicularly 0.1-0.2 cun or prick to cause bleeding.

Shanqixue (Ex-CA)

A pair of extra acupuncture points.

Location. Take the distance between the two angles of the patient's mouth at one side to make an equilateral triangle with the vertex angle on the acromphalus. The lower side being horizontal, the two lower angles are the points.

Indication. Hernia and collapse of testicles.

Method. Moxibustion.

Shaochong (H 9)

An acupuncture point.

Location. About 0.1 cun lateral to the corner of the nail on the radial side of the little finger.

Indication. Febrile disease, apoplectic coma, psychosis, epidemic acute conjunctivitis, heat in mouth, palpitation, cardialgia and infantile convulsion.

Method. Puncturing obliquely 0.1-0.2 cun or prick the point to cause little bleeding with the three-edged needle. Applying moxibustion to the point with 3-5 units of moxa cones or for 5-10 minutes.

Shaofu (H 8)

A meridian acupuncture point.

Location. In the palm, between the 4th and 5th metacarpal bones, at the part of the palm touching the tip of the little finger when forming a fist is made.

Indication. Palpitation, chest pain, skin itching, pruritus vulvae, prolapse of uterus, pudenda pain, oliguria, little finger contracture, feverish sensation in the palm, susceptibility to sorrow and fear.

Method. Puncturing perpendicularly 0.2-0.3 cun. Applying moxibustion 1-3 units of moxa cones or 3-5 minutes with warming moxibustion.

Shaohai (H 3)

A meridian acupuncture point.

Location. With the elbow flexed, at the midpoint of the line connecting the medial end of the cubital crease and the medial epicondyle of the humerus.

Indication. Precardial pain, numbness of the arm, hand twitching, amnesia, sudden loss of voice, cheirospasm, axilla and hypochondriac pain, neck pain, manic-depressive psychosis, epilepsy, headache, dizziness.

Method. Puncturing perpendicularly 0.5-0.8 cun. Applying moxibustion 3-5 moxa cones or 5-10 minutes with warming moxibustion.

Shaoshang (L 11)

A meridian acupuncture point.

Location. On the radial side of the distal segment of the thumb, 0.1 cun from the corner of the fingernail.

Indication. Inflammation of the throat, cough, asthma, epistaxis, fullness in the epigastrium, apoplectic coma, vomiting due to heatstroke, febrile disease, infantile convulsion.

Method. Puncturing subcutaneously 0.1 cun to the wrist, or pricking to cause bleeding. Applying moxibustion 4-7 units of moxa cones or 5-10 minutes with warming moxibustion.

Shaoyang Disease

It is one of the syndromes of the six meridians.

Symptoms. Alternate fever and chills, fullness of the chest and hypochondrium, dysphoria, dizziness, vomiting, loss of appetite, bitter taste in the mouth, dry throat, etc.

Pathogenesis. The exogenous affection between the exterior and interior parts of the body.

Therapeutic Principle. Mediation method.

Shaoyangwei (Ex-LE)

An extra acupuncture point.

Location. At the midpoint of the line connecting Taixi (K 3) and Fuliu (K 7).

Indication. Chronic eczema, numbness and paralysis of the lower limbs, beriberi, etc.

Method. Puncturing perpendicularly 0.3-0.5 cun. Applying moxibustion 3-5 units of moxa cones or 5-10 minutes with warming moxibustion.

Shaoyin Syndrome

Symptoms. Occurrence of Shaoyin disease, but with such symptoms of yin excess and yang deficiency as sleepiness, aversion to cold, cold limbs, lienteric diarrhea, clear and long urination.

Therapeutic Principle. Warming and invigorating the heart and kidney.

Shaoze (SI 1)

A meridian acupuncture point.

Location. On the ulnar side of the distal segment of the little finger, 0.1 cun from the corner of the nail.

Indication. Febrile diseases, coma due to apoplexy, acute mastitis, sore throat, corneal opacity, headache, deafness, pain in the posterior-lateral aspect of the shoulder and upper limbs.

Method. Puncture perpendicularly 0.1 cun or prick to cause bleeding. Apply moxibustion 1-3 units of moxa cones or 3-5 minutes with warming moxibustion.

Shapeless Mass

Symptoms. Disturbance in intestines and abdomen with uncertain painful regions, fullness in the chest and abdomen, etc.

Pathogenesis. Emotional depression, impairment of the regulating function of the liver, and blockage of the qi circulation.

Therapeutic Principle. Regulating the flow of qi and alleviating the mass.

Shape of Tongue

Observing the shape of the tongue to diagnose diseases. For example, fine and smooth veins, and a tender, lovely form and color of the body of tongue indicating cold syndrome. Rough veins, aged, dry form and color indicates heat syndrome of excess type. Thin and small tongue of light color indicates insufficiency of qi and blood, etc.

Sheathed Monochoria Herb

It is the whole herb of Monochoria vaginalis (Burm. f.) Presl. (Pontederiaceae).

Effect. Clearing away heat, detoxicating, inducing diuresis and repercussion.

Indication. Dysentery, enteritis, acute tonsillitis, hyperpyrexia, laryngitis, gingivitis, furuncle and edema.

Sheeny Complexion

It is one of ten methods of observation of complexion, refering to radiant and moist complexion. It is the normal complexion of unexhaustion of the vital-qi or the complexion of the patient with mild illness, with favorable prognosis.

Sheep Blood

It is the blood of Capra hircus L. or Ovis aries L. (Bovidae).

Effect. Dissipating blood stasis and arresting bleeding.

Indication. Hemoptysis, epistaxis, metrorrhagia, metrostaxis, postpartum bruise and swelling pain due to ecchymoma.

Sheepear Inula Root

It is the root of Inula cappa DC. (Compositae).

Effect. Dispelling wind, removing cold, relaxing muscles and tendons and activating blood circulation.

Indication. Common cold resulting from wind cold with cough and asthma, rheumatic arthralgia and irregular menstruation.

Sheep Fat

It is the fat of Capra hircus L. or Ovis aries L. (Bovidae).

Effect. Tonifying qi, moistening dryness of the viscera, expelling wind and detoxicating.

Indication. Asthenia consumption, emaciation with sallow complexion, chronic dysentery, erysipelas, carbuncle and tinea.

Sheep Gall

It is the gall of Capra hircus L. or Ovis aries L. (Bovidae).

Effect. Removing heat, detoxicating, improving eyesight and moistening the lung.

Indication. Conjunctival congestion resulting from pathogenic wind-heat, oculopathy, hemoptysis due to tuberculosis, pharyngitis, jaundice and constipation.

Sheep Kidney

It is the kidney of Capra hircus L. or Ovis aries L. (Bovidae).

Effect. Nourishing the kidney-qi and replenishing vital essence and marrow.

Indication. Pain in the loins and back, flaccidity of the lower limbs, due to the kidney deficiency, frequent micturition and diabetes.

Sheep Liver

It is the liver of Capra hircus L. or Ovis aries L. (Bovidae).

Effect. Nourishing the liver and kidney, tonifying vital essence and blood, and improving eyesight.

Indication. Shallow complexion due to blood deficiency, manifested as blurred vision, night blindness, optic atrophy and inactive corneal opacity due to deficiency of liver-yin and kidney-yin.

Sheep Marrow

It is the marrow or spinal cord of Capra hircus L. or Ovis aries L. (Bovidae).
Effect. Nourishing qi, tonifying marrow and moistening the lung.
Indication. Emaciation with sallow complexion, hectic fever, cough, diabetes, carbuncles, conjunctival congestion and opacity.

Sheep Testis

It is the testis of Capra hircus L. or Ovis aries L. (Bovidae).
Effect. Nourishing the kidney, tonifying vital essence and restoring yang.
Indication. Lumbago due to the kidney deficiency, emission, impotence, leukorrhea, frequent micturition, hernia, etc.

Shegong Wound

It is a skin disease.
Symptoms. Stabbing pain in the local area. After a prolonged time, itching externally and painful internally. In the center of the affected position of the stabbing hair, skin rashes like urtica appear in the size of a green gram or a broad bean surrounded by aula. It can even become ulcerated.
Pathogenesis. Stabbing wound of a stab-and-hair worms shegong stab.
Therapeutic Principle. Treating externally mainly.

Shell to Suppress Sthenic Yang

It refers to the medicine from shells, such as oyster, sea-ear shell, tortoise plastron, fresh-water turtle shell, etc.
Effect. Suppress the sthenic yang-qi.
Indication. Syndromes of disturbance of yang-qi, hyperactivity of the liver-yang, etc.

Shencang (K 25)

An acupuncture point.
Location. In the thoracic region, 2 cun lateral to the anterior median line, in the second intercostal space.
Indication. Cough, dyspnea, pain of chest, vomiting, anorexia, etc.
Method. Puncturing obliquely or subcutaneously 0.3-0.5 cun and applying moxibustion to the point with 3-5 units of moxa cones or for 5-10 minutes.
Notice. Deep insertion is inadvisable.

Shendao (GV 11)

A meridian acupuncture point.
Location. On the posterior midline, in the depression below the spinous process of the 5th thoracic vertebra.
Indication. Precordial pain, palpitation due to fright, severe palpitation, insomnia, aphasia due to apoplexy, epilepsy, clonic convulsion, pain in the shoulder and back, cough and dyspnea.
Method. Puncturing obliquely 0.5-1.0 cun. Applying moxibustion 3-5 moxa cones or 5-10 minutes with warming moxibustion.

Shending

A point of massage.
Location. On the tip of the little finger.
Operation. Kneading and rubbing manipulation is used.
Function. Astringing primary qi and consolidating superficial resistance to stop perspiration.
Indication. Spontaneous perspiration, night sweat, infantile metopism, etc.

Shenfeng (K 23)

A meridian acupuncture point.
Location. On the chest, in the 4th intercostal space, 2 cun lateral to the anterior midline.
Indication. Cough, dyspnea, fullness in the chest, vomiting, acute mastitis.
Method. Puncturing obliquely or subcutaneously 0.5-0.8 cun. It is not advisable to puncture deep. Applying moxibustion 3-5

moxa cones or 5-10 minutes with warming moxibustion.

Shenfu (Ex-CA)

An extra acupuncture point.

Location. At the center of the xiphoid process.

Indication. Precordial pain.

Method. Puncturing subcutaneously 0.3-0.5 cun. Applying moxibustion to the point with 3-5 moxa cones or for 5-10 minutes.

Shenjiao (Ex-CA)

An extra acupuncture point.

Location. On the abdomen, 3 cun below the center of the umbilicus.

Indication. Constipation, anuresis, enuresis, morbid leukorrhea, etc.

Method. Puncturing perpendicularly 0.5-1.0 cun. Be cautious in the case of pregnant women. Applying moxibustion point with 3-7 moxa cones for 5-15 minutes.

Shenmai (B 62)

A meridian acupuncture point.

Location. On the lateral side of the foot, in the depression directly below the external malleolus.

Indication. Epilepsy, mania, headache, dizziness, insomnia, lumbago, cold foot, stiff neck.

Method. Puncturing perpendicularly 0.2-0.3 cun. Applying moxibustion 3-5 moxa cones or 5-10 minutes with warming moxibustion.

Shenmen (H 7)

A meridian acupuncture point.

Location. On the wrist, at the ulnar end of the crease of the wrist, in the depression of the radial side of the tendon of the ulnar flexor, muscle of the wrist.

Indication. Cardialgia, anxiety, trance, vexation, amnesia, insomnia, palpitation due to fright, severe palpitation, dementia, epilepsy, feverish sensation in the palms, hematemesis, spitting blood, stool with pus and blood, headache, dizziness, dry throat and anorexia, dyspnea.

Method. Puncturing perpendicularly 0.3-0.5 cun. Moxibustion is applicable.

Shenmen (MA)

An auricular point.

Location. At the upper half of the lateral 1/3 of the triangular fossa which is divided into three equal parts by two curved lines parallel to the anterior border of the helix. The point plays the role to tranquilize and allay excitement, clear heat and alleviate pain.

Indication. Insomnia, dream-disturbed sleep, pain, menopausal syndrome. It is a commonly used auricular point in auriculo-acupuncture anesthesia.

Shenque (CV 8)

A meridian acupuncture point.

Location. On the middle abdomen at the center of the umbilicus.

Indication. Collapse syndrome of apoplexy, cold limbs, epilepsy due to wind pathogen, abdominal pain around the umbilicus, edema and tympanitis, diarrhea, dysentery, constipation, urinary incontinence, five types of stranguria, sterility.

Method. Acupuncture is forbidden. Applying moxibustion 5-15 moxa cones with ginger, salt interposed moxibustion or 15-30 minutes with warming moxibustion.

Shenshu (B 23)

A meridian acupuncture point.

Location. On the low back, below the spinous process of the 2nd lumbar vertebra, 1.5 cun lateral to the posterior midline.

Indication. Seminal emission, impotence, enuresis, frequent micturition, irregular menstruation, soreness and weakness of the waist and knees, blurred vision, deafness, difficulty in urination, edema, cough.

Method. Puncturing perpendicularly 0.5-1 cun. Applying moxibustion 5-7 moxa cones or 5-15 minutes with warming moxibustion.

Shentang (B 44)

A meridian acupuncture point.

Location. On the back, below the spinous process of the 5th thoracic vertebra, 3 cun lateral to the posterior midline.

Indication. Cough, dyspnea, full sensation in the chest and abdomen, pain in the shoulder, rigidity of the back and spinal column.

Method. Puncturing obliquely 0.5-0.8 cun. Applying moxibustion 3-5 moxa cones or 5-15 minutes with warming moxibustion.

Shenting (GV 24)

A meridian acupuncture point on the Back Middle Meridian and the crossing point of the Back Middle Meridian and the Meridians of Foot-taiyang and Yangming.

Location. On the head, 0.5 cun directly above the midpoint of the anterior hairline.

Indication. Headache, dizziness, the redness, pain and swelling of the eye, nyctalopia, rhinorrhea with turbid discharge, epistaxis, epilepsy, opisthotonus.

Method. Puncturing subcutaneously 0.3-0.5 cun. Applying moxibustion 3-5 moxa cones or 5-10 minutes with warming moxibustion.

Shenxi (Ex-LE)

An extra acupuncture point.

Location. At the point 1 cun below Futu (S 32).

Indication. Diabetes and frequent micturition.

Method. Moxibustion is applicable.

Shenzhu (GV 12)

A meridian acupuncture point.

Location. On the back, on the posterior midline, in the depression below the spinous process of the 3rd thoracic vertebra.

Indication. Fever with headache, cough, dyspnea, infantile convulsion, epilepsy, furuncle, lumbodorsal carbuncle.

Method. Puncturing obliquely 0.5-1.0 cun. Applying moxibustion 3-5 moxa cones or 5-10 minutes with warming moxibustion.

Shepherdspurse Herb

It is the whole herb of Capsella bursa-pastoris (L.) Medic. (Cruciferae) with root.

Effect. Dredging the spleen, inducing diuresis, cooling blood arresting bleeding and improving acuity of vision, lowering blood pressure.

Indication. Dysentery, edema, stranguria, hematemesis, hemafecia, metrorrhagia, and bloodshot, hypertension.

Shepherdspurse Seed

It is the seed of Capsella bursa-pastoris (L.) Medic. (Cruciferae).

Effect. Dispelling wind and improving acuity of vision.

Indication. Painful eyes, optic atrophy and oculopathy.

Shexia (Ex-HN)

An extra acupuncture point.

Location. On the lateral borders of lingual surface against the mouth angles when the tongue is stretched out.

Indication. Jaundice, acute laryngeal infection, tonsillitis.

Method. Puncturing perpendicularly 0.1-0.2 cun or pricking to cause bleeding.

Shidou (Sp 17)

An acupuncture point.

Location. On the lateral thoracic region, in the 5th intercostal space, 6 cun lateral to the anterior median line.

Indication. Cough, dyspnea, dysphagia, regurgitation, stomachache, abdominal distention, and edema.

Method. Puncturing obliquely 0.3-0.5 cun, deep needling is forbidden, and applying moxibustion to the point with 3-5 units of moxa cones or for 5-10 minutes.

Shiguan (Ex-CA)

An extra acupuncture point.

Location. On the upper abdomen, 0.5 cun lateral to Jianli (CV 11).

Indication. Dysphagia, vomiting, gastritis, enteritis, dyspepsia, etc.

Method. Puncturing perpendicularly 1-1.5 cun. Applying moxibustion is applicable.

Shiguan (K 18)

A meridian acupuncture point.

Location. On the upper abdomen, 3 cun above the center of the umbilicus, and 0.5 cun lateral to the anterior midline or 0.5 cun lateral to Jianli (CV 11).

Indication. Vomiting, abdominal pain, constipation, abdominal pain after delivery.

Method. Puncturing perpendicularly 0.5-0.8 cun. Applying moxibustion with 5-7 moxa cones or for 10-15 minutes.

Shimen (CV 5)

An acupuncture point.

Location. 2 cun inferior to the center of the umbilicus on the ventral median line.

Indication. Abdominalgia, edema, dysentery, diarrhea, hernia, irregular menstruation, amenorrhea, dysmenorrhea, metrorrhagia, metrostaxis, dysuria and enuresis.

Method. Puncturing perpendicularly 0.5-1.0 cun and applying moxibustion to the point with 3-7 units of moxa cones or for 15-30 minutes.

Shimian (Ex-LE)

An extra acupuncture point.

Location. On the bottom of the heel, at the crossing point of the midline of the sole and the line joining the medial malleolus and lateral malleolus.

Indication. Insomnia, and pain in the sole, etc.

Method. Puncturing perpendicularly 0.3-0.5 cun. Applying moxibustion for 5-15 minutes with warming moxibustion.

Shiny Cinquefoil Herb

It is the root or herb of Potentilla fulgens Wall. (Rosaceae) with root.

Effect. Clearing away heat, relieving inflammation, removing heat from blood to stop bleeding.

Indication. Dysentery, enteritis, stomachache, hemoptysis caused by pulmonary tuberculosis, epistaxis, hemafecia, metrorrhagia, traumatic bleeding, etc.

Shinyleaf Pricklyash Root

It is the root or branch and leaf of Zanthoxylum nitidum (Roxb.) DC. (Rutaceae).

Effect. Eliminating pathogenic wind, dredging meridian, alleviating edema and relieving pain.

Indication. Rheumatic arthralgia, inflammation of the throat, stomachache, traumatic injuries, burns and scalds.

Shiqizhui (Ex-B 8)

One of the extraordinary points.

Location. Inferior to the spinous process of the 5th lumbar vertebra, on the posterior midline.

Indication. Lumbago, paralysis of lower limbs, anal diseases, sciatica, metrorrhagia and metrostaxis.

Method. Puncturing 0.5-1 cun and applying moxibustion to the point with 3-7 units of moxa cones or for 10-15 minutes.

Shisu (Ex-CA)

An extra acupuncture point.

Location. On the lateral side of the chest, on the middle axillary line, in the depression about 1 cun above Yuanye (G 22).

Indication. Fullness in the chest and hypochondrium, lumbago radiating to the abdomen.

Method. Puncturing obliquely 0.1-0.5 cun. Applying moxibustion with 1-3 moxa cones or for 3-5 minutes.

Shiwang (Ex-UE)

An extra acupuncture point.
Location. On the dorsal aspect of the 10 fingers, 0.1 cun directly above the midpoint of the nail roots.
Indication. Coma, high fever, heat stroke, cholera, infantile convulsion, etc.
Method. Pricking the point to cause bleeding with a triangular needle.

Shixuan (Ex-UE11)

It belongs to extraordinary point.
Location. At the ending of each finger, 0.1 cun to the nail. There are 10 such points on both hands altogether.
Indication. Shock, coma, faint, high fever, heliosis, epilepsy, infantile convulsion, tonsillitis.
Method. Puncturing for bleeding with a triangular needle, and applying moxibustion to the point with 1-3 units of moxa cones or for 5-10 minutes.

Short Breath

Symptoms. The breathing with short rapid breath, like asthma without lifting shoulders.
Pathogenesis. The case of deficiency type is mainly caused by weakness and debility or exhaustion of the kidney-yang after attack of disease, while the case of excess type, mainly by stagnation of phlegm and stagnation of qi.

Shortened Tongue

It refers to a shortened and contracted tongue unable to protrude out. A shortened pale and moist tongue refers to stagnation of coldness in the meridians. A reddened, dry, and shortened tongue without tongue coating or with deep dark tongue coating shows a impairment of the body fluid by febrile disease. A plump, greasy and shortened tongue is ascribable to retention of wet-phlegm and consequent numbness of the tongue. The unconscious patient with shortened and stiff tongue is in a critical condition in which the disease has entered pericardium.

Shortness of Breath due to Blood Stasis

Symptoms. Hypochondriac pain, difficult, and short breath, emaciation and weakness, etc.
Pathogenesis. Injury by overload, indignation which injure the liver, and blood stasis which stagnates the meridians.
Therapeutic Principle. Dispersing the depressed liver-qi and regulating the lung-qi, and promoting the blood circulation to dredging blood stasis.

Short-pedicel Aconite Root

It is the root tuber of Aconitum brachypodum Diels. (Ranunculaceae).
Effect. Relieving swelling and pain, dispelling wind and dampness.
Indication. Traumatic injuries, fracture, rheumatic osteodynia, infections on the body surface and snake-bite.

Shortstem Ardisia Root

It is the root or whole plant of Ardisia brevicaulis Diels. (Myrsinaceae).
Effect. Expelling pathogenic wind, clearing away heat, dissipating blood stasis and dissipating subsidence of swelling.
Indication. Swollen and sore throat, toothache due to pathogenic wind-fire, arthralgia and myalgia due to wind-dampness, lumbago, innominate inflammatory swelling, etc.

Short-thrust Needling

An acupuncture point technique.
Indication. Arthralgia with other joint symptoms.
Method. Shaking the handle slightly after inserting the needle, gradually inserting it to the bone, then lifting and thrusting it shortly and quickly.

Shorttube Lyloris Bulb

It is the bulb of Lycoris radiata (L'Her.) Herb. (Amaryllidaceae).

Effect. Expelling phlegm, eliminating diuresis, detoxicating eliminating stagnation, detumescence and inducing vomiting.

Indication. Acute throat trouble, nephritis, pleuritis edema, subcutaneous swelling, furunculosis and scrofula.

Shoudazhijiahou (Ex-UE)

An extra acupuncture point.

Location. On the ulnar side of the thumb, at the end of the transverse crease of the digital joints and the junction of the red and white skin.

Indication. Diseases of intestines and stomach in children, conjunctivitis, pancorneal opacity.

Method. Puncturing perpendicularly 0.1-0.2 cun, or pricking the point to cause little bleeding with triangular needle. Applying moxibustion with 3-5 moxa cones or for 5-10 minutes.

Shouhuai (Ex-UE)

An extra acupuncture point.

Location. On the dorsal side of the wrist, at the high point of the styloid process of radius.

Indication. Finger spasm, toothache.

Method. Apply moxibustion with 3-7 moxa cones or for 5-15 minutes.

Shoulder (MA-SF 4)

An auricular point.

Location. Divide the scapha into 6 equal parts and the 4th and 5th parts are the point.

Indication. Shoulder pain, scapulohumeral periarthritis, gallstones, etc.

Shoulder and Neck Pain

Pathogenesis. Weak constitution, or overburden, attacking of external evil, the impeded of circulation of qi and blood, or deficiency of the kidney and insufficient essence, failure in nourishing the bone and blood stasis due to trauma.

Shounizhu (Ex-UE)

An extra acupuncture point.

Location. On the flexion side of the forearm, 6 cun above the transverse crease of the wrist, between the tendons of m. palmaris longus and m. flexor carpi radialis.

Indication. Hysteria, pain of the forearm, spasm, numbness and arthralgia, etc.

Method. Puncturing perpendicularly 0.5-1.0 cm. Applying moxibustion 3-7 moxa cones or 5-10 minutes.

Shousanli (LI 10)

A meridian acupuncture point.

Location. On the radial side of the dorsal surface of the forearm and on the line connecting Yangxi (LI 5) and Quchi (LI 11), 2 cun below the cubital crease.

Indication. Abdominal distention, vomiting, diarrhea, aphasia, swelling of the cheek, scrofula, paralysis, numbness and pain of the hand and arm and optic diseases.

Method. Puncturing perpendicularly 0.5-0.8 cun. Applying moxibustion 3-5 moxa cones or 5-10 minutes.

Shouwuli (LI 13)

A meridian acupuncture point.

Location. On the lateral side of the upper arm and on the line connecting Quchi (LI 11) and Jianyu (LI 15), 3 cun above Quchi.

Indication. Spasm and pain in the elbow and arm, scrofula, cough with spitting blood, somnolence and yellow body.

Method. Avoiding the artery, puncturing perpendicularly 0.5-0.8 cun. Applying moxibustion with 3-5 moxa cones.

Shouxin (Ex-UE)

An extra acupuncture point.

Location. On the palm, at the midpoint of the line connecting the midpoint on the metacarpophalangeal articulation of the middle finger and Daling (P 7).

Indication. Epilepsy due to the dog bite.
Method. Moxibustion is applicable.

Shrubalthea Bark

It is the root bark or stem bark of Hibiscus syriacus L. (Malvaceae).
Effect. Clearing away heat promoting urination, cooling blood to stop bleeding, poisoning parasites in the intestines and relieving itching.
Indication. Cough, hemoptysis, icterus, gonorrhea, skin scabies, tinea, leukorrhagia, dysentery, etc.

Shrub Lespedeza Stem or Leaf

It is the stem or leaf of Lespedeza bicolor Turcz. (Leguminosae).
Effect. Clearing away heat, moistening the lung, inducing diuresis and treating stranguria.
Indication. Cough caused by the lung-heat, pertussis and gonorrhea.

Shuaigu (G 8)

A meridian acupuncture point.
Location. On the head, directly above the ear apex, 1.5 cun above the hairline, directly above Jiaosun (TE 20).
Indication. Hemilateral headache, vomiting, infant convulsion.
Method. Puncturing subcutaneously 0.5-0.8 cun. Applying moxibustion with 1-3 moxa cones or for 3-5 minutes.

Shufu (K 27)

A meridian acupuncture point.
Location. On the chest, below the lower border of the clavicle, 2 cun lateral to the midline.
Indication. Cough, asthmatic breath, pain in the chest, vomiting, loss of appetite.
Method. Puncturing obliquely or subcutaneously 0.5-0.8 cun. Applying moxibustion with 3-5 moxa cones or for 5-10 minutes.

Shugu (B 65)

A meridian acupuncture point.

Location. On the lateral side of the foot, below the tuberosity of the 5th metatarsal bone, at the junction of the red and white skin.
Indication. Mania, headache, stiffness of the neck, vertigo, pain of the back and the lower limbs.
Method. Puncturing perpendicularly 0.3-0.5 cun. Applying moxibustion 3-5 moxa cones or 5-10 minutes.

Shuidao (S 28)

A meridian acupuncture point.
Location. On the lower abdomen, 3 cun below the center of the umbilicus and 2 cun lateral to the anterior midline.
Indication. Distention and pain of the lower abdomen, hernia, dysmenorrhea, dysuria.
Method. Puncturing perpendicularly 0.5-1.2 cun. Applying moxibustion with 5-7 moxa cones or for 10-20 minutes.

Shuifen (CV 9)

A meridian acupuncture point.
Location. On the upper abdomen and the anterior midline, 1 cun above the center of the umbilicus.
Indication. Abdominal pain and distention, borborygmus, diarrhea, regurgitation, edema, stiffness of the lumbar and spine.
Method. Puncturing perpendicularly 0.5-1.0 cun. Be cautious in pregnant women. Applying moxibustion with 3-7 moxa cones or for 5-15 minutes.

Shuigou (GV 26)

A meridian acupuncture point.
Location. On the face, at the junction of the upper 1/3 and middle 1/3 of the philtrum.
Indication. Coma, syncope, summer-heat diseases, epilepsy, acute or chronic infantile convulsion, facial edema due to pathogenic wind, trismus, jaundice, diabetes, cholera, stiffness and pain of the back.

Method. Puncturing obliquely upward 0.3-0.5 cun or press and nip with nails. Moxibustion is not applicable.

Shuiquan (K 5)

A meridian acupuncture point.
Location. On the medial side of the foot, posterior and inferior to the medial malleolus, 1 cun directly below Taixi (K 3), in the depression of the medial side of the tuberosity of the calcaneum.
Indication. Irregular menstruation, dysmenorrhea, prolapse of uterus, difficult urination, blurring of vision, abdominal pain.
Method. Puncturing perpendicularly 0.3-0.5 cun. Applying moxibustion 3-5 moxa cones or 5-10 minutes with warming moxibustion.

Shuitu (S 10)

A meridian acupuncture point.
Location. On the neck on the anterior border of the sternocleidomastoid muscle, at the midpoint of the line connecting Renying (S 9)and Qishe (S 11).
Indication. Cough and dyspnea due to reversed flow of lung-qi, asthma, sore throat, swelling of the shoulder, scrofula.
Method. Puncturing perpendicularly 0.3-0.4 cun. Applying moxibustion with 1-3 moxa cones or for 5-10 minutes.

Shuwei (Ex-LE)

An extra acupuncture point.
Location. On the sole, on the upper edge of the midline of the heel.
Indication. Scrofula.
Method. Moxibustion.

Sibai (S 2)

A meridian acupuncture point.
Location. On the face, with the eyes looking straight forward, directly below the pupil, in the depression of the infraorbital foramen.
Indication. Redness, itch, pain and swelling of the eye, epiphora, ache of the head, dizziness, deviation of the mouth and eye.

Method. Puncturing perpendicularly or obliquely 0.2-0.3 cun. Moxibustion is not applicable.

Siberian Clematis Stem

It is the stem branch of Clematis sibirica (L.) Mill. (Ranunculaceae).
Effect. Clearing away heart-fire, promoting diuresis, relieving stranguria, dispelling damp-heat and activating blood circulation.
Indication. Urethritis, acute cystitis, urinary infection, hematuria, difficulty and pain in urethra, amenorrhea, scanty lactation aphthae, and sore throat, etc.

Siberian Cocklebur Fruit

It is the fruit of Xanthium sibiricum Patr. et Widd. (Compositae).
Effect. Clearing the nasal passage, expelling wind-dampness and arresting pain.
Indication. Headache, rheumatic arthralgia, spasm of limbs, etc.

Siberian Cocklebur Herb ⊛ S-5

It is the stem leaf of Xanthium sibiricum Patr. et Widd. (Compositae).
Effect. Dispelling pathogenic wind, clearing away heat and detoxicating.
Indication. Headache and arthralgia caused by wind-dampness manifested as spasm of limbs, thin nasal discharge, leprosy, cutaneous pruritus, etc.

Siberian Elm Bark

It is the root phloem of Ulmus pumila L. (Ulmaceae).
Effect. Promoting diuresis for stranguria and subduing swelling.
Indication. Dysuria, stranguria with turbid urine, edema, deep-rooted carbuncles, erysipelas, scabies, tinea, etc.

Siberian Elm Fruit or Seed

It is the fruit or seed of Ulmus pumila L. (Ulmaceae).
Effect. Clearing away damp-heat and destroying parasites.

Indication. Leukorrhea, infantile malnutrition with fever, emaciation, etc.

Siberian Filbert Seed

It is the kernel of Corylus heterophylla Fisch ex Bess (Betulaceae).
Effect. Regulating the middle-energizer, inducing appetite and digestion and improving acuity of vision.
Indication. Weakness during convalescence, anorexia, fatigue, blurred vision, etc.

Siberian Solomonseal Rhizome ⊛ S-6

It is the rhizome of Polygonatum kingianum Coll. et Hemsl., and Polygonotum sibiricum Red. or P. cyrtonema Hua (Liliaceae).
Effect. Moistening the lung, nourishing yin, replenish the spleen and stomach, and nourishing the vital essence of the lung.
Indication. Dry-cough caused by deficiency of the lung, soreness of waist, dizziness, lassitude in feet due to deficiency of the kidney essence and dry mouth, fatigability, poor appetite, constipation, etc.

Sichuan Chinaberry Fruit

It is the ripe fruit of Melia toosendan Sieb. et Zucc. (Meliaceae).
Effect. Promoting flow of qi to arrest pain, destroying parasites and curing tinea.
Indication. Pain in the hypochondrium, gastric and abdominal pain, hernial pain, and also abdominal pain due to parasitic infestation, scabies, etc.

Sidu (TE 9)

A meridian acupuncture point.
Location. On the dorsal side of the forearm and on the line connecting Yangchi (TE 4) and the tip of the olecranon, 5 cun distal to the tip of the olecranon, between the radius and ulna.
Indication. Sudden hoarseness of voice, sudden deafness, toothache, short breath, obstruction of the throat, pain in the forearm.
Method. Puncturing perpendicularly 0.5-1 cun. Applying moxibustion with 3-5 moxa cones or for 5-10 minutes.

Siegesbeckia Herb

It is the aerial parts of Siegesbeckia orientalis L., S. pubescens Mak. or S. glabrescens Mak. (Compositae).
Effect. Eliminating pathogenic wind and dampness, activating obstruction in the meridians, clearing away heat and detoxicating.
Indication. Arthralgia due to wind-dampness, numbness of the limbs, suppurative infections on the body surface and eczema.

Sifeng (Ex-UE 10)

A set of extra acupuncture points.
Location. Four points on each hand, on the palmar side of the 2nd to 5th finger at the center of the proximal interphalangeal joints.
Indication. Infantile malnutrition pertussis, ascariasis, etc.
Method. Pricking with a three-edged needle and squeeze out a small amount of yellowish viscous fluid.

Sihengwen

A massage point.
Location. At the cross striation of the first finger joints of the index, middle, ring and little fingers on the palm.
Operation. Pushing or nipping-kneading is applied.
Function. Clearing away heat of zang-fu, harmonizing qi and blood and relieving distention and dispersing accumulation of pathogen.
Indication. Disharmony between qi and blood, dyspnea and gastro-intestinal diseases.

Silktree Albizzia Bark ⊛ S-7

It is the bark of Albizzia julibrissin Durazz. (Leguminosae).

Effect. Sedateness, allaying excitement and relieving the depressed liver, promoting blood circulation, and relieving swelling and pain.

Indication. Melancholia, restlessness, palpitation, insomnia and forgetfulness due to emotional stress; traumatic injuries, carbuncles and other pyogenic skin diseases, etc.

Silktree Albizzia Flower

It is the flower of Albizzia julibrissin Durazz. (Leguminosae).

Effect. Sedateness, allaying excitement, and relieving the depressed liver.

Indication. Melancholia, irritability due to vexation, fidgetiness, insomnia, etc.

Silkworm Cocoon

It is the cocoon of Bombyx mori L. (Bombycidae).

Indication. Regurgitation, hemafecia, hematuria and carbuncle.

Silkworm Excrement

It is the solid feces excreted by Bombyx mori L. (Bombycidae).

Effect. Dispelling pathogenic wind and eliminating dampness, clearing away heat to promote blood circulation, regulating the function of the stomach and promoting digestion.

Indication. Rheumatic arthralgia, tetraplegia, eczema, blood stasis, and vomiting due to retention of pathogenic dampness.

Silkworm Pupa

It is the worm of Bombyx mori L. (Bombycidae).

Indication. Infantile malnutrition with fever and diabetes.

Silkworm Slough

It is the slough of Bombyx mori L. (Bombycidae).

Effect. Stopping bleeding, metorrhayia and leukorrhea.

Indication. Leukorrhea, hematemesis, metrorrhagia, metrostaxis, hemachezia and perleche.

Silverfish

It is the whole insect of Lepisma saccharina L. (Lepismatidae).

Effect. Inducing diuresis, treating stranguria, dispelling wind and detoxicating.

Indication. Stranguria, dysuria, infantile epilepsy and carbuncles scabies.

Silvervine Fleece-flower Root

It is the root tuber of volubile plant polygonum subertii L. Henry (Polygonaceae).

Effect. Astringing, stopping dysentery and relieving inflammation.

Indication. Dysentery, digestive trouble, internal hemorrhage, furuncles at their initial stages, etc.

Siman (Ex-CA)

An extra acupuncture point.

Location. On the lower abdomen, 2 cun below the center of the umbilicus and 1.5 cun lateral to the anterior midline.

Indication. Menoxenia, sensation of gas rushing, sterility, etc.

Method. Moxibustion.

Siman (K 14)

A meridian acupuncture point.

Location. On the lower abdomen, 2 cun below the center of the umbilicus and 0.5 cun lateral to the anterior midline.

Indication. Irregular menstruation, uterine bleeding, sterility, persistent postpartum lochia, lower abdominal pain, emission, enuresis, hernia, constipation, edema.

Method. Puncturing perpendicularly 0.8-1.2 cun. Applying moxibustion with 3-5 moxa cones or for 5-10 minutes.

Simultaneous Disorders of both Defence Phase and Nutrient Phase

Symptoms. Fever higher at night, vexation, insomnia, delirium, faint eruptions, deep red tongue proper, etc. as well as chills, headache, general pain.

Pathogenesis. Pathogenic heat is attacking the nutrient system while the defense system syndrome still exists.

Therapeutic Principle. Clearing up the nutrient system and relieving exterior syndrome.

Simultaneous Treatment of Superficiality and Origin of Disease

A therapeutic principle. When the incidental and fundamental disease are acute and severe at the same time or not too urgent, they should be treated at the same time.

Simultaneous Use of Sweating and Purging

It refers to the method in which the disease involving both exterior and interior is treated with the medicine of relieving superficial syndrome by means of diaphoresis and relieving constipation by purgation.

Indication. Pathogenic factor attacking the exterior of the body and interior excess.

Sishencong (Ex-HN 1)

A set of extra points.

Location. Four points on the vertex of the head, 1 cun anterior, posterior, and lateral to Baihui (GV 20).

Indication. Apoplexy, headache, dizziness, epilepsy and neurasthenia, etc.

Method. Puncturing subcutaneously 0.3-0.5 cun. Applying moxibustion with 1-3 moxa cones or for 3-5 minutes.

Sitting Drugs

It refers to the pills, lozenges, tablets, or drug powder wrapped with gauze. They are put into the vagina, or the anus to treat some diseases.

Indication. Gynecological disease, pruritus vulvae, etc.

Sixangular Dysosma Rhizome and Root

It is the root or rhizome of Dysosma pleiantha (Hance) Woods. (Berberidaceae).

Effect. Clearing away heat, detoxicating, dissipating phlegm and resolving masses, removing blood stasis.

Indication. Subcutaneous swelling or abscess, furuncle, scrofula, traumatic injuries and snake bite.

Six Evils

It refers to six exogenous factors, which cause the exopathic disease. They are wind, cold, summer-heat, dampness, dryness and fire. If the occurrence of the six natural factors is too excessive or insufficient or unreasonable, they will affect the body function and become evil causing disease.

Six Fu-organs

It refers to the gallbladder, stomach, large intestine, small intestine, urinary bladder and tri-energizer. Their common physiological functions are to digest and absorb food and transport waste products.

Six Fu-organs Qi

It refers to the property of dysfunction of activity of qi in six fu-organs. If in the gallbladder, it indicates anger; in the stomach, it indicates adverse rising of qi; in both large and small intestines, it indicates diarrhea; in the urinary bladder, it indicates enuresis, and in the lower-energizer, it indicates water.

Six Kinds of Natural Factors

1. It refers to wind, cold, summer-heat, dampness, dryness, and fire (heat). 2. It refers to six vital substances of the body:

qi, blood, body fluid, essential fluid, essence, and vessels.

Sizhukong (TE 23)

A meridian acupuncture point.
Location. On the face, in the depression of the lateral end of the eyebrow.
Indication. Headache, blurred vision, redness and pain of the eye, toothache, epilepsy.
Method. Puncturing subcutaneously 0.5-1.0 cun. Moxibustion is not applicable.

Skin Areas

It refers to the twelve skin areas where the twelve regular meridians and their collaterals travel. Painful region and the area of the referred pain, abnormal color of the skin, rash and sensitive points are related to the skin areas.

Skin Fluid

One of edema diseases.
Symptoms. Slow onset, general pitting edema with finger trace, abdominal distention like a drum.
Pathogenesis. Usually caused by the fluid-spilling skin.
Therapeutic Principle. Nourishing the spleen and activating yang to induce diuresis.

Skin Needle

It is a therapeutic apparatus with certain short needles fixed on one end of the handle. It also refers to the seven-star needle, plum needle, and bound needle. Apply spring-like pricking to the point with the strength of the wrist during manipulation.

Skin Numbness

Symptoms. Urticaria and rubella, painless when scratched with the sensation of insect crawling.
Pathogenesis. Invasion of wind, cold and dampness into the skin.
Therapeutic Principle. Expelling wind and enriching blood.

Sleepiness after Meal

Symptoms. Mental fatigue after meal, dim complexion, sleepiness and somnolence, fullness sensation of the stomach and abdomen, etc.
Pathogenesis. Retention of food in the stomach, attack of the spleen by deep-rooted pathogens, dysfunction of the spleen in transport.
Therapeutic Principle. Strengthening the spleen and invigorating qi.

Sleeplessness due to Deficiency of Heart Blood

Symptoms. Dysphoria with feverish sensation in the chest, palms and soles, dryness of the mouth and tongue, frightened in sleep, etc.
Pathogenesis. Overstrain of the heart and the exhaustion of the heart blood.
Therapeutic Principle. Nourishing and enriching the blood to calm the mind.

Sleeplessness due to Deficiency of Heart-qi

Symptoms. Insomnia, liability to awake, palpitation, lassitude, aversion to cold, etc.
Pathogenesis. Deficiency of the heart-qi and the disorder of mental activities.
Therapeutic Principle. Supplementing qi and nourishing the heart to calm the mind.

Sleeplessness due to Liver-fire

Symptoms. Dysphoria, and irritability, frequent hypochondriac distention, frequent panic during sleep, insomnia and dreaminess sleep.
Pathogenesis. Disturbance of the heart by fire-transmission from the depressed liver resulting in dysphoria.
Therapeutic Principle. Purging fire from the liver, and nourishing the heart to calm the mind.

Slender Falsenettle Herb

It is the whole herb of Boehmeria gracilis C.H.Wright (Urticaceae).

Effect. Removing heat, detoxicating, expelling pathogenic wind, relieving itching and eliminating diuresis.
Indication. Cutaneous pruritus and noxious dampness.

Slight-constipation of Yang
It refers to slight accumulation of heat in the interior.
Symptoms. Fullness in the epigastrium, poor appetite and hard feces.
Therapeutic Principle. Dispelling heat and dissipating obstruction.

Slight Emission
Symptoms. Urination with a little sperm, mild pain of penis, or some sperm after micturition.
Pathogenesis. Unconsolidation of the kidney-qi.
Therapeutic Principle. Tonifying the kidney.

Slippery Phlegm
It refers to phlegm which is easy to cough up.
Pathogenesis. The spleen-dampness.
Therapeutic Principle. Dispelling dampness to reduce phlegm.

Slow-moving Stool due to Stickiness
Symptoms. Yellow stool like soya-sauce, difficulty with excretion due to stickiness.
Pathogenesis. Damp-heat accompanied by stagnation obstruction of the intestinal tract.

Slow Pathogenic Wind
Referring to a critical disease.
Symptoms. Tiredness of both feet, edema of leg, or numbness of legs without edema, and even violent palpitation.
Pathogenesis. Invasion of meridians and collaterals by pathogenic wind and water.
Therapeutic Principle. Dispersing wind and removing toxic materials, and regulating qi and blood.

Slow-rapid Reinforcing-reducing Method
One of the reinforcing-reducing methods in acupuncture therapy. Reinforcing and reducing are differentiated by the speed of inserting and withdrawing the needle. Slow insertion and rapid withdrawal is reinforcement; rapid insertion and slow withdrawal is reduction.

Sluggish Complexion
It is one of ten methods of observing the complexion; the said complexion is usually seen in the chronic disease. It indicates the deep accumulation of the pathogenic factor; the disease is difficult to cure, with unfavourable prognosis.

Smallflower Galinsoga Herb
The whole herb of Galinsoga parviflora Cav. (Compositae).
Effect. Relieving inflammation, arresting bleeding and relieving pain.
Indication. Tonsillitis, laryngopharyngitis, toothache, hemicrania acute icterohepatitis, traumatic bleeding, etc.

Smallflower Seaberry Herb
The whole herb of Haloragis micrantha R. Br. (Haloragaceae).
Effect. Clearing away heat, relieving cough catharsis, promoting blood circulation and detoxicating.
Indication. Difficulty with urine and feces, heat stranguria, dysentery with bloody stool, constipation, irregular menstruation, traumatic injuries, scald, etc.

Smallfruit Fig Aerial Root
The aerial root of Ficus microcarpa L. (Moraceae).
Effect. Dispelling pathogenic wind, clearing away heat, promoting blood circulation and detoxicating.
Indication. Influenza, bronchitis, stomach pain, tonsillitis, conjunctivitis, osteodynia due to pathogenic wind dampness,

epistaxis, stranguria complicated by hematuria, traumatic injuries, etc.

Smallfruit Fig Leaf

The leaf of Ficus microcarpa L. (Moraceae).

Effect. Promoting blood circulation to dissipate blood stasis and clearing away heat to regulate dampness.

Indication. Bronchitis, influenza, chin cough, tonsillitis, bacillary dysentery, bloodshot eyes, toothache, traumatic injuries, etc.

Smallfruit Rose Root or Leaf

The root or the tender leaf of Rosa cymosa Tratt. (Rosaceae).

Effect. Dissipating blood stasis, arresting bleeding, subduing swelling and detoxicating.

Indication. Irregular menstruation, diarrhea, abdominalgia, hysteroptosis, proctoptosis, hemorrhoids, superficial infections and traumatic bleeding.

Small Intestinal Abscess

Symptoms. Abdominal pain, distention and fullness, or sound of water when turning the body, or sores around the umbilicus, fever, and anorexia.

Pathogenesis. Improper diet, blockage in the intestines and the stomach, blockage of transportation and transformation, stasis of qi and blood.

Therapeutic Principle. Clearing away heat and toxic material, removing abdominal obstruction and purging away the heat.

Small Intestine (MA-SC)

An auricular point.

Location. The middle 1/3 of the superior aspect of the helix crus.

Indication. Indigestion, palpitations, etc.

Small Intestine in Charge of Receiving and Digesting Food

Referring to the main functions of the small intestine which are receiving food preliminarily digested from the stomach and digesting it further for separating the refined matter from the scum.

Small Intestine Meridian

It starts from the ulnar end of the 5th finger, goes up along the palmar ulnar border and comes out from the area where the styloid process of ulna is located, then, passes through the elbow along the lateral posterior border of the upper arm, gets to the back of the shoulder joint, goes round scapular region and intersects at the shoulder, Dazhui (GV14). It goes forward, comes to the supraclavicular fossa, deep into the body cavity, connects with the heart, along the esophagus through the diaphragm, arrives at the stomach and goes downward to small intestine. Its branch comes to the outer canthus from the supraclavicular fossa along the lateral neck and through the cheek. Then, it goes back into the ear. Another branch is separated from the cheek, goes up to the inner canthus, Jingming (B 1) through the area below the eye, and connects with the Bladder Meridian.

Small Leaf Desmodium Herb

The whole herb of Desmodium microphy Hum. (Thunb.) DC. (Leguminosae).

Effect. Clearing away heat, inducing diuresis and detoxicating.

Indication. Urinary lithiasis, cholecystiits, chronic gastritis, chronic trachitis, infantile dyspepsia and malnutrition, carbuncles, deep-rooted carbuncles, hemorrhoids, toothache, etc.

Small Polemonium Root

The root of Polemonium liniflorum V. Vassil. (Polemoniaceae).

Effect. Eliminating phlegm, arresting bleeding and tranquilizing the mind.

Indication. Acute and chronic bronchitis, hemoptysis, hematuria, epistaxis, hemafecia, menorrhagia and insomnia.

Smothery Polypnea

Symptoms. Shortness of breath and fullness in chest and hypochondrium.

Pathogenesis. Attack of excessive fluid into the lung and phlegm due to splenic dampness, obstruction of pulmonary qi and edema.

Snake Head-like Infection

Symptoms. At the beginning numbness and itching on the end of the finger, followed by stabbing pain, swelling distention, snake head-like form, aversion to cold, fever. Long resistance to treatment.

Pathogenesis. Injury and infection of toxins.

Therapeutic Principle. Clearing away heat and toxic materials.

Snow Lotus Herb

The herb of Saussurea laniceps Hand.-Mazz., S. involucrata Kar. et Kir., S. medusa Maxim. (Compositae) with flower.

Effect. Removing cold, tonifying yang, regulating menstruation and arresting bleeding.

Indication. Impotence, lassitude of the loins and knees, metrorrhagia, leukorrhea, irregular menstruation, rheumatic arthritis and traumatic bleeding.

Soda-apple Nightshade Herb

The whole herb of Solanum surattense Burm. f. (Solanaceae).

Effect. Astringing lung to relieve cough and asthma, removing obstruction and pain.

Indication. Dyspnea, chronic bronchitis, bronchitis, stomachache, rheumatalgia, scrofula, pustule of cold nature, proctoptosis, etc.

Soft Tissue Swelling of Lower Limb

Symptoms. Tight and bright of skin, thickening, pachylosis, pain, rather severe swelling, fever with chills, etc.

Pathogenesis. Retention of wind-dampness and heat, together with phlegm stagnancy.

Therapeutic Principle. Removing obstruction in the meridians to promote circulation, softening hard masses, and removing dampness by diuresis.

Solar Dermatitis

Symptoms. Erythema on the exposed parts of the skin, swelling, even blisters, burning heat, itching and stabbing pain. In the severe case, aversion to cold, fever, nausea, etc.

Pathogenesis. Caused by the scorching sunshine.

Therapeutic Principle. Clearing away heat, removing summer-heat and detoxicating.

Sole Pain

Symptoms. Pain at the yongquan (K 1) along the Kidney Meridian in the center of the sole.

Pathogenesis. Deficiency and affection of dampness of the kidney.

Soliloquy

Referring to the case in which the patient is basically conscious, but mutters to himself. It is usually found in hysteria, senile psychosis.

Pathogenesis. Insufficiency of the heart-qi, and failure to warmly nourish the heart and mentality.

Somnolence

Symptoms. Patients sleep now and then, no matter whether it is during the day or at night, and after awaking when called soon falling into sleep.

Pathogenesis. Deficiency of yang-qi or deficiency of the spleen and excessive wetness.

Therapeutic Principle. Supplementing qi and warming yang, or invigorating the spleen and eliminating dampness.

Somnolence due to Gallbladder-heat

Symptoms. Mental depression, lethargic state resembling drunk, sleepiness, distress of the chest, bitter taste, blurred vision, etc.

Pathogenesis. Excessive-heat of gallbladder, phlegm in chest and diaphragm, stagnation in zang and fu, and conflict between yin and yang.

Therapeutic Principle. Dispelling gallbladder-heat, and resolving phlegm for resuscitation.

Songaria Cynomorium Herb

The flesh stem of Cynomorium songaricum Rupr. (Cynomoriaceae).

Effect. Tonifying the kidney, supplement essence, moistening the bowels and relieving constipation.

Indication. Impotence, seminal emission, sterility, debility of extremities, chronic constipation of the aged, etc.

Sore Throat due to Wind-Heat Pathogen

Symptoms. Pain and swelling of the throat, chills, fever, profuse and viscous sputum, obstructed feeling in throat, dysphagia.

Pathogenesis. Pathogenic wind-heat attacking the lung, and heat evil cauterizing the lung system.

Therapeutic Principle. Expel wind and clear away heat to relieve sore throat.

Source of Development

It has two meanings:

1. The five zang organs, whose common function of generating essence and vital energy, are the source of development.
2. It refers to the spleen and stomach. They furnish acquired essence. The normal functions of the five-zang and six fu organs, extremities and skeleton depend on digesting and absorbing food, transportation and transformation of food essence by the spleen and stomach and nourishing of essential substances.

Sour Flavor

The drugs with sour flavor have the effects of inducing astringency and arresting discharge. They can be used for syndromes of incessant and excessive loss of the body fluid or vital essence such as hyperhidrosis, chronic diarrhea, emission, enuresis, leukorrhagia, and hemorrhage.

Sour Taste

Symptoms. Frequent sour taste in the mouth.

Pathogenesis. Upward invasion of the liver-heat, or hepatic qi attacking the spleen, food accumulation and indigestion.

Soybean

The seed of Glycine max (L.) Merr. (Leguminosae) with yellow coating.

Effect. Invigorating the spleen and stomach, relieving epigastric distention, moistening dryness and promoting diuresis.

Indication. Diarrhea, abdominal malnutrition, poisoning during pregnancy, suppurative infections on the body surface and traumatic injuries, etc.

Soybean Milk

The pressed milk from the seed of Glycine max (L.) Merr. (Lequminosae).

Effect. Clearing away heat from the lung and resolving sputum, restoring qi, moistening dryness.

Indication. Cough due to deficiency type, dyspnea due to phlegm fire, constipation and stranguria with turbid urine.

Soybean Oil

The fatty oil pressed from the seed of Glycine max (L.) Merr. (Leguminosae).

Effect. Expelling intestinal parasites and lubricating the intestines.

Indication. Intestinal obstruction and constipation.

Sparrow Tongue

Referring to the syndrome of new growth of uvula on the tongue in the shape of a sparrow tongue.

Symptoms. Growth of uvula on the tongue, pain at the beginning and then erosion and stench, which may result in reddish swelling in both parotid glands, etc.

Pathogenesis. Overeating of pungent and hot food, which results in the accumulation of toxic heat in the Heart and Stomach Meridians.

Therapeutic Principle. Clearing away the heart-fire and cooling the pleuroperitoneum.

Spasm and Contracture of Muscle

Symptoms. Stiffness of the joints and difficulty in movement, etc.

Pathogenesis. Failure to nourish muscle and tendon and loss of tenacity of it.

Therapeutic Principle. Massage, acupuncture and moxibustion, and physiotherapy, external application of drugs and oral administration of medicine, etc.

Spasm due to Wind-cold

Symptoms. Sudden lockjaw, stiffness of the neck, general feverish, cold feet, etc.

Pathogenesis. Invasion of pathogenic wind-cold into the body which results in obstruction of meridians and collaterals, impeded flow of qi and blood, irregularity of yin and yang leading to yang hyperactivity and failure of yin to nourish tendons.

Therapeutic Principle. Removing wind, dispelling cold, regulating the defensive function and nourishing the vessels to promote the circulation of qi and blood.

Spasm due to Wind-phlegm

Symptoms. Facial hemiparalysis, vibration or spasm of extremities, or even coma, etc.

Pathogenesis. Obstruction of meridians and collaterals due to stagnation or wind-phlegm.

Therapeutic Principle. Dispelling wind, resolving phlegm, invigorating the spleen and nourishing blood.

Spasm of Limbs

Symptoms. The spasm of the limb muscles and inability to flex and extend.

Pathogenesis. The invasion of pathogenic-cold into meridians or consumption of yin fluid by heat, resulting in dryness of blood and myo-atrophy.

Spasm of Lower Abdomen

Symptoms. Subjective uncomfortable sensation of spasm and urgency below the umbilicus.

Pathogenesis. Insufficiency of kidney-yang, dysfunction of the urinary bladder in qi transformation.

Spasm of Muscle

Symptoms. Spasm of muscles of the limbs with pain, difficulty in movement of limbs, aversion to wind and cold, or dry mouth, dizziness.

Pathogenesis. Invasion of pathogenic cold, or impairment of muscles and tendons by heat, or failure in nourishing muscles due to insufficiency of blood, etc.

Therapeutic Principle. Eliminating cold, clearing away heat and nourishing the blood.

Spatholobus Stem

The stem of Spatholobus suberectus Dunn (Leguminosae).

Effect. Tonifying and enriching blood, relaxing muscles and tendons and activating the flow of qi, promoting, blood circulation.

Indication. Irregular menstruation, stagnant menstruation, dysmenorrhea, amenorrhea due to deficiency of blood, aching of joints, numbness of the body and limbs, acroparalysis, arthralgia due to wind-dampness, and leucopenia induced by radio-therapy, etc.

Spermatorrhea

Symptoms. Emission without dreaming, or even worse emission at the sight of a female, frequent emission, aching and cold in lumbar region, pale complexion, lassitude with impotence, spontaneous perspiration, or shortness of breath, pale tongue and white coating, thready and rapid pulse.

Pathogenesis. Unsatisfied sexual intemperance in sexual life, deficiency of the kidney. Sometimes caused by lower-energizer damp-heat.

Therapeutic Principle. Tonify the kidney qi, arrest emission.

Spiked Gingerlily Fruit

The fruit of Hedychium spicatum Ham. (Zingiberaceae).

Effect. Warming up the stomach, removing dampness, regulating flow of qi and promoting digestion.

Indication. Stomachache of stomach-cold type, abdominal distention due to indigestion and periumbilical colic due to invasion of cold.

Spinach

The whole plant of Spinacia oleracea L. (Chenopodiaceae) with root.

Effect. Nourishing the blood, astringing yin fluid, and moistening dryness.

Indication. Epistaxis, hemafecia, diabetes and constipation.

Spiny Date Seed

The ripe seed of Ziziphus jujuba Mill. var. Spinosa (Bunge) Hu ex. H.F. Chou (Rhamnaceae).

Effect. Nourishing the heart, tranquilizing mind and arresting sweating.

Indication. Fidgetiness, insomnia, palpitation due to fright, dreaminess, spontaneous perspiration, night sweat, etc.

Spinyleaf Pricklyash Root

The root or root bark of Zanthoxylum dimorphophyllum Hemsl. var. spinifolium Rehd. et Wils. (Rutaceae).

Effect. Expelling wind, and removing cold, dispelling muscles and tendons to promote blood circulation and relieving pain.

Indication. Rheumatalgia, stomachache, dysmenorrhea, traumatic injuries, traumatic bleeding, constipation, cough due to wind-cold, numbness due to wind-dampness, etc.

Spitting Blood due to Stomach-heat

Symptoms. Spitting blood of fresh or dark purple color with residue of food, epigastric and abdominal distention and pain, foul smell in the mouth, black stool or constipation.

Pathogenesis. Over indulgence of alcohol, greasy and spicy food, leading to the accumulation of the heat in the stomach, or emotional stress leading to injury of the collaterals of the stomach.

Therapeutic Principle. Clear heat from the stomach, and lowering of the adverse flow of stomach-qi to stop bleeding.

Spleen (MA)

An auricular point.

1. **Location.** At the lateral and superior aspect of the cavity of concha.
   Indication. Abdominal distention, chronic diarrhea, constipation, indigestion, stomatitis, dysfunctional uterine bleeding, leukorrhagia, auditory vertigo, anorexia.
2. **Location.** In the center of the back of the ear.
   Indication. Abdominal distention and diarrhea, anorexia.

Spleen Closely Related to Stomach

It refers to one of interrelations of zang-organs and fu-organs. The exterior and interior relationship between the spleen and the stomach is formed by the connections between their meridians. The spleen transports nutrients while the stomach mainly receives and digests water and food. The spleen has the function of ascending while the stomach has the function of descending. The spleen is a yin zang-organ and likes dryness and hates dampness. The stomach is a yang fu-organ and likes dampness but hates dryness. They both cooperate to fulfil the task of digesting, absorbing and transporting water and food essence by means of coordination of yin zang-organ and yang fu-organ, the interdependence between the ascending and the descending, and mutual supplement of the dampness and dryness.

Spleen-cold Syndrome

Symptoms. Distention of the upper abdomen or the chest, contracture of the extremities, inability to eruct, constipation, or diarrhea.

Pathogenesis. Invasion of the Spleen Meridian by the pathogenic cold.

Therapeutic Principle. Warming the spleen to remove cold.

Spleen Collateral

One of the collaterals. It branches from Gongsun (SP 4) point on the Spleen Meridian, posterior to the first phalangeal joint, running to the Stomach Meridian. It branches into the abdominal cavity, and communicate with the intestine and stomach. The excess syndrome of this collateral is marked by abdominal pain. The deficient syndrome is marked by abdominal distention. If there is collateral qi disorders, it leads to vomiting.

Spleen Determining Required Constitution

It means that the growth and development of the body after birth depends upon the food essence absorbed by the spleen-qi and stomach-qi. The normal functions of both the spleen and stomach, especially the spleen, determine the digestion, absorption and transport of water and food. The spleen, therefore, is of great importance for life activities of the human body.

Spleen Distention

Symptoms. Edema, water retention in the stomach and intestines, heaviness sensation in limbs, rapid respiration, restless sleep, etc.

Pathogenesis. Invasion of the spleen by pathogenic cold and dampness, disability to control water due to deficiency of the spleen, retention of the water in the stomach and intestines and water overflowing to the skin.

Therapeutic Principle. Warming the middle-energizer and dispelling cold, invigorating the spleen and promoting diuresis.

Spleen Divergent Meridian

A divergent meridian. It branches from the Spleen Meridian, runs to the anterior thigh, connects with the Stomach Meridian, goes upward to the throat and arrives at the center of tongue.

Spleen Governing Blood

One of main functions of the spleen. It means that the spleen has the function of controlling the blood and keeping it circulating within the vessels. If it loses the function of governing the blood due to the deficiency of the spleen, the chronic hemorrhagic diseases will usually occur.

Spleen-heat Syndrome

Symptoms. Pain or fullness and distention in the abdomen, red lip, dry mouth restlessness, constipation, scanty dark urine, etc.

Pathogenesis. Attack of pathogenic heat on the spleen or excessive intake of heat-producing pungent food.

Therapeutic Principle. Clearing away heat and removing fire, and moisturizing the intestines and smoothing stool.

Spleen Impairment

Symptoms. Yellowish complexion, mental and physical tiredness, desire for lying in bed inappetence, abnormal stools, etc.

Pathogenesis. Improper diet, unbalanced cold and heat, overwork, overthinking, etc. which injure spleen-energy.

Therapeutic Principle. Invigorating the spleen and nourishing the stomach.

Spleen Impairment due to Overstrain

Symptoms. Abdominal distention and fullness, poor appetite, vomiting, acid regurgitation, emaciation, weak limbs, etc.

Pathogenesis. Injury of the spleen due to hunger or overeating, overthinking and overworking.

Therapeutic Principle. Nourishing the spleen and supplementing qi.

Spleen Meridian

It is one of twelve regular meridians. The meridian starts from the tip of the medial side of the great toe. From there it runs along the junction of the red and white skin of the medial aspects, ascends in front of the malleolus, then along the central line of the medial aspect of the calf, ascends in front of the Liver Meridian, goes through the anterior medial aspect of the thigh, and into the abdominal cavity, belongs to the spleen, and communicates with the stomach. From there it goes through the diaphragm, and upwards along the two sides of the throat, reaches the root of the tongue and spreads over its lower surface. The branch of the meridian sprouts from the stomach, goes upwards through the diaphragm, disperses into the heart and connects with the Heart Meridian.

Spleen-qi

There are two meanings.
1. It refers to the functional activities of the spleen in transport and transformation.
2. It means the vital essence in the spleen.

Spleen-qi Deficiency

Symptoms. Abdominal distention aggravated after meals, poor appetite, and loose stool, weakness of extremities, shortness of breath.

Pathogenesis. Irregular diet, overthinking and over-fatigue, or impairment of the spleen-qi due to acute disease.

Therapeutic Principle. Strengthening the spleen and replenishing qi.

Spleen-qi in Charge of Ascending

The spleen has the function of absorbing and ascending the food essence and other nutrients upward to the lung. With the help of both the heart and lung, these substances are turned into qi and blood which nourish the whole body. So the spleen-qi means ascending. In addition, the ascending function of the spleen includes preventing the internal organs from descending.

Spleen-stomach Incoordination

Symptoms. Abdominal distention and pain, poor appetite, nausea, vomiting, diarrhea, etc.

Pathogenesis. Dysfunction of the spleen transport and transformation due to spleen deficiency and disorder for the stomach to receive and digest food.

Therapeutic Principle. Strengthening the spleen and stomach.

Spleen-warm Syndrome

Symptoms. Sticky and sweet taste in the mouth, emaciation, frequent micturition and constipation, etc.and becoming diabetic with the passing of time.

Pathogenesis. Rich and fatty diet and ascending of turbid qi due to the spleen heat.

Therapeutic Principle. Eliminating turbidity with aromatics, accompanied by tonifying the spleen-qi.

Spleen-wind

Symptoms. Perspiration, aversion to wind, lassitude, anorexia, vexation, yellowish skin, etc.

Pathogenesis. Wind attacks the spleen or liver-wind spreads over the spleen.

Therapeutic Principle. Invigorating the spleen and supplementing qi, relieving the depressed liver-qi and stopping the wind.

Spleen-yang

Referring to the function of spleen in transport and its yang-qi acting as warmth in the process of the spleen transporting, distributing and transforming nutrients.

Spleen-yang Deficiency

Symptoms. Abdominal distention pain with preference for warmth and pressing, cold limbs, clear and loose stool, poor appetite, edema and intolerance of coldness, plump and pale tongue with white and slippery fur, deep, slow and weak pulse, etc.

Pathogenesis. Spleen-qi deficiency affects the spleen-yang, making the spleen lose its warmth, or the invasion of pathogenic cold or cold food, thus disturbing the spleen-yang.

Therapeutic Principle. Warming the middle-energizer to invigorate the spleen.

Spleen-yin

1. Referring to the essence fluid (including blood, body fluid, etc.).
2. Referring to the spleen itself, opposite the stomach-yang. The spleen is a zang organ and belongs to yin while the stomach is a fu organ and belongs to yang.

Spleen-yin Deficiency

Symptoms. Anorexia, retching and hiccups, dry mouth and throat, etc.

Pathogenesis. Consumption of both the spleen-yin and stomach-yin due to prolonged illness or febrile disease.

Therapeutic Principle. Nourishing the spleen-yin.

Splenic Constipation

Symptoms. Frequent micturition, constipation, spontaneous perspiration, etc.

Pathogenesis. Spleen deficiency and insufficiency of body fluid.

Therapeutic Principle. Nourishing yin and blood, moisturizing the intestines and relaxing the bowels.

Splenic Diarrhea

Symptoms. Diarrhea, abdominal distention and fullness, vomiting after eating, heaviness of limbs, etc.

Pathogenesis. Accumulation of cold dampness, or the impairment of the spleen by improper diet, dysfunction of the spleen due to deficiency of the spleen-qi.

Therapeutic Principle. Invigorating the spleen, regulating the middle-energizer and stopping diarrhea.

Splenic Shock due to Postpartum Putrid Blood

Symptoms. Vomiting with loss of appetite after delivery.

Pathogenesis. Lochia entering the Spleen Meridian.

Therapeutic Principle. Strengthening the spleen and regulating the flow of qi to remove stasis.

Spontaneous Galactorrhea

Symptoms. Automatic secretion and overflow of milk after delivery without the baby sucking.

Therapeutic Principle. Enriching qi and blood or soothing the liver and clearing away heat.

Spontaneous Perspiration due to Damp

Symptoms. Spontaneous perspiration with aversion to wind, heavy and turbid voice, heaviness sensation in the limbs, and pain in joints, and deterioration in wet weather.

Pathogenesis. Stagnation of damp-evil.

Therapeutic Principle. Tonifying the spleen and qi, dispelling heat and eliminating fire.

Spontaneous Perspiration due to Deficiency of Heart

Referring to sweating, not caused by overstrain and hot weather, when the patient is awake.

Symptoms. Severe palpitation, profuse sweating.

Pathogenesis. Deficiency of heart-qi and blood.

Therapeutic Principle. Invigorating qi and nourishing the heart to arrest sweating.

Spontaneous Perspiration due to Deficiency of Stomach-qi

Symptoms. Pale complexion, lassitude of limbs, and perspiration from the head to the navel.

Pathogenesis. Deficiency of stomach-qi.

Therapeutic Principle. Reinforcing the stomach and arresting sweating.

Spontaneous Perspiration due to Phlegm Syndrome

Symptoms. Spontaneous perspiration, dizziness, oppressing feeling in the chest, nausea, vomiting and spitting sputum and salvia.

Pathogenesis. Internal obstruction of yang-qi due to the stagnation of turbid phlegm.

Therapeutic Principle. Regulating the middle-energizer and dissipating phlegm.

Spontaneous Perspiration due to Yang Deficiency

Symptoms. Aversion to cold spontaneous perspiration, lassitude, etc.

Pathogenesis. Weakness of the defending yang, lowered superficial resistance, disconnection of striae of skin, muscles and viscera.

Therapeutic Principle. Warming yang and consolidating superficial resistance.

Spontaneous Sweating due to Blood-heat

Symptoms. Tidal fever, spontaneous sweating, flushed face, dysphoria, insomnia, feverish sensation in the palms and soles, etc.

Pathogenesis. Hyperactivity of fire due to yin deficiency and heat in the blood system.

Therapeutic Principle. Clearing away fire to invigorate yin, and consolidating superficial resistance to stop sweating.

Spontaneous Sweating due to Qi-deficiency

Symptoms. Sweat with aversion to wind, inclination to catching cold.

Pathogenesis. Weak physique, or long coughing attack and asthma leading to the deficiency of lung-qi, loose muscle and the impairment of defensive function.

Therapeutic Principle. Nourishing qi and strengthening the exterior.

Spreading Hedyotis Herb

The whole plant of Oldenlandia diffusa (Willd.) Roxb. (Rubiaceae).

Effect. Clearing away heat, inducing diuresis, detoxicating and treating boils.

Indication. Acute appendicitis, suppurative infections on the body surface, cancer of the gastrointestinal tract, swollen sore throat, snake bite, etc.

Squarrose-leaved Gentian Herb

The whole herb of Gentiana squarrosa Lede. (Gentianaceae).

Effect. Clearing away heat and detoxicating.

Indication. Furuncle, subcutaneous swelling, scrofula, and bloodshot, swollen and painful eyes, acute appendicitis.

Stagnancy of Liver-qi and Blood

Symptoms. Stuffiness or distending pain in the chest and hypochondrium, relieved by pressing and patting, preference for hot drink, etc.

Pathogenesis. Stagnancy of the liver-qi and blood.

Therapeutic Principle. Promoting the circulation of blood and dispersing blood stagnancy, activating yang and promoting blood circulation.

Stagnated Phlegm

Symptoms. Thick mucous sputum difficult to expectorate, fullness sensation in chest and abdomen, etc.

Pathogenesis. Impairment of seven emotions, disturbance of qi transformation, dysfunction of the spleen in transport, production of sputum resulting from retention of dampness or impairment of purifying and descending function of the lung and stagnation of sputum in the lung.

Therapeutic Principle. Regulating qi by alleviating mental depression and resolving phlegm, invigorating the spleen and promoting the dispersing function of the lung.

Stagnant Heat Retained in the Interior

There are two meanings.

1. It refers to stagnancy of heat pathogen in deep site, failure of heat to be expelled in the exterior, failure of dampness to go down.

   Symptoms. Fever without sweating, difficulty with urination, jaundiced body.

2. It refers to pathogenic heat of Taiyang entering fu organ through meridians, accumulation with blood stasis in lower-energizer.

   Symptoms. Craziness, fullness and hardness in lower abdomen, but normal urine, headache, chills and fever, etc.

Stagnation due to Anxiety

Symptoms. Susceptibility to anxiety, insomnia and amnesia, dim complexion, anorexia, or trance, etc.

Pathogenesis. Accumulation of qi due to anxiety, emotional depression, dysfunc-

tion of the spleen in transport, stagnation of qi with damp phlegm.

Therapeutic Principle. Regulating qi, relieving depressed liver, eliminating phlegm and resolving dampness.

Stagnation due to Deficiency of Spleen and Stomach

Symptoms. Slight fever, loss of appetite, drowsiness, coma, hot in abdomen, cold in foot.

Pathogenesis. Deficiency of the spleen and stomach, further accompanied by improper diet.

Therapeutic Principle. Nourishing and removing stagnancy.

Stagnation of Gallbladder

Symptoms. Bitter taste, hectic fever, timidity with frightening sensation, etc.

Pathogenesis. Insufficiency of qi.

Therapeutic Principle. Regulating the flow of qi to alleviate mental depression, removing heat from the liver and the gallbladder, invigorating qi and tranquilizing the mind.

Stagnation of Liver and Gallbladder

A kind of melancholia.

Symptoms. Acid regurgitation, fullness and distention in the hypochondrium and sighing, etc.

Pathogenesis. Emotional imbalance, stagnation of the liver and gallbladder qi or the impairment of the liver and gallbladder by prolonged disease.

Therapeutic Principle. Regulating the function of the liver and normalizing the function of the gallbladder.

Stagnation of Liver-qi and Deficiency of Spleen

Symptoms. Emotional depression and anger, preference for sighing, distending pain the hypochondrium, fatigue, poor appetite, abdominal distention, loose stool.

Pathogenesis. Emotional depression, failure of the liver to control the qi flow and the failure of the spleen in transport and transformation.

Therapeutic Principle. Relieving the depressed liver and strengthening the spleen.

Stagnation of Nutrient system-qi

Referring to a morbid state of carbuncle and swelling resulting from stagnation of nutrient system-qi circulation in the blood vessels.

Pathogenesis. Invasion of pathogen and toxin which brings about stagnation of nutrient system-qi circulation and is accumulated in the muscle, thus forming blood stasis and heat accumulation.

Stagnation of Qi and Blood in Lung

Symptoms. Chest stuffiness and dysphoria, asthma with vomiting, or stuffiness and pain in the chest and back, etc.

Pathogenesis. Protracted numbness of the skin with the affection by exopathogen or attack of the lung by exopathogen, or excessive sorrow, etc.

Therapeutic Principle. Promoting the dispersing function of the lung and eliminating the pathogenic factors.

Stagnation of Qi in Chest

1. Referring to a morbid condition of the fullness, stuffiness, and pain in the chest.

    Symptoms. Fullness, stuffiness and pain in the chest, with the pain even radiating to the back, dyspnea too severe to lie flat, etc.

    Pathogenesis. Yang deficiency of upper-energizer, turbid phlegm, stasis of the blood, obstruction of the chest yang, disorder of visceral function and obstruction of the meridians.

Therapeutic Principle. Activating yang and clearing obstruction, and regulating qi and eliminating phlegm.

2. Referring to the stagnation of qi in the stomach.

    Symptoms. Fullness and stuffiness in the stomach, poor appetite, stomachache when eating, vomiting now and then.

Starwort Root

The root of stellaria dichotoma L. var. Lanceolata Beg. (Caryophyllaceae).

Effect. Removing asthenic fever and clearing away infantile malnutrition with fever.

Indication. The late stage of febrile disease due to yin deficiency, hectic fever with night sweat due to yin deficiency, fever in children due to malnutrition, emaciation, etc.

Steatomosis

Symptoms. The lipoma body is round and soft of different sizes, mostly appearing on the head, face and back. After breaking, soybean-like residue can be found.

Pathogenesis. Caused by the stagnancy of phlegm qi.

Therapeutic Principle. A surgical operation is applied.

Steeping Cheeks

Symptoms. The infant slobbers.

Pathogenesis. Deficiency of spleen qi or stasis of damp-heat.

Therapeutic Principle. Warm and tonify the spleen-qi, clear away the heat and promote diuresis.

Stemona Root

The root tuber of Stemona sessilifolia (Miq.) Franch. et. Sar., S. japonica (Bl.) Miq. or S. tuberosa Lour. (Stemonaceae).

Effect. Nourishing the lung, eliminating phlegm and relieving cough, destroying lice and parasites.

Indication. Cough in bronchitis, pertussis, cough due to tuberculosis, enterobiasis and lice.

Sterility

A disease.

Referring to cases where, after three or more years of a couple cohabiting, even though the man is healthy, the woman does not become pregnant; or to cases where, after an interval of more than three years after an impregnation, and the woman can no longer become pregnant. It is divided into sterility due to kidney deficiency, to blood deficiency, to retention of cold in the uterus, to blood stasis and due to phlegm-dampness.

Sterility due to Blood Deficiency

Symptoms. Scanty menstruation with pink color, delayed menstrual cycle, emaciation, sallow complexion, fatigue, dizziness and palpitation, pale tongue, deep and thready pulse.

Pathogenesis. Deficiency of the spleen and stomach, or prolonged illness with bleeding and Yin damage leading to insufficiency of Yin-blood and emptiness of the Vital and the Front Middle Meridians with failure to nourish the uterine collaterals.

Therapeutic Principle. Replenish and invigorate the essence and blood, regulate the Vital and the Front Middle Meridians.

Sterility due to Blood Stasis

Symptoms. Inability for intake of sperms, retarded menstruation, astringent excretion of menstrual blood with more blood clots, untouchable abdominal pain, etc.

Pathogenesis. Retention of blood stasis in Vital and Front Middle Meridians and uterine collaterals due to impeded circulation of qi and blood.

Therapeutic Principle. Warming meridians to expel cold and promoting blood circulation to remove stasis.

Sterility due to Kidney Deficiency

Symptoms. Irregular menstruation, with scanty amount and light color, listlessness, dizziness, tinnitus, lassitude in loin and legs.

Pathogenesis. Debilitated constitution and insufficiency of kidney-qi, or prolonged illness and excess of sexual intercourse leading to deficiency of essence and blood.

Therapeutic Principle. Tonify the kidney and regulate the Vital and Front Meridians.

Sterility due to Liver-qi Stagnation

Symptoms. Mental depression, distending pain in the chest, irregular menstruation, etc.

Pathogenesis. Emotional depression and the liver-qi stagnation, leading to disorder of qi and blood, and irregularity of Vital and Front Middle Meridians and effect on the uterus.

Therapeutic Principle. Soothing the liver to remove stasis and enriching blood to regulate menstruation.

Sterility due to Phlegm-dampness

Symptoms. Obesity, dizziness and palpitation, profuse leukorrhea, irregular menstruation, white greasy tongue coating, slippery pulse.

Pathogenesis. Phlegm and dampness resulting from obesity and a fatty diet which obstructs the Vital and Front Middle Meridians and affects uterine fertilization.

Therapeutic Principle. Strengthen the spleen, eliminate dampness and reduce phlegm.

Sterility due to Retention of Cold in the Uterus

Symptoms. Cold pain in lower abdomen, lumbar soreness and lassitude in the legs, delayed menstrual period, diluted and dark menstrual blood, clear and excessive urine, a pale tongue with little coating, a deep and slow pulse.

Pathogenesis. Insufficiency of kidney-yang, failure to warm the uterus; or improper nursing during the menstrual period and wind-cold invading the uterus leading to a cold uterus in which sperm cannot be kept.

Therapeutic Principle. Warm the womb and dispel cold.

Sticky Mouth

Referring to the glutinous feeling in the mouth.

Pathogenesis. Retention of dampness and heat in the spleen.

Therapeutic Principle. Clearing away heat and removing dampness.

Stiffleaf Juniper Cone

The seed of Juniperus rigida Sieb. et Zucc. (Rhamnaceae).

Effect. Expelling wind and removing dampness and inducing diuresis.

Indication. Rheumatic arthralgia and edema.

Stiff Neck

Symptoms. Aching and uncomfortable neck, and difficulty in turning, lifting and lowering the head; in serious cases, pain involving the shoulder, back and upper limb on the affected side and accompanied by tenderness in the cervical part.

Pathogenesis. Improper lying position, or attack of pathogenic wind and cold, or external injury.

Therapeutic Principle. Massage, acupuncture and moxibustion in combination with oral administration and external application of medicine.

Stiff Tongue

Symptoms. Referring to tongue with difficulty in moving freely, often accompanied by unclear and vague speech.

Pathogenesis. Obstruction of collaterals due to the uprising of liver-wind with sputum which blocks at the root of the tongue.

Stimulation Area

The positions for stimulation are not points, but a region. For the needling technique of plum needling the human body is divided into several stimulation regions.

Stirring-up of Deficiency of Wind

Symptoms. Dizziness, trembling of hands and feet, fainting, etc.

Pathogenesis. Impairment of yin due to prolonged illness, severe diarrhea and loss of blood, exhaustion of the body fluid and blood, deficiency of both liver yin and the kidney yin, with failure of the liver yin to control yang and the kidney to nourish the liver.

Therapeutic Principle. Nourishing yin, suppressing hyperactive yang and tranquilizing wind.

Stomach (MA)

An auricular point.

Location. Around the area where the helix crus terminates.

Indication. Gastrospasm, gastritis, gastric ulcer, insomnia, toothache, indigestion.

Stomachache due to Blood Stasis

Symptoms. Fixed or stabbing pain in the stomach with tenderness, even worse after eating. One can even see melena and hematemesis.

Pathogenesis. Obstruction of the meridians and collaterals by blood stasis resulting from lingering stomach disorder or pathological change from qi to blood.

Therapeutic Principle. Promote blood circulation by removing blood stasis to relieve pain.

Stomachache due to Cold Accumulation

Symptoms. Cold and pain in the stomach, aggravation after exposure to cold, poor appetite, cold hands and feet, clear urine and diarrhea, etc.

Pathogenesis. Interior impairment by cold drink, and stagnation of yin-cold.

Therapeutic Principle. Warming the middle-energizer and dispelling cold.

Stomachache due to Improper Diet

Symptoms. Distending pain in the stomach, nausea, vomiting, acid regurgitation, pain relieved by vomiting.

Pathogenesis. Retention of food in the middle-energizer, resulting from improper diet, failure in descending the stomach-qi and dysfunction of the spleen in transport.

Therapeutic Principle. Promoting digestion to remove retention of food.

Stomachache due to Phlegm Retention

Symptoms. Gastric pain, poor appetite, nausea, vomiting, abundant expectoration, dizziness, palpitation, shortness of breath.

Pathogenesis. Dysfunction of the spleen and stomach in transportation leading to accumulation of dampness and further retention of phlegm in the middle-energizer.

Therapeutic Principle. Removing fluid retention and regulating the stomach.

Stomachache due to Stagnation of Liver-qi

Symptoms. Distending pain in the epigastrium, frequent eructation, distention and fullness in the chest and hypochondrium and susceptibility to sigh, etc.

Pathogenesis. Impairment of the stomach by the stagnation of the liver-qi and emotional disorder.

Therapeutic Principle. Relieving depressed liver and regulating the stomach.

Stomachache due to Yin Deficiency

Symptoms. Dull pain in the stomach, dry mouth and throat, constipation.

Pathogenesis. Lingering stomachache, or impairment of yin due to stagnated heat, leading to failure to nourish the stomach.

Therapeutic Principle. Nourish yin and reinforce the stomach to alleviate pain.

Stomach Collateral

Starts from Fenglong (S 40), 8 cun above the external malleolus, and goes to Spleen Meridian. The branch ascends along the anterolateral aspect of the tibia, connects with head and neck, meets the qi of all meridians, and descends to connect with throat.

Stomach Disorder Caused by Lochioschesis

Referring to postpartum lochia retaining and retrograding to disturb the stomach.

Symptoms. Nausea, vomiting, epigastric fullness, abdominal distention and pain, etc.

Therapeutic Principle. Regulating the flow of qi to relieve pain and ensuring proper downward flow of blood.

Stomach Distention

Symptoms. Stomachache, abdominal fullness and discomfort and inappetence, etc.

Pathogenesis. Stomach cold and indigestion.

Therapeutic Principle. Warming middle-energizer to dispel cold and inducing appetite to promote digestion.

Stomach Divergent Meridian

One of the branches of the Twelve Meridian. It emerges from the Stomach Meridian, entering abdominal cavity from the front of thigh, distributing in the spleen, and ascending to the heart. From there, it runs upwards along the pharynx, emerges from the mouth, then ascends to the root of the nose and the infraorbital region, where it connects with the surrounding tissues of the eye, again entering the Stomach Meridian.

Stomach-heat

Symptoms. Burning-pain in gastric cavity, polyorexia, thirst, halitosis, constipation, oliguria with dark urine.

Pathogenesis. Impairment of the stomach by pathogenic heat or eating excessive heat-producing food which result in dry-heat in stomach.

Therapeutic Principle. Clearing away the stomach-heat.

Stomach Meridian

This meridian starts from the side of the nose, Point Yingxiang (LI 20), ascends curving the nose, the left and the right meeting at the root of the nose, running laterally into the inner canthus and meeting the Taiyany Meridian. Then it descends along the lateral side of the nose and enters into the upper gum. Emerging and curving round the lips, it connects with the symmetrical meridian at Chengjiang (CV 24), and runs backwards along the posterior-inferior side of the jaw to Daying (S 5)and then ascends along the jaw, in front of the ear, through Shangguan (G 3). At last, it runs along the hairline and reaches the forehead. The branch starts from the front of Daying (S 5), descends to Renying (S 9)and goes along the throat to Dazhui (GV 14), turns forward into the supraclavicular fossa. Deeply into the body cavity, it descends through the diaphragm, the stomach, and communicates with the spleen. A straight branch from the supraclavicular fossa emerges from the body surface, descends along the medial border of the papilla mamae. Then it makes its descent along the side of the umbilicus and enters into point Qichong (S 30), located in inguen. The branch starting from the pylorus, descends along the inside of the abdominal cavity, and joins the straight branch at point Qichong (S 30).Then it runs downward along the front side of thigh to the knee. Along the anterolateral aspect of the tibia, it goes towards the dorsum o the foot, and then to the lateral side of the tip of the second toe. Another branch divides from the region 3 individual cun below the genu, and descends to the lateral side of the middle toe. The branch sprouting from the dorsum of the foot, Chongyang (S 42), runs forwards into the medial margin of the big toe, point Yinbai (Sp 1), and connects with the Spleen Meridian.

Stomach Wind

1. It is divided into two types. Due to the pathogenic wind attacking the stomach.

   Symptoms. Abdominal distention and diarrhea, hyperhidrosis and aversion to wind.

   Therapeutic Principle. Expelling wind and clearing away cold, warming the middle-energizer and regulating the flow of qi.

2. Occurrence of wind due to the heat accumulated in the stomach.

   Symptoms. Vomiting.

   Pathogenesis. Usually caused by being addictive to sweet and rich fatty diet, resulting in the occurrence of wind syndrome; in the case of pathogenic heat accumulated for a long time.

   Therapeutic Principle. Removing the pathogenic heat and purging the pathogenic fire, and calming the wind to relieve vomiting.

Stony Goiter

Symptoms. Masses in the front of the neck which increase rapidly and are hard like stone, uneven, immovable when they are pushed, accompanied by pain, hoarseness, even difficulty with breathing. It is a thyroid cancer in modern medicine.

Pathogenesis. Stagnation of qi, accumulation of damp-phlegm and blood stasis due to internal emotional injury.

Therapeutic Principle. In the early phase, it is advisable to follow surgical operation and take drugs for resolving phlegm and softening hard masses, relieving stagnation and removing blood stasis through oral administration.

Stony Uterine Mass

It refers to the tumour in a woman's uterus.

Symptoms. Mass in lower abdomen which gradually increases in size, resembling a pregnant uterus.

Pathogenesis. Due to invasion of the pathogenic cold and stagnant blood.

Therapeutic Principle. Promoting the flow of qi by warming the meridian and promoting blood circulation to remove blood stasis.

Storax

The resin obtained from the bark of Liquidambar orientalis Mill. (Hamamelidaceae).

Effect. Inducing resuscitation, removing the pathogens of filth, eliminating phlegm and alleviating pain.

Indication. Sudden faint apoplexy or epilepsy, cold pain, fullness and tightness in the chest and abdomen, respiratory infections.

Strabismus

It refers to one eye or both eyes slanting to the inner or outer canthus, with limitation of eye movement, or even diplopia. It can occur suddenly with fever, headache, nausea, vomiting, etc. These manifestations are caused by the attack of exogenous wind evil. On the other hand, slow onset, dizziness with blurred vision, and tinnitus are caused by deficiency of the liver and kidney.

Therapeutic Principle. Dispel wind and dredge the meridians, tonifying the liver and kidney.

Stranguria Caused by the Disorder of Qi

Symptoms. Distending pain in the lower abdomen and the perineum, short breath, soreness of the waist, mental fatigue.

Pathogenesis. Deficiency of kidney-qi in the aged, causing disturbance of qi transformation in the bladder.

Therapeutic Principle. Strengthen the spleen and remove dampness by diuresis, tonify the kidney and induce astringency.

Stranguria Caused by the Passage of Urinary Stone

A type of stranguria.

Symptoms. Distending and pricking pain in the lower abdomen and penis, dysuria due to the calculi and unblocked by changing posture, severe pain in the loin and abdomen.

Pathogenesis. Downward flow of damp-heat which decoctes the urine to form urolithiasis.

Therapeutic Principle. Dispel damp-heat and relieve stranguria to stop pain.

Stranguria Complicated by Hematuria

Symptoms. Frequent urination with difficulty and pain, blood in urine, slight distention and pain in the lower abdomen.

Pathogenesis. Damp-heat flowing downward to attack the urinary bladder and accumulation of heat attacking the collaterals leading to bleeding.

Therapeutic Principle. Clear heat and promote diuresis, promote stranguria and arrest pain.

Stranguria due to Liver Heat

Symptoms. Dribbling urination with severe pain on micturition, or swelling of vulva, dysphoria, etc.

Pathogenesis. Caused by the stagnation of the liver-fire in the lower-energizer.

Therapeutic Principle. Removing fire from the liver to stop stranguria.

Stranguria due to Overstrain

Symptoms. Dribbling urination, intermittent attacking and attacking in overstrain, accompanied by lassitude in the loin and knees.

Pathogenesis. Prolonged stranguria or over-eating cold food, or debility after chronic illness or overstrain leading to deficiency of the spleen and kidney, the stagnation of dampness.

Therapeutic Principle. For the spleen type, strengthening spleen and nourish qi; for the kidney type, restoring qi and nourishing the kidney.

Stranguria due to Phlegm Stagnation

Symptoms. Dribbling urination and cloudy urine with cough and dyspnea, etc.

Pathogenesis. Stagnation of phlegm.

Therapeutic Principle. Resolving phlegm and eliminating dampness.

Stranguria with Urinary Obstruction

Symptoms. Burning sensation during urination with pain, distending pain in the lower abdomen with intermittent attack, soreness of waist or difficulty in micturition, etc.

Pathogenesis. Damp-heat, stagnancy of qi, deficiency of the kidney and ureterostenosis.

Therapeutic Principle. Eliminating dampness and heat, promoting diuresis and invigorating.

Strengthening Body Resistance to Eliminate Pathogen

A principle of treatment. It is one of the important principles in guiding clinical treatment and referring to strengthening the vital-qi and the resistance of the human body as well as its self-repairing ability to remove pathogenic factors and recover health. Clinically according to excess or deficiency of vital-qi and pathogenic factors, this principle should be applied by strengthening the body resistance before eliminating pathogenic factors or by combination of strengthening the body resistance with elimination pathogenic factors.

Strengthening Yang with Warm Drug in Nature

It refers to the therapeutic principle of excessive phlegm. The drugs of warm or hot nature usually have functions to invigorate yang-qi, strengthen muscles and regulating the fluid passage so as to mediate, warm and activate yang-qi of the internal and external and removing obstruction for dispelling the excessive pathogenic fluid.

Stretch Skin to Open the Striae

One of the methods for needle insertion.

Method. Stretch the skin with the left hand along the suture of tendons and muscles, and insert the needle gently and slowly with the right hand. As a result, a good needling sensation appears without frightening the patient.

Stridor

Referring to bronchial wheezing in the throat due to dyspnea.

Symptoms. Wheezing sound in the throat, short breath with dyspnea, etc. and unable to lie with face upward in serious cases, etc.

Pathogenesis. Retention of phlegm in the lung in combination with affection by exopathogens, improper diet, depressed emotion, and fatigue, which leads to reversed flow of qi due to stagnation of phlegm, and adverse flow of the lung-qi.

Therapeutic Principle. Eliminating pathogenic factors to alleviate symptoms, and removing phlegm to promote the circulation of qi, strengthen the body resistance to consolidate the constitution.

Stringy Stonecrop Herb

The whole plant of Sedum sarmentosum Bunge. (Crassulaceae).

Effect. Clearing away heat and counteract inflammation, detoxicating and inducting diuresis.

Indication. Acute and chronic hepatitis, pharyngitis, tonsillitis, carbuncles, swellings, sores, ulcers, snake bite, burns and scalds, jaundice due to damp-heat, dysuria, etc.

Stuffiness of Nasal Cavity

Symptoms. Stuffy nose that is sometimes mild and sometimes severe, or alternate obstruction of cavities, attack, or even anosmia.

Pathogenesis. Qi deficiency of the lung and spleen, stagnation of pathogenic factors in the nasal cavity, which results in obstruction of meridians and collaterals and unsmooth flow of qi and blood.

Therapeutic Principle. Nourishing the lung and spleen, regulating the circulation of qi and blood, eliminating stagnation and remove blood stasis.

Stuffiness Syndrome of Excess Type

Symptoms. Fullness and distress in the chest and stomach.

Pathogenesis. Accumulation of depression of the liver-qi, retention of pathogenic dampness, stagnation of cold in the spleen and stomach, accumulation of phlegm and food, or lingering of exopathogen in the body.

Therapeutic Principle. Soothing the liver, strengthening the spleen, resolving phlegm and eliminating dampness.

Stuffy Sensation of Deficiency Type

Symptoms. Slight oppressed distention of the chest, anorexia, deficiency of qi in middle-energizer, loose stool, the preference for warmth and aversion to cold, etc.

Pathogenesis. Diet impairment, overstrain, the deficiency and cold of the spleen and stomach, the insufficiency of the heart, kidney, qi and blood.

Therapeutic Principle. Reinforcing and warming the spleen.

Stuffy Stagnation of Qi

Symptoms. Shortness of breath, dyspnea, chest fullness and distress in the chest.

Pathogenesis. Accumulation and stagnation of phlegm and heat in the lung, impairment of the lung's dispersing function and the kidney's governing function of inspiration, due to pathogenic factors or impairment of the seven emotions.

Therapeutic Principle. Facilitating the flow of the lung-qi to relieve asthma, and strengthening the spleen and tonifying the kidney.

Subcortex (MA)

An auricular point.

Location. On the medial side of antitragus.

Effect. It plays the role of replenishing marrow and benefiting the brain, arresting pain and tranquilize.

Indication. Hypoplasia in intelligence, insomnia and dreaminess sleep, tinnitus due to the kidney deficiency, pseudo-myopia, neurasthenia.

Subcutaneous Nodes

Symptoms. Hard and painless fruit pit-like lump inside the skin and outside the membrane.

Pathogenesis. Stagnation of wind, fire, qi, dampness and phlegm.

Therapeutic Principle. Dispelling wind, clearing away fire, promoting the circulation of qi, eliminating dampness, resolving phlegm and relieving stagnation.

Sublingual Cyst

Symptoms. The cyst like a gourd which is smooth, soft, yellowish but not painful. It distends beneath the tongue, causes dysphasia and dysphagia. After ulceration, it runs yellowish mucous substances. Though recovered quickly, it may frequently recur.

Pathogenesis. Phlegm-fire interconnection that results in obstruction under the tongue.

Therapeutic Principle. Before ulceration, borate powder is used to scrub the diseased region. When the cyst is big enough, a knife or needle is used to cut or prick it open to release pus.

Submaxillary Nodes

Symptoms. Single swelling mass in submaxillary region or cervical part, movable when the mass is being pushed. The onset is fast, with clear pain when the mass is being pressed, and seldom becomes suppurative. It usually has no body symptoms.

Pathogenesis. Caused by the infection from the injury or the sore of the head, the face, mouth cavity, etc.

Therapeutic Principle. Expelling wind, clearing away heat, resolving phlegm and subduing swelling.

Subprostrate Sophora Root

The root and rhizome of Sophora tonkinensis Gapnep. (Leguminasae).

Effect. Clearing away heat, detoxicating, relieving sore throat, subduing swelling and relieving pain, antineoplastic.

Indication. Swollen and sore throat, early stage of lung cancer, gingivitis, jaundice, cough due to lung-heat, suppurative infections on the body surface, scabies, etc.

Suchow Mosla Herb

The whole herb of Mosla soochowensis Matsuda (Labiatae).

Effect. Expelling pathogenic factors from exterior the body, regulating the flow of qi and alleviating pain.

Indication. Cold, tonsillitis, gastrelcoma, toothache, etc.

Sudden Death Following Measles

Symptoms. Recovering from measles, the patient suddenly sweats like water all over the body, or from angina pectoris. If suffering from epidemic qi, the patient will die.

Pathogenesis. Lack of primordial qi although all seem normal, in fact, the internal organs are impaired.

Therapeutic Principle. Invigorating primordial qi.

Sudden Diarrhea

There are two types of diseases.

1. Cold type

Symptoms. Sudden diarrhea with watery stool and fecal mass, tenesmus, thin urine, cold limbs, absence of thirst, etc.

Pathogenesis. Pathogenic cold in the spleen.

Therapeutic Principle. Warming the middle energizer and expelling cold.

2. Heat type

Symptoms. Sudden diarrhea with ropy or watery stool, burning pain in anus, thirst, desire for cold drink, dark urine with difficulty on micturition, etc.

Pathogenesis. Impairment of the spleen by pathogenic heat.

Therapeutic Principle. Clearing away heat and purging fire.

Sudden Dyspnea

Symptoms. Sudden shortness of breath, dyspnea, flaring of nares, stuffiness in the chest, etc.

Pathogenesis. Sudden attack by invasion of pathogenic wind or emotional stress, reversed flow of qi with accumulation, or impairment of diet and drinking.

Therapeutic Principle. Expelling pathogenic wind to relieve dyspnea, alleviating asthma, promoting digestion and eliminating retained fluid.

Sudden Loss of Hearing

Pathogenesis. Deficiency of the kidney-qi with the invasion by pathogenic wind in the meridian and collateral to ears.

Therapeutic Principle. Tonifying the kidney to expel pathogenic factor.

Sudden Loss of Vision

Symptoms. The disease progresses rapidly, causing patients to have sudden loss of eyesight. In the case of liver-yang rising, vision loss is accompanied by dizziness and vertigo, vexation, irritability, pain in the hypochondrium and a flushed face. Stagnation of qi and blood is accompanied by a distending pain in the head, dysphoria.

Pathogenesis. Due to rage and hyperactivity of the liver-yang leading to failure of the eye functions, or to qi stagnation and blood stasis leading to the qi and blood being unable to transfer essence to the eyes.

Therapeutic Principle. For the former, remove heat from the liver and improve the acuity of vision. For the latter, promote the circulation of qi and blood, and thus improve activity of vision.

Sudden Lumbar Sprain with Qi Blocked

Symptoms. Pain in the waist immediately after injury, inability to straighten lumbar region, and obvious pressure pain of lumbar muscles on one or both sides.

Cause. Indirect external force, such as hyperpost extension and hyperante flexion, and torsion and bending beyond the normal lumbar movement.

Therapeutic Principle. Acupuncture and moxibustion, and massage, etc.

Sudden Precordial Pain

Pathogenesis. Weakness of the viscera, and invasion of the Heart Meridian by pathogenic cold, heat, and wind, resulting in blockage of meridian and stagnancy of qi and blood.

Therapeutic Principle. Dispelling cold, promoting the flow of qi by warming the meridian, clearing away heat to remove obstruction in the meridian and dispelling wind and dredging the meridian due to wind.

Sudden Scrotal Swelling

Symptoms. Sudden scrotal swelling, pain and cold.

Pathogenesis. Invasion of cold into the Liver Meridian and stagnation of qi and blood.

Therapeutic Principle. Warming the liver and promoting circulation of qi of the Liver Meridian, regulating the flow of qi to

alleviate pain, or giving acupuncture and moxibustion of Dadun (Liv 1) point.

Sudden Spurt of Appetite Prior to Collapse

Symptoms. The patient is suddenly able to eat after failure to do so for a long time, in the long course of the disease or during serious disease. After eating, the condition usually takes a turn for the worse or becomes critical. Prognosis is usually unfavourable.

Therapeutic Principle. Immediately decocting Ginseng, Aconite Root to rescue the yang-qi.

Suffrutescent Securinega Twig

The twig and root of Securinega suffruticosa (Pall.) Rehd. (Euphorbiaceae).

Effect. Promoting blood circulation, relaxing muscles and tendons, strengthening the spleen and tonifying the kidney.

Indication. Lumbago due to pathogenic wind-dampness, numbness of the limbs, impotence, facial palsy, and the sequelae of infantile paralysis, etc.

Suffusion of White

Symptoms. Retention of the blood inside the superficial layer of the white eyeball forming red flakes with a clear boundary. The patient has no subjective symptoms.

Pathogenesis. Retention of heat in the Lung Meridian resulting in bleeding, yin insufficiency of the liver and kidney, hyperactivity of fire due to yin deficiency, or by violent coughing and vomiting that lead to upward attack of the reversed flow of qi.

Therapeutic Principle. The mild case does not need treatment, for the serious case, clear away heat from the lung to cool blood and nourish the liver and kidney.

Suliao (GV 25)

A meridian acupuncture point.

Location. On the face, at the center of the nose apex.

Indication. Nasal obstruction, epistaxis, watery nasal discharge, rhinorrhea, ache rosacea, convulsion, loss of consciousness, etc.

Method. Puncture obliquely upward 0.3-0.5 cun, or prick to cause bleeding. Moxibustion is forbidden.

Sulphur

It is the processed material by refinement of the natural Sulphur or sulphreous ore.

Effect. Externally destroying parasites and relieving itching; internally reinforcing vital function and relaxing the bowels.

Indication. Scabies, tinea, eczema, cutaneous pruritus; shortness of breath, impotence, frequent micturition, cold pain in the loins and knees due to kidney deficiency; and constipation due to cold of deficiency type.

Summer-asthma

Symptoms. Dyspnea, hyperhidrosis, dysphoria, or general fever, etc.

Pathogenesis. Pathogenic summer-heat injures the lung, which impairs the purging and descending function of the lung.

Therapeutic Principle. Eliminating summer-heat and invigorating the flow of qi.

Summer Boil

Symptoms. Vesiculation all over the body, with stinking water inside.

Pathogenesis. Damp-heat pathogen suffusing skin.

Therapeutic Principle. Clearing away heat and eliminating dampness.

Summer Cholera

Symptoms. Severe pain in the chest and abdomen, sudden vomiting and drarrhea, rice watery stool with fetid smell, restlessness, fever, thirst, scanty dark urine, even unconsciousness, etc.

Pathogenesis. Internal injury by rich fatty diet, or the affection by exopathogenic summer-heat and dampness in the middle-energizer.

Therapeutic Principle. Clearing away heat, resolving dampness and expelling turbid pathogen.

Summer Convulsive Disease

Symptoms. It is usually seen in children, characterized by fever and headache, neck rigidity, without perspiration.

Pathogenesis. Caused by affecting pathogenic summer-heat.

Therapeutic Principle. Clearing away summer-heat, and arresting convulsion.

Summer-dampness Malaria

It is one type of malaria caused by pathogenic summer-heat, summer dampness stagnating in Shaoyang Meridians. It can be divided into summer malaria and damp malaria. The former means the case with more severe pathogenic summer-heat than dampness. The latter means the case with more severe dampness than pathogenic summer-heat.

Symptoms. For the former, slight cold and serious heat, tendency to drink due to thirst, spontaneous perspiration, etc. For the latter, fever and chills, heaviness sensation in the limbs, lassitude of limbs, myalgia, and stuffiness and fullness in epigastrium, chest abdomen.

Therapeutic Principle. For the former, clearing away the heat located at Shaoyang Meridians, accompanied by eliminating dampness. For the latter, treating Shaoyang disease by mediation, eliminating dampness and regulating the stomach.

Summer Diarrhea

Referring to diarrhea due to summer heat and damp pathogen injuring intestines and stomach. The disease is divided into two types.

1. For the case with more dampness

   Symptoms. Watery diarrhea, nausea, tongue with greasy fur, etc.

   Therapeutic Principle. Remove dampness and relieve summer-heat.

2. For the case with more heat.

Symptoms. Abdominal pain, diarrhea, excessive thirst, dark urine, spontaneous perspiration, dirty complexion, yellowish greasy coating of tongue, etc.
Therapeutic Principle. Clearing away heat and eliminating dampness.

Summer Dysentery

It is one type of dysentery.
Symptoms. Abdominal pain, diarrhea, fever.
Pathogenesis. Caused by affecting heat pathogen in summer.
Therapeutic Principle. Clearing away heat to stop diarrhea.

Summer Fever

Symptoms. High fever, thirst, vexation, flushed face, spontaneous perspiration, deficiency of qi, etc.
Pathogenesis. Affecting heat pathogen in summer.
Therapeutic Principle. Clearing away heat to protect body fluid. Calming the endopathic wind, and relieve spasm, supplementing qi and promoting the production of body fluid, removing dampness.

Summer Fever with Dampness

It refers to summer fever accompanied by more fever than dampness.
1. Due to summer-heat and dampness obstructing the middle-energizer.
   Symptoms. High fever, vexation, thirst, much perspiration and less urine, feeling of stuffiness in stomach, heaviness sensation in the limbs.
   Therapeutic Principle. Clearing away Yangming stomachheat accompanied by resolving Taiyin spleendampness.
2. Due to summer-heat and dampness fill three-energizer.
   Symptoms. Fever, flushed face, deaf, oppressed feeling in chest, productive cough with blood, feeling of stuffiness in stomach and abdomen, thirst, diarrhea with water, scanty dark urine.
   Therapeutic Principle. Clearing away the damp-heat from tri-energizer.

Summer Filthy Disease

Symptoms. Headache, stuffiness and fullness in epigastrium, fever, perspiration, nausea, thirst, vexation, in serious case, unconsciousness, etc.
Therapeutic Principle. Expelling filth by means of aromatics, eliminating dampness and removing turbidity.

Summer Filthy Infection

Symptoms. Vomiting, nausea, stinking and filthy diarrhea, discontinuous abdominal pain, dizziness, perspiration, etc.
Pathogenesis. Due to affecting filthy and turbid pathogen in summer.
Therapeutic Principle. Clearing away summer-heat, eliminating turbidity, and regulating the functions of the spleen and the stomach.

Summer-heat Spasm

It is divided into two types.
1. **Symptoms.** Muscle twitching and cramps of hands and feet.
   Pathogenesis. Due to invasion of pathogenic summer-heat and wind.
   Therapeutic Principle. Clear away summer-heat and dispel wind.
2. **Symptoms.** Itching all over like needle stabbing or red-swollen skin in summer months.
   Therapeutic Principle. Expelling wind and clearing away collaterals.

Summer Phthisis

It refers to sudden hemoptysis and cough due to pathogenic summer-heat, like consumptive disease.
Symptoms. Fever, sudden hemoptysis, epistaxis, cough with heavy breath. Usually sudden attacks and in the serious case it may result in exhaustion of qi, due to hemorrhea.
Pathogenesis. Summer-heat injuring the lung and yang collaterals.
Therapeutic Principle. Removing pathogenic heat from the blood and expelling toxic material from the body to promote the dispersing function of the lung. If ex-

haustion of qi resulting from hemorrhea occurs, the drugs of invigorating qi and controlling exhaustion should be prescribed at once.

Summer Stranguria

Symptoms. Oliguria with dark urine, dribbling and difficulty in urination, thirsty, fever, fullness and oppressed feeling in the chest, etc.

Pathogenesis. Excessive eating raw and cold food in summer, resulting in excessive fluid retention in the body and its failure to go up and down fluently.

Therapeutic Principle. Supplementing qi and promoting the production of body fluid for the deficiency type; and eliminating dampness and heat for excess type.

Summer Unacclimatization

1. It refers to a syndrome of fever attack in summer.

   Symptoms. Sudden attack of dizziness, headache, fatigue, pedal flaccidity, fever, poor appetite, frequent yawn, vexation, spontaneous perspiration, etc. in the period between spring and summer.

   Pathogenesis. Pathogenic summer heat.

   Therapeutic Principle. Replenishing qi and nourishing yin.

2. It is a kind of consumptive disease, which worsens in spring and summer, and alleviates in autumn and winter.

   Symptoms. Feverish extremities, dysphoria with smothery sensation, spermatorrhoea due to cold, inability to walk due to pedal aching, deficiency distention of lower abdomen, etc.

   Therapeutic Principle. Invigorating the spleen and replenishing qi.

3. It refers to an attack of flaccidity in summer.

   Symptoms. Lassitude of limbs, poor appetite due to emaciation, etc.

   Pathogenesis. Deficiency and weakness of the spleen and stomach.

   Therapeutic Principle. Clearing away summer heat, invigorating the spleen

and replenishing the stomach. If not serious, it will be cured naturally without taking medicine when it gets cool in autumn.

Sun Euphorbia Herb

The whole herb of Euphorbia helioscopia L. (Euphorbiaceae).

Effect. Inducing diuresis, subduing swelling, removing phlegm, relieving cough expelling worms and detoxication.

Indication. Ascites, general edema, cough due to lung-heat, cough with dyspnea due to retention of phlegm, dysentery and lichen simplex chronicus.

Sunk Fontanel

If the infantile fontanel sinks over the age of 6 months, it is a morbid state. It will be more serious when the occiput also sinks.

Symptoms. Yellowish face, tiredness and shortness of breath, loss of appetite, loose stool, cold limbs, pale stagnated superficial venule of the index finger etc.

Pathogenesis. Congenital defect or infantile malnutrition, lack of primary qi, diarrhea and qi-deficiency, failure of spleen qi, to ascend, the fontanel will sink.

Therapeutic Principle. Tonifying primary qi and the spleen, invigorate middle-energizer and qi.

Sunward Melandrium Herb

The whole herb of Melandrium apricum (Turcz.) Rohrb. (Caryophyllaceae).

Effect. Promoting blood circulation, regulating menstruation, strengthening the spleen and inducing diuresis.

Indication. Irregular menstruation, alactation, infantile dyspepsia and malnutrition, etc.

Superficial Collaterals

Referring to the collaterals lying just beneath the skin. In the clinic, diseases can be diagnosed through changes in their location, color and lustre.

Superficial Puncture

A needling technique, the modern intradermal needle therapy developed from it.

Indication. Diseases of muscular spasm due to cold.

Method. Puncture obliquely and shallowly from the side of the affected area.

Superficial Thrombophlebitis

Symptoms. Local veins are painful and swelling. Along the veins hard things like ropes can be felt, with clear pressed pain. Erythema appears on the skin near the veins for about 1-3 weeks, then gradually subdues. But the things left like ropes will stay for a long time.

Pathogenesis. External attacking of pathogenic damp-heat, stagnancy of qi and blood stasis, blockage of meridians and collaterals.

Therapeutic Principle. Promoting blood circulation to remove blood stasis, clearing away heat and promoting diuresis or the anaphase, removing obstruction in the meridians to subdue swelling.

Superior Triangular Fossa (MA)

An auricular point.

Location. On the interior superior border of the triangular fossa.

Effect. Calm the liver to stop wind.

Indication. Hypertension.

Suppurative Infection behind Ear

It refers to the phlegm infected between the ear wrinkles.

Symptoms. There are two types.

1. Reddish swelling with a head, easy to ulcerate. It has cheesy pus and is a favourable case.
2. Dark purple without brightness, sunken and hard, headache uneasy to ulcerate belonging to the serious case.

   Pathogenesis. The wind pathogens together with gallbladder-fire.

Therapeutic Principle. At the beginning of the disease, it is advisable to follow the therapeutic principle of clearing away heat from the liver; in pus forming, expelling from within and detoxicating; in those with general deficiency of qi, replenishing and restoring qi and blood.

Suppurative Osteomyelitis

It is a pyogenic disease with pathogens deeply adhering to the bone.

Symptoms. It is usually found in children, mostly in the long bones of the limbs, local swelling adhering to the muscle and bone, immovable by pushing, pain penetrating the bone, many watery pus after ulceration, difficulty in healing. It may form sinus to injure the muscle and bone.

Pathogenesis. Improper treatment and nursing for furuncle and boil to let the remaining toxins and excessive internal damp-heat go deeply inside and linger in the muscle and the bone, or by external injury, particularly open fracture with additional affection of pathogens.

Therapeutic Principle. At the beginning, removing stagnation and obstruction in the meridians. After the formation of pus, regulating the nutrient and expelling toxin. After ulceration regulating qi and blood, clearing away heat and resolving dampness.

Suppurative Otitis Media

Symptoms. The auricular membrane perforation and internal purulence.

Pathogenesis. Outward invasion of pathogenic heat due to fire sufficiency of the liver and gallbladder, dampness retention due to splenic deficiency which flows upward to invade the auricular canal and orifice, and insufficiency and loss of primordial qi of the kidney, which causes stagnation of pathogenic toxin.

Therapeutic Principle. Clearing away heat from the liver, detoxicating and subduing swelling, or strengthening the spleen, excreting dampness and nourishing qi and blood to promote pus discharge, reinforcing the kidney to invigorate the primordial qi and eliminating dampness to resolve turbid discharge.

Suqarcane

The stem stalk of Saccharum sinensis Roxb. (Gramineae).

Effect. Removing heat, promoting the production of the body fluid, and moistening dryness.

Indication. Thirst due to consumption of body fluid, dysphoria, regurgitation, vomiting, cough due to dryness of the lung, constipation, ect.

Swallow Wort Rhizome

The rhizome and root of Cynanchum stauntonii (Decne.) Schltr. ex Levl. and Cynanchum glaucescens (Decne.) Hand.-Mazz. (Asclepiadaeae).

Effect. Dispelling phlegm, maintaining the descend the adverse-rising energy and relieving cough.

Indication. Obstruction of the lung-qi, unsmooth expectoration with profuse phlegm, and dyspnea.

Swallowwort Root

The root or rhizome of Cynanchum atratum Bge. and C. versicolor Bge. (Asclepiadaceae).

Effect. Lowering asthenic fever, removing heat from the blood, inducing diuresis, relieving stranguria, detoxicating.

Indication. Prolonged fever in consumptive diseases, cough due to the lung-heat, postpartum fever, suppurative infections on the body surface, swollen sore throat, snake bite, stranguria due to heat, stranguria with blood, etc.

Swamp Mahogany Leaf

The leaf of Eucalyptus robusta Sm. (Myrtaceae).

Effect. Clearing away dampness-heat and detoxication.

Indication. Common cold, acute enteritis, dysentery, acute and chronic pyelitis, subcutaneous swelling, scalds, etc.

Sweating due to Overstrain

Symptoms. Heavy sweating with slight overstrain.

Pathogenesis. Deficiency of the spleen and qi.

Therapeutic Principle. Nourishing qi and strengthening the spleen.

Sweating from Forehead

Much sweating from the forehead only.

Pathogenesis. Failure of stagnated heat inside to escape which results in its going up along the meridians and sweating from the forehead as seen in yin and yang syndrome with blood stasis and damp-heat.

Sweating in Shock

Symptoms. Pearl-like sweating, profuse perspiration with sticky sweat, cold limbs and faint pulse on the verge of death.

Pathogenesis. Dissociation of yin and yang on the verge of exhaustion of yang-qi, or yang kept externally by yin-excess in the interior and profuse sweating due to exhaustion of yang.

Therapeutic Principle. Recuperating depleted yang and treating yang exhaustion.

Sweating Syndromes

Symptoms. Spontaneous sweat, night sweat, perspiration after shivering and so on. It is divided into deficiency type and excess type.

Pathogenesis. Resulting from qi deficiency, yin deficiency, yang deficiency, pathogenic fire, conflict between the vital energy and the pathogenic factor, etc.

Therapeutic Principle. For deficiency type: nourishing qi and yin, consolidating superficial resistance to arrest sweating; for excess type: removing heat from the liver, removing dampness to restore normal functioning of yin, etc.

Sweet Broomword Herb

The whole herb of Scoparia Back Middlelcis L. (Scrophulariaceae).

Effect. Clearing away heat and removing toxic substances, promoting diuresis and subduing swelling.

Indication. Cough due to the lung-heat, sore throat, diarrhea due to summer-heat, beriberi, edema, infantile measles, eczema, and drug poisoning.

Sweet Flavor

Referring to a kind of herbs with sweet flavor.

Effect. Nourishing, normalizing the functions of stomach and spleen, relieving spasm, etc.

Indication. For syndrome of deficiency type, with such herbs as pilose asiabell root and prepared rehmannia root; for incooperation between the spleen and the stomach, with such herbs as germinatedel barley, and hawthorn fruit; for reliving spasm with pain, with harmonized in properties of different drugs, such as Licorice Root, malt extract, etc.

Sweetgum Fruit

The fruit of Liquidambar formosana Hance (Hamamelidaceae).

Effect. Expelling pathogenic wind, removing obstruction in the meridians, inducing diuresis and removing dampness.

Indication. Pantalgia of limbs, edema, amenorrhea, hypogalactia, carbuncle, hemorrhoids complicated by anal fistula, scabies, etc.

Sweet Orange Peel

The peel of Citrus sinensis (L.) Osbeck (Rutaceae).

Effect. Activating qi circulation, resolving phlegm, strengthening the spleen and removing stagnancy.

Indication. Cough with profuse phlegm due to common cold, vomiting, poor appetite, gastrointestinal distention, diarrhea with borborygmus, acute mastitis, etc.

Sweet Osmanthus Flower

The flower of Osmanthus fragrans Lour. (Oleaceae).

Effect. Resolving phlegm and dissipating blood stasis.

Indication. Cough due to retention of phlegm, toothache, bloody defecation.

Sweet-scented Oleander Leaf or Bark

The leaf or bark of Nerium indicum Mill. (Apocynaceae).

Effect. Exerting a tonic effect on the heart, eliminating diuresis, resolving sputum to relieve asthma and relieving pain.

Indication. Palpitation and slow pulse with irregular intervals due to deficiency of the heart-yang, dyspnea with cough, epilepsy, traumatic injuries, ect.

Sweet Wormwood Herb

The whole plant of Artemisia annua L. (Compositae).

Effect. Lowering asthenic fever, clearing away heat from the blood, relieving summer-heat and preventing the recurrence of malaria, eliminating phlegm, relieving cough.

Indication. Various types malaria epidemic febrile diseases at the later stage marked by nocturnal fever, abatement of fever without sweating or lingering slight fever, chronic bronchitis, dizziness and headache, dysuria, etc.

Swelling and Pain of Glans Penis

Pathogenesis. Caused by the down-ward flow of damp-heat in the Liver Meridian.

Therapeutic Principle. Eliminating the dampness and heat from the Liver Meridian.

Swelling and Pain of the Throat due to Excessive Heat

Symptoms. Sore throat, high fever, thirst, dark urine, yellowish and greasy tongue coating.

Pathogenesis. Excessively pungent diet which leads to the upward stomach-fire burning the body fluid to form phlegm, which accumulates to cause fire.

Therapeutic Principle. Clear stomach heat and relieve sore throat.

Swelling and Pain of the Throat due to Heat of Deficiency Type

Symptoms. Slight redness and swelling of the throat with slight pain, dry mouth and tongue, flushed face and red lips, fever in the palm and sole, red tongue.

Pathogenesis. Consumption of kidney-yin, failure of the yin-fluid to ascend to nourish the throat, causing flaring-up of deficiency-fire which burns the throat.

Therapeutic Principle. Nourish yin to reduce pathogenic fire.

Swelling around Anus

Symptoms. Flat wart-like blocks projecting out, itching, painful, watery, stinking, dirty, and it is also a contagious disease.

Pathogenesis. Infection of toxins due to dirty sexual intercourse, and by damp invasion of lower energizer.

Therapeutic Principle. Removing heat from blood and detoxicating.

Swelling of Eyelid

Symptoms. Swelling of the eyelid like a ball without crimson and pain.

Pathogenesis. Splenic deficiency with dampness interspersed.

Therapeutic Principle. Reinforcing the spleen and replenishing qi together with removing dampness.

Swelling Palate of Infant

Symptoms. Swelling palate like carbuncle, difficulty for the tongue to stretch out and draw back and for the mouth to be closed, inability to suck, and even inability to cry due to swelling obstructing in the pharynx.

Pathogenesis. Dirt in the mouth or heat in the stomach.

Therapeutic Principle. Dispelling stomach heat. The affected parts can also be stabbed by the prismatic needle.

Swelling with Bearing-down Pain of One Testis

Pathogenesis. Phlegm-dampness, blood stasis and the excess of liver-fire. Some of the syndromes are secondary after parotitis.

Therapeutic Principle. Eliminating dampness and resolving phlegm, promoting blood circulating to remove blood stasis, and clearing away the liver-fire.

Swollen and Painful Hand

Symptoms. Swollen and painful hand with sensation of breaking off, or pain in the upper arm, elbow and wrist.

Pathogenesis. Phlegm retention due to deficiency of the spleen, wind-heat and wind-damp invading meridians with phlegm, the blocking of qi in meridians of hand and arm.

Therapeutic Principle. Strengthening the spleen, expelling pathogens, dispersing phlegm, and removing obstructions in meridians.

Swollen Vulva during Pregnancy

Symptoms. Vulval swelling with water retention in the lower part of the body.

Pathogenesis. Yang deficiency of the spleen and kidney.

Therapeutic Principle. Warming yang and strengthening the spleen.

Sword Bean

The ripe seed of Canavalia gladiata (Jacq.) DC. (Leguminosae).

Effect. Sending down the abnormally ascending qi, expelling phlegm to relieve dyspnea and stopping vomiting.

Indication. Hiccups due to cold of deficiency type, abdominal distention and vomiting.

Sword Brake Herb

The whole herb of Pteris ensiformis Burm. (Pteridaceae).

Effect. Clearing away heat, promoting diuresis, eliminating pathogenic heat from the blood and detoxicating.

Indication. Dysentery, liver disease, enteritis, sore throat, stranguria, metrorrhagia, metrostaxis, traumatic injuries, parotitis, fulminant carbuncle, eczema, etc.

Sycosis

Symptoms. At the beginning red papular eruptions from millet-size to soybean-size on the mandible can be seen, heating, itching and slight pain in parts, yellowish water flowing out after ulceration and soaking in stretches.

Pathogenesis. Stagnation of damp-heat of the spleen and the stomach in the skin and also the affection of pathogenic wind.

Therapeutic Principle. Removing pathogenic heat from blood, expelling wind and removing dampness.

Symblepharon

Symptoms. Adhesion of the palpebral margin to the black of the eye and difficulty in rotating the eyeball.

Pathogenesis. Upward attack of wind-heat, blood gushing due to heat and dryness, and stagnation of qi and blood, often found in serious trachoma, or it is caused by burn and introduction of corrosive substances into the eye.

Therapeutic Principle. Clearing away heat and expelling wind, and dissipating blood stasis.

Sympathetic (MA-AH 7)

An auricular point, at the end of the inferior antihelix crus.

Indication. Palpitations, spontaneous perspiration, gastrointestinal spasm, angina pectoris, colic of urethral calculus, one of the common points for auriculo-acupuncture anesthesia.

Symptom Complex of Premenstrual Tension

It refers to a complex occurring a week before menstruation.

Symptoms. Dysphoria, liability to anger, somnolence, dizziness, headache, distending pain of the breast, sore throat, hoarseness, oppressed feeling in the chest, sore waist, distending abdomen, edema, diarrhea, arthralgia, urticaria, and sudden relief or full recovery with the coming of menstruation.

Pathogenesis. Disorder of the liver and kidney leading to impairment of Vital and Front Middle Meridians.

Therapeutic Principle. In the case of stagnation of the liver-qi, soothing the liver and removing stagnation; in the case wof insufficiency of the kidney-yin, replenishing yin and nourishing the kidney.

Syncope

Symptoms. Fever, fullness in the chest and phlegm excess, sudden cold of hand and feet, lockjaw, coma, recovering very soon, etc.

Pathogenesis. Invasion of warm-heat into the body.

Therapeutic Principle. Purgation, expelling heat and detoxifying.

Syncope due to Deficiency of Blood

Symptoms. Pale complexion, cold limbs, palpitation, shortness of breath, or even sudden fainting and unconsciousness, etc.

Pathogenesis. Deficiency of blood and malnutrition of the brain due to loss of blood, postpartum, metrorrhagia, metrostaxis and the impairment of overstrain, etc.

Therapeutic Principle. Invigorating qi and enriching blood.

Syncope due to Excess of Heat

Symptoms. Fever with headache, burning sensation in the chest and abdomen, thirst with fondness of drink, constipation and dark urine, dysphoria at the initial stage, then unconsciousness, cold limbs.

Pathogenesis. Excessive pathogenic heat and stagnation of yang-heat inside the body.

Therapeutic Principle. Revive the faint by inducing resuscitation.

Syncope due to Immoderate Drinking

Symptoms. Cold limbs after drinking alcohol, shaking hands and feet, unconsciousness, etc.

Pathogenesis. Addiction to alcohol or acute alcoholism.

Therapeutic Principle. Neutralizing the toxic effect of alcohol, waking the patient from unconsciousness.

Syncope due to Injury

Symptoms. Lethargic state and unconsciousness.

Cause. Disorder of consciousness and unconsciousness by injury.

Therapeutic Principle. It is a critical internal injury and should be treated properly in time. For the qi-blockage type: inducing resuscitation; for the blood-stasis type: removing blood stasis to induce resuscitation; for the blood-deficiency type: invigorating qi, strengthening the body and recuperating depleted yang.

Syncope due to Phlegm

Symptoms. Sudden syncope, wheezing sound in throat, or vomiting saliva with foam, asthma, white greasy tongue coating.

Pathogenesis. The blockage of qi resulting from phlegm.

Therapeutic Principle. Restore consciousness and remove phlegm.

Syncope due to Summer-heat

Symptoms. Sudden faint, fever, cold limbs, raucous breath as wheezing, slight trismus or dry mouth.

Pathogenesis. Sudden attack by heat pathogen in summer.

Therapeutic Principle. Removing heat from the heart to resuscitate, without using the drugs, cold and cool in nature, abruptly.

Syncope for Lack of Yin-fluid

Symptoms. Tinnitus, deafness, blindness, and even sudden syncope.

Pathogenesis. Consumption of yin-fluid due to the interior heat, mainly resulted from deficiency of yin essence, excessiveness of yang qi, and in addition attack of summer-heat.

Therapeutic Principle. Nourishing kidney essence.

Syncope Resulting from Disorder of Qi

A type of syncope, divided into two types: of excess and deficiency.

1. Due to occasional anger.

   Symptoms. Sudden fainting in strong people accompanied by lockjaw, fists, shortness of breath, cold limbs, thin and whitish coating, deep and taut pulse.

   Therapeutic Principle. Wake the faint by inducing resuscitation.

2. Due to weakness of the body, tiredness, and fright.

   Symptoms. Pale complexion, fatigue and terror, shallow breathing, sweating, cold limbs, pale tongue, deep and feeble pulse.

   Therapeutic Principle. Recuperate depleted and rescue the patient from collapse.

Syndrome due to Retention of Phlegm and Saliva

Symptoms. Unbearable pain in the chest, back and hypochondrium, which is pulling and burning, cold and numb hands and feet, etc.

Pathogenesis. Phlegm and saliva stagnated in the heart and diaphragm due to deficiency of the lung, spleen and kidney, excessive phlegm and saliva retained in the heart and diaphragm, and stagnation of qi circulation.

Therapeutic Principle. Invigorating the spleen, dispersing the phlegm and activating qi circulation.

Syndrome of Exterior Deficiency and Interior Excess

Symptoms. Aversion to wind, spontaneous sweat, fullness in gastric cavity, fullness and excess of phlegm and saliva, constipation, etc.

Pathogenesis. Exopathogen invading interior, insufficiency of defense energy, stagnation of qi in the stomach and intestine, and the retention of phlegm.

Therapeutic Principle. Eliminating pathogenic factors and consolidating superficial resistance.

Syndrome of Exterior Excess and Interior Deficiency

Symptoms. Aversion to cold, fever, anhidrosis, shortness of breath, listlessness, poor appetite, lassitude, palpitation and lumbago, etc.

Pathogenesis. Deficiency of vital energy with the affection of exopathogen, or erroneous administration of purgatives before unrelieved exterior syndrome resulting in the damage of vital energy.

Therapeutic Principle. Strengthening the body resistance and relieving exterior syndrome.

Syndrome of Liver Heat

Symptoms. Dizziness, lassitude, dryness of throat with thirst, stuffiness in the chest and hypochondriac distention, or insomnia, irritability or liability to fight, etc.

Pathogenesis. Fire-transmission by stagnation of the liver-qi, or hyperactivity of yang due to the liver yin deficiency resulting in hypofunction in dispersing and purging, internal disturbance of pathogenic heat.

Therapeutic Principle. Relieving the depressed liver and nourishing the liver-yin.

Syndrome of Lung Meridian

Symptoms. Tightness and stuffiness in the chest, pain in supraclavicular fossa, cough with dyspnea, vexation and heat in palm, etc.

Pathogenesis. Abnormal qi of the Lung Meridian.

Therapeutic Principle. Promoting the dispersing function of the lung to send down abnormally ascending qi.

Syndrome of Pain in Chest and Abdomen

Symptoms. Intermittent pain epigastrium without fixed spot, etc.

Pathogenesis. Debility, attack by pathogens which invade the meridian and collaterals and enter the chest and abdomen.

Therapeutic Principle. Restoring qi and eliminating pathogenic factors.

Syndrome with Cloudy Urine

Symptoms. Turbid urine which is white like rice-washed water, dysuria, or distending sensation of the lower abdomen, burning sensation of urethra with difficulty in urination, or lassitude in loin and legs, dizziness and tinnitus, etc.

Pathogenesis. Deficiency of primordial qi of the lower-energizer, failure to arrest discharges, or improper diet, dysfunction of the spleen in transport, accumulation of dampness and production of heat, failure to separate the useful from the waste, or impairment of meridians and collaterals due to fire of deficiency type.

Therapeutic Principle. Nourishing the kidney, clearing away heat, removing dampness and invigorating the spleen.

Syndrome with Dyspnea due to Phlegm Retention

Symptoms. Often seen in infants, dyspnea with tide-sounding wheezing.

Pathogenesis. The abnormal rising of functional activities of qi due to the phlegm retention in the lung.

Therapeutic Principle. Clearing away the phlegm retention quickly.

Syphilitic Skin Lesions

Symptoms. At the beginning, fever, headache, arthralgia, and sore throat, and afterwards flushing in the skin patch like rubella or like red beans embedded in the skin. When rash granulates faster, the interior contents are projected in the exterior. At the late stage, syphilis invades marrow, joints or viscera.

Pathogenesis. Invasion of syphilis by means of sexual contact.

Therapeutic Principle. Clearing blood and detoxicating.

T

Tabasheer

It is the lump material by coagulating the secretory juice from the dried stalk of Bambusa textilis McClure (Gramineae).

Effect. Clearing away heat, eliminating phlegm, clearing heart-fire and tranquilizing mind.

Indication. Convulsion due to heat-phlegm, apoplexy, accumulation of phlegm, infantile convulsion, night cry, etc.

Tablet Moxibustion

A type of indirect moxibustion.

Function. Warm the middle-energizer to dispel cold and promote flow of qi and blood circulation.

Method. Apply to the point a tablet made of drugs pungent in flavor, warm and fragrant in property, with a moxa-stick placed on a point for moxibustion. When applied in the clinic there are various methods of moxibustion, such as pepper-cake moxibustion and fermented soybean-cake moxibustion, etc.

Tachypnea due to Exopathogen Wind-cold

Symptoms. Dyspnea with cough, copious watery phlegm, stuffy nose with clear nasal discharge, aversion to cold.

Pathogenesis. Wind-cold attacks exterior the skin, results in obstruction of the lung-qi and its adverse flow.

Therapeutic Principle. Dispersing wind and expelling cold to arrest wheezing.

Tadpole

It is the frog juveniie of Rana limnocharis Boie. R. plancyi Lataste or R. nigromaculata Hallowell (Ranidae).

Effect. Clearing away heat and detoxicating.

Indication. Carbuncles, sores and other pyogenic infections on the body surface caused by noxious heat, etc.

Taibai (Sp 3)

An acupuncture point.

Location. At the medial margin and the junction of the reddish and whitish skin, posterior and inferior to the first metatarsophalangeal joint of the great toe.

Indication. Stomachache, abdominal distention, diarrhea, vomiting, constipation, dysentery and beriberi.

Method. Puncture perpendicularly 0.3-0.5 cun and apply moxibustion to the point with 3-5 moxa cones or for 5-10 minutes.

Taichong (Liv 3)

An acupuncture point.

Location. On the excavation posterior to the space of the 1st and 2nd metatarsal bones on the dorsum of the foot.

Indication. Headache, vertigo, tinnitus, hernia, irregular menstruation, metrorrhagia and metrostaxis, amenorrhea, dysuria, infantile convulsion, epilepsy and jaundice.

Method. Puncture perpendicularly 0.5-0.8 cun and apply moxibustion to the point with 3-5 units of moxa cones or for 5-10 minutes.

Taixi (K 3)

An acupuncture point.

Location. At the excavation between the medial malleolus and achilles tendon, parallel to the tip of the medial malleolus.

Indication. Sore throat, toothache, deafness, hemoptysis, dyspnea, diabetes, insomnia, seminal emission, impotence, frequent micturition, irregular menstruation, beriberi.

Method. Puncture perpendicularly 0.5-1 cun and apply moxibustion to the point with 3-5 units of moxa cones or for 5-10 minutes.

Taiyang (Ex-HN5)

It is one of the extraordinary points.

Location. In the temple, about 1 cun lateral to the midpoint of the line connecting the end of the eyebrow and the outer canthus.

Indication. Headache, migraine, common cold, vertigo, toothache, swelling pain.

Method. Puncturing perpendicularly 0.3-0.4 cun or subcutaneously 0.5-1 cun or prick to cause little bleeding with triangular needle.

Taiyang and Shaoyang Complication

It refers to a case in which shaoyang syndrome occurs before taiyang disease subsides.

Symptoms. Epigastric fullness, neck rigidity, and dizziness.

Pathogenesis. Insufficient vital-qi, serious pathogenic affection, loss of treatment, or erroneous treatment.

Therapeutic Principle. Puncturing Dazhui (GV 14) and Feishu (B 13) to relieve the pathogen in taiyang, and puncturing Ganshu (B 18) to relieve pathogen in shaoyang.

Taiyang Headache

1. It refers to headache caused by taiyang disease due to attack of exogenous cold.
   Symptoms. Headache, aversion to cold.
   Therapeutic Principle. Relieving the exterior syndrome with drugs pungent in flavor and warm in property.
2. It refers to the headache located at the part where Taiyang Meridian passes.
   Symptoms. Ache from the back of the head to vertex of the head and then to the neck.

Therapeutic Principle. Relieving the exterior syndrome with drugs pungent in flavor and warm in property, and arresting pain.

Taiyi (S 23)

An acupuncture point.

Location. At the upper abdomen, 2 cun superior to the center of the umbilicus, 2 cun to the anterior median line.

Indication. Stomachache, abdominal distention, psychosis, beriberi and dysphoria.

Method. Puncture perpendicularly 0.8-1.2 cun and apply moxibustion to the point with 3-5 units of moxa cones or for 5-10 minutes.

Taiyin (Ex-LE)

An extra acupuncture point.

Location. Directly above the medial malleolus, in the depression of the posterior border of the medial aspect of tibia, two points in all in the left and right lower limbs.

Indication. Beriberi.

Method. Moxibustion with 3-7 moxa cones.

Taiyin Headache

Symptoms. Headache, profuse phlegm and heaviness sensation in the limbs, abdominal fullness and pain.

Pathogenesis. The retention of phlegm-dampness in the spleen which prevents lucid yang from rising to the head.

Therapeutic Principle. Removing dampness and phlegm.

Taiyin Syndrome

It is one of the syndromes of the six meridians.

Symptoms. Abdominal pain and distention, vomiting, diarrhea, anorexia, or usually vomiting clear and watery saliva, diarrhea.

Pathogenesis. Hypofunction of the spleen and accumulation of cold and dampness, deficiency of the spleen-yang, and excessive cold-dampness in the interior, dysfunction in transferring and transforming.

Therapeutic Principle. Warming and invigorating the spleen and stomach, and dispelling cold and drying dampness.

Taiyuan (L 9)

An acupuncture point.

Location. On the radial side of the transverse crease of the wrist, at the pulsation of the radial artery.

Indication. Cough, dyspnea, pain and fullness in the chest, cardialgia, palpitation, facial edema due to attack of pathogenic wind on head, swelling sore throat, febrile disease without sweating, palmar heat.

Method. Avoiding the radial artery, puncture perpendicularly 0.3-0.5 cun and apply moxibustion to the point for 3-5 minutes. Apply moxibustion 3-5 moxa cones or 5-10 minutes with warming moxibustion.

Taking off Clothes

Referring to an acupuncture technique, which induces sweat.

Operation. Puncture points on the Hand and Foot-taiyin Meridians with the reinforcing method.

Indication. Two kinds of excess heat syndromes: exterior heat due to excess yang qi, and internal heat caused by deficient yin qi, both of which cause patients to feel as if they were carrying charcoal fire in their arms.

Taking Qi from Defence System

It refers to the method technique of reinforcing, or waiting for qi in the superficial area and then pressing it down to the deep area.

Talcum

It is the talc mineral of monoclinic system, comprising mainly hydrous magnesium silicate.

Effect. Inducing diuresis for treating stranguria, clearing away summer-heat,

eliminating dampness and arresting secretion.

Indication. Dysuria, dribbling and painful micturition, summer-heat with excessive thirst, diarrhea, oppressed feeling in the chest due to damp-warm, exudative wound, eczema, miliaria, ect.

Tall Rattlesnake Plantatain Herb

It is the whole herb of Goodyera procera (Ker-Gawl.) Hook. (Orchidaceae).

Effect. Expelling wind, eliminating dampness, tonifying blood and relaxing muscles.

Indication. Wind-cold-damp arthralgia and hemiplegia.

Talon Needling

An ancient needling technique.

Operation. A needle is thrust directly to the muscle (the boundary between muscles or muscle layers), lifted to the skin and then pricked obliquely right and left like the talons of a chicken.

Indication. Numbness and pain of the muscle.

Tamarind Fruit

It is the fruit of Tamarindus indica L. (Leguminosae).

Effect. Clearing away summer-heat and dissipating food stagnancy.

Indication. Inappetence due to summer-heat, vomiting during pregnancy, infantile dyspepsia, malnutrition, etc.

Tangerine Leaf

It is the leaf of Citrus reticulata Blanco (Rutaceae).

Effect. Dispelling the depressed liver-qi, promoting flow of qi, subduing swelling and dissipating stasis.

Indication. Pain in the hypochondrium, nodules of breast and mass in the abdomen, acute mastitis.

Tangerine Peel

It is the fruit peel of Citrus reticulata Blanco (Rutaceae).

Effect. Regulating flow of qi, normalizing the function of the spleen and stomach, eliminating dampness and dissipating phlegm.

Indication. Abdominal distention, belching, nausea and vomiting, oppressed feeling in the chest, loose stool; cough, profuse sputum, adverse flow of qi.

Tangerine Pith

It is the vascular bundle in the orange peel and endocarp of Citrus reticulata Blanco (Rutaceae).

Effect. Invigorating the spleen and promoting flow of qi eliminating dampness and resolving phlegm.

Indication. Stagnation of phlegm in the meridians, fullness and distention of the chest and abdomen, anorexia, vomiting and diarrhea.

Tangerine Seed

It is the seed of Citrus reticulata Blanco (Rutaceae).

Effect. Promoting flow of qi, eliminating stagnation to stop pain.

Indication. Hernia, painful and swollen testis, distending pain of the breast nodules.

Tanzhong (CV 17)

Location. On the anterior midline, at the level with the 4th intercostal space.

Indication. Cough, asthma, pain in the chest, palpitation, insufficient lactation, vomiting, dysphugia.

Method. Puncture subcutaneously 0.3-0.5 cun. Moxibustion is applicable.

Taodao (GV 13)

An acupuncture point.

Location. On the back, in the excavation inferior to the spinous process of the 1st thoracic vertebra on the posterior median line.

Indication. headache, fever, malaria, common cold, cough, rigid nape, dyspnea, hectic fever due to yin-deficiency, pain in the chest, aching pain in the spine.

Method. Puncture obliquely upward 0.5-1 cun. Moxibustion is applicable.

Taperleaf Japanese Spiraea Twig and Leaf

It is the whole herb of Spiraea japonica L. f. var. acuminata Franch. (Rosaceae).

Effect. Restoring menstrual flow, relaxing the bowels and inducing diuresis.

Indication. Irregular menstruation, amenorrhea, abdominal distention due to constipation and dysuria.

Tarsitis of Newborn

Symptoms. The newborn's eyes are swelling and erosional.

Pathogenesis. Washing unclean afterbirth, and something dirty entering the eyelids.

Therapeutic Principle. Clearing away heat and detoxifying.

Tatarian Aster Root

It is the root or rhizom of Aster tataricus L. f. (Compositae).

Effect. Eliminating phlegm and relieving cough, nourishing the lung to keep the adverse qi downward.

Indication. Cough, reversed flow of qi, unsmooth expectoration, chronic cough with blood in the phlegm due to the lung deficiency and many other kinds of cough.

Tawny Sweat

Symptoms. Edema of the head-face and extremities, fever, aching of the body with heaviness, difficult urination.

Pathogenesis. Obstruction of nutrient and defensive system because of profuse sweating or excessive retention of damp-heat in the interior.

Therapeutic Principle. Regulating nutrient and defence system, invigorating yang and reinforcing yin.

Tea-seed Oil

It is the oil expressed from the seed of Camellia oleifera Abel. (Theaceae).

Effect. Clearing away heat and dissipating dampness, destroying parasites and detoxicating.

Indication. Abdominal pain due to eruption disease, acute ascaris, intestinal obstruction, scabies, and burns.

Teeth Clenching

Symptoms. Grinding of the upper teeth with the lower ones during sleeping, making noisy sounds.

Pathogenesis. Stomach-heat, attack of pathogenic wind upon muscles and tendons, and malnutrition due to parasitic infestation.

Teeth Observation

It is one of the diagnostic methods including observation of teeth and gums, not only for the diagnosis of local illness, but also for finding clues in detecting diseases of internal organs, such as pathogenic changes of kidney and stomach.

Temple (MA)

An ear point, also known as Sun (MA).

Location. At the middle of the lateral aspect of the antitragus.

Indication. Migraine.

Tendon Exhaustion

Symptoms.
1. Deficient type: muscular contracture and spasm, pain of fingers, lassitude, and inability to stand for a long-time, even curled-up tongue and ascended testes and purple lips and nails.
2. Excess type: muscular contracture, dark blue nails, pain in soles of feet, dry mouth with heat sensation, irritability and distending pain in the hypochondrium, etc.

Pathogenesis. Yin deficiency of the liver and kidney, the fire transformed from the depressed liver-qi and the impairment of tendon and muscle by the liver-fire.

Therapeutic Principle. Nourishing the liver and kidney for the former, and clearing away fire from the liver for the latter.

Tendon Failure

Referring to the impairment and failure of tendon and muscle.

Symptoms. Nervousness and fear, purple lips and nails, etc.

Pathogenesis. The qi failure of the Liver Meridian.

Therapeutic Principle. Tonifying the liver and kidney, relieving muscular spasm and tranquilizing the mind.

Tenesmus

It refers to the frequent urge to defecate, but bowels opening only a little with great effort.

Pathogenesis. Prolonged dysentery which injures yin-blood, and deficiency of qi which causes lucid yang going down.

Teniasis

Symptoms. Abdominal pain, borborygmus, diarrhea, and repeated vomiting with pus and blood.

Therapeutic Principle. Dissipating mass and destroying parasites.

Tense Cough

Symptoms. Continuous cough, obstruction in breath.

Pathogenesis. The attacking of the pathogenic wind and cold which leads to the impairment of the purifying and descending functions of the lung, and the abnormal rising of the lung qi.

Therapeutic Principle. Dispelling wind and cold, and releasing the flow of the lung qi to relieve cough.

Terebinthaceous Hogfennel Root

It is the root of Peucedanum terebinthaceum (Fisch.) Fisch. ex Turcz. (Umbelliferae).

Effect. Expelling pathogenic factors from exterior the body, relieving cough and asthma.

Indication. Cough and especially intractable cough during pregnancy.

Tetanus Neonatorium

Symptoms. Trismus with cyanotic lips, lockjaw. In serious cases, convulsion of limbs and opisthotonus.

Pathogenesis. Unclean instruments used in cutting the umbilical cord, or improper nursing and attack by pathogenic wind, cold, water and dampness.

Therapeutic Principle. Clearing and activating meridians and collaterals, and expelling pathogenic wind and spasmolysis.

Tetany due to Indigestion

Symptoms. Fullness of abdomen and borborygmus, lower fever in the afternoon, restlessness during sleep, dysphoria, even spasm of the extremities and constipation or loose stool with sour and foul smell.

Pathogenesis. Immoderate drinking and eating resulting in heat from the stagnant food.

Therapeutic Principle. Harmonizing the liver and spleen, clearing away heat and nourishing the stomach.

Tetraplegia after Apoplexy

Symptoms. Paralysis and disability of limbs, lassitude in loin and knees, or disturbance of consciousness.

Pathogenesis. The deficiency of qi and blood, the deficiency of liver-yin and kidney-yin, the stagnation of phlegm and blood stasis after apoplexy.

Therapeutic Principle. Invigorating qi and dissipating blood stasis, tonifying the liver and kidney, activating the meridians and collaterals.

The Liver and kidney have the same origin

It is one of the theories on the relationship between five zang organs. The essence of life stored in the kidney and the blood stored in the liver. They have a relationship of mutual nourishing and transformation. The liver-yin and the kidney-yin are restricted, coordinated and balancing each other.

Thelorrhagia

Symptoms. Bleeding from the nipple, without pain. In some cases, a bean-sized round soft and movable mass can be felt in the mammary areola.

Pathogenesis. Impairment of the liver and spleen due to stagnated anger and anxiety, failure of keeping the blood flowing within the vessels.

Therapeutic Principle. In the case of excessive liver-fire, soothing the liver and regulating the circulation of qi, clearing away pathogenic heat from the blood. In the case of failure of keeping the blood flowing within the vessels due to deficiency of the spleen, invigorating the spleen and nourishing the blood. When the treatment is inefficient, operation should be applied.

Theory of Meridians and Collaterals

It is the theory to study the physiological functions, pathological changes of the system of the meridians and collaterals and their relationship with the zang-fu organs. It is one of the important components of the theoretical system of TCM.

Therapeutic Principles

Selection of treatment based on the differential diagnosis, they are also directive rules for guiding the establishment in a therapy and prescription of a recipe. The principle of treatment is usually searching for the primary cause of a disease in treatment, strengthening the body resistance and eliminating pathogenic factors, harmonizing yin and yang and treating in accordance with seasonal conditions, local conditions and the physique of an individual.

Thick Leaf Croton Root

It is the root of Croton crassifolius Geisel. (Euphorbiaceae).

Effect. Expelling wind, removing dampness, relaxing muscles and tendons, and activating the flow of qi and blood.

Indication. Gastralgia, flatulence, rheumatic arthralgia and traumatic injuries.

Thick Sputum

Symptoms. The phlegm adheres to the pharynx, inability of expectoration and swallow accompanied by dry mouth, cough with dyspnea, etc.

Pathogenesis. Accumulation of fire and stagnation of qi, obstruction of the lung-qi, and failure in distribution of body fluid for a long time.

Therapeutic Principle. Relieving stagnation and removing fire, moistening the lung and clearing away phlegm.

Thinleaf Crazyweed Root

It is the root of Oxytropis leptophylla (Pall) DC. (Leguminosae).

Effect. Clearing away heat and detoxicating.

Indication. Tinea capitis and scrofula.

Thinleaf Milkwort Root

It is the root of Polygala tenuifolia Willd. (Polygalaceae).

Effect. Relieving mental distress, tranquilizing the mind, dispelling phlegm to induce resuscitation, removing carbuncles and dissolving lumps.

Indication. Palpitation, insomnia and forgetfulness; epilepsy cough with profuse sputum; carbuncles, poisoning swelling.

Thin Nasal Discharge

Symptoms. Sudden attacks, itching of nasal cavity, persistent sneezing, and stuffy nose with clear nasal discharge.

Pathogenesis. Deficiency of the lung-qi, resulting in invasion of wind and cold into the nasal orifice.

Therapeutic Principle. Expelling cold and releasing the flow of the lung-qi.

Thin White Coating of Tongue

A tongue picture.

Symptoms. Dim and pale complexion, weariness, dizziness, palpitation, short breath, etc.

Pathogenesis. Deficiency of both qi and blood, malnutrition of the tongue body.

Thirst and Urination

Symptoms. Dry mouth, excessive thirst, over-drinking with immediate passing of urine.

Pathogenesis. Improper medicine taken as a child, or intemperance in sexual life, consumption of kidney-qi, accumulation of heat in lower-energizer, and the deficient kidney failing to control water.

Therapeutic Principle. Nourishing yin and the kidney.

Thirst due to Hemorrage

Symptoms. Thirst, profuse perspiration, fatigue, poor appetite, restlessness, dizziness, palpitation, etc.

Pathogenesis. Hemoptysis, epistaxis, bloody stool, bleeding after delivery and other hemorrhage, or over-exertion resulting in impairment of the stomach, which leads to the deficiency of body fluid and blood, or deficiency of qi which is unable to consolidate body fluid.

Therapeutic Principle. Strengthening the spleen, nourishing blood, and nourishing yin to produce body fluid.

Thirteen Ghost Points

It refers to the thirteen points commonly used to cure mental diseases, such as depressive psychosis, insanity etc.

The points are called respectively: Shuigou (GV 26), Shaoshang (L 11), Yinbai (Sp 1), Daling (P 7), Shenmai (B 62), Fengfu (GV 16), Jiache (S 6), Chengjiang (CV 24), Laogong (P 8), Shangxing (GV 23), Huiyin (CV 1) of the male, Yumentou (Ex) of the female, Quchi (LI 11) and Haiquan (Ex-HN 11).

Thoracic Vertebrae (MA)

An auricular point.

Location. There are five equal shares from the incisure of helix to the branching point of the upper and lower crus of helix, the middle two fifths is the point.

Function. Strengthen the spine and benefit marrow.

Indication. Pain in the chest and hypochondriac region, mastitis, insufficient lactation, and distention and pain in the breast before the menses.

Thorowax Root

It is the root or whole plant of Bupleurum chinense DC., and B. Scorzonerifolfium Willd. (Umbelliferae).

Effect. Reducing fever, soothing the liver and regulating the circulation of qi, invigorating vital function and elevating spleen yang.

Indication. Alternate chills and fever, fullness and pain in the chest and hypochondrium, bitter taste, dry throat, headache and dizziness, irregular menstruation, etc.

Those Stored in Five Zang Organs

A theory in TCM. Since the mental activities of human beings are based on vital essence and energy, the abnormal mental state is associated with dysfunction of zang-fu organs. The heart, lung, liver, spleen, and kidney store the mind, spirit, mood, idea and memory respectively.

Thready Pulse

It refers to the pulse feels thin and soft, like silk thread, feeble yet always perceptible on pressing, more obvious than indistinctive pulse. It indicates deficiency of both qi and blood, internal injury caused by overstrain and damp syndrome.

Threatened Abortion due to Anger

Symptoms. Oppressed feeling in the chest, pain in the hypochondrium, abdominal distention, soreness in the waist, and even vaginal bleeding.

Pathogenesis. Frequent anger and qi stagnation. The fire from qi stagnation goes down to disturb vital and Front Middle Meridians.

Therapeutic Principle. Soothing the liver and clearing away heat to prevent abortion.

Threatened Abortion due to Kidney Deficiency

Pathogenesis. Deficiency of the kidney, failing to hold the fetus.

Therapeutic Principle. Invigorating the kidney to prevent abortion.

Three Contraindications for Fetus and Delivery

Referring to drug contraindications during pregnancy and post-delivery. The doctor is not permitted to make prescriptions containing the medicines of diaphoresis, purgative and diuretic.

Three Different Ways of Needling

Referring to needling bleeding to discharging qi and to applying moxibustion.

Method. Puncture to cause bleeding for treating diseases in the nutrient phase; puncture superficially to dispel pathogenic factors for treating diseases in the defensive phase and apply moxibustion for treating numbness and pain due to severe cold evil.

Three-edged Needle

A kind of needle which is made of stainless steel with a thicker cylinder-shape needle handle and a triangular prim body, the end of which has three sharp blades.

Function. Puncture certain points or superficial blood vessels to let out a little blood for therapeutic purposes.

Indication. Febrile disease, inflammation, heat stroke, coma. Be careful when applying it to those who are weak, with anemia, hypotension, or pregnant women. Contraindicated for those with hemorrhagic tendency, angioma, hemophilia.

Three-fingered Pinching Manipulation

It is one of pinching methods.

Operation. Grip the limb with thumb, index and middle fingers, and squeeze forcefully in opposite directions.

Function. Relaxing muscles and tendons, promoting blood circulation, relieving stagnation of qi and eliminating obstruction in the collaterals.

Indication. Muscular tension and spasm, injury of soft tissues, and topoalgia.

Three Guan of Fingers

A massage point.

Location. The faces of the three sections of the index finger.

Function. Pushing them are invigorating qi, promoting the blood circulation and diaphoresis.

Three Hand Yang Meridians

It refers to the Large Intestine Meridian of Hand-yangming, the Small Intestine Meridian of Hand-taiyang, and the Tri-energizer Meridian of Hand-shaoyang.

Pathogenesis. Running in the lateral aspect of the upper extremities in the Twelve Meridians. The Three Hand Yang Meridians all start from the hand by way of lateral aspect of the upper extremities to the head.

Three Hand Yin Meridians

It refers to Lung Meridian of Hand-taiyin, the Heart Meridian of Hand-shaoyin and the Pericardium Meridian of Hand-jueyin.

Pathogenesis. Running in the medial aspect of the upper extremities. The Three Hand Yin Meridians start from the internal organs in the chest by way of the medial aspect of the upper extremities to the hand.

Three Insertions and One Lifting

A needling method, generally used in heat-producing needling.

Operation. Needle the three layers, one after the other, from the superficial through the middle to the deep layer little by little and lift the needle from the deep to the superficial layer all at one time. Do this repeatedly. This method embodies the re-inforcement principle of slow insertion and quick withdrawal to get qi from the defensive phase.

Three Methods to Treat Blood Troubles

It refers to three major methods to treat all kinds of blood troubles: enriching the blood, promoting blood circulation and removing pathogenic heat from blood are used to treat blood deficiency, blood stasis and blood-heat respectively.

Three Methods to Treat Qi-disorders

It refers to three major methods to treat all qi disorders, such as invigorating qi and sending down abnormally ascending qi is used to treat adverse qi flow, and the administration of drastic drugs is used to remove stagnation and obstruction of qi circulation, etc.

Three Syndromes of Timely Purgation of Yangming

Referring to the three syndromes caused by transmission of acute febrile disease to Yangming fu organ disease.

Symptoms. 1. Fever and much sweating in Yangming disease; 2. The patient suffered from febrile disease for six or seven days with dim eyesight, difficulty in defecation, slight fever; 3. Fullness and pain in abdomen, and continuous diaphoresis. Those three should be timely purged.

Three Treatments for Metrorrhagia

Referring to the three methods of treating metrorrhagia at its primary, intermediate, and at the late stage.

Method. At the primary stage, adopting hemostasis to arrest bleeding; at the intermediate, clearing away heat from blood to disperse its source; and at the late stage, enriching blood to restore its routine.

Three Yang

1. It refers to the Urinary Bladder Meridians of Foot-taiyang, the Stomach Meridians of Foot-yangming, and the Gall Bladder Meridians of Foot-shaoyang. 2. It is the general term for taiyang, shaoyang, and yangming.

Three Yang Meridians of Foot

A collective term referring to the Stomach Meridian of Foot-yangming, the Gallbladder Meridian of Foot-shaoyang and the Urinary Bladder Meridian of Foot-taiyin.

Location. They all run along the lateral lower extremities. The Stomach Meridian runs along the anterior border, the Gallbladder, along the midline, and the Urinary bladder, along the posterior border. They all travel from the head, through the neck, back, and the lower extremities and arrive at the foot.

Three Yang Meridians of Hand

A collective term for the Large Intestine Meridian of Hand-yangming, the Small Intestine Meridian of Hand-taiyang and the Triple-energizer Meridian of Hand-shaoyang.

Location. They run from hand to head, distributing in the lateral part of the upper extremities.

Three Yin

1. It refers to the Spleen Meridian of Foot-taiyin, the Liver Meridian of Foot-jueyin, and the Kidney Meridian of Foot-shaoyin; 2. Only refers to the Spleen Meridian of Foot-taiyin.

Three Yin Meridians of Foot

A collective term for referring to the Spleen Meridian of Foot-taiyin, the Liver Meridian of Foot-jueyin, and the Kidney Meridian of Foot-shaoyin.

Location. They all run along the medial aspect of the lower limb. They all go along the lower part of the shank and the back of foot, with the Liver Meridian along the anterior border, with the Kidney Meridian along the posterior border and with the spleen along the midline. They cross at the area 8 cun above the medial malleolus then, the Spleen Meridian runs along the anterior border, the Liver Meridian along the midline, and the Kidney Meridian still along the posterior border. They all run from the foot, through lower extremities and the abdomen, arriving at the chest.

Three Yin Meridians of Hand

A general term for the Lung Meridian of Hand-Taiyin, the Heart Meridian of Hand-shaoyin and the Pericardium Meridian of Hand-jueyin.

Location. They run from chest to hand, distributing in the medial part of the upper extremities.

Throat Infection

It generally refers to an acute infectious disease of larynx. It is often found in infants.

Symptoms. Sudden swelling and pain in the throat, suppuration in purplish-red or yellowish-white, either covered with tunica albuginea that cannot be wiped out or accompanied by high fever and reddish spot-like patches dotting the skin.

Pathogenesis. Heat accumulation in the lung and stomach, and repeated attacks by pathogenic factors of epidemic diseases.

Therapeutic Principle. Clearing away heat to nourish yin, and detoxicating and relieving sore throat.

Throat Inflammation with Whitish Surface

Referring to inflammation of the throat whose surface is white.

Symptoms. Whitish region of inflammation, feverish sensation, slow pulse, etc.

Pathogenesis. Affection of pathogenic cold in the lung and stomach.

Therapeutic Principle. Dispelling cold to relieve sore throat and activating collaterals and detoxicating.

Throat-pain during Pregnancy

Symptoms. Red and swelling throat.

Pathogenesis. Original fire hyperactivity due to yin deficiency, upward attack of the fetal qi after pregnancy, or affection by seasonal exopathic factors and upward attack of heat in the lung and stomach.

Therapeutic Principle. Clearing away heat and purging intense heat.

Throat Tinea

Symptoms. Dryness, itching, slight pain of the throat with reddish venules all over and projecting spots on the surface which erode and ulcerate as time passes, tidal fever, night sweat, hoarseness, etc.

Pathogenesis. Yin insufficiency of the liver and kidney, and flaring up of deficient fire; or by intense heat accumulation in the stomach that fumigates the lung and results in damage to the lung-yin.

Therapeutic Principle. Nourishing yin to reduce pathogenic fire.

Thrush

It is a kind of oral ulcer, mostly found in the newborn.

Symptoms. Multiple white exudative patches in shape of goose mouth all over the oral mucosa and surface of the tongue.

Pathogenesis. Weakness of the spleen and stomach of children, and the flaming-up of the stomach fire.

Therapeutic Principle. Clearing away heat, removing fire, or nourishing yin.

Thrusting Once and Lifting Thrice

A needling technique.

Operation. Inserting the needle directly into the required depth and then lift it to the subcutaneous level according to a deep, medium and superficial sequence. No matter whether we insert or lift it, just twirl and rotate, or lift and thrust the needle on the basis of the above-mentioned sequence.

Thrusting while Pushing the Needle

A needling technique.

Operation. After getting the acupuncture feeling, the needle is pressed down. This is a reinforcing method.

Thunbery Grape Stem and Leaf

It is the stem and leaf of Vitis thunbergii Sieb. et Zucc. (Vitaceae).

Effect. Eliminating dampness, inducing diuresis and detoxicating.

Indication. Stranguria, dysentery, numbness, epilepsy, nodules of breast, eczema, etc.

Thunder-headache

Symptoms. Headache, painful swelling in the face or aversion to cold and high fever, and thundering sound in the head.

Pathogenesis. Pathogenic wind, or disturbance of the upper part of the body by phlegm and heat.

Therapeutic Principle. Clearing away heat, resolving phlegm, dispelling wind, and raising the lucid-yang to dissolve lumps.

Thyme Herb   ⊛ T-1

It is the whole herb of Thymus serpyllum L. (Labiatae).

Effect. Warming the middle-energizer to dispel cold, expelling pathogenic wind and relieving pain.

Indication. Abdominal pain with vomiting and diarrhea, anorexia, cough due to wind-cold, swollen and sore throat, tooth-ache, etc.

Tianchi (P 1)

An acupuncture point.

Location. In the thoracic region, 1 cun lateral to the nipple in the 4th intercostal space.

Indication. Hypochondriac pain, vexation and oppressed feeling in the thoracic diaphragm, cough, scrofula, and swelling and pain in armpit.

Method. Puncturing obliquely 0.3-0.5 cun and apply moxibustion to the point with 1-3 units of moxa cones or for 3-5 minutes.

Tianchong (G 9)

An acupuncture point.

Location. 0.5 cun posterior to Shuaigu (G 8) and above posterior border of the auricular radicle on the head, 2 cun within the hairline.

Indication. Headache, palpitation, psychosis. Gingivitis and goiter.

Method. Puncture transversely 0.5-0.8 cun and apply moxibustion to the point with 3-5 units of moxa cones or for 5-10 minutes.

Tianchuang (SI 16)

An acupuncture point.

Location. 3.5 cun lateral to the Adam apple, at the posterior border of the sternocleidomastoid muscle, in the exterior cervical region.

Indication. Headache, tonsillitis, tinnitus, deafness, lockjaw from apoplexy, goiter, etc.

Method. Puncture perpendicularly 0.5-1 cun and apply moxibustion to the point with 3-5 units of moxa cones or for 5-10 minutes.

Tiancong

It is one of the extraordinary points.

Location. 3 cun interior or superior to the front hairline on the median cephalic line.

Indication. Headache, stuffy nose, etc.

Method. Puncture subcutaneously 0.5-1 cun and apply moxibustion to the point with 1-3 units of moxa cones or with a moxa stick for 5-10 minutes.

Tianding (LI 17)

An acupuncture point.

Location. In the lateral cervical region, at the posterior border of the sterno-cleidomastoid muscle, lateral to the Adam apple, at the middle on the connecting line between Futu (LI 18) and Quepen (S 12).

Indication. Obstruction of air passage, laryngitis, swelling sore throat, dysphagia and thyroma.

Method. Puncture perpendicularly 0.5-0.8 cun and apply moxibustion to the point with 3-5 units of moxa cones or for 5-10 minutes.

Tianfu (L 3)

A meridian acupuncture point.

Location. On the medial side of the upper arm and on the radial border of the biceps muscle of the arm, 3 cun below the anterior end of the axillary fold.

Indication. Dyspnea, epistaxis, hematemesis, irregular menstruation, edema, goiter, pain in the medial side of the upper arm.

Method. Puncture perpendicularly 0.3-0.5 cun. Apply moxibustion 3-5 moxa cones or 5-10 minutes with warming moxibustion.

Tianheshui

A massage point.

Location. On the straight line from Zongjing to Quze (P 3) in the very middle of the forearm.

Operation. Pushing method is mostly used.

Effect. Clearing away pathogenic heat and relieving exterior syndrome, removing fire from heart, and eliminating dysphoria.

Indication. All kinds of pyretic syndrome.

Tianjing (TE 10)

A meridian acupuncture point.

Location. On the lateral side of the upper arm, in the depression 1 cun to the tip of the olecranon with the elbow fixed.

Indication. Migraine, pain in the hypochondriac region, neck and nape, shoulder and back, and deafness, scrofula, epilepsy.

Method. Puncture perpendicularly 0.5-1.0 cun. Apply moxibustion 3-7 moxa cones or 5-15 minutes with warming moxibustion.

Tianliao (TE 15)

An acupuncture point.

Location. In the scapular region, midway between Jianjing (G 21) and Quyuan (SI 13), at the superior angle of the scapula 1 cun above Quyuan (SI 13).

Indication. Fever without sweating, irritable fullness sensation in chest, sore shoulder and backache, rigid nape, and pain in supraclavicular fossa.

Method. Puncture perpendicularly 0.5-0.8 cun and apply moxibustion to the point with 3-7 units of moxa cones or for 5-15 minutes.

Tianmen

A massage point.

Location. On the straight line from the region between the eyebrows to the anterior hairline.

Operation. Pushing method is mostly applied.

Indication. Common cold, fever, infantile night crying, headache, etc.

Tianquan (P 2)

A meridian acupuncture point.

Location. On the medial side of the arm, 2 cun below the anterior end of the axillary fold, between the long and short heads of the biceps muscle of the arm.

Indication. Precardial pain, fullness in the chest and hypochondrium, cough, pain in the chest, back and medial aspect of the upper arm.

Method. Puncture perpendicularly 0.5-0.8 cun. Apply moxibustion 3-5 moxa cones or 5-10 minutes with warming moxibustion.

Tianrong (SI 17)

A meridian acupuncture point.

Location. On the lateral side of the neck, posterior to the mandibular angle, in the depression of the anterior border of the sternocleidomastoid muscle.

Indication. Tinnitus, deafness, swelling and pain of the throat, swelling of the check, vomiting with salivation.

Method. Puncture perpendicularly 0.5-0.8 cun. Apply moxibustion 3-5 moxa cones or 5-10 minutes with warming moxibustion.

Tianshu (S 25)

A meridian acupuncture point.

Location. On the middle abdomen, 2 cun lateral to the center of the umbilicus.

Indication. Abdominal pain, vomiting, borborygmus, mass in the abdomen, dysentery, diarrhea, constipation, dysmenorrhea, irregular menstruation, and edema.

Method. Puncture perpendicularly 0.8-1.2 cun. Apply moxibustion 5-7 moxa cones or 10-20 minutes with warming moxibustion.

Tiantu (CV 22)

A meridian acupuncture point.

Location. On the neck, at the anterior midline, and the center of the superasternale fossa.

Indication. Cough, asthma, spitting with blood and pus, swelling and pain of the throat, sublingual contracture, sudden loss of voice.

Method. First, puncture perpendicularly 0.2-0.3 cun, then slowly insert the needle downwards along the posterior aspect of the sternum and the anterior aspect of the trachea 0.5-1 cun. Apply moxibustion 3-5 moxa cones or 5-10 minutes with warming moxibustion.

Tianxi (Sp 18)

A meridian acupuncture point.

Location. On the lateral side of the chest, in the 4th intercostal space, 6 cun lateral to the anterior midline.

Indication. Pain in the chest and hypochondrium, cough, acute mastitis and insufficient lactation.

Method. Puncture subcutaneously or obliquely 0.5-0.8 cun. Apply moxibustion 5-10 minutes with warming moxibustion.

Tianyou (TE 16)

A meridian acupuncture point.

Location. On the lateral side of the neck, directly below the posterior border of the mastoid process, at the level of the mandibular angle, and on the posterior border of the sternocleidomastoid muscle.

Indication. Dizziness, headache, edema of face, blurred vision, sudden loss of hearing and stiffness of the nape.

Method. Puncture perpendicularly 0.5-1 cun. Apply moxibustion 1-3 moxa cones or 3-5 minutes with warming moxibustion.

Tianzhu (B 10)

A meridian acupuncture point.

Location. On the nape, in the depression of the lateral border of the trapezius and 1.3 cun lateral to Yamen (GV 15) the midpoint of the posterior hairline.

Indication. Headache, stiffness of the nape, dizziness, pain, redness and swelling of the eyes, stuffy nose, swelling of the throat, pain in the shoulder and back, flaccid lower limbs.

Method. Puncture perpendicularly or obliquely 0.5-0.8 cun. Moxibustion is applicable.

Notice. Avoid deep or upward needling.

Tianzhugu

A massage point.

Location. On the straight line from the middle of the posterior hairline to the Dazhui (GV 14) point.

Operation. Pushing method is mostly applied.

Function. Regulating the middle energizer, decreasing the adverse flow of qi, clearing away pathogenic heat and relieving pain.

Indication. Vomiting, fever, exopathic affection, etc.

Tianzong (SI 11)

A meridian acupuncture point.

Location. On the scapula in the depression of the center of the subscapula fossa, at the level of the 4th thoracic vertebra.

Indication. Pain in the scapular region, pain in lateral posterior aspect of the elbow and arm, shortness of breath and acute mastitis.

Method. Puncture perpendicularly or obliquely 0.5-1.5 cun. Apply moxibustion 3-5 moxa cones or 3-5 minutes with warming moxibustion.

Tiaokou (S 38)

An acupuncture point.

Location. On the anterior lateral side of the shank, 2 cun below Shangjuxu (S 37), a transverse length of the middle finger to the anterior border of the tibia.

Indication. Numbness, aching and pain of knee and leg, beriberi, edema of dorsum of foot and diarrhea.

Method. Puncture perpendicularly 1-1.5 cun and apply moxibustion to the point with 3-5 units of moxa cones or for 5-10 minutes.

Tiber Milkwort Root

It is the root of Polygala crotalarioides Buch-Ham. (Polygalaceae).

Effect. Supplement the heart, tranquilizing the mind and removing sputum.

Indication. Palpitation due to blood deficiency, insomnia, dreaminess and cough with scanty sputum.

Tidal Fever after Measles

Symptoms. Tidal fever, irregular defecation, marasmus, cough with weakness, spontaneous perspiration and night sweet.

Pathogenesis. Measles toxin and pathogenic heat which impair qi and body fluid, and lack qi yin.

Therapeutic Principle. Replenishing yin and clearing away heat.

Timely Purgation to Preserve Yin

A treatment.

Indication. High fever, thirst, abdominal distention and pain, constipation.

Method. Prevent loss of body fluid by using drastic purgatives, bitter in taste and cold in property to empty the bowels and clear away accumulated heat.

Timidness

Symptoms. Timidity with frightening sensation like being caught.

Pathogenesis. Stagnation of the liver-qi due to rage, or sudden fright and deficiency of gallbladder-qi.

Tinea

Symptoms. The injured skin which assembles together and gradually spreads, and itching limitlessly.

Pathogenesis. The attacking of wind, heat and dampness into the skin and muscle.

Therapeutic Principle. Destroying parasites and clearing away heat, and excreting dampness and sterilizing.

Tinea Capitis

Symptoms. Appearing mostly among children, at the beginning with greyish, white spots of scraps on the skin of the head. Gradually, enlarging into stretches. The hairs are dry and easy to break. With passing of the the time, the hair will drop and leave psilotic spots, or with itching. It is mostly cured naturally up to adolescence.

Pathogenesis. The attacking and accumulation of pathogenic wind in the striae of skin, or by contact infection.

Therapeutic Principle. Treating mainly externally.

Tinea Circinata

Symptoms. It usually appears on the face, the neck, the trunk and the limbs, etc. At the beginning, coin-like erythemas appear with clear borders, covered with thin scales, followed by healing naturally in their centers. Around these centers, such changes can be found as papular eruptions, vesicles, pustular, crusts and scales.

Pathogenesis. The external affection of wind, dampness and heat, or the infection due to the contact with the pig and the dog, etc.

Therapeutic Principle. Clearing away heat and drying dampness, destroying parasites and relieving itching.

Tinea Manus

Symptoms. At the beginning small blisters appearing on the palm, itching, followed by breaking of the blisters, rising and removal of white skin in succession. Then the whole skin of the hand becomes rough, thick, hard, dry, painful, and bleeding. In further development it will cause the nails to become thick, dark-grey and brittle.

Pathogenesis. The stagnation of pathogenic wind-dampness.

Therapeutic Principle. Clearing away wind and dampness, detoxcation and destroying parasites can be applied to smear or soak.

Tinea Pedis

Symptoms. There are two kinds, dryness and dampness. In the damp syndrome, at the beginning, small itching chickenpoxes appear. After breaking, water flows out, or there is erosion between the toes. In the dry syndrome, there is dryness and itching between the toes, pachylosis, desquamation of skin, wrinkles and laceration of skin.

Pathogenesis. Downward flow of damp-heat in the spleen and the stomach meridians, or by the contact with poisonous pathogenic factors.

Therapeutic Principle. Clearing away heat, excreting dampness, and detoxicating.

Tinea Ungues

It refers to onychomadesis.

Symptoms. Itches of the nails at the beginning, followed by gradual thickening and deforming of the nails, and grey, white, nail surface without shine.

Pathogenesis. The lingering and spreading of tinea on the hand and the foot.

Therapeutic Principle. Soaking the sick nails with vinegar, and oral administration of the drug nourishing the blood and expelling wind.

Tinea Versicolor

Symptoms. At the beginning, pea-sized spots appear on the skin, in the color of slight red, red purple, or brown yellow, followed by turning into stretches, with small thin chaff-like scales on the top, slightly bright. They will turn into grey-white stretches shortly before healing.

Pathogenesis. The attacking of wind-dampness or summer-heat and dampness.

Therapeutic Principle. Treating externally.

Tinggong (SI 19)

Location. Anterior to the tragus and posterior to the condyloid process of the mandible, in the depression formed when the mouth is slightly open.

Indication. Tinnitus, deafness, otorrhea, toothache, depressive psychosis, mania, epilepsy, etc.

Method. Puncture perpendicularly 1-1.5 cun when the mouth is open. Moxibustion is applicable.

Tinghui (G 2)

An acupuncture point.

Location. On the face, anterior to the intertragal notch, on the posterior border of the condyloid process of the mandible,

in the depression formed when the mouth is open.

Indication. Deafness, headache, mumps, toothache, epilepsy, vomiting, clonic convulsion, wry mouth and eye, etc.

Method. Puncture perpendicularly 0.5-1.0 cun with the mouth open and apply moxibustion to the point for 3-5 minutes.

Tinnitus due to Blood Deficiency

Symptoms. Tinnitus, restlessness, dizziness, dim eyesight, more severe while overstrain, pale face, poor appetite, etc.

Pathogenesis. Deficiency of the liver, kidney essence and blood, impairment of external acoustic meatus.

Therapeutic Principle. Nourishing yin and blood, regulating the function of liver and inducing resuscitation.

Tinnitus due to Kidney Deficiency

Symptoms. Tinnitus, soreness of waist, flushing of zygomatic region, dry mouth, heat sensation in palms and soles, etc.

Pathogenesis. Deficiency of the kidney and insufficiency of vital essence and energy.

Therapeutic Principle. Replenishing essence and tonifying the kidney.

Tinnitus due to Phlegm-fire

Symptoms. Tinnitus, sometimes obstruction like deafness, feeling of oppression in the chest, abundant expectoration and bitter taste, difficulty in urination and defecation.

Pathogenesis. Flaming up of phlegm-fire.

Therapeutic Principle. Eliminating sputum and clearing away fire.

Tinnitus due to Qi Deficiency

Symptoms. Tinnitus, yellowish and pale face, tiredness and poor appetite, loose stool, etc.

Pathogenesis. Deficiency of qi and blood, deficiency of assembled meridians.

Therapeutic Principle. Invigorating the spleen and replenishing qi.

Toad Skin

It is the skin of Bufo bufo gargarizans Cantor or B. Melanostictus Schneider (Bufonidae)

Effect. Clearing away heat, detoxicating, and inducing diuresis to alleviate edema, inducing resuscitation and relieving pain.

Indication. Carbuncles, pyogenic, tumor, infantile malnutrition, chronic bronchitis, sore throat.

Toad Venom

It is the white secretion from the postauricular and skin gland of Bufo bufo gargarizans Cantor and B. melanostictus Schneider's retroauricular gland (Bufonidae) after collecting and drying.

Effect. Detoxicating, subduing swelling, alleviating pain, cardiotonic, hypertensive and stimulating respiration.

Indication. Carbuncle, swelling and sore throat, acute filthy disease, vomiting, diarrhea, hemorrhagic shock and respiratory failure, etc.

Toe (MA)

An auricular point.

Location. On the external superior angle of the superior crus of antihelix.

Indication. Pain of the toe and paronychia.

Tokyo Violet Herb

It is the herb of Viola yedoensis Mak. (Violaceae) with root.

Effect. Clearing away heat and detoxicating.

Indication. Furuncle, superficial infection, dysentery, conjunctival congestion due to excessive liver-heat, scrofula, snakebite, etc.

Tomato

It is the fresh fruit of Lycopersicon esculentum Mill. (Solanaceae).

Effect. Promoting the production of body fluid to quench thirst, strengthening the stomach and promoting digestion.

Indication. Thirst and poor appetite.

Tongli (Ex-LE)

An extra acupuncture point.

Location. On the dorsum between the 4th and 5th metatarsal tones, 2 cun above the joint of the little toe.

Indication. Metrorrhagia and metrostaxis, menorrhagia.

Method. Puncture obliquely 0.3-0.5 cun. Apply moxibustion 2-7 moxa cones.

Tongli (H 5)

An acupuncture point.

Location. On the palmar side of the forearm, 1 cun superior to the transverse crease of the wrist, at the radial border of the ulnar carpal flexor muscular tendon.

Indication. Palpitation, dizziness, swelling sore throat, cough, vomiting, metrorrhagia, metrostaxis, pain of arm and wrist.

Method. Puncture perpendicularly 0.3-0.5 cun and apply moxibustion to the point with 1-3 moxa cones or for 3-5 minutes.

Tongtian (B 7)

A meridian acupuncture point.

Location. On the head, 4 cun directly above the midpoint of the anterior hairline and 1.5 cun posterior to Chengguang (B 6).

Indication. Headache, dizziness, nasal obstruction with running nose, epistaxis, stuffiness of the neck.

Method. Puncture subcutaneously 0.3-0.5 cun. Apply moxibustion 1-3 moxa cones or 3-5 minutes.

Tongue-bleed

Symptoms. Tongue bleeding, distending pain in hypochondrium, vexation and thirst, dry mouth with bitter taste, etc.

Pathogenesis. Accumulation of heat in the Heart Meridian, or exuberance of the liver-fire, or flaring-up of fire of deficiency type of the spleen and Kidney Meridians, tongue bleeding, distending pain in hypochondrium, vexation and thirst, dry mouth with bitter taste.

Therapeutic Principle. Clearing away heat, purging the liver of pathogenic heat, nourishing yin and removing heat from blood.

Tongue Coating

It is something on the tongue like mosses.

Function. Diagnosing.

Method. When a patient's tongue is observed, attention should be paid to changes in the color, thick or thin fur, moisture or dryness, shape and distribution, in order to differentiate the nature of illness, the degree of seriousness of pathogenic factors, and degree of consumption of the body fluid.

Tongue Color

Function. Diagnosing.

Method. Inspecting of the proper color of the tongue. A light red tongue with moisture is normal. A pale, red, crimson, purple, bluish tongue, or a tongue with ecchymosis reflects some pathological changes.

Tongue Erosion

1. **Symptoms.** Whitish spots and ulceration in the margin, bitter taste, tendency to anger, scanty dark urine.

   Pathogenesis. Damp-heat in the liver and stomach.

   Therapeutic Principle. Clearing away damp-heat from the liver and gallbladder.

2. **Symptoms.** Ulceration and swelling of the lingual surface or the body of the tongue with the result of dysphagia.

   Pathogenesis. Caused by fumigating and steaming of the noxious heat in the heart and spleen.

   Therapeutic Principle. Clearing away toxic heat from the heart and spleen.

Tongue Mien

It is one of the inspections of tongue.

Method. 1. A proper red and moist tongue, with sensitive activity, indicating sufficiency of qi, blood, and yin fluid. 2. A dim, dry, thin and small tongue with ineffective activity, indicating exhaustion of qi, blood and yin fluid, and indicating a serious case.

Tongue Reflecting Spleen

Function. Tongue reflects the functional activities and pathologic changes of the spleen and stomach. A pale tongue with white greasy fur indicates stagnant dampness in the spleen, while a red tongue with dry thick yellow fur indicates excess of the stomach-fire.

Tongue Serving as Sprout of Heart

It refers to the relation between the tongue and the heart.

Function. Diagnosing.

Method. The pathologic changes of the heart can be learned by observing the tongue, e.g. the red tip of the tongue and erosive painful tongue show flaring-up of the heart-fire while a stiff and tremulous tongue and aphasia indicates disturbance of the spirit.

Tongue Tip

It has relation to the heart and lung.

Function. Heart and lung diseases can be diagnosed by observing the tongue tip, e.g. red or ulcerous and painful tongue tips show the patient is suffering from exterior syndrome of wind-heat and excess of the heart-fire.

Tongue with Tortoise-vein Fur

A tongue picture.

Function. Diagnosing.

Method. There are two type of manifestations. The excess type: there are fissures like the curve of tortoise-shell on the surface of the tongue. A fissured tongue, proper red tongue, erosion of the whole oral cavity, swollen cheek and tongue, thirst, and vigorous and forceful pulse caused by extremely excessive heart-fire. The deficiency type: a fissured tongue with light color, or with white speckles, broken tongue surface without skin, no thirst, and feeble pulse.

Tongziliao (G 1)

A meridian acupuncture point.

Location. On the face, 0.5 cun lateral to the outer canthus, in the depression on the lateral border of the orbit.

Indication. Headache, redness and pain of the eye, photophobia, epiphora induced by wind, myopia, internal oculopathy.

Method. Puncturing subcutaneously or obliquely 0.3-0.5 cun, or pricking to bleed.

Tonic Convulsion

Symptoms. Fever without sweat, chill, rigidity of the neck, shaking the head and lockjaw, contracture of the extremities or clonic convulsion.

Therapeutic Principle. For the patient with superficial syndrome, inducing diaphoresis to relieve superficial syndrome, and promoting the production of the body fluid and dredging the meridians.

Tonifying before Attacking Pathogens

It refers to the therapy for tonifying deficiency and then eliminating the pathogenic factors. It usually applies to patients if vital qi is too deficient so that removing pathogenic factors will result in the impairment of the vital qi.

Tonsill (MA)

An auricular point, located in the 8th section.

Indication. Acute tonsillitis and pharyngitis.

Tonsillitis

Symptoms. Swelling and hardness in the pharyngeal tonsils.

Pathogenesis. In infants, affection of exopathogen that stagnates at the throat and fails to disperse. In adults, stagnation of liver-fire and thick sputum, qi stagnation and blood stasis and constant overstrain.

Therapeutic Principle. Clearing away fire from the liver, expelling sputum and relieving sore throat.

Tonsillitis with Log-like Tongue

Symptoms. Tonsillitis on one side, swollen and purplish-red tongue and profuse phlegm and saliva.

Pathogenesis. Heat-toxin in the Heart Meridian, or insidious febrile disease due to over-drinking, resulting in upward attack of the heat-toxin.

Therapeutic Principle. Acupuncture the point Jinjin (Ex-HN 12), Yuye (Ex-HN 13) and then prick the tonsil to bleeding with a three-edged needle.

Toothache Caused by Fire of Deficiency Type

Referring to toothache due to flaring up of fire of deficiency type.

Symptoms. Toothache, red lips and flushing of zygomatic region dry and sore throat, red tongue and scant saliva.

Pathogenesis. General debility in advanced age, deficiency of kidney-yin, and flaring up of deficient fire.

Therapeutic Principle. Nourishing yin to reduce pathogenic fire.

Toothache due to Excess Heat

Symptoms. Severe toothache, foul breath, thirst, constipation, yellowish tongue coating.

Pathogenesis. Heat in the large intestine and stomach leading to stagnated fire moving upward along the meridians.

Therapeutic Principle. Clearing away heat to stop pain.

Toothache due to Wind-fire Pathogen

Symptoms. Toothache with gingival swelling, accompanied by chills and fever, thin and whitish tongue coating.

Pathogenesis. Pathogenic wind attacking the meridians, stagnating in Yangming and then transforming into fire, leading to the flame-up of the accumulated fire along meridians.

Therapeutic Principle. Dispelling wind and clearing away heat to alleviate pain.

Toothleaf Goldenray Root
❀ T-2

It is the root or rhizome of Ligularia dentata (A. Gray) Hara. (Compositae).

Effect. Regulating flow of qi and promoting blood circulation, relieving pain and cough and dispelling phlegm.

Indication. Traumatic injuries, painful back and legs, cough with asthma, hemoptysis, etc.

Tortoise Meat

It is the meat of Chinemys reevesii (Gray) (Testudinidae).

Effect. Replenishing the vital essence and enriching blood.

Indication. Hectic fever due to consumptive disease, hemoptysis due to chronic cough, dysentery with bloody stool, hematochezia.

Tortoise Plastron

It is the plastron of Chinemys reevesii (Gray) (Testudinidae).

Effect. Nourishing yin and suppressing hyperactive liver-yang, reinforcing the kidney to strengthening the bones, nourishing the blood and reinforcing the heart, regulating menstruation and relieving metrorrhagia.

Indication. Consumption of yin due to febrile disease, dizziness, vexation, hemoptysis, night sweat, seminal emission, infantile metopism, insomnia, amnesia, menorrhagia and leukorrhagia, etc.

Toulinqi (G 15)

An acupuncture point.

Location. 0.5 cun within the anterior hairline directly above the pupil, in the midpoint of the line between Shenting (GV 24) and Touwei (S 8).

Indication. Headache, dizziness, corneal opacity, delacrimation, stuffy nose, infantile epilepsy, upward turning of the eyeball, apoplexy, unconsciousness, etc.

Method. Puncture obliquely 0.3-0.5 cun and apply moxibustion to the point for 3-5 minutes or 1-3 units of moxa cones.

Touqiaoyin (G 11)

An acupuncture point.

Location. On the head, posterior and superior to the postauricular mastoid process, at the junction of the middle and lower third of the distance between Tianchong (G 9) and Wangu (G 12).

Indication. Headache, vexation, tinnitus, deafness, earache, sore throat, stiffness of the tongue, etc.

Method. Puncture 0.3-0.5 cun horizontally along the skin and apply moxibustion to the point for 3-5 minutes or 1-3 units of moxa cones.

Touwei (S 8)

An acupuncture point.

Location. Lateral to the head, 0.5 cun above the hairline of the corner of the forehead, 4.5 cun lateral to the midline of the head.

Indication. Headache, vertigo, ophthalmalgia, blurred vision, dyspnea, vexation and fullness in the chest.

Method. Puncture 0.5-1.0 cun horizontally along the skin. Moxibustion is forbidden.

Toxin-scraping Method

Operation. Scrape both sides of the patient's spine slightly downward, using a glossy-edged copper or coin with a piece of sesame oil. Gradually, scrape forcefully till purplish red spots or plaques come out. Then, use a sterilized three-edged needle to prick the spots or plaques to let out purplish black blood to eliminate the filthy toxin.

Indication. Acute diseases of excessive heat caused by infection of filthy pathogens that invade the muscular surface.

Trachea (MA-IC 2)

An auricular point.

Location. Between the orifice of the external auditory meatus and Heart (MA).

Indication. Cough and dyspnea.

Traction and Counter-traction

A massage Method. It means pulling and tracting.

Operation. Fix the one end of the limb or the joint and pull the other end. It is applied to joints such as those of the head, neck, shoulder, wrist, and finger.

Effect. Treat the joint malposition and injury of muscles and tendons.

Tragic Apex (MA)

An ear point.

Location. At the tip of the upper prominence on the border of the tragus.

Function. Clearing away heat and arresting pain.

Indication. Fever and pain.

Trance

It refers to absent-mindedness and flurry and accompanied by dyspnea, tiredness, greyish complexion.

Pathogenesis. Mostly visceral injury due to emotional stress and invasion of exopathogen, which results in insufficiency of the heart-qi and deficiency of the heart blood.

Trance due to Summer-heat

Referring to the mild case of sunstroke.

Symptoms. Feeling sleepy, unwillingness to speak, etc.

Pathogenesis. The invasion of the summer-heat into the body.

Therapeutic Principle. Expelling heat and clearing fever.

Tranquilization

It refers to a method of tranquilizing the mind.

Indication. Emotional distress and restlessness, palpitation, insomnia, epilepsy induced by terror, madness, dysphoria and anger. This method includes tranquilization with heavy material and tranquilizing the mind by nourishing the heart.

Transformation between Yin and Yang

A theory in TCM. It is one of the principal contents of the yin-yang theory. Under certain circumstances, yin and yang transforms into each other, i.e. yang can be transformed into yin and vice versa. A disease of heat nature in the extreme may show symptoms of pseudo-cold or vice versa, a transformation between yin and yang.

Translocation of Muscle and Tendon

Symptoms. Pain caused by ecchymoma, translocation of muscle tendon and ligament felt by touching.

Pathogenesis. Transposition of muscle and tendon due to the action of external force fail to fulfil their duties, leading to difficulty in joint movement.

Therapeutic Principle. Manual reduction in combination with physiotherapy, massage, hot compression, steaming and washing with medicinal herbs, etc.

Transmission from Exterior to Interior

A theory in TCM. The transmission of yang Meridian and yin Meridian which are exterior and interior, such as exterior syndrome of taiyang to interior syndrome of Shaoyin, Yangming Meridian to Taiyin Meridian, and shaoyang Meridian to Juyin Meridian.

Transmission of Epidemic Febrile Disease Directly to Pericardium

Symptoms. Heat, retraction of the tongue, cold limbs, delirium or confusion, deep red, fresh and moist tongue, etc.

Pathogenesis. Warm pathogen invading the pericardium directly instead of transmitting in an ordinary order to middle-energizer from the lung.

Therapeutic Principle. Removing heat from the heart to restore consciousness.

Transmitting to Origin

A theory in TCM. Referring to transmission of pathogen from Meridian to the original organs. For example, in taiyang disease, if the pathogen is in meridian with symptom, such as headache, fever, spontaneous perspiration, and the conditions mentioned above cannot be relieved after six or seven days, extreme thirst and drinking, immediate vomit after drinking occur, it means that pathogen has entered urinary bladder and it is the syndrome of transmitting to the original organs.

Trauma of Kidney

Symptoms. Aching pain in waist, mental fatigue and asthenia, dizziness and tinnitus, or emission and impotence, etc.

Pathogenesis. Mainly ascribable to sexual strain, loss of essence and impairment of the kidney.

Therapeutic Principle. Tonifying the kidney and replenishing essence.

Traumatic Cataract

Symptoms. Turbidity of lens and visual disturbance in varying degrees.

Pathogenesis. Cephalic or ocular vibration and contusion, or sharp instrument injury of lens in the ocular region.

Therapeutic Principle. When the lens is not entirely turbid yet with some visual acuity remaining at its early stage. Clearing away heat from the liver and promoting blood circulation to remove blood stasis, while operative therapy is applicable when the nebula is settled down and the cataract is obsolete with only light sensation left.

Traumatic Injury

It is a general term for injury.

Symptoms. Pain and swelling, bleeding, bone fracture, joint dislocation in the affected parts, or injuries of the internal organs.

Cause. Knives and spears, fall and stumble, contusion, stabbing and abrasion, sport injuries, etc.

Therapeutic Principle. Subduing swelling, eliminating blood stasis, promoting the circulation of qi, arresting bleeding, relaxing muscles and tendons, and relieving pain.

Treating Diarrhea with Purgatives

It is one of the therapeutic methods to treat diarrhea of excessive type with purgatives.

Indication. Stagnation of food, abdominal pain, fecal impaction due to heat with watery discharge, metrostaxis due to accumulation of blood stasis, frequent, quick and painful micturition due to damp-heat in the urinary bladder.

Therapeutic Principle. Relieving constipation by purgation, clearing away heat and purging fire, promoting blood circulation and dissipating blood stasis and removing damp-heat in the bladder.

Treating Different Diseases with the Same Therapeutic Principle

Method. When the same pathologic changes occur in the course of different diseases, the same therapy can be used to treat them, e.g. for the diarrhea due to spleen deficiency, prolapse of the anus or prolapse of the uterus, etc. the same treatment of tonifying the interior and faciliating qi may be employed because their pathogenesis is sinking of qi of middle-energizer though they are different diseases.

Treating Disease Contrary to Routine

The remedy coincides with the false symptoms of the disease, contrary to the remedy for heat symptoms. Actually, it is directed to the cold nature of the disease itself.

Treating Excess with Reducing Methods

A treatment principle in acupuncture and moxibustion. It refers to treating syndromes of excessive pathogenic factors by reducing methods, which means using reducing methods for excess syndromes to make pathogenic factors weaken.

Treating Primary in Chronicity

A therapeutic principle. This principle is opposite to that of treating the incidental in an urgent situation. Causal treatment must be given according to the basic cause of a disease when the incidental is relatively mild.

Treating Shaoyang Disease by Mediation

A treatment.

Symptoms. Alternate chills and fever, fullness in the mouth, dry throat, margins of eyelids.

Indication. Shaoyang syndrome due to affection by heat exopathogen in half exterior and half interior.

Therapeutic Principle. Therapy of administering the prescription with the action of regulating the function of Shaoyang Meridians to treat shaoyang disease.

Treating Symptoms in Emergency Cases

A principle of treatment. When some symptoms are vital, expectant treatment should be given first. Then, when such symptoms are improved, the principle of the therapy must be treating the root cause of a disease.

Treating the Same Disease with Different Methods

It refers a therapeutic principle in certain conditions.

Application. Treatment of the same disease should be varied with different conditions such as the patient's constitution, seasonal changes, geographical localities, or kinds of pathogenic factors, development and pathogenesis of the disease.

Treating Upper Pathogen with Light Drugs of Mild Action

A treatment method.

Application. When the pathogen is in the lung of the upper-energizer, it is advisable to using light drugs with lifting action to suit the drugs to the disease, and cure it properly.

Treatment in Accordance with Local Conditions

A principle of treatment.

It refers to making up a prescription in accordance with the geographical features of different localities. Different geographical conditions, climate and customs and habits determines that people in different areas have different physiological functional activities and features of their pathological changes are different; therefore, treatment and prescription should be different to people in different areas.

Treatment in Accordance with Physique of Individual

A principle of treatment.

It refers to making up therapy according to the age, sex, constitution, and life-style of a patient.

Treatment in Accordance with Seasonal Conditions

A principle of treatment.

It refers to making up therapy according to the climatic variations in different seasons.

Treatment of Excess Syndrome with Purgation and Reduction

A therapeutic principle.

Application. All excess syndromes can be treated with the method of purgation and reduction to eliminate the pathogenic factors, including reduction in acupuncture.

Treatment of Yin Hyperactivity by Supplementing Source of Fire

A therapeutic principle. It is also called reinforcing yang to eliminate pathogenic factors yin in nature, treating the syndrome caused by yin hyperactivity.

Indication. The syndrome of insufficiency of the kidney-yang resulting from excess of yin-cold because yang deficiency cannot control yin.

Trembling Method

A form of needling method.

Operation. Vibrating the needle handle with small amplitude and high frequency to strengthen the needling response.

Application. In the clinic, it is commonly used when the needle is inserted to the depth of a certain point to be needled and the needling sensation is obtained, though very weak.

Tremella

It is the sporophore of Tremella fuciformis Berk. (Tremellaceae).

Effect. Nourishing yin, moistening the lung, reinforcing the stomach and promoting the production of the body fluid.

Indication. Cough due to consumption, bloody sputum and thirst due to asthenia heat.

Tremor Capitis

It refers to shaking of head uncontrollably, a symptomatic manifestation of many diseases.

Pathogenesis. General debility in the aged, deficiency of the liver and kidney; or insufficiency of blood and qi after suffering from severe or long-standing illness, which leads to failure in nourishing muscles and tendons.

Tremor of Tongue

A tongue picture. A light red or pale tongue with the body of tongue trembling slightly, indicating deficiency of both the heart and the spleen, wind due to deficiency of blood. A deep red tongue with the body of tongue shivering indicates wind due to extreme heat. A deep red tongue with the body of tongue trembling and projecting can be seen in alcoholism.

Trichosanthes Fruit   ✇ T-3

It is the ripe fruit of Trichosanthes kirilowii Maxim. and Trichosanthes rosthornii Harms (Cucurbitaceae).

Effect. Clearing away heat from the lung, dissipating sputum, promoting circulation of flow of qi to soothe chest oppression, moistening the bowels to relieve constipation.

Indication. Cough due to the lung-heat with thick sputum, feeling of fullness and stuffiness in the chest, carbuncles of breast and dryness of the intestines with constipation.

Trichosanthes Peel

It is the ripe fruit peel of Trichosanthes kirilowii Maxim. and Trichosanthes rosthornii Harms (Cucurbitaceae).

Effect. Clearing away heat, dissipating phlegm, promoting circulation of flow of qi to soothe chest oppression.

Indication. Cough due to phlegm-heat, fullness in the chest and pain in the hypochondrium.

Trichosanthes Root

It is the dried stem root of Trichosanthes kirilowii Maxim. (Cucurbitaceae).

Effect. Clearing away heat, promoting the production of body fluid, relieving thirst, detoxication, subduing swelling and promoting the drainage of pus. An injection prepared from it is used for artificial abortion.

Indication. Excessive thirst due to febrile diseases, dry mouth with cracked lips, diabetes, cough due to lung-heat, hemoptysis due to lung dryness, and suppurative infections on the body surface.

Tri-diabetes due to Essence of Life Deficiency

Symptoms. Drinking a lot and always feeling hungry, polyuria and gradual emaciation.

Pathogenesis. Consumption of yin essence.

Therapeutic Principle. Nourishing yin and producing the body fluid.

Tri-energizer

It is a general term for the upper-, middle- and lower-energizer, and regarded as one of the six-organs. It is the largest one outside all the viscera and bowels within the body cavity.

Function. Governing the qi activities and making the passage of water unblocked.

Tri-energizer Carbuncle

Referring to the carbuncle appearing at Shimen (CV 5).

Symptoms. At the beginning it is an indistinct pain, slight swelling, alternate attacks of chills and fever, difficulty in urination and defecation.

Pathogenesis. The integration of damp-heat with coldness.

Therapeutic Principle. Same as peri-appendicular abscess.

Tri-energizer Constipation

Referring to the constipation due to disorder of tri-energizer.

Symptoms. Constipation, abdominal distention, anorexia and fullness in the chest, etc.

Pathogenesis. The disturbance in qi transformation of tri-energizer and slow transportation of the intestines.

Therapeutic Principle. Smoothing functional activities of qi.

Tri-energizer Cough

Referring to the cough due to disorder of tri-energizer.

Symptoms. Cough, shortness of breath, fullness in the chest, and abdominal distention, etc.

Pathogenesis. Qi damaged by protracted cough, and the invasion of pathogenic factors into tri-energizer.

Therapeutic Principle. Regulating functional activities of qi and dredging tri-energizer.

Tri-energizer Disease

Symptoms. Abdominal distention and fullness, oliguria, even fullness in the chest and dyspnea, etc. for the excess syndrome; while cold sensation in the abdomen, diarrhea, discharge of urine, shortness of breath, even straining distention in the lower abdomen and gastroptosia, etc. for the deficiency syndrome.

Pathogenesis. Disorder of upper-energizer, middle-energizer and lower-energizer in qi transformation and obstruction of water passage.

Therapeutic Principle. Dispersing function of tri-energizer and regulating the functional activities of qi.

Tri-energizer Distention

Symptoms. Distention of abdomen without stuffiness, edema of the whole body due to the disease of tri-energizer and the stagnation of qi function.

Pathogenesis. Stagnation of liver-qi or yang deficiency of the spleen and kidney, etc.

Therapeutic Principle. Warming and invigorating the spleen and kidney, and regulating qi and blood.

Tri-energizer Meridian of Hand-shaoyang

It is one of the twelve meridians.

Course. It starts from the lateral end of the fourth finger, along which it comes to the dorsal carpus and goes upward along the median line on the lateral side of the upper limbs to the shoulder, goes ahead and comes to the greater supraclavicular fossa, distributes at Shanzong, scatters in the pericardium and passes through the diaphragm, which are, in turn, called upper-, middle- and lower-energizer. Its branch is separated from Shanzhong, goes upward to the shoulder through the supraclavicular fossa, and intersects at Dazhui (GV 14) both on the right and left, keeps on going up to the lateral side of the neck, along the auricularis posterior and comes out from the epiotic corner, and then flexes to the area below the orbit through the cheek. Another branch is separated from auricularis posterior, enters the ear, comes out from auricularis anterior, through the upper border of zygomatic arch, intersects the former branch at the cheek, gets to the outer canthus and connects with the Gallbladder Meridian of Foot-shaoyang.

Tri-energizer Stagnancy

Symptoms. Dry mouth and anorexia due to the stagnation of functional activities of tri-energizer qi and the failure of fluid to go upward.

Pathogenesis. The stagnation of liver-qi or the combined accumulation of phlegm and stagnancy, etc.

Therapeutic Principle. Soothing the liver and regulating the circulation of qi, and dissipating sputum and promoting blood circulation.

Trifoliate-orange Immature Fruit

It is the immature fruit of Poncirus trifoliata (L.) Rat. (Rutaceae).

Effect. Promoting the circulation of qi and relieving pain, dispersing stagnated hepatic qi.

Indication. Stagnation of the liver-qi, tuberculosis of breast, hernial pain, indigestion.

Tri-impairment due to Dryness-heat

It refers to three types of impairment due to dry and pathogenic heat.

1. The upper-impairment: thirst, cracked lips, vexation, restlessness due to impairment of the lung by dryness-heat.
2. The middle-impairment: emaciation with polyphagia caused by the impairment of the stomach due to dryness heat.
3. The lower-impairment: frequent dribbling urination like oil, due to the impairment of the small intestine and bladder.

Triquetrous Tadehagl Herb

It is the whole herb of Desmodium triquetrum (L.) DC. (Leguminosae).

Effect. Clearing away heat, removing toxic material, dispelling phlegm removing stagnancy and destroying parasites.

Indication. Common cold, sore throat, hemoptysis due to the lung disease, enteritis, dysentery, arthralgia due to wind-dampness, vomiting during pregnancy, infantile malnutrition, sores, etc.

Tri-yang Malaria

It belongs to a mild malaria.

Symptoms. The mild malaria with its pathogens located superficially and leads to early and frequent attacks, generally, once daily. The attacks usually occur during the day.

Pathogenesis. It refers to invasion of malarial pathogens into yang meridians.

Therapeutic Principle. Treating shaoyang diseases by mediation and relieving exterior syndrome to eliminate pathogenic heat of the interior.

True Apoplexy

Symptoms. Sudden coma, inability of recognition during coma, deviation of eye and mouth, hemiplegia, and inability to speak, with stiff tongue. It is different from an apoplexic stroke which is due to the interior wind.

Pathogenesis. A disease due to an attack by external wind.

Therapeutic Principle. Dispelling wind, and promoting and activating excretion for the case with both constipation and dysuria.

True Indigo Leaf and Stem

It is the leaf and stem of Indigofera tinctoria L. (Leguminosae).

Effect. Clearing away heat and detoxicating, dissipating blood stasis and arresting pain.

Indication. Encephalitis B, parotitis, swelling due to sores, hematemesis, etc.

True Qi

1. It refers to vitality qi, i.e. dynamic force of all vital functions, originating from the combination of the original qi inherited and the acquired energy derived from food and air.
2. It refers to primordial-qi, which is the most essential and important qi in the body and acts as the primary motive force for the life activities.

True Yin

It is also called kidney-yin opposite to kidney-yang.

Effect. It is the material basis of vital function of the kidney. The kidney stores congenital essence of life which nourishes and moistens the other zang-fu organs and tissues.

Tsaoko

It is the dried ripe fruit of Amomum tsaoko Crevost et Lem. (Zingiberaceae).

Effect. Removing dampness and warming the middle-energizer and dispelling phlegm.

Indication. Epigastric and abdominal distention, pain and vomiting due to accumulation of cold-dampness in the spleen and stomach.

Tuangang (Ex-B)

An extra acupuncture point.

Location. On the sacral portion, 2.0 cun directly below Xiaochangshu (B 27).

Indication. Constipation, difficulty in urination, pain in the loin, etc.

Tuberculate Speranskia Herb

It is the whole herb of Speranskia tuberculata (Bge.) Baill. (Euphorbiaceae).

Effect. Expelling pathogenic wind, relaxing muscles, subduing swelling, eliminating dampness, dissipating blood stasis and destroying parasites, relieving pain.

Indication. Rheumatic arthralgia, spasm of muscle and joint, cold-damp beriberi, scabies, tinea and pyogenic infections.

Tuberculosis of Bones and Joints

Symptoms. At the beginning, the affected region is slightly painful, without redness and heat, followed by articular moving disturbance, severe pain in movement. In the metaphase, the affected region swells gradually, with the formation of pus, and fever in the afternoon. In the last phase, the pus is diluted; the opening of the sore will sink, with fever, night sweat, swelling joints in the affected region, rigidity or paralysis. It is difficult to heal.

Therapeutic Principle. Invigorating the liver and kidney, clearing and activating the meridians and collaterals, dispelling cold, resolving phlegm and nourishing qi and blood.

Tuberculosis of Breast

1. It refers to the mammary tuberculous disease.

   Symptoms. A chronic disease course. At the beginning, it has one or several masses like plums, with unclear borders, which are connected by skin and muscle.

Pathogenesis. Deficiency of yin fluid of both the lung and the kidney, or stagnation of liver-qi to transform fire to burn the body fluid into phlegm.

Therapeutic Principle. Relieving the depressed liver, nourishing yin and resolving phlegm.

2. It refers to infantile malnutrition due to excessive feeding.

Symptoms. Malnutrition due to infantile dyspepsia, yellowish face, thin and bony body.

Pathogenesis. Weakness of the spleen and the stomach, difficult consumption of breast milk.

Therapeutic Principle. Regulating the spleen and the stomach and improving breast milk.

Tuberculosis of Epididymis

Referring to the cold abscess appearing in the region of the testis.

Symptoms. Distending pain of testis, induration on the epididymis, thickening of spermatic cord with nodes like strings of pearls. Afterwards formation of pus and ulceration with such symptoms as low fever and night sweat, etc.

Pathogenesis. Mostly caused by downward flow of turbid phlegm due to the impaired liver-kidney essence and empty and deficient meridians and collaterals.

Therapeutic Principle. Nourishing yin to clear away heat, removing dampness and resolving phlegm, removing obstruction in the meridians and resolving mass.

Tuberculosis Point

It is one of the extra acupuncture points.

Location. 3.5 cun lateral to the lower border of the spinous process of the 7th cervical vertebrae.

Indication. Pulmonary tuberculosis and other tuberculosis.

Method. Puncture perpendicularly 0.5-1 cun and apply moxibustion to the point for 5-10 minutes or 3-7 units of moxa cones.

Tuberculous Peritonitis

It has two types. 1. The acute type, where the patient may die within a few days. 2. The chronic type, where the condition may last several years.

Symptoms. Swelling limbs, emaciation, cough with dyspnea, edema of the abdomen, exhaustion of strength, heaviness in the joints, restlessness and infectious property.

Pathogenesis. Affection by parasites.

Therapeutic Principle. Nourishing deficiency and destroying parasites.

Tuckahoe

It is the sclerotium of the fungus Poria cocos (Schw.) Wolf (Polyporaceae).

Effect. Promoting diuresis, removing dampness, invigorating the spleen and tranquilizing the mind.

Indication. Edema, dysuria, leukorrhagia, lassitude, anorexia, loose stool, palpitation and insomnia.

Tufted Bracketplant Herb

It is the whole plant of Chlorophytum comosum (Thunb.) Bak. (Liliaceae).

Effect. Arresting cough, eliminating phlegm, subduing swelling, detoxicating, promoting blood circulation and knitting bones.

Indication. Tracheitis, cough with profuse phlegm, suppurative infections on the body surface, swelling and pain of hemorrhoid, fracture or burns.

Tumor

Symptoms. A localized mass appearing on the body surface, developing slowly, usually with no subjective symptoms, chronic and difficult in subsidence.

Pathogenesis. The staying of blood stasis, phlegm retention and turbid qi in the tissue of the body surface. The common ones are tumors due to disorder of qi, angioma, fleshy tumor, tumorous varix, bone tumor, and steatoma.

Therapeutic Principle. Promoting the circulation of qi, resolving masses, dissipating blood stasis with potent drugs subduing swelling, resolving phlegm and softening hard masses, etc.

Tumor due to Disorder of Qi

Symptoms. Multiple tumors appearing between skins. The mass is superficial, soft, and elastic, just like gas in the tumor. After it is pressed it will spring up with the lifting of the hand.

Pathogenesis. The injury of lung-qi due to overstrain and the additional affection of external pathogens.

Therapeutic Principle. Promoting the dispersing function of the lung, regulating qi, alleviating mental depression and resolving mass.

Tung Oil

It is the oil squeezed from the seed of Aleurites fordii Hemsl. (Euphorbiaceae). It is for external use.

Indication. Burns and scalds, frost bite, scabies and tinea.

Tunzhong (Ex-B)

An extra acupuncture point.

Location. On the buttocks. Draw an equilateral triangle with the line connecting the greater trochanter of the femur and the node of sciatic as the base, and the point is at the apex of the triangle.

Indication. Sciatica, hemiparalysis of the lower limbs, urticaria, etc.

Method. Puncture perpendicularly 1.5-2.5 cun. Apply moxibustion 3-7 moxa cones or 5-15 minutes with warming moxibustion.

Turbidity

1. It refers to turbidity of urine.

   Symptoms. Turbid urine with blood that is called red turbidity, and turbidity urine with white, but without blood, that is called white turbidity.

   Pathogenesis. Damp-heat that goes downward, with white turbidity when dampness is in excess of heat, and with red turbidity when heat is in excess of dampness.

   Therapeutic Principle. Mainly removing dampness and heat.

2. It refers to the disease of seminal turbidity.

   Symptoms. A constant dripping of turbid discharge from the penile orifice with clear urine. It is divided into white turbidity and bloody turbidity, according to whether there is blood in the discharge or not.

   Therapeutic Principle. Purging pathogenic fire if it belongs to fire excess, in excreting dampness if it belongs to downward flow of damp-heat into the seminal vesicle and in calming the heart, and reinforcing the kidney if it belongs to insufficiency of the heart and kidney.

Turbid Urine

Symptoms. Turbid, white-colored urine and no painful or unsmooth feeling with urination.

Pathogenesis. The dysfunction of the spleen in transportation due to a fatty and sweet diet, which thereafter produces heat and dampness, or the remaining evil of damp-heat accumulating in the lower-energizer after illness which fails to separate the clear substance from the turbid one.

Therapeutic Principle. Clearing away heat and removing dampness by diuresis for the onset of the illness. For those suffering from deficiency of both the spleen and kidney due to chronic illness, it is advisable to follow treatment of nourishing the spleen, kidney and consolidating kidney qi.

Turbid Urine due to Impairment of Heart

Symptoms. Severe palpitation, mental aberration, panic, dysphoria, insomnia, nocturnal emission, reddish and whitish turbid urine, etc.

Pathogenesis. The heart impaired by excessive anxiety.

Therapeutic Principle. Nourishing the heart to calm the mind.

Turbid-urine Stranguria

Symptoms. Frequent urination with pain, turbid urine, or mucous pus-like discharge shedding out of the urethra.

Pathogenesis. Downward flow of damp-heat and turbid phlegm, which oozes into urinary bladder.

Therapeutic Principle. Excreting dampness, resolving phlegm, clearing away heat and detoxicating.

Turmeric Root   ✿ T-4

It is the root tuber of Curcuma aromatica Salisb. and Curcuma zedoara (Berg) Rosc. or Curcuma longa L. or Curcuma kwangsiensis S. Lee et. C. F. Liang. (Zingiberaceae).

Effect. Promoting blood circulation to remove blood stasis, relieving pain, soothing depressed liver, clearing away heat in the blood and heart, eliminating phlegm, and normalizing the gallbladder to treat jaundice.

Indication. Distending pain in hypochondrium, irregular menstruation, dysmenorrhea and masses in the abdomen, stuffiness and fullness in the chest and upper abdomen, traumatic injury, epilepsy, psychosis, hematemesis, hematuria, etc.

Turnip

It is the root and leaf of Brassica rape L. (Cruciferae).

Effect. Promoting digestion, breaking wind, removing dampness and detoxicating.

Indication. Dyspepsia, jaundice, diabetes, pathopyretic sore, furuncle and acute mastitis.

Turnip Seed

It is the seed of Brassica rapa L. (Cruciferae).

Effect. Improving acuity of vision, clearing away heat and inducing diuresis.

Indication. Optic atrophy, blurring of vision, jaundice, dysentery and dysuria.

Turtledove

It is the meat of Streptopelia orientalis (Latenm) (Columbidae).

Effect. Tonifying qi, improving eyesight and strengthening muscles and bones.

Indication. Various consumptive diseases, hiccups, etc.

Tussive Blood due to Visceral Injury

Symptoms. Cough with spitting of blood or tussive phlegm with blood filaments, etc.

Pathogenesis. Mostly caused by heat accumulation in the lung and stomach, upward flaring of the liver-fire to invade the hung, fire hyperactivity due to yin deficiency, or failure of qi in charge of blood circulation, etc.

Therapeutic Principle. Clearing away heat from the liver, purging fire to arrest bleeding, nourishing yin, replenishing qi, strengthening the power of qi as commander in charge of blood circulation, and invigorating the spleen to nourish blood.

Twelve Meridians

A general term for the Twelve Meridians of the human body, that is, the three yin meridians of hand (the Lung Meridian of Hand-taiyin, the Heart Meridian of Hand-shaoyin, the Pericardium Meridian of Hand-jueyin); the three yang meridians of hand (the Large Intestine Meridian of Hand-yangming, the Small Intestine Meridian of Hand-taiyang, the Tri-energizer Meridian of Hand-shaoyang); the three yin meridians of foot (the Spleen Meridian of Foot-taiyin, the Kidney Meridian of Foot-shaoyin, the Liver Meridian of Foot-jueyin), and the three Yang meridians of foot (the Stomach Meridian of Foot-yangming, the Bladder Meridian of Foot-taiyang, the Gallbladder Meridian of Foot-shaoyang). These are the major trunks of the system of the meridians and collaterals, thus named the Regular Meridians or the Twelve Regular Meridians. Each meridian pertains to certain zang or fu organs; the yin meridians pertain to zang organs linking up the fu, and the yang meridians pertain to the fu organs linking up the zang, connecting exteriorl the head, face, trunk and limbs, integrating the interior and exterior parts of the body into and organic whole, and becoming the leading transportation passage of qi and blood.

Twelve Muscle Regions

Referring to the connecting part of the meridian system in the human body. The tendons and muscles of the whole body are divided into three yins and three yangs of foot and hand, namely, the Twelve Muscle Regions. The functions of the Twelve Muscle Regions rely on the nourishing action of qi, blood in the meridians and are coordinated by the twelve regular meridians. Their main function is to bind the bones to make possible the flex-stretch movement of the joints.

Twelvestamen Melastoma herb

It is the whole herb of Melastoma dodecandrum Lour. (Melastomataceae).

Effect. Promoting blood circulation, clearing away heat to cool blood, detoxicating, subduing swelling.

Indication. Dysmenorrhea, postpartum abdominal pain, metrorrhagia, leukorrhea, hemafecia, dysentery, nephritis, subcutaneous swelling, furuncle and bleeding wound.

Twinleaf Zornia Herb

It is the whole plant of Zornia diphylla Pers. (Leguminosae).

Effect. Clearing away heat, detoxicating and eliminating blood stasis.

Indication. Convulsion due to high fever, diarrhea, common cold, dysentery, infantile dyspepsia, sore throat, furuncle and mastitis, etc.

Twirling

One of the basic techniques of acupuncture.

Operation. The body of the needle is taken as a longitudinal axle. Twirl the needle clockwise and anti-clockwise repeatedly after the needle is inserted to a certain depth. The angle and frequency of twirling vary with the condition of the disease and acupoints. The amount of stimulation will be greater with more twirling degrees and faster frequency. The degree of twirling is generally no more than 360. It is used to obtain a needling reaction and make the needling reaction conduct, or employ the reinforcing and reducing method.

Notice. Do not twist the needle in only one direction when twirling, so as to prevent the body of the needle from winding the muscle fiber, and avoid pain and difficulty in withdrawing the needle.

Twisting Finger

A massage method, one of the self-massage methods.

Operation. Pinch and twist the finger joint from above to below alternately with the thumb and index.

Indication. Health care of the upper limbs.

Twisting Manipulation

A massage method.

Operation. Pinch the finger joint or a certain part of skin with the whorled surface of the thumb and index finger, and twist it as if twisting a thread.

Function. Regulating qi and blood and relaxiation joints.

Indication. Aching pain, swelling and inconvenient flexing-extending of the interphalangeal joint.

Typical Malaria

Symptoms. Intermittent chill and high fever. Headache, flushed face, thirst, and ending in sweating all over the body.

Pathogenesis. Invasion of malarial pathogen hiding in half exterior and half interior part of the body and struggling with the nutrient system and defense system.

Therapeutic Principle. Eliminating malarial pathogen to prevent relapse of malaria, regulating the interior and exterior.

U

Umbilical Carbuncle

It refers to the acute suppurative disease appearing in the position of navel.

Symptoms. Umbilical swelling, pain, tenderness, slight red. In the phase of pus formation, it is accompanied by body syndrome, or flowing of stinking mucus, from the navel. Fistula may remain unhealed for a long time.

Pathogenesis. Caused by damp-heat in the heart and the spleen, or accumulation of fire-toxin in the navel, blood stasis and toxic stagnancy.

Therapeutic Principle. Clearing away fire, detoxicating, tonifying the spleen and stomach, or treating with an operation.

Umbilical Cord around the Shoulder

Symptoms. Difficult labor.

Pathogenesis. Umbilical cord winding around the fetal neck or shoulders.

Therapeutic Principle. A well-experienced midwife is needed in this case.

Umbilical Warming

A kind of indirect moxibustion.

Indication. The common diseases of obstetrics and gynecology.

Method. Take Faeces of Flying Squirrel 6g, Dahurian Angelica Root 6g, salt 6g and a little Musk, and grind them into powder, mix some buckwheat flour with water and shape it into a circle, and put the circle on the navel. Place the medical powder in the circle and put the ignited moxa cone over the medical powder until the patient feels warm.

Uncaria Stem with Hooks

It is the stem leaf of Uncaria rhynchophylla (Miq.) Jacks. and other plants of the uncaria genus with hooks (Rubiaceae).

Effect. Calming the liver and clearing away heat, expelling wind and relieving spasm improving visual acuity, lowering blood pressure.

Indication. Epidemic febrile diseases, convulsion, dizziness, and headache caused by hyperactivity of the liver-yang or heat in the Liver Meridian, etc.

Uncinate Spikmoss Herb

It is the whole herb of Selaginella uncinata (Desv.) Spring (Selaginellaceae).

Effect. Clearing away heat, inducing diuresis, detoxicating, removing blood stasis and hemostasis.

Indication. Hepatitis, dysentery, edema, bronchitis, cough with hemoptysis, urethritis, retropharyngeal abscess, hemorrhoid complicated by anal fistula, traumatic injuries, scalds, etc.

Uncoated and Smooth Tongue

Symptoms. The tongue coating is suddenly coming off completely or partly, and the tongue is smooth and glossy.

Pathogenesis. The sudden disappearance of tongue coating is caused by the insufficiency of the stomach-qi. The rear part peeling of the tongue is caused by the impairment of stomach-qi though pathogenic factor attacks the interior superficially. The front part peeling of the tongue is caused by the retention of indigested food in the stomach and intestines, and phlegm obstruction. The central part peeling of the tongue is caused by the impairment of the stomach-qi, or deficiency of yin and blood.

Unconsciousness

Symptoms. Abnormal mentality, coma and delirium, sometimes somnolence.

Pathogenesis. Heat and dampness in the qi system forming phlegm to impair pericardium and collaterals and disturb mind.

Unconsolidation of Kidney-qi

Symptoms. Pale complexion, lassitude loin and legs, tinnitus and deafness, frequency of micturition, and spermatorrhea and prospermia, etc.

Pathogenesis. Mostly caused by excess of sexual intercourse, insufficiency of the kidney-yang, or chronic disease involving kidney and failure of nourishment.

Therapeutic Principle. Reinforcing the kidney to stop emission, and arresting essence to invigorate yang.

Unification of Mindwill and Qi

A term in Qigong, referring to the state in which the mind is concentrated on the respiration and the circulation of the internal qi to reach the unification of vitality and qi.

Uniformity of Liver and Tendon

A theory in TCM. It refers to a close physiological relation between the liver and tendon. Muscle tendon and aponeurosis hold joints together to maintain the normal movement by means of the liver blood nourishment. Sufficient liver blood results in strong tendon and nimble joints. The malnutrition of the tendons and meridians due to deficiency of the liver blood.

Uniform Reinforcing-reducing

A needling technique.

Indication. The diseases that can hardly be identified as deficiency-type nor can be diagnosed as excess-type, or that possess either deficiency syndrome accompanied with an excess one, or vice versa.

Method. 1. A reinforcing-reducing skill by which a soft manipulation is applied with a small stimulating amount; 2. A needling skill of reducing first and reinforcing next, by which pathogenic factors are eliminated and healthy energy is supported for regulation of yin and yang; 3. A needling skill also designated as regulating skill by which reinforcing and reducing are not separated into subdivisions. In the clinic, uniform reinforcing-reducing mainly refers to twirling, rotating, lifting, and thrusting with medium intensity.

Unproductive Cough

It is a type of cough.

Symptoms. Dry cough without sputum, dry mouth and dry throat, or feverish sensation in the palm and sole, etc.

Pathogenesis. Hyperactivity of fire due to yin deficiency, or impairment of body fluid by fire stagnancy, or impairment of the lung by pathogenic dryness.

Therapeutic Principle. Nourishing yin, moistening dryness, clearing away lung-heat and relieving cough.

Unripeness and Ripeness

A moxibustion term. Unripeness means little moxibustion or moxibustion with mild fire; ripeness refers to much moxibustion or moxibustion with strong fire. The ripeness is also subdivided into slight ripeness and great ripeness.

Unsteadiness of Heart-qi

Symptoms. Dysphoria, palpitation, susceptible to terror, vexation, insomnia. It is usually accompanied with listlessness, tiredness, tender tongue, and feeble pulse.

Pathogenesis. Caused by mental overstrain, or deficiency of the heart-blood, or the heart-qi due to fright.

Unusual Dysentery

It refers to the unusual dysentery.

Symptoms. Slight dysentery but with coma and delirium, dry and obstructive throat, choking and dyspnea. The disease develops rapidly, and can become a crisis.

Pathogenesis. The excess of yang pathogen which invades upward into the lung and downward into the intestines.

Therapeutic Principle. Removing the excessive yang pathogen and regulating yin.

Upper Cold and Lower Heat

It refers to a jumbled morbid condition in which symptoms of cold, such as aversion to cold, nausea, vomiting and whitish tongue coating occurring in the upper part of the body exist with symptoms of heat, such as abdominal distention, constipation and scanty dark urine simultaneously appearing in the lower. That means different diseases in both upper and lower parts of the body respectively.

Upper Dantian

A term in Qigong, one of the three Dantians.

Location. 3 cun inside the acupoint Yintang (Ex-HN3) between the two eyebrows. It is the site used for storing the brain vitality and for training the mind to return to void.

Function. Mind concentration on upper Dantian will develop intelligence, keep the spirit fresh and vigorous, improve the hearing and eyesight, and activate the potential energy of the human body.

Upper Deficiency and Lower Excess

It refers to a jumbled morbid condition with deficiency of genuine qi in the upper part of the body and preponderance of pathogenic factors in the lower, such as cardiac palpitation due to deficiency of blood, accompanied by dysentery due to damp-heat, abdominal pain, diarrhea with red and white stool many times a day and yellowish greasy tongue coating.

Upper Disease Affecting the Lower

A pathogenesis. It refers to the spread of pathogenic changes of deficiency from an upper organ to another lower organ, such as from the lung to the heart, the stomach, the liver, or the kidney.

Upper Dysphagia

Symptoms. An uneasy feeling of a cord being tightly wound around the throat or something clogging in the throat, and which can neither be spat out nor swallowed.

Pathogenesis. Impairment of the liver by melancholy and functional disturbances of the liver.

Therapeutic Principle. Soothing the liver and regulating the circulation of qi.

Upper-energizer

Location. It is the upper portion of tri-energizer from the throat to the diaphragm.

Function. Distribution of the nutrients throughout the body to nourish the skin, muscles and joints and regulation of the sweat pores.

Upper-energizer Dysfunction

A pathogenesis theory. It refers to disturbance of the upper-energizer function in qi transformation. It includes dysfunction of the heart to circulate blood and failure of the lung to distribute liquid.

Upper-energizer in Charge of Receiving

It refers to the main function of the upper-energizer through inhaling air and ingesting food.

Upper-energizer Resembling a Sprayer

The upper-energizer can spread water and food essence from the middle-energizer throughout the body just like fog and evenly spreading mist.

Upper Excess and Lower Deficiency

It refers to yin deficiency of the kidney and the liver with yang hyperactivity in the upper body. Distress and weakness of the loins and knees, and nocturnal emission, indicating deficiency in the lower, as well as hypochondriac pain, headache, dizziness, bloodshot eyes and irritability, indicating hyperactivity of the liver-yang in the upper. It also refers to a complicated morbid condition with deficiency of genuine-qi in the lower part of the body and a preponderance of pathogenic factors in the upper.

Upper Heat and Lower Cold

A jumbled case with heat symptoms in the upper part of the body and cold symptoms in the lower part of the body.

Symptoms. Irritable feverish sensation in the chest, frequent desire for vomiting, abdominalgia with preference to warmth, loose stool, etc.

Pathogenesis. Mainly caused by excess of yang in the upper and excess of yin in the lower.

Therapeutic Principle. Clearing away heat in the upper and warming the lower, regulating the stomach and decreasing the ascending qi.

Upper Magpie Bridge

A term in Qigong.

Method. According to traditional Chinese medical theory, the link between the Front Middle Meridian and Back Middle Meridian of the human body will discontinue after birth; their original links are called magpie bridges (upper and lower magpie bridges). The upper one is located at Yintang (Ex-HN3) and Biqiao. In Qigong drill, when the essence qi flows up to Yintang and Biqiao, the tongue tip should be raised against the lower hard palate to direct the essence qi down to the Front Middle Meridian.

Upper Root of Auricle (MA)

An ear point, also called Yuzhong (MA), Spinal Cord 1 (MA).

Location. Extreme superior border of the ear root.

Indication. Headache, abdominal pain, asthma and epistaxis.

Upper Stony Cellulitis on both Sides of Neck

Symptoms. Masses on both sides of the neck shaped like a plum, with normal skin color, hard as a stone, without fever, slightly painful, enlarging gradually, and difficult to subdue, to ulcerate and to heal.

Pathogenesis. Stagnancy of qi and blood due to the stagnation of the liver-qi.

Therapeutic Principle. Smoothing the liver and resolving masses.

Upper Syncope and Lower Exhaustion

Symptoms. Coma and unconsciousness.

Pathogenesis. Resulting from divorce of yin-qi and yang-qi while exhaustion refers to the exhaustion of genuine yin and yang in the lower part of the body.

Up Rising of Lung-qi

Symptoms. Cough, excessive phlegm, shortness of breath, and chest distress, etc.

Pathogenesis. It resembles the impairment of the normal function of clarifying and sending down the lung-qi, while asthmatic cough and reversed flow of qi in the former is more serious than that in the latter. It is the further development of the latter.

Therapeutic Principle. Decreasing the adverse flow of qi and prevent asthma.

Upset

Symptoms. Irritability accompanied by insomnia and dreaminess sleep, or aphtha and redness of the tongue tip, etc.

Pathogenesis. Disturbing the heart by the pathogenic heat.

Up-stirring of Liver-wind

Symptoms. Dizziness, feeling heavy in the head, convulsion and trembling of hands and feet.

Pathogenesis. Resulting from dysfunction of the liver due to excess liver-yang and disturbance of liver functions by which the liver stores and regulates blood, the condition of the liver has its specific body opening in the eyes. Pursuant to the pathogenesis, it can be divided into several types, such as wind syndromes due to hyperactivity of the liver-yang, excess of pathogenic heat, yang excess and yin deficiency, and blood deficiency.

Therapeutic Principle. Tranquilizing liver-wind, clearing away heat to expel wind, nourishing yin to calm the wind, and nourishing blood to calm wind.

Upward Adverse Flow of Pathogens

Symptoms. Feeling of fullness in the chest, retching, vexation, borborygmus, diarrhea and dyspepsia.

Pathogenesis. The therapy of purgation is misused to treat exterior syndrome caused by exopathogenic factor, so that the stomach-qi is insufficient and the exopathogen is not expelled and moves upward in the body.

Therapeutic Principle. Regulating the stomach, strengthening the middle-energizer and disintegrating masses and anti-diarrhea.

Upward Floating of Deficiency Yang

Symptoms. Tidal fever, delicate and red complexion, dry mouth without thirst.

Pathogenesis. Yang is floating upward due to the consumption of essence and blood, and lack of the foundation upon which yang-qi depends.

Upward Flow of Fetal Qi

Symptoms. Distending fullness in the chest and hypochondrium, dyspnea and dysphoria.

Pathogenesis. A constitution with insufficient yin malnutrition of the Liver Meridian, disturbance of qi circulation due to original yin deficiency and severe kidney-yin deficiency when kidney water collects to nourish the fetus after pregnancy.

Therapeutic Principle. Soothing the liver, strengthening the spleen and promoting qi circulation.

Upward Invasion of Hyperactive Liver-qi

It is one of upward invasion qi.

Symptoms. Invasion of qi from the lower abdomen to the chest and pharynx, abdominal pain, and alternative chill and fever.

Pathogenesis. Emotional depression, hepatic stagnation and upward invasion of qi and fire in the Liver Meridian.

Therapeutic Principle. Soothing the liver and clearing away heat, regulating the stomach to decreasing the adverse flow of qi.

Ureter

An auricular point.

Location. Between Kidney (MA) and Bladder (MA-SC 8).

Indication. Colic pain of the ureter calculus.

Urethra (MA)

An auricular point.

Location. On the helix and on the level of the lower border of the inferior antihelix.

Indication. Enuresis, frequent urine, urgency of urination, urodynia, retention of urine.

Urinary Bladder

A term of massage.

Location. At ventral knuckle of the proximal little finger.

Indication. Enuresis, urinary retention.

Urinary Bladder Collateral

Course. It branches from Feiyang (B58) 7 cun above lateral malleolus, and runs into the Kidney Meridian.

Symptoms. For the excess syndrome, nasal obstruction, headache, pain in the back. For the deficient syndrome, running nose or nasal bleeding.

Urinary Bladder Divergent Meridian

It is one of twelve divergent meridians.

Course. It derives from Urinary Bladder Meridian, into the popliteal fossa; One branch enters into the anus at 5 cun below sacrum, connecting the bladder internally, distributing in the spleen, and ascending along two sides of spinal column to the heart, and distributing into the heart. The direct branch ascends from the two sides of spinal column, emerges from neck, and again distributes into Bladder Meridian.

Urinary Bladder Dysfunction

Symptoms. Distention and fullness in the lower abdomen, pain and tenderness, difficulty in urination, watery nasal discharge, etc.

Pathogenesis. Pathogenic wind, cold and dampness in the urinary bladder for a long time, obstruction of qi activities.

Therapeutic Principle. Warming and clearing. If it is caused by the damp-heat stagnated in the urinary bladder, expelling the damp-heat.

Urinary Obstruction

Symptoms. It is an acute case marked by the complete ceasing of urine.

Therapeutic Principle. Clearing away heat and inducing diuresis for patients with damp-heat of the bladder; clearing away heat of lung and inducing urine for patients with excessive lung heat; regulating qi and promoting urine for patients with live-qi depression and qi stagnation; lifting clear substance, decreasing turbid substance, alleviating qi and inducing urine for patients with deficiency of middle-energizer; warming and strengthening kidney-yang for patients with deficiency of kidney-yang.

Urine

It is a sort of fluid produced by the functional activities of the kidney, tri-energizer, and urinary bladder. This is closely related to clearing the inspired air and descending function of the lung, to promoting water metabolism of the spleen, to clearing and regulating water passage of tri-energizer and to separating purity from turbidity of the small intestine. The evacuation of urine is of important influence to the metabolism of the body fluid.

Urolithic Stranguriaa

A sort of stranguriaa.

Symptoms. Difficulty in urination with pain involving the lower abdomen. In case of micturition with stone, relief of the pain with dark of bloody urine. It is similar to vesical calculus.

Pathogenesis. The heat accumulation in the lower-energizer which steams the urine and impurity.

Therapeutic Principle. Clearing away the heat and removing the stone.

Uroschesis

A name of syndromes.

Symptoms. Difficulty in urination, difficult dribbling urination and even blocked urination. In the clinic, there are two kinds of uroschesis: excess syndrome and deficiency syndrome.

Ursine Seal's Penis and Testes

It is the dried penis and testes of Callorhinus ursinus (L.) or Phoca vitulina (L.).

Effect. Promoting sexual potency and suppliment the kidney.

Indication. Impotence, cold penis and testes, tiredness of the loins and knees, aversion to cold, cold limbs, cold pain in the abdomen caused by deficiency of both the kidney-yang and the kidney essence.

Urticaria

Symptoms. The local rising edema of the skin, appearing suddenly and subduing quickly, without leaving any signs. It can be divided into two kinds, red and white.
Pathogenesis. They are caused by wind-cold or by wind-heat respectively.

Urticaria

Symptoms. Like rubella with broken tops, sometimes healing, and sometimes attacking, and similar to rash measles.
Pathogenesis. The attacking of wind-dust into the skin and muscle due to the deficiency and looseness of muscular striae.
Therapeutic Principle. Dispelling wind and consolidating superficial resistance. Attention should be paid to skin cleaning to prevent further attacks.

Using Drug in Meridian of Sore

It is one of the treatments for sores.
Method. Using the different medicinal guide pursuant to which position the meridian and collateral of the sore belongs to. By using these guides, the drugs can directly reach the affected positions and are likely to be more effective.

Using Medicine of Warm Nature to Treat Pseudo-heat

It is one of the therapies contrary to the routine. It refers to treating cold syndrome with medicines of warm and hot nature, e.g. yin cold syndrome keeps heat externally. If medicines of warm or hot properties are taken, cold syndrome may be kept externally, otherwise cold syndrome can't be kept externally.

Uterine Collateral

1. It refers to "Uterine collaterals".
2. A term of massage locality.
   Location. On the whorled surface of the proximal knuckle of the ring finger.

Uterine Prolapse

Referring to weighing down of the uterus, or even prolapse from the vaginal orifice.

Symptoms. Tenesmus of the uterus or even prolapse from the vaginal orifice together with the vaginal wall or bladder and rectum.

Pathogenesis. Multi-production, dystocia, and overstrain during delivery, with injury to the uterine collaterals and the kidney-qi, leading to unfastening of the uterus.

Therapeutic Principle. Enriching qi and sending it up. For the patient with kidney deficiency, tonifying the kidney and enrich qi; for the patient with dampness-heat in the lower energizer, clearing away heat and promoting diuresis.

Uterus Meridian

It refers to meridians and collaterals distributed in uterus, including the Front Middle Meridian and the Vital Meridian. The uterus meridian governs the menses and pregnancy.

Uvula Hematoma

Symptoms. Swollen and red uvula, hard, and covered or wrapped all over with whitish membrane, with purplish bloody vesicle on the uvula tip, difficulty in lingual contraction, obstruction of the throat, difficult swallowing and breathing, and irritable tight sensation in the chest.

Pathogenesis. Subjective burning sensation of stomach-fire and upward invasion of the isthmus of fauces by heat accumulation of the spleen and stomach, or traumatic injury.

Therapeutic Principle. Clearing away heat and detoxicating, or applying insufflation of powdered drug to the diseased part if blood is shedding from the swollen part.

V

Vacillating Qi
Symptoms. Dysphoric fullness accompanied by restlessness, deficient flatulence due to yang deficiency of the spleen and kidney, etc.
Pathogenesis. Disorder of the five viscera which leads to qi distention in the tri-energizer.
Therapeutic Principle. Dispersing the depressed liver-qi, regulating circulation of qi and eliminating the distention.

Vaginal Discharge due to Noxious Dampness
Symptoms. A large quantity of fetid and various colored vaginal discharge which looks like rice-water or pus, fever, abdominal pain, scanty dark urine, etc.
Therapeutic Principle. Clearing away heat and toxic material and decreasing dampness to relieve leukorrhagia.

Vaginal Fetor
Symptoms. Unbearable fetor from the vagina accompanied by leukorrhagia, or cold sensation in the vagina.
Therapeutic Principle. For the patient with pathogenic cold in the uterus, warming the meridians to expel cold and eliminating dampness to get rid of fetor; for the patient with downward flow of dampness-heat from the Liver Meridian, clearing away heat from the liver to promote diuresis.

Valve-like Tongue Coating
A tongue condition.
Symptoms. Tongue coating bulging, assuming valve in shape, burned black, and black yellow in color, and even greasy coating.

Pathogenesis. Usually caused by steaming by fire of excessive type in zang-fu organs. It can be seen in pestilence, damp-warm syndrome, etc.

Variation of Complexion Reflecting Condition of Qi
The skin color of face is the exterior sign of vital essence and energy of the viscera. All the vital-qi of the viscera will run upward to the face. So, it can reflect the prosperity or decline of the vital-qi and the essence of the viscera. Bright and moist complexion indicates sufficient vital essence and energy of the viscera. Pale and dim complexion indicates deficient vital essence and energy of the viscera.

Variegated Leaf Begonia Herb
It is the whole herb of Begonia cathayana Hemsl.
Effect. Subduing inflammation, clearing away heat, detoxicating and dissipating blood stasis.
Indication. Fire burns and scalds, carbuncles, sores, furuncle, swellings, and ecchymosis and pain caused by traumatic injuries.

Vascular Nevus
Symptoms. Small red nevus appear on the skin, which usually appear on the face, the neck, the trunk, rising above the skin, with a smooth surface. They are red or purple red, soft and will fade when pressed, bleed when broken by touching.
Pathogenesis. Mostly congenital or caused by the blood stasis in the minute collaterals due to the excess of liver-fire.
Therapeutic Principle. The disease is similar to vascular hemorrhoid. Removing

pathogenic heat from blood, regulating the nutrient phrase and dissipating blood stasis. External treatment is mainly adapted.

Velutinous Cinquefoil Leaf

It is the root of Potentilla griffithii Hook. f. var. velutina Card. (Rosaceae).

Effect. Promoting digestion and activating flow of qi, cooling blood to dissipate stasis.

Indication. Stomachache due to dyspepsia, dysentery, metrorrhagia, hemorrhoidal bleeding etc.

Ventilating Lung and Resolving Phlegm

It refers to a treatment for exopathogenic wind-cold with productive cough by using diaphoretics, expectorants, and antitussives.

Symptoms. Cough with white clear sputum, aversion to cold, fever without sweating, nasal obstruction, itching of throat, thin white tongue coating.

Pathogenesis. Affection of pathogenic wind and cold, impairment of body surface and the lung in keeping pure and descendant.

Therapeutic Principle. Diaphoresis relieving superficies, releasing pulmonary qi, dissipating sputum and relieving cough.

Vertigo

It is the collective term for vertigo and dizziness.

Symptoms. Dim eyesight, faint vision, blurred vision, rotating sensation of oneself or surrounding, and inability to stand firmly.

Pathogenesis. Usually caused by hyperactivity of the liver-yang, insufficiency of qi and blood, and the stagnation of phlegm in the middle-energizer-yang.

Therapeutic Principle. Calming the liver, subdue hyperactivity of the liver yang, clearing away the liver fire to stop the wind, eliminating dampness and phlegm, strengthening the spleen and stomach, promoting blood circulation or clearing away heat in meridians.

Vertigo and Trembling

Symptoms. Vertigo accompanied by shaking of head and trembling of limbs.

Pathogenesis. Up-stirring of the liver-fire.

Therapeutic Principle. Calming the liver and suppressing the yang hyperactivity of the liver.

Vertigo Caused by Summer-dampness

Symptoms. It is classified into damp-heat and cold-dampness. The first one is manifested by fever, spontaneous perspiration, dysphoria, thirst, feeble and rapid pulse; the second one by cold, heaviness and pain of the body, feeble and slow pulse.

Pathogenesis. The attack of pathogenic dampness in summer.

Therapeutic Principle. For the former, clearing away summer-heat and eliminating dampness. For the latter, removing dampness and expelling cold.

Vertigo due to Attack of Pathogenic Wind on Head

It refers to dizziness and giddiness.

Symptoms. Dizziness and giddiness, epigastric pain, fullness and choking sensation in the chest and abdomen, pressing with sound of water.

Pathogenesis. Accumulation of wind-type phlegm in the chest, failure of the lucid yang to rise.

Therapeutic Principle. Emetic therapy.

Vertigo due to Cold-dampness

Symptoms. Dizziness, aversion to cold, heaviness and pain in the limbs, anhidrosis and contracture, slow and tense pulse.

Pathogenesis. Reversed damp-pathogen in the interior, and the stagnation of the pathogenic cold.

Therapeutic Principle. Dispelling dampness and cold.

Vertigo due to Common Cold

It refers to dizziness or the syndrome of head wind.

Symptoms. Dizziness, accompanied by aversion to wind and spontaneous perspiration, etc.

Therapeutic Principle. Eliminating wind and dispersing cold.

Vertigo due to Deficiency Phlegm

It is a kind of vertigo.

Symptoms. Heavy sensation of the head, dizziness, dim eyesight, lassitude, and drowsiness.

Pathogenesis. Insufficiency of the spleen and the stomach, phlegm accumulation due to stagnation of the body fluid.

Therapeutic Principle. Strengthening the spleen and tonifying the kidney, and dissipating phlegm.

Vertigo due to Excess of Liver-fire

It is a kind of vertigo.

Symptoms. Dizziness and headache, flushed face like burning flame, bitter taste in mouth and conjunctival congestion, red tongue.

Pathogenesis. The deficiency of kidney-fluid and emotional upset.

Therapeutic Principle. Clearing away liver-fire for cases with excessive fire; nourishing yin to decrease the fire in cases with deficiency of yin.

Vertigo due to Fluid Retention

Symptoms. Dizziness, blurred vision, lassitude, cephalic heaviness, oppressed feeling in the chest, vomiting of phlegm and saliva from time to time, or poor appetite, drowsiness.

Pathogenesis. Fluid retention in the region below the heart or in the diaphragm.

Therapeutic Principle. Activating yang and promoting diuresis.

Vertigo due to Kidney Deficiency

Symptoms. Dizziness and giddiness, insomnia and hyperhidrosis amnesia, emission, tinnitus, weakness of the loins and legs etc.

Pathogenesis. Usually caused by insufficiency of kidney essence, which leads to failure to nourish the brain.

Therapeutic Principle. Tonifying the kidney and nourishing yin, warming the kidney and restoring yang.

Vertigo due to Loss of Blood

Symptoms. All kinds of bleeding such as hematemesis, epistaxis, metrorrhagia or metrostaxis, injury, etc., accompanied by dizziness with dim eyesight, pale complexion, palpitation, and spontaneous perspiration. Prostration with cold limbs in the serious case.

Pathogenesis. Profuse bleeding resulting in the loss of nutrition of the brain.

Therapeutic Principle. Nourishing the blood and invigorating qi.

Vertigo due to Pathogenic Dryness-fire

Symptoms. Dizziness, fever, dysphoria, thirst, insomnia, unsmooth and dark urine.

Pathogenesis. Affection by seasonal pathogenic dryness-fire or cold due to pathogenic factors, leading to impairment of body fluid and malnutrition of the liver and lung.

Therapeutic Principle. Clearing away heat and moistening, and nourishing yin and moistening the lung.

Vertigo due to Pathogenic Wind

Symptoms. Dizziness, blurred vision, hiccups, or even cold limbs, which attacks unexpectedly, and is accompanied with pain of limbs, etc.

Pathogenesis. Weakness and insufficiency of qi and blood, due to invasion of pathogenic wind onto the head.

Therapeutic Principle. Consists mainly in strengthening the body resistance to dispelling pathogenic wind.

Vertigo due to Phlegm-fire

Symptoms. Dizziness, distention and heaviness of the head and eyes, upset and palpitation, nausea with phlegm and saliva, bitter taste, reddish urine, yellowish tongue coating.

Pathogenesis. The stagnation of phlegm with fire, which goes up to disturb lucid yang.

Therapeutic Principle. Eliminating phlegm and purging fire.

Vertigo due to Phlegm Retention

Symptoms. Dizziness, eyelid margins, excessive phlegm, chest tightness and nausea, dyspnea, etc.

Pathogenesis. Disturbance of the upper orifices by phlegm.

Therapeutic Principle. Strengthening the spleen and removing dampness, lowering the adverse flow of qi and stopping vomiting.

Vertigo due to Qi Deficiency

Symptoms. Dizziness, which becomes serious when moving and occurs immediately after overwork. It is accompanied by lassitude, pale face, palpitation, insomnia.

Pathogenesis. Qi deficiency.

Therapeutic Principle. Chiefly tonifying qi.

Vertigo due to Qi Retention

Symptoms. Vertigo, irritability, red face and sensation of distention in the head.

Pathogenesis. Depressed emotions, reversing flow of qi, unsoomthness of zang-qi and the abnormal rising of qi.

Therapeutic Principle. Relieving the depressed emotion, promoting the circulation of qi, and tranquilizing the mind.

Vertigo due to Wind-cold

Symptoms. There are two kinds. For the dizziness due to wind pathogen, headache

with the forehead involved, pain in the joints, fever and polyhidrosis, dyspnea, and dizziness with restlessness. For the dizziness due to cold pathogen, marked by fever without sweating, aversion to cold and muscular contracture, headache and general pain, and frequent dizziness.

Pathogenesis. Invasion of pathogenic wind-cold.

Therapeutic Principle. Dispelling the wind for the former. Dispelling the cold for the latter.

Vertigo during Menstruation

Symptoms. Cyclic and repeated attacks of dizziness following menstruation.

Pathogenesis. Malnutrition of the head and eye due to blood and qi insufficiency and yin deficiency of the liver and kidney, or stagnation of phlegm-dampness and failure of lucid yang to rise.

Therapeutic Principle. Invigorating qi to produce blood, nourishing yin and suppressing hyperactive yang, or strengthening the spleen and dissipating phlegm.

Vertigo during Pregnancy

Symptoms. Dizziness during the second and third trimester of pregnancy.

Pathogenesis. Insufficiency of essence and blood, and hyperactivity of liver-yang due to original weakness of visceral-qi and severe deficiency after pregnancy.

Therapeutic Principle. Invigorating the spleen, nourishing yin and calming the liver to suppress yang.

Vertigo of Deficiency Type

Symptoms. Vertigo aggravated on moving, onset upon exertion, lightsome pale complexion, listlessness, insomnia and dreaminess, cold limbs, emission and tinnitus.

Pathogenesis. The deficiency of qi, blood, yang or kidney. Vertigo aggravated on moving, onset upon exertion, lightsome pale complexion, listlessness, insomnia and dreaminess, cold limbs, emission and tinnitus.

Therapeutic Principle. Replenishing qi, tonifying blood, warming yang and reinforcing the kidney.

Vertigo with Unsteadiness Sensation

Symptoms. Dim-sighted vision, dizziness, and vibrating and unstable sensation in head, often accompanied by blindness, deafness.

Pathogenesis. It belong to the clinical manifestations of the liver and gallbladder diseases usually resulting from deficiency of the liver-yin and kidney-yin and hyperactivity of the liver-yang.

Vesicles of Tongue

Symptoms. The white vesicles appear on and under the tongue. If the syndrome is due to the flaring-up of fire of deficiency of the spleen and the kidney, white vesicles will appear under the tongue, with different size, and five or six in connection. The color may be red, yellow. If the syndrome is due to the accumulation of heat in the heart and the spleen, the white vesicles will appear on the tongue, with five or six in connection, which are painful, itching and ulcerate.

Therapeutic Principle. For the former, replenishing the vital essence and removing heat. For the latter, clearing away the heat-fire.

Vesiculated Dermatitis of Eyelid

Symptoms. Redness of the eyelid with blisters or even local ulceration thereon. It is often accompanied by pain and itching.

Pathogenesis. Heat accumulation in the spleen and stomach, and repeated affection of pathogenic wind with heart-fire that goes upward to attack the eyelid.

Therapeutic Principle. Clearing away heat and purging fire.

Vibrating Ear

A massage manipulation. It is one of self-massage manipulations.

Operation. Press the two ears heavily with the two palm centers and then make a fast and rhythmic push-press about 30 times.

Function. Tranquilizing the mind.

Indication. Insomnia and dreaminess.

Vibration Manipulation

A massage manipulation.

Operation. The stimulation whose frequency is higher and the intensity is alternate acts on the body continuously to cause local vibration. It covers shaking and vibrating manipulations.

Vibration Needling

An acupuncture point manipulation.

Operation. After the insertion of the needle, hold the handle of the needle with the thumb, index and fingers of the right hand and vibrate it gently and rapidly to induce the needle sensation for therapeutic purpose as a kind of auxilliary technique coupled with other manipulations.

Vigorous Reinforcing and Reducing Method

A form of needle manipulation contrary to the mild reinforcing and reducing method. It refers to vigorous and strong stimulative skill of reinforcing and reducing, like methods of setting the mountain on fire and penetrating heaven coolness etc.

Villose Ardisia Root

It is the root or whole herb of Ardisia villosa Roxb. (Myrsinaceae).

Effect. Expelling wind, dissipating dampness, promoting blood circulation and relieving pain.

Indication. Pain due to pathogenic wind-dampness, swelling and pain due to traumatic injuries, hematemesis due to cough, abdominal pain due to cold, etc.

Villosulous Veronicastrum Herb

It is the stem leaf or root of Veronicastrum axillare (Sieb. et Zucc.) Yamazaki or

Veronicastrum villosulum (Miq.) Yamazaki (Scrophulariaceae).

Effect. Inducing diuresis, removing blood stasis, subduing swelling and detoxicating.

Indication. Edema, dysuria, hepatitis, irregular menstruation, furuncle, subcutaneous swelling due to skin and external diseases, traumatic injuries, burns, scald, etc.

Villous Amomum Fruit   ⊛ V-1

It is the dried ripe fruit of Amomum villosum Lour or A. longiligulare T. L. Wu. (Zingiberaceae).

Effect. Dissipating dampness, regulating qi, warming the middle-energizer and preventing abortion.

Indication. Accumulation of dampness in the middle-energizer and stagnation of qi in the spleen and stomach.

Vinegar

It is the liquid acetic acid, which is made from rice, wheat, sorghum, and distillers' grains.

Effect. Promoting digestion, dissipating blood stasis, arresting pain, detoxicating, destroying parasites, etc.

Indication. Postpartum faint due to blood stasis, mass beside umbilicus, mass in the abdomen, jaundice, tawny sweat, hematemesis, epistaxis, hemafecia, pruritus in the pudendum, suppurative infections on the body surface.

Violent Sweating

It refers to the manifestation in which pestilence and epidemic febrile disease will relieve by sweating.

Symptoms. Suddenly extreme restlessness, feeling uneasy whether sitting or lying, then profuse sweating, fever subsiding and normal pulse.

Pathogenesis. Violent struggle between pathogenic factor and vital-qi due to excessive pathogenic factors but failure of vital-qi to exhaust.

Virulent Heat Pathogen

1. A cause of disease. It is one cause of epidemic febrile disease and is mostly seen in spring and winter. It can bring out such disease as acute febrile disease caused by virulent heat pathogen.

2. A disease.

   Symptoms. Besides the symptoms of epidemic febrile disease, it possesses such manifestations as local red and swollen pain, erosion and diabrosis, for instance, infection with swollen head, scarlet fever etc.

   Pathogenesis. Caused by affection with virulent heat pathogen.

   Therapeutic Principle. Clearing away heat and toxic materials.

Visceral Stagnation

It is a general designation of stagnancy syndrome due to emotional stress. It covers several types due to anger, anxiety, melancholy, grief, terror, fear, etc.

Viscera-state Theory

A term in TCM. It is the theory studying the functional laws of the zang-fu or of the human body and their interrelationship.

Theory. Pursuant to this theory, the five zang organs are considered as the center, which are coordinated by the six fu organs, and qi, blood and the body fluid are considered as the substantial base. One zang organ and the other one, the zang organ and its corresponding fu organ, one fu organ and the other one are closely connected by the meridians and collaterals. The zang-fu organs are connected with the five sense organs, the nine orifices, limbs, and skeletons into an organic whole.

Viscid Germander Herb

It is the whole herb of Teucrium viscidum Bl. (Labiatae.).

Effect. Promoting circulation of blood and qi, clearing away heat from blood, dissipating blood stasis, relieving swelling and detoxicating.

Indication. Hematemesis, hemoptysis, hematochezia, arthrorheumatism, traumatic injuries, subcutaneous swelling, hemorrhoid.

Visual Hallucination

Symptoms. The illusion appears in one's vision.

Pathogenesis. Stagnation phlegm-fire, mental disorder due to heat or interior consumption of essential energy.

Vital Essence and Energy

It generally refers to the essential substances to maintain the life activities, such as essential substance for reproduction, extract obtained from food and water, nourishing qi, defending qi.

Vitality

1. In generally, it refers to life processes of the human body, including the interior signs of physiology and pathology in nature. 2. In a narrow sense, it refers to mentality, consciousness, and thinking.

Vitality with Stomach-qi

It is the principle of prognoticating disease. In the serious case, if the patient can still eat or the pulse is mild, it indicates that his stomach-qi still exists and his vitality is good. In this case, the patient is likely to recover.

Vital-qi

1. It refers to genuine qi, the combination of the inborn primordial energy and the acquired energy derived from food and the air, generally denoting the vital function, including functional activities, ability of resisting against diseases, and ability of recovery from a disease.

2. It refers to the normal climate conditions in the four seasons, say springwarm, summer-heat, autumn-cool, and winter-cold.

Vital-qi Prevailing over Pathogenic Factors

It refers to a disease which is improved and cured in the struggle between pathogenic factors and vital-qi. Such result is often seen in patients whose vital-qi is not deficient and who have the ability to resist pathogenic factors or who are correctly treated in time.

Vital Syndrome of Apoplexy

It refers to critical syndrome of apoplexy.

Theory. It has been thought in the ancient time that apoplexy with mouth open indicated failure of the heart, apoplexy with incontinence of urine showed failure of the kidney, apoplexy with hands relaxed demonstrated failure of spleen, apoplexy with eyes closed suggested failure of liver, and apoplexy with snore denoted failure of the lung. All the above are considered as critical syndromes. Of the five syndromes, if only one occurs, there are chances of being cured.

Vitiligo

Symptoms. Skin injury of white spots, white hair on the affected region, clear boundary, deep color of the surrounding skin, no pain and itching, no infectivity.

Pathogenesis. Deficiency of blood, which cannot moisten the meridians and collaterals, and attacks of toxins into the lung.

Therapeutic Principle. Nourishing the blood and moistening the lung, clearing and activating the meridians and collaterals.

Vitreous Opacity

Symptoms. Ocular disease characterized by subjective sensation of mosquito or fly-like blackish shadow, dancing and floating in front of the eye, or even by blurred vision.

Pathogenesis. Internal accumulation of damp-heat, upward attack of turbid qi, or yin deficiency of the liver and kidney, and fire burning blood and collaterals.

Therapeutic Principle. Dispelling phlegm, promoting diuresis, nourishing yin and purging fire.

Viviparous Bistort Rhizome

It is the rhizome of Polygonum viviparum L. (Polygonaceae).

Effect. Hemostasis, promoting blood circulation and stopping diarrhea.

Indication. Hematemesis, epistaxis, metrorrhagia, dysentery, leukorrhagia, traumatic injuries, etc.

Vomit due to Disorder of Qi

Symptoms. Sensation of fullness in the chest and diaphragm, vomiting after dieting, relief after vomiting.

Pathogenesis. Depressed emotions, impairment of the descending function of the stomach, disorder of qi and adverse rising of the stomach qi.

Therapeutic Principle. Descending qi and normalizing the stomach.

Vomiting

Symptoms. Food or phlegm floating upwards from the stomach. There are two types of syndromes: the deficiency and excess.

Pathogenesis. For the excess syndrome, the six pathogens due to exogenous pathogenic factor, retention and accumulation of phlegm, indigestion with prolonged retention of food in the stomach and intestines, disorder of emotion, and reversed disturbance in the middle energizer. For the deficiency syndrome, deficiency and cold in the spleen and stomach, or deficiency of stomach yin which cannot regulate the stomach and calm the adverse-rising qi.

Therapeutic Principle. For the former, regulating the stomach and calming the adverse rising qi, finding out the cause and curing the disease. For the latter, warming the middle-energizer and strengthening the spleen, or nourishing the stomach yin.

Vomiting and Diarrhea

It refers to the condition of illness in which the infant vomits and also has diarrhea.

Pathogenesis. The pathogenic dampness disturbs the spleen or improper diet, which leads to disorder of the stomach-qi and depression of the spleen-qi.

Therapeutic Principle. Regulating the stomach to relieve vomiting and strengthening the spleen and eliminating dampness.

Vomiting and Diarrhea due to Cold

It is a type of cholera morbus, referring to cold type.

Symptoms. Vomiting of watery fluid or rice washed like water, less fetor, slight pain in abdomen, aversion to cold, cold limbs, black or violet lips and nails.

Pathogenesis. Usual deficiency of yang-qi, internal injury due to raw or cold food and affection by exopathic cold-dampness evil.

Therapeutic Principle. Warming the middle-energizer to dispel cold and dampness.

Vomiting and Diarrhea due to Latent Summer-heat

Symptoms. Sudden vomiting and diarrhea, dysuria, yellow or red defecation.

Pathogenesis. The infantile vomiting and diarrhea in autumn is due to summer-heat retaining in the intestines, and stomach with infection of exterior pathogens in autumn, disorder of the stomach and the intestines.

Therapeutic Principle. Clearing away summer-heat, detoxifying and regulating the intestines and the stomach.

Vomiting before Diarrhea

Symptoms. Fever, contracture of elbows and arms, shortness of breath, chest rightness and vexation, vomiting at first then diarrhea after food-intake, etc.

Pathogenesis. Accumulation of summer-heat and dampness in middle-energizer.

Therapeutic Principle. Clearing away heat and dissipating dampness, and discharging the dregs and turbid pathogenic factors.

Vomiting Blood due to Excessive Drinking

A disease and a syndrome.

Symptoms. Cough, thoracic pain, hematemesis, etc.

Pathogenesis. Mainly the excessive heat of alcohol injuring the stomach. The heat involving the lung leads to cough with dyspnea. The blood overflowing with qi causes vomiting blood.

Therapeutic Principle. Clearing away stomach-heat, removing blood heat and removing blood stasis.

Vomiting Caused by Intestinal Parasitosis

It refers to vomiting due to intestinal parasites interfering with the stomach. There are two types: cold type and heat type.

1. **Symptoms.** Vomiting with thin discharge, intermittent abdominal pain, pale and green complexion.

   Pathogenesis. Cold pathogens affecting the meridian of the stomach, forcing the parasites upwards and interfering with the stomach.

   Therapeutic Principle. Warming the stomach to quieten the parasites.

2. **Symptoms.** Vomiting with thin saliva, intermittent abdominal pain, flushed face and red lips.

   Pathogenesis. Excess fire of the stomach, leading to irritated parasites interfering with the stomach.

   Therapeutic Principle. Clearing heat from the stomach to kill the parasites.

Vomiting due to Accumulation of Phlegm

Symptoms. Distending pain in hypochondrium, vomit with sputum and lassitude.

Pathogenesis. Spleen deficiency, which leads to stagnation phlegm-dampness, and adverse rising of gastric qi.

Therapeutic Principle. Warming stomach and dispersing coldness, and eliminating phlegm to decrease the up-going qi.

Vomiting due to Cold

One of the syndromes of infantile vomiting.

Symptoms. Vomiting with milk and undigested food or sialemesis, cold limbs, pale tongue with white coating.

Pathogenesis. Due to cold of the deficient type in the stomach.

Therapeutic Principle. Regulate the middle-energizer to stop vomiting.

Vomiting due to Cold Milk

Symptoms. Cold limbs, no thirst, etc.

Pathogenesis. Cold milk is hurting the stomach.

Therapeutic Principle. Warming middle-energizer to dissipating the stagnation.

Vomiting due to Cold of Insufficiency Type

Symptoms. Vomiting after improper diet with intermittent condition, pale complexion, lassitude, dry mouth without preference to drink, cold limbs, loose stools, pale tongue.

Pathogenesis. Due deficiency of the spleen and stomach, dysfunction of the middle-yang and failure of the stomach-qi to descend.

Therapeutic Principle. Invigorating the spleen and stomach. Acupuncture treatment, and moxibustion is applicable.

Vomiting due to Damp-heat

Symptoms. Vomiting, upset, fever and foul breath, yellowish and swollen complexion, fullness and nausea.

Pathogenesis. Damp-heat in the intestines and stomach.

Therapeutic Principle. Clearing away heat and dispersing dampness, regulating the stomach-qi and arresting vomiting.

Vomiting due to Exogenous Diseases

It refers to the symptom of vomiting appearing in the course of exogenous diseases.

Pathogenesis. Many reasons: the failure to descend the stomach-qi due to attacks of fire-toxin into the interior; blocking of the qi of the bowels due to the impaction of toxic heat; also the failure to descend the stomach-qi due to the insufficiency of the stomach-qi.

Vomiting due to Exopathogen

A type of vomiting.

Symptoms. For the cases with cold, sudden and violent vomiting, vomiting with some clear fluid and thin saliva, desire for warmth and fear of chill, loose stool accompanied by aversion to cold, fever, headache, white tongue coating. For the cases with heat, frequent vomiting, vomiting straight after eating or drinking, eructation with sour-bitter bile or fetid odor due to heat, thirst, desire for cold drinks, aversion to heat, dry stools, accompanied by headache, fever, red tongue.

Pathogenesis. Wind, cold, summer-heat and damp pathogens, and filthy and turbid qi invading the stomach, leading to failure of the stomach-qi to descend and the adverse flow of stomach-qi.

Therapeutic Principle. Relieving the exterior syndrome and regulating the spleen and stomach acupuncture.

Vomiting due to Gallbladder-heat

Symptoms. Cholemesis, bitter taste in mouth and conjunctival congestion, vexation and restlessness, fullness in chest and hypochondrium.

Pathogenesis. Production of heat due to long-time stagnation of gallbladder-qi, internal disturbance of the middle-energizer by pathogenic heat, failure of the stomach-qi to descend.

Therapeutic Principle. Regulating flow of qi, clearing away heat and decreasing the adverse flow of qi.

Vomiting due to Heat

A type of infantile vomiting.

Symptoms. Infantile vomiting with foul smell, fever, thirst, flushed face and dysphoria, feverish sensation in the palms and soles, red tongue with yellowish coating, slippery pulse.

Pathogenesis. Infantile dyspepsia transforming into heat, or summer-heat affecting the stomach in summer and autumn, adverse rising of the stomach-qi.

Therapeutic Principle. Clearing pathogenic heat to promote digestion.

Vomiting due to Improper Diet

A type of vomiting.

Symptoms. Vomiting with sour and rotten discharge, abdominal distention, eructation and anorexia. The condition gets worse after eating, and better after vomiting; loose stool, or constipation with foul smell, thick and greasy tongue coating.

Pathogenesis. The accumulation of food leading to the adverse-rising of the stomach qi.

Therapeutic Principle. Promoting the flow of qi, relieving stagnancy of undigested food.

Vomiting due to Intestinal Parasitosis

A disease and syndrome. It refers to vomiting caused by ascaris.

Symptoms. Nausea, pain in the stomach and vomiting sour fluid, which temporarily stops when eating food, and becomes serious in hunger, etc.

Therapeutic Principle. Regulating stomach and expelling parasites.

Vomiting due to Liver-qi

A type of vomiting.

Symptoms. Vomiting, acid regurgitation, frequent eructation, distending pain in the chest and hypochondrium, red border of the tongue with thin and greasy coating.

Pathogenesis. The disorder of liver qi, resulting in transverse attack on the stomach.

Therapeutic Principle. Relieving the depressed liver and regulating the stomach.

Vomiting due to Retained Food

Symptoms. Infantile vomiting with undigested food or yellow and sour water, sallow complexion.

Pathogenesis. Retention of food in the stomach.

Therapeutic Principle. Promoting digestion and dissipating stagnancy, and regulating the spleen and stomach.

Vomiting due to Stomach-cold

Symptoms. Immediate vomiting when attacked by cold, aversion to cold and preference to warmth, anorexia, cold limbs, clear urine and watery stool.

Pathogenesis. Failure of middle-energizer yang, weakness of the spleen and the stomach, adverse rising of the stomach-qi.

Therapeutic Principle. Warming the middle-energizer and strengthening the spleen, regulating the stomach and lowering ascending qi.

Vomiting during Menstruation

Pathogenesis. Retention of water after drinking, or impairment by over-eating and retention of food due to weak stomach.

Therapeutic Principle. In the former case, warming the middle-energizer and dispelling fluid retention; in the latter case, dissipating food retention and promoting digestion.

Vomiting during Pregnancy

Symptoms. Nausea and vomiting of the pregnant woman.

Pathogenesis. Dysfunction of the stomach resulting from blood collection to nourish the fetus, and the upward flow of the sufficient qi of Vital Meridian.

Therapeutic Principle. There is no need for treatment in the mild case. The serious vomiting that makes intake of food impossible is due to a disease called pernicious vomiting. It should be treated by pursuant to the condition of the disease.

Vomiting in Children due to Fright

One type of vomiting in children.

Symptoms. Watery vomits, pallor, listlessness, low fever, anorexia or slight intermittent convulsion of the four limbs, taut and thready pulse, pale tongue with whitish and greasy coating.

Pathogenesis. Fright, causing the adverse flow of qi followed by the regurgitation of food.

Therapeutic Principle. Tranquilizing the mind and arresting vomiting.

Vomiting Milk in Newborn

Symptoms. The newborn infant's vomiting, or vomiting when drinking milk.

Pathogenesis. Swallowing the dirty fluid when born, not clearing the mouth or excessive cold-heat, failure to descending the stomach-qi.

Vomiting of Bilious Fluid

Symptoms. Vomiting of bitter fluid.

Pathogenesis. Seasonal exogenous pathogen attacking the Shaoyang and Yangming Meridians or impairing the Liver and Gallbladder due to anger.

Vomiting of Black Fluid

Symptoms. Vomiting black fluid from the stomach.

Pathogenesis. The insufficiency of stomach fluid.

Vomiting of Clear Fluid

Symptoms. Vomiting only water without any food.

Pathogenesis. Phlegm-dampness, excessive fluid, accumulation of cold in middle-energizer, indigestion, or parasites.
Therapeutic Principle. Dissipating phlegm-dampness and regulating the stomach.

Vomiting of Deficiency Type

Symptoms. Intermittent vomiting, it occurs all at once as the patient smells food or eats something slightly cold; or eating in the morning while vomiting in the evening, and vice versa.
Pathogenesis. Weakness of the spleen and stomach or decline of fire from the gate of life.
Therapeutic Principle. Warming and reinforcing the spleen and kidney, and regulating the stomach and arresting vomiting.

Vomiting of Excess Type

Symptoms. Sudden vomiting, fullness and oppressed feeling in epigastrium, eructation and salivation, constipation, etc.
Pathogenesis. Invasion of the stomach by exopathogens, retention of phlegm, reversed flow of qi and fire stagnancy, indigestion, etc.
Therapeutic Principle. Eliminating pathogens, removing pathogenic factor, relieving ascending qi and promoting digestion.

Vomiting of Milk and Diarrhea with Green Stool

Symptoms. Vomiting of milk, diarrhea and passing dark green stool in infants.
Pathogenesis. Infection of cold pathogens and disorder of the liver and the spleen.
Therapeutic Principle. Tonifying the liver and strengthening the spleen.

Vomiting of Milk and Diarrhea with Yellow Stool

Symptoms. The infant is vomiting milk with diarrhea and passing yellow stool with foul smell.
Pathogenesis. Improper feeding, and heat stagnating in stomach.

Therapeutic Principle. Regulate the stomach and clearing the large intestine.

Vomiting Right after Eating

Symptoms. Vomiting right after eating, also a symptom of dysphagia.
Pathogenesis. The heat accumulation in the stomach, or phlegm stagnation and food retention.

Vulval Pain

Symptoms. Painful sensation in the vulva, which may be accompanied with vulval injury or swelling.
Pathogenesis. Stagnation of the liver-fire in the vaginal gateway, which impedes the circulation of qi and blood and causes pain.
Therapeutic Principle. For the patient with heat stagnation of the Liver Meridian, soothing the liver to clear heat; for the patient with downward flow of damp-heat, clearing away heat to promote diuresis; for the one with affection by wind-cold, expelling wind and cold.

Vulval Perspiration

Symptoms. Perspiration in the vulval area, or in some cases accompanied by dampness and itching.
Pathogenesis. Downward flow of dampness-heat.
Therapeutic Principle. Clearing away heat and promoting diuresis.

Vulvar Lump

Symptoms. Silkworm cocoon-like lumps which have grown out of one or both sides of the vaginal gateway.
Pathogenesis. Local trauma, or infection of pathogenic toxin.
Therapeutic Principle. Clearing away heat of the liver and detoxication or dissipating phlegm and eliminating dampness. Operation is applicable when necessary.

Vulvar Swelling

Symptoms. Distending swelling of the vulva and vagina, accompanied with pain, leukorrhagia, itching, etc.

Pathogenesis. Invasion of pathogenic wind and interference of qi and blood with each other,

Therapeutic Principle. Expelling wind to subdue swelling and relieve pain; for the patient with downward flow of damp-heat, clearing away heat and promoting diuresis.

W

Wagging Tongue

Referring to sticking out of the tongue, long and relaxed tongue in children, presenting febrile disease, extreme deficiency of vital-qi, when the central nervous system is involved, belonging to critical condition. It is also being seen in congenital dementia children.

Waibagua

A massage point.
Location. Around the Wailaogong (Ex-UE 8) on the dorsum of the hand and opposite to the Neibagua point.
Operation. Arc-pushing.
Function. Relieve the chest stiffness and regulating qi, dissipating stagnancy to disperse accumulation of pathogen.
Indication. Chest distress, abdominal distention, constipation, etc.

Waidingchun

An extra acupuncture point.
Location. 1.5 cun lateral to Dazhui (GV 14).
Indication. Asthma, cough and bronchitis.
Method. Puncture obliquely 0.5-1 cun in the direction of the spine, and apply moxibustion to the point with 3-5 units of moxa cones or for 5-10 minutes.

Waiguan (TE 5)

An acupuncture point.
Location. 2 cun above to the transverse crease of the wrist dorsum, between the ulna and radius.
Indication. Febrile disease, headache, deafness epidemic acute conjunctivitis, rigid nape, hypochondriac pain, sore elbow and brachialgia, pain of fingers, and shivering of hand.

Method. Puncture perpendicularly 0.5-1 cun and apply moxibustion to the point with 3-5 units of moxa cones or for 5-10 minutes.

Waihuaijian (Ex-LE 9)

An extra acupuncture point.
Location. On the lateral side of the foot, at the tip of the lateral malleolus.
Indication. Convulsion, beriberi, toothache, spasm of the toes, hemiplegia, etc.
Method. Prick to cause bleeding. Moxibustion is applicable.

Waihuaiqianjiaomai (Ex-LE)

An extra acupuncture point.
Location. On the dorsum of the ankle joint, at the junction of the middle and lateral one-quarter of the line connecting the two tips of the medial and external malleolus.
Indication. Anemogenous toothache.
Method. Moxibustion.

Waihuaishang (Ex-LE)

An extra acupuncture point.
Location. 3 cun above the tip of the lateral malleolus.
Indication. Muscular spasm leading to the inability to move.
Method. Moxibustion.

Waijinjinyuye (Ex-HN)

An extra acupuncture point.
Location. 1.5 cun straight above Lianquan (CV 23), 0.3 cun external to the point.
Indication. Aphasia and salivation due to apoplexy muscular paralysis or spasm of tongue, aphtha ulcer.
Method. Puncture obliquely 0.5-1.0 cun toward the direction of the tongue root.

Wailaogong (Ex-UE 8)

An extra acupuncture point.

Location. On the dorsum of the hand, contrary to Laogong (P 8), between the 2nd and 3rd metacarpal bones and 0.5 cun proximal to the metacarpophalangeal joint.

Indication. Indigestion, diarrhea, loose stool, acute and chronic infantile convulsion, stiff neck, failure of fingers to stretch, numbness of fingers and palm, itching.

Method. Puncture perpendicularly or obliquely 0.3-0.5 cun. Apply moxibustion 1-3 moxa cones or 4-5 minutes with warming moxibustion.

Wailing (S 26)

A meridian acupuncture point.

Location. On the lower abdomen, 1 cun below the center of the umbilicus and 2 cun lateral to Yinjiao (CV 7).

Indication. Abdominal pain, hernia, dysmenorrhea, umbilical and abdominal pain due to hanging feeling of the heart.

Method. Puncture perpendicularly 0.8-1.2 cun. Apply moxibustion 5-7 moxa cones or 10-20 minutes with warming moxibustion.

Waiqiu (G 36)

An acupuncture point.

Location. At the anterior border of the fibula, parallel to Yangjiao (G 35), 7 cun above to the tip of the external malleolus.

Indication. Headache, rigid nape, fullness sensation in chest and hypochondrium, flaccidity and numbness of lower limb, hepatitis, epilepsy, and beriberi.

Method. Puncture perpendicularly 1-1.5 cun and apply moxibustion to the point with 3-5 units of moxa cones or for 5-10 minutes.

Waiting for QI

An acupuncture point term, referring to waiting for the needling sensation at a proper depth after insertion of the needle.

Method. Stop puncturing to wait for qi; changing the depth or direction of the insertion if the sensation does not appear and properly applying the lifting and thrusting method, etc. It is divided into two forms: waiting for qi in the superficial area, and waiting for qi in the deep area.

Walking Maiden-hair Herb

It is the whole herb of Adiantum caudatum L. (Adiantaceae).

Effect. Clearing away heat and detoxication, promoting diuresis and subduing swelling.

Indication. Mammary abscess, impetigo, edema, etc.

Wangu (G 12)

An acupuncture point on the Gallbladder Meridian of Foot-shaoyang.

Location. On the head, in the excavation posterior and inferior to the opisthotia mastoid process.

Indication. Headache, sore throat, dental caries, swelling cheek, toothache, laryngitis, rigidity and spasm of neck and nape, and psychosis.

Method. Puncture obliquely 0.3-0.5 cun and apply moxibustion to the point with 3-5 units of moxa cones or for 5-10 minutes.

Wangu (SI 4)

An acupuncture point.

Location. On the dorsal ulnar side of the hand at the junction of the red and white skin between the base of the 5th metacarpal bone and the triangular bone.

Indication. Rigidity of the head and neck, nephelium, pain in the arm, corneal opacity, jaundice, febrile diseases, malaria, diabetes, convulsion, contracture of the fingers, pain in the wrist.

Method. Puncture perpendicularly 0.3-0.5 cun and apply moxibustion to the point for 5-10 minutes or for 3-5 units of moxa cones.

Warm-dryness Syndrome

It refers to a seasonal disease caused by warm and dryness in autumn.

Symptoms. Headache, fever, dry cough without phlegm or cough with thin and sticky phlegm, dry sore-throat, fullness and pain in the chest, redness of both the tip and sides of the tongue with thin, dry and white fur, etc.

Therapeutic Principle. Dispelling the wind and heat with mild diaphoretic pungent in taste and cool in property and moistening the lung.

Warm Hands and Feet

1. It refers to feverish palms and soles. The symptom is usually seen in outward steaming of pathogenic heat in Yangming disease.

   Therapeutic Principle. Clearing away heat.

2. It refers to the subjective feeling of warm hands and feet, which is usually seen in deficiency of the spleen-yang, wind-cold due to affection by exopathogen, and stagnation of exopathogen in Taiyang disease.

   Therapeutic Principle. Warming the middle-energizer to dispel cold and relieving exterior syndrome simultaneously.

Warming Emaciated with Qi

A principle of treatment. It refers to the emaciated patient, due to insufficiency of the yang-qi, who should be treated with warming nourishing drugs to reinforce vital energy, and to strengthen the functions of the zang-fu organs and promote the recovery from the disease.

Warming Over-exhausted Patient

A principle of treatment. The exhausted and debilitated patients should be treated with the drugs of sweet flavor and warm natured tonics for the sake of invigoration.

Warm Needle Moxibustion

A form of moxibustion.

Operation. After inserting the needle into the body, heating the needle by burning mugwort stick on the handle of the needle.

Function. Regulate the flow of qi; promote blood circulation and the flow of qi by warming the meridian.

Indication. Pain along the spinal column, cold-pain of the extremities and abdomen, loose stool, abdominal distention caused by the stagnation of pathogenic cold in the meridian and impeded circulation of blood and qi.

Warm Pathogen

A general term for various pathogens causing acute febrile diseases, which belong to warm and damp pathogen among exopathogens, such as wind-heat pathogen, damp-heat pathogen, dry-heat pathogen, virulent heat pathogen, etc.

Wasps Flying into Hole

A massage method for children.

Operation. Knead the nostrils of the sick child with the tips of the index and middle finger.

Function. Inducing diaphoresis.

Indication. Fever with anhidrosis.

Wasp's Nest

It is the honeycomb of Polistes mandarinus saussure or the honeycomb with bee pupae (Vespidae).

Effect. Eliminating toxic substances, destroying parasites, expelling the wind and arresting pain, skin and external diseases and pyogenic infections, toothache, obstinate skin diseases, mammary abscess, tinea pain due to pathogenic wind-dampness and cancer.

Water Asthma

Symptoms. Cough, dyspnea, croup, thin sputum and spittle, pain in the chest and hypochondrium or body swollen, vomiting.

Pathogenesis. The accumulation of sputum in the lungs.

Therapeutic Principle. Dispelling the retention of fluid in the body and clarifying lung-qi.

Water Chestnut

It is the flesh of Trapa bispinosa Roxb. (Hydrocaryaceae).

Effect. Clearing away summer heat, relieving restlessness, quenching thirst, replenishing qi and nourishing the spleen.

Indication. Heatstroke, extreme thirst and retention of food due to deficiency of the spleen.

Water Furuncle

Symptoms. Black spot in the middle, which is hard and painful, with red surroundings, and the flowing out blood water after breaking.

Pathogenesis. Noxious heat of skin and muscle.

Therapeutic Principle. The same as furuncle.

Water Insufficiency Leading to Excess of Fire

1. It refers to the failure of the kidney (water) to restrain the activity of the heart (fire), leading to exuberance of the latter.

   Symptoms. Dysphoria, dizziness, tinnitus, insomnia, red tongue tip.

2. It refers to the fire from the gate of life.

   Symptoms. Consumption of the kidney-yin and excess of the fire from the gate of life resulting in loss of teeth and aching, increased sexual libido and nocturnal emission.

Water-like Menstruation

Referring to pale and water-like menstrual blood.

Pathogenesis. Deficiency of both qi and blood.

Therapeutic Principle. Enriching qi and nourishing blood.

Water Melon   ⊛ W-1

It is the pulp of Citrullus vulgaris Schrad. (Cucurbitaceae).

Effect. Clearing away summer-heat, relieving restlessness, quenching thirst and promoting diuresis.

Indication. Summer-heat with excessive thirst, consumption of body fluid due to excessive heat, dysuria, inflammation of the throat and aphthae.

Water Melon Kernel

It is the seed of Citrullus vulgaris Schrad. (Cururbitaceae).

Effect. Clearing away heat from lung, moistening the intestines, regulating stomach and quenching thirst.

Indication. Cough caused by the lung-heat, constipation due to dryness of the bowels, consumption of the body fluid and thirst.

Water Melon Peel

It is the peel of Citrullus vulgaris Schrad. (Cucurbitaceae).

Effect. Clearing away heat, relieving summer-heat, quenching thirst and inducing diuresis.

Indication. Summer-heat syndrome with extreme thirst, oliguria, edema and canker sores.

Water-paste Pill

A kind of dosage form, made of finely powdered drugs with cold boiled water, wine, vinegar, or some drug juices. Usually they are made into small size pills like green beans. It is a relatively common dosage form.

Water Peper

It is the whole herb of Polygonum lapathifolium L. var. sealicifolium Sibth. (Polygonaceae).

Effect. Eliminating swelling to relieve pain.

Indication. Swelling sore, abdominal pain due to dysentery.

Waterplantain Ottelia Herb

It is the whole herb of Ottelia alismoides (L.) Pers. (Hydrocharitaceae).

Effect. Clearing away heat, eliminating phlegm, arresting cough and inducing diuresis.

Indication. Asthma, cough, edema, ulcerative carbuncle, etc.

Water Soaking Stomach

Symptoms. Beating in the region of the stomach, and cold limbs.

Pathogenesis. Deficiency of the stomach-qi, insufficiency of splenogastric yang and resulting in water retention in the interior.

Watery Diarrhea

Symptoms. Distending abdomen, diarrhea as if there was water flooding in serious cases.

Pathogenesis. Weakness of the spleen and stomach, failure to separate the waste from the useful, retention of dampness, water passing through the intestine and inability to prohibit and arrest it.

Therapeutic Principle. Strengthening the spleen, eliminating dampness and stopping diarrhea.

Watery Stool with Indigested Food

Symptoms. Abdominal pain, preferring warmness and pressing, abdominal distention, poor appetite, clear urine.

Pathogenesis. Affection of the spleen and stomach by cold pathogen and dysfunction of the spleen in transporting.

Waxgourd Peel

It is the peel of Benincasa hispida (Thunb.) Cogn. (Cucurbitaceae).

Effect. Inducing diuresis and eliminating swelling.

Indication. Edema.

Waxing and Waning of Yin and Yang

It is one of the principal contents of the yin and yang theory. It refers to that yin and yang, opposing and depending on each other for existence, are not stagnant but in a dynamic state. Increase or excess of the one is usually associated with decrease or deficiency of the other. If the wane and wax of yin and yang change beyond the physiological limit, yin or yang excess or deficiency occurs, imbalance between yin and yang in a dynamic state appears and thus resulting in a disease.

Weakness and Emaciation due to Dysentery

Symptoms. Weakness and emaciation, diarrhea with yellow-whitish jelly, tenesmus, emaciation, pale tongue with whitish coating.

Pathogenesis. Dysentery in the case of deficiency of the spleen and stomach, insufficiency of qi and blood, prolonged dysentery.

Therapeutic Principle. Nourishing qi and invigorating the spleen.

Weakness Metrorrhagia

Referring to metrorrhagia due to qi and blood deficiency and debility of Vital Meridian and Front Middle Meridian.

Therapeutic Principle. Restoring qi to remove stasis for the incessant metrorrhagia with dark clots, and enriching qi and blood for profuse metrorrhagia with deficiency and emaciation.

Weeping Forsythia Fruit
⊛ W-2

It is the fruit of Forsythia suspensa (Thunb.) Vahl (Oleaceae).

Effect. Clearing away heat, detoxicating, treating carbuncles and resolving masses.

Indication. Exopathic diseases or epidemic diseases with the syndromes of fever and headache, high fever, restlessness, unconsciousness, mammary abscess, suppurative infections on the body surface, heat gonorrhea, dysuria and scrofula, etc.

Weibao (Ex-CA)

An extra acupuncture point.

Location. On the lateral abdomen, 1 cun below Weidao (G 28), in the depression inferior to the anterior superior iliac spine.

Indication. Hysteroptosis.

Method. Puncture 0.5-1.0 cun Perpendicularly. Apply moxibustion 3-5 moxa cones or 5-10 minutes with warming moxibustion.

Weicang (B 50)

An acupuncture point.

Location. Inferior and 3 cun lateral to the spinous process of the twelfth thoracic vertebra.

Indication. Stomachache, abdominal distention, indigestion, pain in the back spine, edema, and dysentery.

Method. Puncture obliquely 0.5-0.8 cun and apply moxibustion to the point 5-7 moxa cones or for 10-20 minutes.

Weicui (Ex-B)

An extra acupuncture point.

Location. 3 cun directly above the tip of the coccyx.

Indication. Infantile malnutrition, dyspepsia, abdominal pain, diarrhea and prolapse of anus.

Method. Puncture subcutaneously 0.5-1 cun. Apply moxibustion 3-7 moxa cones with warm needling.

Weidao (G 28)

A meridian acupuncture point.

Location. On the lateral side of the abdomen, anterior and below the anterior iliac spine, 0.5 cun anterior and inferior to Wushu (G 27).

Indication. Pain in the waist and hip, pain in the side of the lower abdomen, prolapse of the uterus, hernia, irregular menstruation and edema.

Method. Puncture 0.8-1.5 cun obliquely in the anterior-inferior direction. Apply moxibustion to the point for 5-10 minutes or 3-5 units of moxa cones.

Weigong (Ex-CA)

An extra acupuncture point.

Location. On the lateral abdomen. 1 cun obliquely below the depression inferior to the anterior superior iliac spine.

Indication. Hysteroptosis, hernia pain, dysfunction of the intestines.

Method. Puncture 0.5-1.0 cun perpendicularly. Apply moxibustion 5-10 minutes with warming moxibustion.

Weiguanxiashu

An extra acupuncture point.

Location. 1.5 cun lateral to the space between the spinous processes of the 8th and 9th thoracic vertebrae.

Indication. Diabetes, dry throat, abdominalgia, vomiting, intercostal neuralgia, etc.

Method. Puncture obliquely 0.3-0.5 cun and apply moxibustion to the point with 5-7 units of moxa cones or for 10-20 minutes.

Weiling

A massage point.

Location. In the suture between the 2nd and 3rd metacarpal bones.

Operation. Nipping is used.

Function. Causing resuscitation, restoring consciousness and tranquilizing convulsion.

Indication. Acute syndrome, such as convulsion, spasm, etc.

Weiqionggu (Ex-B)

An extra acupuncture point.

Location. On the caudal and sacral region, three points in total, one point is 1 cun above the lower tip of the coccyx, and the other two are 1 cun on each side of the above point.

Indication. Lumbago, pain in the caudal and sacra region, stranguria, constipation, enuresis, hemorrhoid, etc.

Method. Apply moxibustion 3-5 moxa cones or 5-10 minutes with warming moxibustion.

Weishu (B 21)

A meridian acupuncture point.

Location. On the back, below the spinous process of the 12th thoracic vertebra, 1.5 cun lateral to the posterior midline.

Indication. Pain in the chest and hypochondrium, stomachache, abdominal distention, cough, short breath, dysuria, edema, vomiting and diarrhea, irregular menstruation, leukorrhea.

Method. Puncture perpendicularly 0.5-0.8 cun. Apply moxibustion 5-7 moxa cones or 10-20 minutes with warming moxibustion.

Weiwanxiashu (Ex-B 3)

Location. 1.5 cun lateral to the interspace below the spinous process of the 8th thoracic vertebra.

Indication. Diabetes, stomach disorders, abdominal pain, vomiting, intercostal neuralgia.

Method. Puncture obliquely 0.5-0.8 cun. Moxibustion is applicable.

Weiyang (B 39)

A meridian acupuncture point.

Location. At the lateral end of the popliteal crease, medial to the tendon of the biceps muscle of the thigh or 1 cun lateral to Weizhong (B 40).

Indication. Stiffness and pain in the waist and along the spine, distention and fullness of the lower abdomen, difficulty in urination, spasm and pain in the legs and feet.

Method. Puncture perpendicularly 0.5-1.0 cun. Apply moxibustion 3-5 moxa cones or 5-10 minutes with warming moxibustion.

Weizhong (B 40)

A meridian acupuncture point.

Location. At the midpoint of the transverse crease of the popliteal fossa, between the tendons of the biceps muscle of the thigh and the semitendinous muscle.

Indication. Lumbago, contracture of the popliteal tendon, flaccidity and numbness

of the lower limbs, hemiplegia, abdominal pain, vomiting epilepsy, difficulty in urination, night sweat, erysipelas, back carbuncle.

Method. Puncture perpendicularly 0.5-1 cun, or prick to cause little bleeding. Apply moxibustion 3-5 moxa cones or 5-10 minutes with warming moxibustion.

Wenliu (LI 7)

An acupuncture point.

Location. On the radial side of the anterior arm dorsum, on the line connecting Yangxi (LI 5) and Quchi (LI 11), 5 cun above Yangxi.

Indication. Headache, edema of the face, sore of mouth, tongue and throat, wry mouth and eye, aching and contracture of the shoulder and arm, furuncle, borborygmus, epistaxis, abdominal pain, etc.

Method. Puncture perpendicularly 0.5-1 cun and apply moxibustion to the point for 5-10 minutes or 3-5 units of moxa cones.

Wet Beriberi

Symptoms. Edema of feet and shanks, numbness and pain of toes, which gradually develops upwards, heaviness, soreness and weakness of legs, weakness of the footsteps. In cases due to cold-dampness, aversion to cold in legs, preference for warmth; in cases due to damp-heat, burning sensation of the legs and preference for cool, or fever with chills, scanty urine, white and greasy coating.

Pathogenesis. Attack of dampness to the lower limbs leading to blockage of the meridians and collaterals.

Therapeutic Principle. Dredging the meridians and collaterals and clearing away heat and dampness.

Wheat-awn Needle

A needling instrument. It is made of stainless steel wire. The body of the needle is long and thin like the wheat awn, with a variety of length of 15 cm, 20 cm, 45 cm, etc. It is applied to deep, subcutaneous or transverse pricking technique.

Whisking Manipulation

A massage method.

Operation. Skim over the massage operating area of the skin gently, with finger straightened naturally, like whisking and flicking the dust. It is applied to the back.

Function. Inducing, conducting qi and tranquilizing the mind.

Indication. Hyperactivity of the liver-yang and insomnia.

White and Smooth Tongue

A tongue picture.

Symptoms. The tongue is light colored, with smooth tongue surface without fur, with severe deficiency of both qi and blood.

Pathogenesis. Failure in nourishing tongue body and meridians and collaterals due to serious deficiency and declining of both qi and blood.

White Boil

Symptoms. It appears under the stony nose. At the beginning it is like a millet, with a red root and a white head, numb or painful itching. And then chill, heaviness in the head, which is like exogenous febrile disease, anorexia, and dyspnea.

Therapeutic Principle. The same as that of furuncle.

White Duck Meat

It is meat of Anas domestica L.

Effect. Nourishing yin and invigorating the stomach, promoting diuresis and subduing swelling.

Indication. Hectic fever caused by consumption, cough and edema.

White Fur Tongue with Black Tip and Root

A tongue picture, referring to tongue with black fur in the tip and root, and white fur in the middle.

Symptoms. High fever with pseudo-cold symptoms in the spleen and stomach.

Pathogenesis. Extreme heat in the heart and kidney.

White Fur Tongue with Grey Tip and Yellow Root

It is refer to that the tongue fur is mainly white, with grey fur in the tip and yellow fur in the root. The tongue picture indicates damp-heat syndrome.

White Mustard Seed

It is the ripe seed of Brassica alba L. Boiss. (Cruciferae).

Effect. Warming the lung, eliminating sputum, promoting flow of qi, dispersing lumps, dredging the meridians and relieving pain.

Indication. Cough, asthma, fullness in the chest, costalgia, arthralgia of extremities, numbness and pain of the extremities.

White Peony Root

It is the root of Paeonia lactiflora pall. (Ranunculaceae).

Effect. Enriching blood, astringing yin, calming and soothing the liver-yang and alleviating pain.

Indication. Irregular menstruation, dysmenorrhea, metrorrhagia, night sweat, pain in the hypochondrium, stomach and abdomen, spasm and pain in the extremities, headache and vertigo.

White Urine

A symptom, referring to dark urine drops on ground, infantile, will solidify like white paste.

Pathogenesis. Impairment of the spleen due to galactic diet, retention of damp-heat in the interior, and food essence pouring into urinary bladder.

White Urine and Defecation

Symptoms. The infantile urine is like rice-washed water, or the urine is scanty; the defecation is white or like fish jelly.

Pathogenesis. Damp heat in the spleen and stomach or stagnant damp-heat.
Therapeutic Principle. Regulating the spleen, subduing the stagnant damp-heat, and moderating in diet.

Whitish Menstruation

Symptoms. Whitish menstrual blood, dysphoria with feverish sensation and sallow complexion.
Pathogenesis. Deficiency of both qi and blood.
Therapeutic Principle. Tonifying qi and blood and activating menstruation.

Whooping in Children

It refers to the infantile dyspnea due to excessive sputum.
Symptoms. Chest fullness, panting, profuse sputum and poor appetite.
Pathogenesis. Latent pathogenic sputum accompanied by the affection of wind and cold, and stagnancy of the sputum in the lungs.
Therapeutic Principle. If the patient has no exterior cold, eliminating phlegm, depressing upward-reverse flow of qi. If the patient has exterior cold, inducting diaphoresis to remove fluid.

Whorlleaf Stonecrop Herb

It is the whole herb of Sedum verticillatum L. (Crassulaceae).
Effect. Detoxicating, subduing swelling and stopping bleeding.
Indication. Injury, innominate inflammation, snake bite.

Wideleaf Osbeckia Root

It is the root or fruit branch of Osbeckia crinita Benth. ex C. B. Clarke (Melastomataceae).
Effect. Tonifying human body and strengthening the kidney and arresting to stop bleeding.
Indication. Cough with hematemesis due to consumption, dysentery, flaccidity and weakness in legs, incontinence of urine and leukorrhea.

Wide Vaginal Orifice

Symptoms. The relaxation of the vaginal orifice, accompanied by subjective cold sensation, leukorrhagia, or sexual anesthesia.
Pathogenesis. Original yang deficiency of the spleen and kidney, traumatic injury during delivery, either of which causes failure of the Belt Meridian to control the external genitalia with the result of the relaxation of the urogenital trigone, due to invasion of pathogenic wind-cold.
Therapeutic Principle. Fumigating and washing the diseased part with herbs which are able to strengthen yang for astringency and expel cold from the meridians.

Wildginger Herb

It is the whole herb of Asarum heterotropoides Fr. Schmidt var. mandshuricum (Maxim.) Kitag. or A. sieboldii Miq. (Aristolochiaceae).
Effect. Dissipating exogenous evils from the body surface to expel cold, relieving pain, warming the lung, removing fluid retention from the interior and clearing the nasal passage, waking up from unconsciousness.
Indication. Headache, cough, and dyspnea with sputum, toothache, nasosinusitis, dyspnea and exterior syndromes due to affection by wind-cold exopathogens.

Wild Mint Herb

It is the stalk leaf of Mentha haplocalyx Briq. (Labiatae).
Effect. Expelling wind-heat, clearing away heat, improving eyesight, relieving sore throat and promoting skin eruption, alleviating itching.
Indication. Headache, fever, common cold of wind-heat type or epidemic febrile diseases at the early stage; conjunctival congestion and swollen and sore throat due to exopathogenic wind-heat; incomplete eruption of measles at the early stage of measles; chest tightness, distend-

ing pain in the hypochondrium due to stagnation of the liver-qi, etc.

Wile Lily Bulb

It is the whole herb of Crotalaria sessiliflora L. (Leguminosae).
Effect. Clearing away heat, promoting diuresis, and detoxication.
Indication. Dysentery, sores, furuncle and infantile malnutrition.

Wilford Swallowwort Root

It is the root tuber of Cynanchum wilfordii (Maxim.) Hemst. (Asclepiadaceae).
Effect. Nourishing yin, supplement the kidney, strengthening the spleen and promoting digestion.
Indication. Consumptive disease, internal injury, dysentery, malnutrition, stomachache, leukorrhea, scabies, and tinea.

Williams Elder Twig   ⊛ W-3

It is the twig of Sambucus williamsii Hance. (Caprifoliaceae).
Effect. Dispelling wind, eliminating stagnation, inducing diuresis, promoting blood circulation to stop pain.
Indication. Rheumatic arthralgia and myalgia, lumbago, edema, urticaria, hemoptysis, hepatitis, dysentery, traumatic fracture.

Willowleaf Cotoneaster

It is the whole herb of Cotoneaster salicifolius Franch. (Rosaceae).
Effect. Expelling wind and removing heat.
Indication. Hoarseness due to dry cough, jaundice due to dampness accumulated in the spleen, hematochezia, scanty urine, etc.

Wind

1. It refers to one of the six pathogenic factors, also called pathogenic wind.
2. The name of a syndrome marked by dizziness, aversion to wind-cold, fever, fainting, convulsion, numbness, unfixed diseased location, etc.

Wind Arthralgia

A type of arthralgia.
Symptoms. Heaviness and pain of the body, the spasm of limbs, migratory arthralgia, or numbness of limbs, etc.
Pathogenesis. The stagnation of qi and blood due to the invasion of pathogenic wind-cold-dampness into meridians and collaterals, joints and muscles.
Therapeutic Principle. Expelling wind, clearing away cold and eliminating dampness, activating collaterals and arresting pain.

Wind-cold

1. It refers to the wind and cold combined as a pathogenic factor.
2. Syndrome caused by attack of wind and cold in combination, clinically shows severe aversion to cold, light fever, headache, pain all over the body, stuffy and running nose.

Wind-cold Asthma

A type of asthma.
Symptoms. Headache, ache all over, aversion to cold, no sweat, cough and asthma with rale, tachypnea and raucous breathing, etc.
Pathogenesis. The superficial stagnation of wind-cold which accumulates in the lung.
Therapeutic Principle. Expelling wind, removing cold and relieving asthma.

Wind-cold Attack of Lung

Symptoms. Stuffy nose, sneezing, profuse watery nasal discharge, headache, anhidrosis, aversion to cold with light fever.
Pathogenesis. Invasion of the skin muscles and the lungs by wind-cold pathogens which affects the lung's function of dispersing defending qi.
Therapeutic Principle. Expelling cold with the warm pungent as well as relieving the exterior syndrome and promoting the dispersing function of the lung.

Wind-cold Cough

Symptoms. Cough with whitish thin sputum, stuffy running nose, aversion to cold, or headache, aching pain of joints, fever with anhidrosis.

Pathogenesis. The invasion of wind-cold into the lung, the failure of lung-qi to disperse.

Therapeutic Principle. Expelling wind-cold and releasing the lung-qi.

Wind-cold Edema

Symptoms. Fever with aversion to cold, edema of both the head and body, perspiration due to pathogenic wind domination or anhidrosis due to pathogenic cold domination.

Pathogenesis. Exterior deficiency, pulmonary heat, cold attack of the body surface with stagnation forming inside.

Therapeutic Principle. Expelling wind and cold, relieving exterior syndrome and inducing diuresis.

Wind-cold Headache

Symptoms. Headache extending to the nape and back, aversion to wind and cold, soreness and pain in joints, stuffy and running nose, etc.

Pathogenesis. The invasion of external wind-cold.

Therapeutic Principle. Expelling wind and removing cold.

Wind-cold Lumbago

Symptoms. Lumbago with stiff lumbar vertebra, or the leg and knee pain, the alternate attacks of chills and fever, cold sensation of the lumbar region.

Pathogenesis. Invasion of wind-cold into the lumbar region.

Therapeutic Principle. Expelling wind and removing cold.

Wind-cold Type Common Cold

Symptoms. Fever, aversion to cold, stuffy nose and watery nasal discharge, cough, headache and pain of the body, etc.

Pathogenesis. Invasion of wind-cold.

Therapeutic Principle. Relieving exterior syndrome and expelling cold.

Wind Convulsion

Symptoms. Superduction, opisthotonus, trembling switching limbs, fever at night, general itching, etc.

Pathogenesis. The liver fire and phlegm stagnancy due to wind movement.

Therapeutic Principle. Relieving the liver, calming endopathic wind and causing vomiting endopathic wind phlegm.

Wind-dampness Headache

Symptoms. Headache, heaviness of the body and limbs, chest fullness, abdominal distention, nausea, anorexia, dryness of the mouth without thirst.

Pathogenesis. The invasion and upper covering of pathogenic wind.

Therapeutic Principle. Expelling wind and subduing dampness.

Wind Diarrhea

Symptoms. Headache, fever, aversion to wind, spontaneous sweating, watery diarrhea, or indigestion of foodstuff, hematochezia, etc.

Pathogenesis. Wind invading intestines and stomach.

Therapeutic Principle. Expelling wind and inducing diarrhea, and promoting the function of spleen and stomach.

Wind-dryness

Symptoms. Headache, fever and chills, anhidrosis, stuffy nose, dry throat and lips, dry skin, dry cough, chest and hypochondrium pain.

Pathogenesis. The combination of wind with dryness. It usually occurs in dry autumn.

Therapeutic Principle. Relieving exterior syndrome and moistening dryness.

Wind Dysentery

Symptoms. Blood or blood clots in stool diarrhea, aversion to cold, stuffy nose, painful body with dark color, watery stool, diarrhea followed by dysentery, etc.

Pathogenesis. Pathogenic wind injuring the spleen and stomach.

Therapeutic Principle. Expelling wind and clearing the intestines and promoting the circulation of qi and blood.

Wind Edema

Symptoms. Sudden onset, fever with aversion to wind, edema of the face and limbs, joint pain, dysuria.

Pathogenesis. The invasion of pathogenic wind into the skin, the failure of lung-qi to dredge water passages and the retention of water-dampness which spreads over the skin.

Therapeutic Principle. Dispelling wind, releasing the lung and inducing diuresis.

Wind-fire Rotating Inside

It refers to pathological mechanism of occurrence of wind syndrome in case of excessive heat. If excessive heat occurs in the Liver Meridian, with fire and wind stirring up each other, a rapid and taut pulse will occur, even spasm of hand and foot.

Wind-fire Toxin

Symptoms. Local pain, numbness, reddish swelling, local necrosis with dark color, fever, headache and jaundice. In the severe case, heart failure and apnea may appear.

Pathogenesis. A pathogenic toxin coming from poisonous snake bite, the effect of the combination of neuro-toxin and blood circulating toxin. It mainly paralyses muscles and respiratory muscle. It produces many kinds of toxic actions on cardiopathy and blood circulation system.

Therapeutic Principle. Promoting blood circulation to dispel wind, removing heat from the blood, bandaging, expelling of toxin, and detoxicating. In the case of heart failure and respiratory failure, it is necessary to carry out emergency treatment.

Wind-flushed Face

Symptoms. Flushed and itching face at the beginning, followed by the burning and swelling.

Pathogenesis. Caused by the ascending of blood and qi, and the affection of wind-heat, which are stagnated in the muscle and skin.

Therapeutic Principle. Clearing pathogenic heat from blood and detoxation.

Wind from Bowels

Symptoms. Gas existing in intestines, usually eliminated from anus.

Pathogenesis. Dryness evil gathering in the stomach and intestine, insufficiency of body fluid in intestinal track, accumulation of stercoroma in the interior, and indigestion due to deficiency of the spleen.

Therapeutic Principle. Clearing away dryness-heat, smoothing visceral function and strengthening both spleen and stomach.

Wind-heat Attack of Lung

Symptoms. Aversion to cold and running a fever, cough, yellow and thick sputum difficult to be coughed out, red tongue, throat sore, dry mouth and thirst, and in the severe case, asthma, and restlessness.

Pathogenesis. The lung fails to dominate both dispersing and descending resulting from exopathogen of wind-heat or heat transmission of wind-cold.

Wind-heat Cough

Symptoms. Cough with sticky phlegm, fever, perspiration and aversion to wind, yellowish nasal discharge, dry mouth and sore throat, thin yellowish fur.

Pathogenesis. The invasion of pathogenic wind-heat into the lung, the impairment of purifying and descending function of the lung.

Therapeutic Principle. Expelling wind, clearing away heat and promoting the lung-qi.

Wind-heat Deafness

A type of deafness.

Symptoms. Deafness, tinnitus, headache and stuffy nose, etc.

Pathogenesis. The attack of pathogenic wind-heat on meridians and collaterals, the disturbance of upper orifices.

Therapeutic Principle. Dispelling wind and clearing away heat, opening orifices with aromatic drugs.

Wind-heat Headache

Symptoms. Distending pain in the head, fever with aversion to wind, or stuffy running nose, conjunctivitis and flushed face, thirst, constipation and dark urine.

Pathogenesis. The attack of pathogenic wind and heat on the upper-energizer.

Therapeutic Principle. Expelling wind and clearing away heat.

Wind-heat Lumbago

Symptoms. Lumbago and stiffness with foot and knee involved, thirst.

Pathogenesis. Invasion of pathogenic wind-heat into the Kidney Meridian.

Therapeutic Principle. Expelling wind and clearing away heat.

Wind-heat Pathogen

Symptoms. Epidemic fever, slight chill, cough, thirst, redness along the tongue margin, yellowish and thin coating of the tongue, dry mouth, bloodshot eye, sorethroat. The disease usually occurs in winter or spring.

Pathogenesis. The wind and the heat are combined as a pathogenic factor.

Wind of Deficiency Type

Symptoms. Dizziness, tremor, or wringing of hands and feet, syncope, etc.

Pathogenesis. Deficiency of blood and deficiency of yin.

Therapeutic Principle. Nourishing yin to calm the endopathic wind.

Wind-phlegm Headache

Symptoms. Headache, vertigo, with tendency to close eyes, heaviness and tiredness of the body, chest fullness, nausea, or greenish-yellow cheeks and sticky sputum, etc.

Pathogenesis. The disturbance of upper orifices by wind pathogen together with phlegm.

Therapeutic Principle. Dissipating wind, eliminating phlegm and opening orifices.

Wind-phlegm Vertigo

Symptoms. Dizziness, headache, the contracture of the shoulder and back, heaviness of the body, somnolence, chest tightness, palpitation, vomiting and sticky sputum, etc.

Pathogenesis. The upper accumulation of wind-phlegm, the obstruction of lucid yang.

Therapeutic Principle. Dispelling wind and dissipating phlegm; clearing obstruction in the meridians to relieve convulsion if such symptoms appear as vertigo, annoyance, paralysis, convulsion etc.

Wind Stagnation

Symptoms. Headache, stiffness of the nape and back, numbness of the skin, stuffy nose, heaviness sensation in the limbs, and high fever with chilliness.

Pathogenesis. The invasion of pathogenic wind.

Therapeutic Principle. Dispelling the wind evil.

Wind Stirring Inside

Symptoms. Vertigo, convulsion, coma, facial distortion, and involuntary staring.

Pathogenesis. Dysfunction of the zang-fu organs, qi and blood disorder and malnutrition of muscles.

Wind-syndrome Caused by Hyperactivity of Liver-yang

Symptoms. Dizziness, headache, numbness of limbs, trembling of hands and feet, even sudden syncope, unconsciousness, facial hemiparalysis and hemiplegia.

Pathogenesis. Hepatic and renal yin deficiency and failure of restriction the reversed excessive liver-yang.

Therapeutic Principle. Calming the liver, and suppressing yang hyperactivity of the liver to relieve wind.

Wind Syndrome Resulting from hepatic stagnation Depression

Symptoms. Vertigo, tremor, numbness of the extremities, convulsion, etc.

Pathogenesis. The liver depression causes heat and fire syndrome which exhausts the liver blood resulting in the various wind symptoms.

Wind-toxin in Toe

Symptoms. The affected toe is unbearably, severely painful. In the severe case, aversion to cold, high fever, aching pain of limbs, later, projecting pterygium, pain like being cut, etc.

Pathogenesis. External attacking of pathogenic toxins or local infection of toxins.

Therapeutic Principle. Clearing away heat, detoxication, subduing swelling and dissipate stasis.

Wind-transmission

Severe damage of the blood and essence in the course of febrile disease may result in pathogenic wind.

Symptoms. Vertigo, tremor, convulsion and rigidity of limbs and even sudden faint.

Wind Type Epilepsy

1. **Symptoms.** Shaking of hand and foot, fever and clonic convulsion, lockjaw with shaking head, excessive flow of saliva and unconsciousness, etc.

   Pathogenesis. The original deficiency, heat retention, the invasion of pathogenic wind, or the heat of the Liver Meridian.

   Therapeutic Principle. Enriching blood, nourishing the liver and relaxing muscles and tendons.

2. **Symptoms.** The edema of the body and face, or aphasia secondary to epilepsy.

   Pathogenesis. The deficiency of qi and blood, the incomplete elimination of heat, or the stagnation of wind-cold in the collaterals of the heart.

   Therapeutic Principle. Tonifying qi and blood, clearing the remained heat, or dissipating the pathogen.

3. It refers to the clonic convulsion caused by the invasion of pathogenic wind.

   Therapeutic Principle. Dispelling wind and relieving convulsion.

4. **Symptoms.** The disability of the hand and foot just like paralysis. The deviation of the eyes and mouth.

   Pathogenesis. The invasion of pathogenic wind into collaterals when they are empty.

   Therapeutic Principle. Nourishing blood, dispelling wind and relieving obstruction in the collaterals.

Wind Type Syncope

1. **Symptoms.** Fever, spontaneous perspiration, restlessness, no relief of restlessness though spontaneous sweating.

   Pathogenesis. Wind pathogen affecting Taiyang, Shaoyin being involved, then reversed flow of qi in Shaoyin.

2. **Symptoms.** Pain in back, frequent eructation and yawn, etc.

   Pathogenesis. Wind invading the stomach and upward adverse flow of the liver-qi.

3. **Symptoms.** Spontaneous perspiration.

   Pathogenesis. Interior adverse flow of qi due to striae of skin being loose and affection by wind pathogen.

Wind Vertigo

Symptoms. The vertigo, usually accompanied by spontaneous perspiration with aversion to wind.

Pathogenesis. Wind pathogen.

Therapeutic Principle. Dissipating wind.

Wind-warm

1. It refers to the wind and warm combined as a pathogenic factor occurring usually in winter and spring.
2. Syndrome caused by wind-warm pathogen referring to fever, cough and excessive thirst etc.

Wind-warm Convulsion

It refers to an acute febrile disease, usually found in children.

Therapeutic Principle. In the mild case, the wind and warm pathogenic factor is attacking superficially. Relieving the exterior syndrome with drugs pungent in flavor and cool in property. For impairment of consciousness and delirium, clearing heat from the heart to restore consciousness.

Wind-warm Cough

Symptoms. Choking cough, aphonia, head distention and sore throat, etc.

Pathogenesis. The invasion of wind-warm pathogen into the lung.

Therapeutic Principle. Expelling the pathogenic factor with drugs of mild action and cool property.

Wind-weed Rhizome   ✿ W-4

It is the rhizome of Anemarrhena asphodeloides Bge. (Liliaceae).

Effect. Clearing away heat, purging fire, replenishing yin essence and moistening the viscera.

Indication. Epidemic febrile diseases with high fever, excessive thirst; toothache due to the stomach fire, cough due to the lung-heat, dry cough due to deficiency of yin, hyperactivity, night sweat, diabetes, constipation.

Wine

A kind of Chinese medicine drink, made from rice, wheat, millet, sorghum and others from leaves.

Effect. Promoting blood circulation, preventing pathogenic cold, and helping drugs to take effect quickly and fully.

Indication. Chronic rheumatism due to wind-cold, muscular spasm, obstruction of qi in the chest and pain due to abdominal cold.

Wingystem Veronicastrum Herb

It is the whole herb of Veronicastrum cauloptera (Hance) Yamazaki (Scrophulariaceae).

Effect. Clearing away heat, detoxicating, subduing swelling, promoting regeneration of the tissue and resting pain.

Indication. Dysentery, sore throat, acute conjunctivitis, carbuncles, skin ulceration, eczema and scalds.

Winter Daphne Flower

A kind of chinese medicine. It is the flower of Daphne odora Thunb. (Thymelaeaceae).

Effect. Dispelling pathogenic wind and arresting pain.

Indication. Swollen and sore throat, toothache and rheumatalgia.

Wintersweet

It is the flower bud of Chimonanthus praecox (L.) Link.

Effect. Relieving summer-heat and promoting the production of the body fluid.

Indication. Polydipsia due to febrile disease, depression, hypochondriac and epigastric pain, globus hystericus, chest distress, cough scalds and burns.

Winter-warm Syndrome

A febrile-disease occurring in winter.

Symptoms. Headache, anhidrosis, fever, cough and pharynx pain.

Therapeutic Principle. Relieving the exterior syndrome with drugs pungent in flavor and cool in property.

Wiping Forehead

A massage method.

Operation. Rubbing the forehead with flat of the index, middle and ring finger of the right and left hand alternately till it feels

hot, or with the thumbs pressing the temples and the remaining four fingers lightly bent, rubbing the forehead from the middle to the frontal eminence with the radial side of the index fingers repeatedly.
Function. Tranquilizing the mind.
Indication. Insomnia, dreaminess and forgetfulness.

Wiping Manipulation

A massage method.
Operation. Rub the skin of the affected part up and down or right and left with the whorled surface of one or two thumbs.
Function. Regulating the circulation of qi and promoting the blood circulation.
Indication. Dizziness, headache, stiffness and pain of the nape, etc.

Withdrawing

An acupuncture point method, referring to the method of withdrawing the needle.
Operation. Lift the needle slowly from the deep portion to the subcutaneous portion, retain it until qi gets unhurried and withdraw it quickly when doctor feels no tension and dragging sensation around the needle.

Withered Bone and Reduced Marrow

Symptoms. Lassitude loin and knee, difficulty in standing upright, atrophic and flaccid muscles of the lower limbs.
Pathogenesis. High fever burning yin fluid, overwork for a long time, insufficiency of the kidney-essence, flaming of the kidney fire, and inability to promote essence and produce marrow.

Wolfberry Fruit   ✿ **W-5**

It is the ripe fruit of Lycium barbarum L. (Solanacecae).
Effect. Tonifying the liver and kidney, nourishing the vital essence, improving eyesight and moistening the lung.
Indication. Dizziness, blurred vision, ringing in the ear, hypopsia, soreness of the

loins, weakness of the knees, spermatorrhea, diabetes, phthisic cough due to yin deficiency, etc.

Wolf's Mile Herb

It is the whole herb of Euphorbia humifusa Willd. (Euphobiaceae).
Effect. Clearing away heat, cooling blood, detoxicating, arresting bleeding, activating blood, inducing diuresis and subduing inflammation.
Indication. Dysentery due to noxious heat, diphtheria, pharyngitis, infantile dyspepsia, enteritis, subcutaneous swelling, snake bite, jaundice, hemafecia, hematuria, uterus bleeding traumatic injuries, etc.

Wood Restricting Earth

1. The liver and spleen physiology is expounded in accordance with the wood and earth properties in the theory of TCM. According to the theory of the fire elements, the liver restricts the spleen.
2. Pathologically, hyperfunction of the liver (wood) may affect the physiological function of the spleen and stomach.

Wrenching Manipulation

A massage method.
Operation. Pinch the skin with the fingers and wrench it repeatedly so that the local skin gets dark red. It is often applied to the shoulder, neck, wrist, and back.
Function. Eliminating pathogenic wind.
Indication. Stagnation of the shoulder-nape and waist-back.

Wringing Manipulation

A massage method.
Operation. Grip the skin of the affected part, pulling and releasing, with the flexed index and middle finger, or the thumb and flexed middle finger, which are opened like pincers. To cause local congestion until the skin turns red and purple.
Function. Expelling wind and eliminating cold, decreasing fever and relieving pain.

Indication. Heat stroke, affections due to pathogenic wind and cold, car sickness and sea sickness.

Wrinkled Giant Hyssop Herb
⊛ W-6

It is the above-ground part of Agastache rugosa (Fisch. et Mey.) O. Ktze. (Labiatae).
Effect. Removing dampness, relieving summer-heat and arresting vomiting.
Indication. The disturbance of middle-energizer due to accumulation of dampness, anorexia, nausea and vomiting and damp-warm syndrome in the summer.

Wrist (MA-SF 2)

An auricular point.
Location. On the 2nd from top to bottom of the six equal parts of the scapha area.
Indication. Diseases of the wrist and stomachache.

Wrist-Ankle Needling

It refers to the method of puncturing the six specific points above the joint of wrist or ankle in order to treat diseases.
Location. Two transverse fingers breadth to the upper wrist and upper ankle, and applicable for diseases on every part of the body.
Indication. Functional disorders and neuralgia.
Method. Puncture subcutaneously towards the upper 1.4 cun. It is unnecessary for the needling feeling to appear. Retain the needle in the point for more than half and hour.

Wry Mouth

It refers to the symptom of mouth deviating to one side.
Pathogenesis. The blockage of meridians by pathogenic wind and phlegm.

Wry Tongue

It refers to the tongue deviating to one side while stuck out.
Pathogenesis. Up-stirring of liver or an attack of the meridians by pathogenic wind.

The tongue picture occurs simultaneously with facial hemiparalysis or hemiplegia. Usually seen in apoplexy.

Wuchu (B 5)

An acupuncture point.
Location. On the head, 1 cun directly superior and 1.5 cun lateral to Shangxing (GV 23).
Indication. Headache, dizziness, blurred vision, stuffy nose, epistaxis, infantile convulsion, epilepsy, etc.
Method. Puncture subcutaneously 0.3-0.5 cun and apply moxibustion to the point with 1-3 units of moxa cones or for 3-5 minutes.

Wuhu (Ex-UE)

An extra acupuncture point.
Location. On the dorsum of the hand, at the highest points of the 2nd and 4th metacarpal bones at their small ends.
Indication. Finger muscular contructure.
Method. Apply moxibustion to the point with 3-5 moxa cones.

Wujingwen

A massage point.
Location. On the cross striation of the interphalangeal joints in the distal ends of the thumb, index, middle, ring and little finger on the palm.
Operation. Pushing method.
Indication. Abdominal distention, alternate attacks of chills and fever, etc.

Wushu (G 27)

A meridian acupuncture point.
Location. On the lateral side of the abdomen, anterior to the anteriosuperior iliac spine, 3 cun below the level of the umbilicus.
Indication. Prolapse of uterus, leukorrhea with reddish discharge, irregular menstruation, hernia, pain in the lower abdomen, constipation, lumbosacral pain.
Method. Puncture perpendicularly 1-1.5 cun and apply moxibustion to the point

with 3-5 units of moxa cones or for 5-10 minutes.

Wuyi (S 15)

An acupuncture point point.

Location. In the thoracic region, in the second intercostal space, 4 cun to Zigong (CV 19) at the anterior median line.

Indication. Cough with dyspnea, thoracic and hypochondriac pain, spitting of pus and blood, acute mastitis, etc.

Method. Puncture perpendicularly 0.2-0.3 cun, or obliquely 0.3-0.5 cun and apply moxibustion to the point with 3-5 units of moxa cones or for 5-10 minutes.

Wuzhijie

A massage point.

Location. At the first articulations of the five fingers on the dorsum of the hand.

Operation. Nipping and kneading manipulations.

Function. Calming convulsion and tranquilizing the mind, eliminating the phlegm and activating meridians.

Indication. Infantile convulsion, cough with dyspnea, chest distress, restlessness.

X

Xenophthalmia

Symptoms. Dryness and uneasy feeling of the eye, presence of foreign objects in the eye. It is mostly accompanied with photophobia, lacrimation, conjunctival congestion with itching and pain.

Pathogenesis. Wind-heat, liver-fire, hyperactivity of fire due to yin deficiency, or introduction of foreign bodies into the eye.

Xiabai (L 4)

An acupuncture point.

Location. On the internal side of the arm, at the radial border of the brachial biceps of the arm, 4 cun inferior to the end of the anterior axillary crease; or 1 cun directly below Tianfu (L 3) transverse crease.

Indication. Cough, vexation, dyspnea, cardialgia, dysphoria with fullness sensation, epistaxis, and pain of external side of forearm.

Method. Puncture perpendicularly 0.5-1 cun and apply moxibustion to the point with 3-5 units of moxa cones or for 5-10 minutes.

Xiachengjiang (Ex-HN)

An extra acupuncture point.

Location. 1 cun lateral to Chengjiang (CV 24), at the mental foramen of the mandible.

Indication. Jaundice, facial paralysis, toothache, deep-rooted sore at the mouth and lips, ulceration of the gums, prosopalgia.

Method. Puncture perpendicularly 0.3-0.5 cun.

Xiaguan (S 7)

Location. On the face, anterior to the ear, in the depression between the zygomatic arch and mandibular notch. The point is located when the mouth is closed.

Indication. Toothache, facial pain, deafness, lockjaw and loosening of temporomandibular joint, deviation of the mouth and eye, dizziness.

Method. Puncture perpendicularly 0.3-0.5 cun, or subcutaneously 0.5-1 cun. Apply moxibustion to the point for 5-10 minutes. Close the mouth while the point is being selected.

Xiajishu (Ex-B 5)

An extra acupuncture point.

Location. On the low back and on the posterior midline, below the spinous process of the 3rd lumbar vertebra.

Indication. Abdominal pain, lumbago, diarrhea, cystitis and enteritis.

Method. Puncture obliquely 0.5-1.0 cun. Apply moxibustion 3-7 moxa cones or 5-15 minutes with warming moxibustion.

Xiajuxu (S 39)

A meridian acupuncture point.

Location. On the anterior lateral side of the leg, 3 cun below Shangjuxu (S 37), one middle finger breadth, from the anterior crest of the tibia.

Indication. Lower abdominal pain, breast abscess, impairment pain and paralysis of the lower extremities, diarrhea bloody and mucous stool.

Method. Puncture perpendicularly 0.5-1.0 cun. Apply moxibustion 5-7 moxa cones or 5-15 minutes with warming moxibustion.

Xiakunlun

An extra acupuncture point.

Location. Anterior to the achilles tendon, 1 cun inferior to the tip of the exterior malleolus.

Indication. Arthralgia due to cold, lumbago, migraine, hemiplegia and heaviness and pain in the foot.

Method. Puncture perpendicularly 0.3-0.5 cun. Apply moxibustion 5-7 moxa cones or 10-15 minutes with warming moxibustion.

Xialian (LI 8)

An acupuncture point.

Location. On the upper radial segment of the back of the forearm, 4 cun inferior to the cross striation of the elbow on the connecting line between Yangxi (LI 5) and Quchi (LI 11).

Indication. Headache, dizziness, abdominalgia, sore elbow and brachialgia.

Method. Puncture perpendicularly 0.5-1 cun and apply moxibustion to the point with 3-5 units of moxa cones or for 5-10 minutes.

Xialiao (B 34)

An acupuncture point.

Location. On the 4th posterior sacral foramen of the sacral region.

Indication. Abdominalgia, constipation, dysuria, morbid leukorrhea and lumbago.

Method. Puncture perpendicularly 1-1.5 cun and apply moxibustion to the point with 5-7 units of moxa cones or for 5-15 minutes.

Xiangqiangxue

An extra acupuncture point.

Location. On the dorsal aspect of the hand, in the depression posterior to the 2nd and 3rd metacarpophalangeal articulations.

Indication. Stiffness of the nape.

Method. Puncture 0.5-0.8 cun perpendicularly.

Xiangu (S 43)

An acupuncture point.

Location. On the dorsum of the foot, in the excavation inferior to the junction between the second and third metatarsal bones.

Indication. Facial edema, painful chest and hypochondrium, redness and swelling and pain of the eyes, borborygmus with diarrhea, abdominal distention, swelling and pain of dorsum of foot, febrile disease, etc.

Method. Puncture perpendicularly 0.3-0.5 cun and apply moxibustion to the point with 3-7 units of moxa cones or for 5-15 minutes.

Xiaochangshu (B 27)

An acupuncture point.

Location. In the sacral region, 1.5 cun to the sacral median line and parallel to the first posterior sacral foramen.

Indication. Abdominal pain, diarrhea, dysentery, hematuria, hemorrhoid, seminal emission, morbid leukorrhea.

Method. Puncture perpendicularly or obliquely 0.8-1.2 cun and apply moxibustion to the point with 3-7 units of moxa cones or for 5-15 minutes.

Xiaoerjixiongxue (Ex-CA)

An extra acupuncture point.

Location. On the intercostal depressions between each two ribs of the 2nd, 3rd and 4th ribs, 2.5 cun lateral to the anterior midline, six points in all on both sides.

Indication. Pigeon chest in children.

Method. Apply moxibustion 3 moxa cones or 5-10 minutes with warming moxibustion.

Xiaoershixian (Ex-CA)

An extra acupuncture point.

Location. On the upper abdomen, 7.5 cun above the umbilicus, on the anterior midline.

Indication. Infantile epilepsy.

Method. Apply moxibustion 3-5 moxa cones or 5-10 minutes with warming moxibustion.

Xiaoershuijing (Ex-UE)

An extra acupuncture point.

Location. 0.3 cun directly above the radial end of the transverse crease of the elbow.

Indication. Infantile fright during sleep, pain in the elbow and arm, etc.

Method. Apply moxibustion 1-3 moxa cones or 3-5 minutes with warming moxibustion.

Xiaogukong (Ex-UE 6)

An extra acupuncture point.

Location. At the center of the proximal interphalangeal joint on the dorsal side of the little finger.

Indication. Ophthalmaphthy, deafness, inflammation of the throat and pain in the finger.

Method. Apply moxibustion to the point with 3-5 moxa cones.

Xiaohai (SI 8)

An acupuncture point.

Location. The elbow bent. In the excavation between olecranon and the medial epicondyle of the humerus.

Indication. Swelling of the cheek, pain in the nape, headache, tinnitus and scrofula.

Method. Puncture perpendicularly 0.3-0.5 cun and apply moxibustion to the point for 5-10 minutes.

Xiaohengwen

A massage point.

Location. At the cross striation of metacarpophalangeal joints of the index, middle, ring and little finger on the palm.

Operation. Pushing and nipping manipulations are mostly used.

Function. Reducing fever, relieving distention, dissipating blood stasis and stagnancy.

Indication. Aphthae, abdominal distention, chapped lips.

Xiaoli (Ex-B)

An extra acupuncture point.

Location. On the back. Take the perimeter of the neck at the position level to the Adam's Apple, measure from Dazhui (GV 14) straight down to the point at the further end of the length and 0.5 cun lateral to it.

Indication. Scrofula.

Method. Moxibustion.

Xiaoluo (TE 12)

An acupuncture point.

Location. On the lateral side of the arm, at the middle on the connecting line between Qinglengyuan (TE 11) and Naohui (TE 13), 3 cun above Qinglengyuan.

Indication. Headache, dizziness, rigid nape, toothache, pain of shoulder and back.

Method. Puncture perpendicularly 0.8-1.2 cun and apply moxibustion to the point with 3-7 units of moxa cones or for 5-15 minutes.

Xiaotianxin (Ex-UE)

An extra acupuncture point.

Location. At the midpoint of the junction between the big thenar eminence and small thenar eminence on the palmar side.

Indication. Infantile convulsion and spasm, high fever and coma, dark urine and dysuria, angina pectoris, and rheumatic heart disease.

Method. Puncture perpendicularly 0.3-0.5 cun.

Xiaozhijian (Ex-LE)

An extra acupuncture point.

Location. At the tip of the little toe, two points on both feet.

Indication. Headache, dizziness and diabetes.

Method. Puncture 0.1-0.2 cun with a filiform needle. Moxibustion is applicable.

Xiaozhijian (Ex-UE)

An extra acupuncture point.

Location. At the tip of the little finger, two points on both hands.

Indication. Jaundice, swelling of the scrotum, diabetes and whooping cough.

Method. Puncture perpendicularly 0.1-0.2 cun. Apply moxibustion 3-7 moxa cones.

Xiaozhizhaowen (Ex-UE)

An extra acupuncture point.

Location. On the dorsal aspect of the little finger, at the root of the nail, two points on both hands.

Indication. Inflammation of the throat.

Method. Prick to cause little bleeding.

Xiashangxing (Ex-HN)

An extra acupuncture point.

Location. 3 cun lateral to the place, 1 cun posterior to the anterior hairline of the head.

Indication. Nasal polyp.

Method. Moxibustion.

Xiawan (CV 10)

An acupuncture point.

Location. At the middle of the abdomen 2 cun above the umbilicus.

Indication. Abdominal pain and distention, diarrhea vomiting, lump glomus.

Method. Puncture perpendicularly 1-1.5 cun and apply moxibustion to the point with 3-7 moxa cones or for 10-15 minutes.

Xiaxi (G 43)

An acupuncture point.

Location. On the external side of the dorsum of the foot, between the 4th and 5th toe, at the junction between the reddish and whitish skin posterior to the border of the digital web.

Indication. Headache, dizziness, deafness, blood-shot eyes, swelling and pain of hypochondrium, hip, knee and dorsum of foot.

Method. Puncture Perpendicularly 0.3-0.5 cun and apply moxibustion to the point with 1-3 units of moxa cones of for 3-5 minutes.

Xiayao (Ex-B)

An extra acupuncture point.

Location. On the sacral region, in the depression between the 2nd and 3rd sacral crest.

Indication. Chronic enteritis, chronic dysentery, and difficult labor, etc.

Method. Apply moxibustion 3-5 moxa cones or 5-10 minutes with warming moxibustion.

Xielei

A massage point.

Location. On the way from both axillae to the Tianshu (S 25).

Operation. Foulage and rub manipulation.

Function. Regulating qi, dissipating phlegm, dispelling stuffiness in the chest and dissipating mass in the abdomen.

Indication. Chest distress, cough with asthma, infantile malnutrition, hepatosplenomegaly.

Xietang (Ex-CA)

An extra acupuncture point.

Location. On the side of chest, in the depression 2.0 cun below the armpit.

Indication. Endocarditis, fullness in the chest and hypochondrium, dyspnea, liver diseases and pleuritis.

Method. Apply moxibustion 3-5 moxa cones or 5-10 minutes with warming moxibustion.

Xiguan (Liv 7)

A meridian acupuncture point.

Location. On the medial side of the leg, posterior and inferior to the medial epicondyle of the tibia, 1 cun posterior to Yinlingquan(S 9), at the upper end of the medial head of the gastrocnemius muscle.

Indication. Swelling and pain of the knee joint, disturbance due to pathogenic cold and dampness, severe and migratory arthralgia, flaccidity and numbness of legs.

Method. Puncture perpendicularly 0.8-1.0 cun. Apply moxibustion 3-5 moxa cones or 5-10 minutes with warming moxibustion.

Ximen (P 4)

An acupuncture point.

Location. On the palmar side of the forearm, on the connecting line between Quze (LI 11) and Daling (P 7), 5 cun superior to the transverse crease of the wrist.

Indication. Cardialgia, palpitation, epistaxis, vomiting of blood, furuncle and hemorrhoid.

Method. Puncture perpendicularly 0.8-1.2 cun. Apply moxibustion 3-5 moxa cones or for 5-10 minutes.

Xingjian (Liv 2)

A meridian acupuncture point.

Location. On the instep of the foot, between the 1st and 2nd toe, at the junction of the red and white skin proximal to the margin of the web.

Indication. Profuse menstruation, amenorrhea, dysmenorrhea, leukorrhagia, vaginal pain, enuresis, stranguria, hernia, pain and fullness in the chest and hypochondrium, cough, diarrhea, headache, dizziness, optic atrophy, apoplexy, epilepsy, insomnia, swelling knee, swelling and pain on the back of foot.

Method. Puncture perpendicularly 0.5-0.8 cun. Apply moxibustion 3-5 moxa cones or 5-10 minutes with warming moxibustion.

Xinglong (Ex-CA)

An extra acupuncture point.

Location. On the upper abdomen, 1 cun above the umbilicus and 1 cun lateral to the Shuifen (CV 9).

Indication. Cold feeling in the heart, mass accumulated due to uprising attack of qi.

Method. Puncture perpendicularly 0.5-1.0 cun. Apply moxibustion 3-5 moxa cones or 5-10 minutes with warming moxibustion.

Xinhui (GV 22)

An acupuncture point.

Location. On the head, 2 cun directly above midpoint of the anterior hairline, 3 cun anterior to Baihui (GV 20).

Indication. Headache, dizziness, rhinorrhea, rhinalgia, rhinophyma, epilepsy, infantile convulsion, etc.

Method. Puncture subcutaneously 0.3-0.5 cun and apply moxibustion to the point for 5-10 minutes or 3-5 units of moxa cones.

Xinshe (Ex-HN)

A meridian acupuncture point.

Location. On the nape, on the lateral border of the trapezius muscle, 1.5 cun below the posterior hairline.

Indication. Occipital headache, rigid neck and back, stiff-neck, pain in the scapular area.

Method. Puncture perpendicularly 0.5-1.0 cun. Moxibustion is applicable.

Xinshu (B 15)

An acupuncture point.

Location. On the back, 1.5 cun lateral to the posterior midline, below the spinous process of the 5th thoracic vertebra.

Indication. Palpitation, cardialgia, cough, spitting of blood, insomnia, seminal emission, night sweating, psychosis and epilepsy.

Method. Puncture obliquely 0.5-0.8 cun and apply moxibustion 3-5 moxa cones or for 5-15 minutes.

Xiongtang (Ex-CA)

An extra acupuncture point.

Location. On the chest, between the two nipples, at the bilateral side of the sternum.

Indication. Cough, dyspnea, hemoptysis, palpitation, severe palpitation, pain in the breasts, etc.

Method. Apply moxibustion 3-5 moxa cones or 5-10 minutes with warming moxibustion.

Xiongtonggu (Ex-CA)

An extra acupuncture point.

Location. On the chest, 2 cun below the nipples.

Indication. Cardiac pain, hypochondriac and mastitis, etc.

Method. Moxibustion is applicable.

Xiongxiang (Sp 19)

An acupuncture point.

Location. On the lateral side of the chest, in the third intercostal space, 6 cun to the anterior median line.

Indication. Fullness and pain in the chest and hypochondriac region and pain radiating to the back, and cough with dyspnea.

Method. Puncture obliquely 0.3-0.5 cun and apply moxibustion to the point with 3-5 units of moxa cones or for 5-10 minutes.

Xipang (Ex-LE)

An extra acupuncture point.

Location. At both ends of the popliteal transverse crease, two points on each leg, four points in total for two legs.

Indication. Lumbar pain, soreness of the feet to stand for a long time.

Method. Puncture perpendicularly 0.5-1.0 cun. Apply moxibustion 3-5 moxa cones or 5-10 minutes with warming moxibustion.

Xi Points

A kind of name of the classified meridian acupuncture points, referring to the places where the meridian qi is deeply converged. Most of them are located below the elbow or knee. Each of the Twelve Regular Meridians and the Meridians of Yinqiao, Yangqiao, Yinwei and Yangwei has a Xi point, 16 in all. The Xi points are used in treating acute disorders in the clinic, e.g., for spitting blood Kongzui (L 6) is cooperated; for cardialgia Ximen (P 4) is cooperated.

Xishang (Ex-LE)

An extra acupuncture point.

Location. On the upper part of the knee, a pair of points located in the two depressions, lateral to the tendon of muscle,

rectus femoris, superior to the kneecap, four points in two legs.

Indication. Inflammation of the knee joint.

Method. Puncture perpendicularly 0.5 cun. Apply moxibustion 3-7 moxa cones or 5-15 minutes with warming moxibustion.

Xiwai (Ex-LE)

An extra acupuncture point.

Location. At the knee, at the end of the lateral aspect of the transverse crease of the cubital fossa, at the anterior edge of the biceps muscle.

Indication. Pain in the knee joint, ulcer of the lower limbs.

Method. Apply moxibustion for sores.

Xixia (Ex-LE)

An extra acupuncture point.

Location. At the knee, at the patellar ligament, at the lower edge of the tip of the patella.

Indication. Pain in the tibia.

Method. Apply moxibustion 1-3 moxa cones or 3-5 minutes with warming moxibustion.

Xiyan (Ex-LE 5)

An extra acupuncture point.

Location. A pair of points at the extensor side of the knee joint, in the two depressions lateral to the patellar ligament with the medial one called Neixiyan (Ex-LE 5), and the lateral one Waixiyan (Ex-LE 5), 4 points in total.

Indication. Knee pain, pain and heaviness in the leg and foot, beriberi, leg numbness.

Method. Puncture obliquely towards the knee joint 0.5-0.7 cun, or penetrate from Neixiyan to Waixiyan or vice versa.

Xiyangguan (G 33)

An acupuncture point.

Location. Lateral to the knee, 3 cun above Yanglingquan (G 34), in the depression of the external epicondyle of femur.

Indication. Swelling and pain in the knees, spasm of the popliteal muscle, numbness of the legs.
Method. Puncture perpendicularly 1.0-1.5 cun and apply moxibustion to the point for 5-15 minutes with moxa stick.

Xuan Edema

Symptoms. Edema of the head and face, even lower limps, sometimes accompanied by headache and dizziness, fever, little and unsmooth urine and stool, etc.
Pathogenesis. Attack of cold-damp of excessive fluid, which results in impairment of purifying and descending function of tri-energizer and overflow of fluid-dampness.
Therapeutic Principle. Soothing lung qi and inducing diuresis.

Xuanji (CV 21)

A meridian acupuncture point.
Location. On the chest and on the anterior midline, 1 cun below Tiantu (CV 22).
Indication. Cough, asthma, fullness and pain in the chest, inflammation of the throat, swelling of the throat, indigestion.
Method. Puncture subcutaneously 0.3-0.5 cun. Apply moxibustion to the point for 5-10 minutes or 3-5 units of moxa cones.

Xuanli (G 6)

An acupuncture point.
Location. At the temporal corner, at the crossing point of the lower 1/4 and upper 3/4 of the line, between Touwei (S 8) and Qubin(G 7).
Indication. Migraine, pain of the outer canthus, tinnitus, toothache, epilepsy, etc.
Method. Puncture subcutaneously 0.3-0.5 cun and apply moxibustion to the point for 3-5 minutes or 1-3 units of moxa cones.

Xuanlu (G 5)

A meridian acupuncture point, on the Gallbladder Meridians of Foot-shaoyang, the crossing point of Hand and Foot Shaoyang Meridian and Yangming Meridians.

Location. On the head, in the hair above the temples, at the midpoint of the curved line connecting Touwei (S 8) and Qubin (G 7).
Indication. Migraine, swelling of the face, pain in the outer canthus, toothache.
Method. Puncture subcutaneously 0.5-0.8 cun towards the posterior aspect. Apply moxibustion 1-3 moxa cones or 3-5 minutes with warming moxibustion.

Xuanming (Ex-HN)

An extra acupuncture point.
Location. At the midpoint of the frenum of the upper lip in the mouth.
Indication. Epilepsy, coma and delirium, and infantile convulsion, etc.
Method. Puncture perpendicularly 0.1-0.2 cun.

Xuanshu (GV 5)

An acupuncture point.
Location. Below the spinous process between the 1st and 2nd lumbar vertebra.
Indication. Stiffness and pain in the lumbar spine, abdominal pain and distention, dyspepsia, indigestion dysentery, proctoptosis.
Method. Puncture obliquely upward 0.5-1.0 cun and apply moxibustion to the point for 5-10 minutes or 3-5 units of moxa cones.

Xuanzhong (G 39)

A meridian acupuncture point.
Location. On the lateral side of the leg, 3 cun above the tip of the external malleolus, on the anterior border of the fibula.
Indication. Hemiplegia, stiffness and pain in the neck, fullness of the chest, abdominal distention, pain in the hypochondriac region, beriberi, and swelling below the axilla.
Method. Puncture perpendicularly 0.5-0.8 cun. Apply moxibustion to the point for 5-10 minutes or 3-5 units of moxa cones.

Xuehai (Sp 10)

A meridian acupuncture point.

Location. With the knee flexed, on the medial side of the thigh, 2 cun above the superior medial corner of the patella, on the prominence of the medial head of the quadriceps muscle of the thigh.

Indication. Irregular menstruation, metrorrhagia and metrostaxis, amenorrhea, dribbling of urine, urticaria and eczema, etc.

Method. Puncturing perpendicularly 1.0-1.5 cun. Apply moxibustion 3-5 moxa cones or 5-10 minutes with warming moxibustion.

Xuemen (Ex-CA)

An extra acupuncture point.

Location. On the upper abdomen, 4 cun above the umbilicus, 3 cun lateral to Zhongwan (CV 12).

Indication. Clots in the woman's abdomen, stomachache, indigestion and acute gastritis, etc.

Method. Puncture perpendicularly 0.5-1.0 cun. Apply moxibustion 3-5 moxa cones or 5-15 minutes with warming moxibustion.

Y

Yamen (GV 15)

An acupuncture point.

Location. At the posterior midline of the nape, 0.5 cun directly superior to the middle of the posterior hairline.

Indication. Dumbness, aphonia, psychosis, epilepsy, headache, rigid nape, epistaxis and swollen tongue.

Method. Puncture perpendicularly or obliquely downward 0.5-1 cun.

Notice. Deep or obliquely upward puncture is prohibited. Moxibustion is prohibited.

Yang

A theory in TCM. It refers to the male or positive principle, the active or functional aspect of an effective position, the things or properties opposite to those of yin. Yang and yin oppose and contain each other. As for the human body, the back and the lateral extremities are considered as yang. As for the zang-fu organs and meridians, six fu-organs and yang meridians are considered as yang.

Yang Aspect of Yin

A theory in TCM. It refers to that the yin may be subdivided into yang and yin, i.e. either yin or yang can be still divided into another pair of yin and yang, e.g. the back of the body is of yang nature and the front of the body is of yin nature, but in the front of the body, the chest is the yang aspect of yin and the abdomen is the yin aspect of yin, because they are in the upper and lower part respectively.

Yangbai (G 14)

An acupuncture point.

Location. On the forehead, when the patient looks straight forward, 1 cun superior to the eyebrow, directly above the pupil.

Indication. Headache, dizziness, rigidity and spasm of neck, irritated epiphora with tear, pain of outer canthus, tremor of eyelids.

Method. Puncture subcutaneously 0.3-0.5 cun and apply moxibustion to the point with 1-3 moxa cones or 3-5 minutes.

Yang Blood

Symptoms. Bleeding from the gum.

Pathogenesis. Excessive heat in interior of Yangming Meridian, abnormal flow of blood.

Therapeutic Principle. Clearing away heat from the stomach and promoting the production of the body fluid.

Yangchi (TE 4)

An acupuncture point.

Location. On the transverse crease of the dorsum of the wrist, in the depression on the ulnar side of the tendon of the common extensor muscle of the fingers.

Indication. Pain of wrist and shoulder, sore elbow, brachialgia, headache, epidemic acute conjunctivitis, deafness, rigid nape, dry mouth, and diabetes.

Method. Puncture perpendicularly 0.3-0.5 cun and apply moxibustion to the point with 3-5 units of moxa cones or for 5-10 minutes.

Yang Dampness

It is one type of damp-warm syndrome.

Symptoms. Chills and fever, persistent fever after sweating, heavy sensation of the body, joint pain, etc.

Pathogenesis. Disturbance of the exterior due to pathogenic dampness and change of dampness into heat.

Therapeutic Principle. Eliminating dampness and clearing away heat.

Yang Deficiency

Symptoms. Pale complexion, intolerance to cold and cold extremities, lassitude, loose stool, copious and clear urine.

Pathogenesis. Congenital defect, malnutrition due to improper diet, internal injury due to over-fatigue, or by chronic diseases leading to the damage of yang-qi.

Therapeutic Principle. Warming and recuperating the kidney-yang.

Yang deficiency of the Spleen and Kidney

Symptoms. Anasarca, chronic diarrhea before dawn, aching of the loins. Weakness of the knees and cold body, aversion to cold, etc.

Pathogenesis. Usually due to failure of the insufficient kidney yang to warm the spleen, the prolonged deficiency of spleen yang makes it unable to transport and transform the essence of food and water.

Therapeutic Principle. Warming and invigorating the spleen and kidney.

Yang Deficiency Syndrome

Symptoms. Pallor complexion, shortness of breath, intolerance of cold, cold limbs, loose bowels, mental fatigue and asthenia.

Pathogenesis. Caused by congenital defect, impairment of yang qi by chronic illness or severe diseases.

Therapeutic Principle. Warming yang and invigorating qi. For the severe syndrome, recuperating depleted yang, rescuing the patient from collapse.

Yang Depletion in Exogenous Febrile Disease

It refers to the yang depletion during the febrile disease.

Symptoms. Pale complexion, aversion to cold, drowsiness, spontaneous perspiration, cold limbs, etc.

Therapeutic Principle. Reviving yang and rescuing the patient from collapse.

Yang Deriving from Yin

A theory in TCM. It refers to the yang existing with yin as its prerequisite, e.g. yang fails to grow without yin. As for the human body, the production of yang-qi holding energy and dynamic force must be on the material basis of yin holding essence of life, blood, and body fluid.

Yang Edema

Symptoms. Edema appears on the eyelids or face first, then edema of limbs, abdomen, back and even the whole body.

Pathogenesis. Affection by pathogenic wind, retention of fluid and pathogenic dampness in the body and damp-heat, which lead to abevacuation of excessive fluid in the body and invasion of the skin.

Therapeutic Principle. Dispelling wind, promoting the dispersing function of the lung, clearing away heat and eliminating diuresis.

Yang Epilepsy

Symptoms. Convulsive seizures accompanied by fever, sweating, flushed face, trismus or crying, superduction of the eyes, shaking of the head, etc.

Therapeutic Principle. Using the drugs cold and cool in property.

Yang Excess

It refers to a pathogenic state in which the body is in an exuberance of yang.

Symptoms. High fever, sweating, dyspnea, restlessness, thirst, red tongue with yellow fur, etc.

Pathogenesis. Mostly caused by heat pathogens, fire transforming from five emotions in excess or stagnated qi, blood stasis, indigestion.

Yang Exhaustion

1. It refers to a pathogenic process.
   Symptoms. Prostration, profuse sweating, hallucination, illusion or other psychic disorders.
   Pathogenesis. Excessive consumption of yang-qi with preponderance of yin.
2. It refers to collapse of the male during or after sexual intercourse.

Yang Floating due to Yin Deficiency

Symptoms. Headache, dizziness, flushed face, heat sensation in the chest, palms and soles, afternoon fever, night sweat, hemoptysis, insomnia, dry and sore throat, nocturnal emission.

Pathogenesis. Deficiency of vital essence, blood or body fluid lead to breakdown of the equilibrium between yin and yang, failure of yin to restrict yang and floating up of yang-qi due to yin deficiency and consumption of the body fluid.

Yangfu (G 38)

An acupuncture point.

Location. 4 cun superior to the external malleolus, on the lateral side of the leg.

Indication. Migraine, sore throat, pain in the supraclavicular fossa, pain in inferior axilla, scrofula, chest and hypochondriac pain, pain of back and leg, beriberi, and malaria.

Method. Puncture perpendicularly 1-1.5 cun and apply moxibustion to the point with 3-5 moxa cones or for 5-10 minutes.

Yanggang (B 48)

An acupuncture point.

Location. 3 cun lateral to Zhongshu (GV 7) below the spinous process of the 10th thoracic vertebra.

Indication. Jaundice, borborygmus, diarrhea, abdominal pain, dysphagia and diabetes.

Method. Puncture obliquely 0.5-0.8 cun. Apply moxibustion to the point with 3-5 moxa cones or for 5-15 minutes.

Notice. Deep puncture is prohibited.

Yanggang (Ex-B)

An extra acupuncture point.

Location. 1 cun lateral to Mingmen (GV 4).

Indication. Diabetes, jaundice, hematochezia, hemorrhoid, lumbago, enuresis, emission.

Method. Puncture perpendicularly 0.5-1.0 cun. Apply moxibustion 3-7 moxa cones or 5-15 minutes with warming moxibustion.

Yanggu (SI 5)

An acupuncture point.

Location. On the ulnar border of the transverse crease of the wrist, in the depression between the ulnar styloid process and the triangular bone.

Indication. Headache, dizziness, deafness, toothache, swelling of the neck and jaw, rigid tongue, redness, swelling and pain of the eyes, hypochondriac, pain of lateral side of arm and wrist, ravings due to epilepsy, verruca from scabies.

Method. Puncture perpendicularly 0.3-0.5 cun and apply moxibustion to the point with 3-5 moxa cones for 5-10 minutes.

Yang Jaundice

Symptoms. Bright yellow coloration of the skin and eyes, fever, thirst, abdominal distention, vomiting, pain in the hypochondrium, impeded stool, scanty dark urine, etc.

Pathogenesis. Caused by the accumulation of pathogenic damp-heat steaming the liver and gallbladder, and leading to a disorder in the dispelling and purging functions and overflow of bile.

Therapeutic Principle. Clearing away heat, eliminating dampness and normalizing the function of the liver and gallbladder.

Yangjiao (G 35)

A meridian acupuncture point.

Location. On the lateral side of the leg, 7 cun above the tip of the external malleolus, on the posterior border of the fibula.

Indication. Distention, fullness and pain in the chest and hypochondrium, swollen face, mania, pain in the knee and thigh, flaccidity and numbness of the lower limbs.

Method. Puncture perpendicularly 1-1.5 cun and apply moxibustion to the point with 3-5 moxa cones or for 5-10 minutes.

Yang Kept Externally

Symptoms. The patient appearing with symptoms of interior true cold and exterior pseudo-heat, such as high body fever with preference for warmth, thirst but no desire for drinking water.

Pathogenesis. Excessive yin-cold in the body and floating-up of asthenic yang.

Therapeutic Principle. Clearing away heat with drugs cold in nature.

Yanglao (SI 6)

An acupuncture point.

Location. On the ulnar side of the posterior surface of the forearm, in the depression on the radial side, proximal to the small head of the ulnar.

Indication. Blurred vision, numbness and pain of the shoulder, back, wrist and arm, redness and swelling in the elbow region.

Method. Puncture perpendicularly or obliquely 0.3-0.5 cun and apply moxibustion to the point for 5-10 minutes or 3-5 moxa cones.

Yanglingquan (G 34)

An acupuncture point.

Location. On the lateral side of the leg, in the depression anterior and inferior to the small head of the fibula.

Indication. Flaccidity and numbness of lower limb, pain of knee, hypochondriac pain, vomiting, jaundice, constipation, beriberi.

Method. Puncture perpendicularly 1-1.5 cun and apply moxibustion to the point with 3-5 moxa cones or for 5-10 minutes.

Yang Macule

A kind of spots. It refers to macule of excessive heat nature.

Symptoms. Fever with excessive thirst, red macule, red tongue with yellow fur, etc.

Pathogenesis. Consumption of Nutrient system-blood by pathogenic heat.

Therapeutic Principle. Clearing away heat, relieving heat from blood, eliminating pathogens and letting out of skin rashes.

Yangming Fu disease

Symptoms. Tidal fever in the afternoon, aversion to heat preference cold, thirst, constipation, distention or pain with fullness and rigidity in the abdomen, eruption, jaundice, dyspnea.

Pathogenesis. Accumulation of pathogenic heat in the stomach and large intestine complicated by dryness-excess.

Therapeutic Principle. Purging and expelling the pathogenic heat.

Yangming Headache

1. It refers to headache of febrile disease caused by disorder of Yangming Meridian.

    Symptoms. Headache, fever, and aversion to heat.

    Therapeutic Principle. Clearing away heat, dispelling wind and relieving pain.

2. It refers to headache occurring along Yangming Meridian.

    Symptoms. Frontal headache often connected to the eyeball.

    Therapeutic Principle. Expelling wind, activating meridian and relieving pain.

Yangming Meridian Disease

Symptoms. Fever without chills, extreme thirst with the desire for drinking, sweating, aversion to heat, etc.

Therapeutic Principle. Clearing away heat and preserving fluid.

Yang Occluding in Yin

An acupuncture point manipulation term.

Indication. Diseases with fever prior to cold.

Method. First insert the needle in the deep region with a quick lifting and slow thrusting movement six times, lift the needle to the shallow layer when patient feels slight coolness, withdraw the needle to the superficial area and slowly lift nine times. Retain the needle for a while when slight warmth is felt, then withdraw the needle.

Yang-qi

A theory in TCM. It is the opposite of the yin-qi, and a generalized term for one aspect of the two opposites. It refers to the function of zang-fu organs, qi of six fu organs defending qi. It represents qi that moves outside, surface, rising, excess, increasing and lighting.

Yangqiao Meridian

One of the Eight Extra Meridians.
Course. It starts from the lateral surface of the heel Shenmai (B 62), goes along the lateral malleolus to the posterior border of the fibula, ascends along the lateral surface of the thigh, crosses the other meridians to the shoulder, passes through the neck to reach the angle of the mouth, then enters the inner canthus, where it meets the Yinqiao Meridian, goes along the Meridian of Foot-Taiyang to the forehead, and at last meets the Meridian of Foot-shaoyang at Fengchi (G 20).

Yang Summer-heat Syndrome

One type of disease during summer.
Symptoms. Headache, irritability, high fever, thirst, profuse sweating, dyspnea, etc.
Pathogenesis. Affection by summer-heat pathogen during a long walk or in the burning sun.
Therapeutic Principle. Clearing away summer-heat.

Yang Syndrome

It refers to excessive heat syndromes manifested by disease.
Symptoms. Fever with chilliness, headache and pantalgia, extreme thirst and desire to drink, flushed face, shortness of breath, abdominal pain with tenderness, constipation or diarrhea, scanty dark urine.
Therapeutic Principle. Relieving exterior syndrome and reducing fever, purgation and mediation therapies.

Yang Type of Edema

Symptoms. At the beginning, swelling of the face and head, then of the whole body, severe swelling of the area above the loin, lustrous skin, oliguria, aversion to cold, fever, cough, short breath.
Pathogenesis. Obstruction of the lung-qi, blockage of tri-energizer causing failure to clear and regulate the water passages to make the body fluid metabolize to the urinary bladder.
Treatment Principle. Clearing away heat, dispelling cold and wind, and inducing diuresis. Acupuncture is applicable.

Yang Wane and Yin Wax

A theory in TCM. It refers to the state in which yang wanes and yin waxes. As to physiological functions of a human body, various functional activities, yang, must consume certain nutritious substances, yin, a process also called yang wane and yin wax.

Yangwei (Ex-HN)

An extra acupuncture point.
Location. At the root of the auricle, at the tight tendons appearing in the back of the ear while pulling the ear forward by hand, at the same level as Ermen (TE 21).
Indication. Tinnitus, deafness, otitis media, etc.
Method. Puncture perpendicularly 0.1-0.2 cun. Apply moxibustion 1-3 moxa cones or 3-5 minutes with warming moxibustion.

Yangwei Meridian

One of the Eight Extra Meridians. Originates on the lateral surface of the heel, goes upward across the lateral malleolus, ascends along the Meridian of Foot-shaoyang to the hip joint, then along the posterior surface of the hypochondrium, goes from the posterior surface of the armpit to the shoulder and the forehead, then to the posterior surface of the nape and finally meets the Back Middle Meridian.

Yangxi (LI 5)

An acupuncture point.

Location. On the radial side of the wrist dorsum. When the thumb is held up, it is in the depression between the tendons of the short extensor and long extensor muscles of the thumb.

Indication. Headache, congestive eyes, toothache, diseases in the wrist joint, epilepsy, insanity.

Method. Prick perpendicularly 0.5-0.8 cun and apply moxibustion to the point for 5-10 minutes or 3-5 moxa cones.

Yankou (Ex-HN)

An extra acupuncture point.

Location. On the junction of the red and white skin lateral to two corners of the mouth.

Indication. Mania, deviated mouth and eyes, infantile spasm and trigeminal neuralgia.

Method. Puncture subcutaneously 0.3-0.5 cun.

Yaomu (Ex-B)

An extra acupuncture point.

Location. On the low back, 3 cun straight down from Shenshu (B 23).

Indication. Diabetes, frequent urination.

Method. Apply Moxibustion to the point with 3-7 moxa cones or 5-15 minutes with warming moxibustion.

Yaoqi (Ex-B 9)

An extra acupuncture point.

Location. 2 cun directly above the tip of the coccyx, in the depression at the sacral horn.

Indication. Epilepsy, headache, insomnia, constipation.

Method. Puncture subcutaneously upward 2-3 cun horizontally along the skin.

Yaoshu (GV 2)

An acupuncture point.

Location. On the posterior midline of the sacro-posterior, just at the sacral hiatus.

Indication. Stiffness and pain in the lower back, irregular menstruation, diarrhea, epilepsy, stranguria with turbid urine, hemafecia, paralysis of the lower extremities.

Method. Puncture obliquely upward 0.5-1.0 cun and apply moxibustion to the point for 5-15 minutes or 3-7 moxa cones.

Yaotongdian (Ex-UE 7)

A set of extra acupuncture points.

Location. On the dorsum of each hand, between the 2nd, 3rd, 4th and 5th metacarpal bones lateral to the midpoint of the cross striation and the metacarpophalangeal articulation, two points on each side.

Indication. Acute lumbar sprain, headache, infantile acute or chronic convulsion, etc.

Method. Puncture 0.3-0.5 cun obliquely toward the palm.

Yaoyan (Ex-B7)

An extra acupuncture point.

Location. On the low back, below the spinous process of the 4th lumbar vertebra, in the depression 3.5 cun lateral to the posterior midline.

Indication. Tuberculosis, lumbar pain, pain in the lower abdomen, orchitis, lumbar muscle strain, contusion of soft tissue in the lumbar region.

Method. Puncture obliquely 0.5-0.7 cun. Apply moxibustion 5-7 moxa cones or 10-20 minutes with warming moxibustion.

Yaoyangguan (GV 3)

An acupuncture point.

Location. On the midline of the lower back, in the depression of below the spinous process of the 4th lumbar vertebra.

Indication. Pain in the lumbosacral region, paralysis of the lower extremities, irregular menstruation, leukorrhea, hemafecia, emission, impotence, etc.

Method. Puncture obliquely upward 0.5-1.0 cun and apply moxibustion to the point for 5-15 minutes or 3-7 moxa cones.

Yaoyi (Ex-B 6)

An extra acupuncture point.

Location. On the lower back, below the spinous process of the 4th lumbar vertebra, in the depression 3.5 cun lateral to the posterior midline.

Indication. Metrorrhagia in women, lumbago, muscular spasm along the spinal column.

Method. Puncture obliquely 0.5-0.7 cun. Apply moxibustion to the point with 3-5 moxa cones or 5-10 minutes.

Yatongxue

An extra acupuncture point.

Location. Between the third and fourth metacarpophalangeal articulation on the palm.

Indication. Toothache.

Method. Puncture perpendicularly 0.3-0.5 cun.

Yawn

Symptoms. Stretching oneself and exhaling when tired or overworked.

Pathogenesis. Qi asthenia, yang exhaustion, and insufficiency of the kidney-qi.

Yellow Angledpwig Magnoliavine Root or Stem

It is the root, lianoid stem and leaf of Schisandra propinqua (Wall.) Baill. var. sinensis Oliv. (Magnoliaceae).

Effect. Promoting blood and qi circulation, relieving pain, and dissipating blood stasis.

Indication. Traumatic injuries, numbness due to pathogenic wind-dampness, pain in the muscles and bones, hematemesis, amenorrhea, abdominal distention, subcutaneous swelling, etc.

Yellow Bedstraw Herb

It is the whole herb of Galium verum L. (Rubiaceae).

Effect. Clearing away heat, detoxicating, subduing swelling, promoting blood circulation and relieving itching.

Indication. Hepatitis, swelling and pain due to tonsillitis, furuncle, sores, urticaria, traumatic injuries and pain due to stagnation of both blood and qi in female.

Yellow Dog's Kidney

It is the penis and testicle of the Canis familiaris L. (Canidae).

Effect. Tonifying the kidney, strengthening yang and warming up the uterus.

Indication. Impotence and coldness of the genitals due to the kidney-yang deficiency, aversion to cold, cold limbs, soreness of the lions, frequent micturition, leukorrhagia, etc.

Yellowish Mass

It is one of the eight masses.

Symptoms. Masses of accumulated blood and qi under the right rib, lassitude of the limbs, hard lower abdomen, stabbing pain in the vulva that spreads to the waist and back, abnormal menstruation, and dark-yellowish leukorrhagia.

Pathogenesis. Pathogenic wind invades and stagnates in the vagina before the restoration of blood, qi and visceral functions because of menstruation or abortion.

Therapeutic Principle. Soothing the liver, clearing away heat, and regulating the flow of qi to relieve pain.

Yellowish Nail

Symptoms. Yellowish complexion and eyes, bitter taste and dry tongue, rigidity of body, pain of limbs, and difficulty in walking.

Pathogenesis. Seasonal pathogenic evil, improper diet, damp-heat or cold dampness stagnating in the middle-energizer, and as a result the bile flowing in an abnormal way.

Therapeutic Principle. Dispelling dampness, inducing diuresis, or moxibustion.

Yellowish Purulent Ear

Symptoms. Yellowish pus discharging from the ear.

Pathogenesis. Fire sufficiency in the liver and gallbladder, and outward invasion of pathogenic heat.

Therapeutic Principle. Clearing away heat from the liver, detoxication and relieving swelling.

Yellowish Swelling

Symptoms. Yellowish color of the skin, facial edema and swollen feet, nausea, vomiting yellowish fluid, fatigue and weakness, parasites in stool, etc.

Pathogenesis. Malnutrition due to parasitic, indigestion, or overstrain.

Therapeutic Principle. Strengthening the spleen, nourishing blood, removing dampness by diuresis to cure jaundice, and killing internal parasites and subduing stagnancy.

Yellow Tongue Fur

A tongue picture.

Function. Diagnosis.

Application. Yellow tongue fur indicates heat syndrome often seen in affection by exopathogen and wind-heat syndrome. Yellow, thick, and dry fur can be seen in impairment of body fluid due to internal heat. Deep fur with prickles indicates extreme heat. Yellow and greasy fur shows stagnation of heat and dampness in the interior.

Yellow Tongue Surrounded with White Fur

A tongue picture.

Function. Diagnosis.

Application. The center of the white tongue fur becomes yellow, caused by superficial pathogen entering the interior and transforming into heat. If disturbance in qi transformation occurs in urinary bladder, excessive fluid accumulates in chest, with syndromes such as excessive thirst, polydipsia, and vomiting due to drinking water.

Yemen (TE 2)

1. An acupuncture point.

   Location. On the dorsum of the hand, between the 4th and 5th finger, when the fist is clenched, in the depression anterior to the metacarpophalangeal joint, 0.5 cun proximal to the margin of the web.

   Indication. Headache, epidemic acute conjunctivitis, deafness, swelling sore throat, pain in the back shoulder and elbow, swelling and pain of hand dorsum.

   Method. Puncture perpendicularly 0.3-0.5 cun and apply moxibustion to the point with 1-3 moxa cones or for 3-5 minutes.

2. An extra acupuncture point.

   Location. At the midline of axilla, 1 cun below the axillary fossa.

   Indication. Headache, congestive eyes, ocular pain, tinnitus, sore throat, pain in arms.

   Method. Puncture perpendicularly 0.3-0.5 cun.

Yerbadetajo Herb

It is the whole herb of Eclipta prostrata L. (Compositae).

Effect. Nourishing liver and kidney, arresting bleeding by clearing heat from blood.

Indication. Dizziness and blurred vision due to deficiency of liver-yin and kidney-yin, tinnitus, premature grey hair, hematemesis, epistaxis, hematuria, metrorrhagia, metrostaxis.

Yexiaxue (Ex-CA)

An extra acupuncture point.

Location. On the middle axillary line of the lateral part of the chest, 1.5 cun directly below the axillary fossa.

Indication. Eructation, hiccups, fullness and oppressive feeling in the chest and diaphragm, bromhidrosis, intercostal neuralgia.

Method. Puncture obliquely 0.3-0.5 cun. Apply moxibustion 3-5 moxa cones or 5-10 minutes with warming moxibustion.

Yifeng (TE 17)

An acupuncture point.

Location. Posterior to the earlobe, in the depression between the mastoid process and the angle of jaw.

Indication. Tinnitus, sudden deafness, deviation of the eye and mouth, swelling of the cheek, toothache, sudden loss of voice.

Method. Puncture perpendicularly 0.5-1.0 cun and apply moxibustion to the point for 5-10 minutes or 1-3 moxa cones.

Yiming (Ex-HN 14)

An extra acupuncture point.

Location. On the nape, posterior to the ear, 1 cun posterior to Yifeng (TE 17).

Indication. Myopia, hyperopia, night blindness, headache, tinnitus, dizziness, insomnia, cataract, glaucoma, atrophy of the visual nerve, parotitis, mental disorder, etc.

Method. Puncture obliquely or subcutaneously 0.5-0.8 cun. Moxibustion is applicable.

Yin and Yang Imbalance

A pathogenesis. It refers to the pathological state of the organism in which the yin and yang sides lose their balance and coordination. The balance and coordination is influenced by some pathogenic factors leading to relative yin and yang excess or deficiency, mutual damage, and exhaustion and repellence between yin and yang.

Yin and Yang in Equilibrium

A theory in TCM. The yin principle flourishes smoothly while the yang principle is their relative kinetic equilibrium. This is the basic condition to promote the normal activities of life.

Yin and Yang Mutual Damage

According to the theory of yin-yang interdependence, this suggests the pathogenesis of the deficiency of both yin and yang due to the pathological change of either side with secondary involvement of the other.

Yin Aspect of Yang

It refers to that yang may be subdivided into yang in yang and yin in yang respectively, e.g. the day is of yang nature and the night is of yin nature, but the period from dawn till noon is the yang aspect of yang; the period from noon till dusk is the yin aspect of yang.

Yinbai (Sp 1)

An acupuncture point on the Spleen Meridian of Foot-Taiyin.

Location. On the medial side of the distal segment of the great toe, 0.1 cun lateral to the corner of the nail.

Indication. Abdominal distention, diarrhea, hematochezia, hematuria, epistaxis, profuse menstruation, infantile convulsion, epilepsy, etc.

Method. Puncture obliquely 0.1-0.2 cun or prick to cause little bleeding and apply moxibustion to the point for 5-10 minutes or 3-5 moxa cones.

Yinbao (Liv 9)

A meridian acupuncture point.

Location. On the medial side of the thigh, 4 cun above the medial epicondyle of the femur, directly above Ququan (Liv 8).

Indication. Irregular menstruation, enuresis, difficulty in urination, and pain in the lumbosacral region extending to the lower abdomen.

Method. Puncture perpendicularly 1-2 cun and apply moxibustion to the point with 3-5 moxa cones or for 5-10 minutes.

Yin Damp Syndrome

Symptoms. Chills, anhidrosis, headache, distress in the chest, heavy sensation in the limbs, etc.

Pathogenesis. Damp pathogen invades the exterior and heat syndrome does not occur.

Therapeutic Principle. Expelling pathogenic factors by means of aromatic drugs pungent in flavor and dispersive in action.

Yin Deficiency

Symptoms. Feverish chest, palms and soles, low or hectic fever, night sweat, thirst, red lips, dry mouth, red or crimson tongue with thin coating, emaciation.

Pathogenesis. Yin is too weak to check yang, relative excess of yang resulting from damage of essence, blood, and body fluid.

Therapeutic Principle. Nourishing yin and clearing away heat.

Yin deficiency of Lung and Kidney

Symptoms. Cough and small amount of sputum, lassitude in the loins and knees, hectic fever and night sweat, emission.

Pathogenesis. Impairment of the lung-yin due to prolonged cough, lung deficiency involving the kidney or the kidney-yin deficiency due to prolonged illness, or excess of sexual intercourse, the kidney deficiency involving the lung.

Therapeutic Principle. Nourishing yin to reduce pathogenic fire both in the lung and kidney.

Yin Disorder due to Yang Excess

A theory in TCM. It refers to the process of yang pathogens invading the body. On the basis of the theory yang in excess makes yin suffer, e.g. endogenous heat (a yang factor) would injure vital essence and body fluid (yin).

Yindu (K 19)

A meridian acupuncture point.

Location. On the upper abdomen, 4 cun above the center of the umbilicus and 0.5 cun lateral to the anterior midline.

Indication. Abdominal distention, borborygmus, abdominal pain, constipation, sterility, pain in the chest and hypochondrium.

Method. Puncture perpendicularly 0.5-0.8 cun. Apply moxibustion 5-7 moxa cones or 10-15 minutes with warming moxibustion.

Yin Edema

A type of edema.

Symptoms. At the beginning the patient presents with pitted edema of the back of feet, gradually extending to the whole body, usually with symptoms of deficiency cold, loose stools, lassitude of limbs, pale complexion, pale tongue with white coating, etc.

Pathogenesis. Dysfunction of the spleen and the kidney, leading to inability to transport and transform water and dampness.

Therapeutic Principle. Strengthen the spleen and warm the kidney, restore yang and remove dampness by diuresis.

Yin Excess

Symptoms. Yin cold syndrome of hypometabolism of body functional activities, insufficient quantity of heat, usually indicating presence of endogenous cold, aversion to cold, cold limbs, diarrhea with watery stool, etc.

Pathogenesis. The infected cold dampness and other yin pathogens, over-eating something raw or cold, the stagnation and obstruction with pathogenic cold inside, resulting in yang being unable to check yin.

Yin Excess Causing Cold Syndrome

Since yin belongs to cold in nature, over-eating cold diet and drinking cold water may bring about cold syndrome such as abdominal pain, diarrhea, chillness, and cold limbs, due to yin excess.

Yin Excess Leading to Yang Deficiency

It refers to yang deficiency due to preponderance of yin.

Symptoms. Aversion to cold, cold limbs, diarrhea, edema and pale tongue.

Pathogenesis. Yang impairment by cold dampness or drugs cold in nature over administered.

Yin Exhaustion

A syndrome, referring to the critical case due to deficiency of yin, blood, body fluid and essence.

Symptoms. Marked emaciation, wrinkled skin, deep eye sockets, restlessness, coma, and delirium.

Pathogenesis. High fever, profuse sweating, excessive vomiting, or diarrhea, hemorrhage and other chronic exhaustion diseases.

Therapeutic Principle. Nourishing yin, promoting the production of the body fluid and nourishing qi.

Yin Fire

It refers to deficiency-fire, or a morbid state due to yin deficiency with resulting of hyperactivity of asthenic fire. The patient may have symptoms such as flushed cheeks, irritability, sore throat, or increased libido.

Yin Fluid

It refers to all nutrient fluid in the body such as essence, blood, body fluid, especially that of the internal organs.

Yingchi (Ex-LE)

An extra acupuncture point.

Location. In the depressions anterior and posterior to the lower edge of medial ankle, two points on each side and four points in total.

Indication. Menorrhagia, leukorrhea with reddish discharge.

Method. Puncture perpendicularly 0.2-0.3 cun. Apply moxibustion 3-7 moxa cones or 5-15 minutes with warming moxibustion.

Yingchuang (S 16)

A meridian acupuncture point.

Location. On the chest, in the 3rd intercostal space, 4 cun lateral to the anterior midline or to Yutang (CV 18).

Indication. Cough, asthmatic breath, distention and pain in the hypochondrium, acute mastitis.

Method. Puncture perpendicularly 0.2-0.4 cun, or medially and obliquely 0.5-0.8 cun. Apply moxibustion 3-5 moxa cones or 5-10 minutes with warming moxibustion.

Yingtu (Ex-CA)

An extra acupuncture point.

Location. On the chest, 6 cun lateral to the middle of sternum, 1 cun below the 6th intercostal space.

Indication. Lack of appetite, fullness of abdomen, borborygmus, diarrhea.

Method. Puncture subcutaneously 0.3-0.5 cun. Apply moxibustion 3-5 moxa cones or 5-10 minutes with warming moxibustion.

Yingu (K 10)

An acupuncture point.

Location. On the medial side of the popliteal fossa, between the muscular tendons of the semi-tendinosus muscle and the semi-membranosus muscle when the knee is flexed.

Indication. Impotence, hernia, irregular menstruation, metrorrhagia, dysuria, psychosis, vulvar dampness and itching.

Method. Puncture perpendicularly 1-1.5 cun and apply moxibustion to the point with 3-5 moxa cones or for 5-10 minutes.

Yingxiang (LI 20)

A meridian acupuncture point.

Location. In the nasolabial groove, beside the midpoint of the lateral edge of the nasal ala.

Indication. Stuffy nose, epistaxis, deviated mouth and eyes, itching of the face, edema of face, nasal polyp.

Method. Puncture perpendicularly 0.1-0.2 cun, or puncture obliquely towards the nose 0.3-0.5 cun.

Notice. Moxibustion is prohibited.

Yin Jaundice

Symptoms. Dim yellow color of the skin and eyes, aversion to cold, lassitude, fullness of stomach, lack of taste, loose stools, pale tongue with whitish and moist or greasy coating.

Pathogenesis. Improper diet or drinking, over-tiredness, leading to impairment of the spleen and stomach, damp stagnancy and qi stagnation, resulting in stagnation of the liver and gallbladder with cholestasis and bile overflowing to the muscle and skin.

Therapeutic Principle. Regulating the spleen and stomach, warming and dissipating cold dampness.

Yinjiao (CV 7)

A meridian acupuncture point.

Location. On the lower abdomen and on the anterior midline, 1 cun below the center of the umbilicus.

Indication. Fullness of the abdomen, edema, diarrhea, hernia, pruritus vulvae, difficulty in urination, cold pain around the navel, metrorrhagia, lochiorrhea, sunken fontanel in infants.

Method. Puncture perpendicularly 0.8-1.2 cun. Apply moxibustion to the point with 3-5 units of moxa cones or for 10-15 minutes.

Notice. Care should be taken in pregnant women.

Yinjiao (GV 28)

A meridian acupuncture point.

Location. Inside the upper lip, at the junction of the labial frenum and upper gum.

Indication. Swollen and painful gums, foul breath, bleeding from the gum, swollen cheek, sore and tinea on the face, manic-depressive disorder.

Method. Puncture upward obliquely 0.2-0.3 cun.

Notice. Moxibustion is prohibited.

Yinjingxue (Ex-CA)

An extra acupuncture point.

Location. In the depression above the urethral opening in male.

Indication. Epilepsy and flaccid constriction of penis.

Yin Kept Externally by Yang Excess in the Interior

Symptoms. High fever with pseudo-cold symptoms, patient may have cold limbs but aversion to heat, thirst, preference for cold drinking, scanty dark urine, constipation, red tongue, yellowish coating, etc.

Pathogenesis. Due to extreme heat inside the body and failure of yang-qi to reach the limbs, resulting from internal stagnation of yang-qi which keeps yin in the exterior by abundant yang in the interior.

Yinlian (Liv 11)

A meridian acupuncture point on the Liver Meridian of Foot-jueyin.

Location. On the medial side of the thigh, 2 cun directly below Qichong (S 30), at the proximal end of the thigh, below the pubic tubercle.

Indication. Irregular menstruation, leukorrhea, pain in the lower abdomen, pain in the medial aspect of thigh, spasm of the lower limbs.

Method. Puncture perpendicularly 0.8-1.0 cun. Apply moxibustion 3-5 moxa cones or 5-10 minutes with warming moxibustion.

Yinlingquan (Sp 9)

An acupuncture point.

Location. On the internal side of the leg, in the depression posterior and inferior to the medial condyle of the tibia.

Indication. Abdominal distention, abdominalgia, edema, jaundice, vomiting, diarrhea, loose stool, dysuria or urinary incontinence, seminal emission, beriberi, pain of the soft tissues surrounding the knee joint.

Method. Puncture perpendicularly 1-2 cun and apply moxibustion to the point with 3-5 moxa cones or for 5-10 minutes.

Yin Macule

Symptoms. Pink spots latent and unnoticed, accompanied by cold limbs, in serious cases diarrhea with undigested food in the stool.

Pathogenesis. Latent cold in the interior of the body, improper diet of cool food, or severe pathogenic cold excessive in the interior, yang kept outside.

Therapeutic Principle. Warming yang and expelling cold, detoxication to relieve rashes.

Yinmen (B 37)

An acupuncture point.

Location. On the posterior side of the thigh, 6 cun inferior to Chengfu (B 36), on the connecting line between Chengfu and Weizhong (B 40).

Indication. Rigidity and pain in the lumbar spine, posterior swelling and pain of thigh, and acute sprain of waist.

Method. Puncture perpendicularly 1-1.5 cun and apply moxibustion to the point for 5-15 minutes with warming moxibustion.

Yinmen (Ex-HN)

An extra acupuncture point.

Location. On the head, 1.8 cun directly above the midpoint of the anterior hairline.

Indication. Jaundice.

Method. Puncture subcutaneously 0.3-0.5 cun.

Yinnangxiahengwen (Ex-CA)

An extra acupuncture point.

Location. At the midpoint of the first transverse crease in the lower part of the scrotum.

Indication. Acute apoplexy, severe case of oppressive feeling in the chest and dysphoria, lockjaw, and severe pain in the abdomen.

Method. Apply moxibustion to the point with 3-5 moxa cones or 5-10 minutes with warming moxibustion.

Yin Occluded in Yang

A needling method, as compared with yang occluded in yin, referring reinforcing followed by reducing.

Indication. Diseases with the symptoms of first feeling cold, then hot.

Method. Apply the needle superficially. First, thrust it rapidly and lift it slowly 9 times. When the patient feels slightly warm, apply the needle in the deep part. Lift it rapidly and thrust it slowly 6 times, retain the needle for a while when the patient feels slightly cold and then withdraw the needle.

Indication. Diseases with the symptoms of first feeling cold, then hot.

Yin Originating from Yang

A theory in TCM. According to the theory of interdependence between yin and yang, yin cannot exist without yang. Yin exists with yang as its prerequisite. In the human body, the substantial transformation of vital essence, blood and body fluid, a yin factor, depends on receiving, transportation, distribution and guardian of vital function, a yang factor.

Yin-qi

A theory in TCM. It is one aspect of the two opposites, as compared with yang-qi. Yin-qi denotes substance, it refers to the qi of five zang-organs, defending qi, it represents qi, which moves internally, downward, restrictedly, weakly and turbidly.

Yinqiao Meridian

One of Eight Extra Meridian.

Course. Branching from the Kidney Meridian of Foot-shaoyin, it begins behind the navicular bone and goes upward to the superior part of the medial malleolus. Running along the medial side of the thigh, it enters the interior pudendum, goes upward along the abdomen, and enters the chest and supraclavicular fossa, then runs anteriorly to Renying (S 9) and reaches the lateral part of the nose, links the inner canthus, and finally converges with the Meridians of Foot-taiyang and Yangqiao.

Yinshi (S 33)

A meridian acupuncture point on the Stomach Meridian of Foot-yangming.

Location. On the anterior side of the thigh, 3 cun above the base of patella on the line connecting the antero-superior iliac process at the antero-lateral thigh.

Indication. Numbness and aching of the knee and leg, paralysis of the lower limbs, lumbago, cold hernia, distention and pain in the abdomen.

Method. Puncture perpendicularly 0.5-1.0 cun. Apply moxibustion 3-5 moxa cones or 5-10 minutes with warming moxibustion.

Yin Summer-heat Syndrome

Symptoms. Fever, headache, anhidrosis, chills, painful limbs, etc.

Pathogenesis. Affection due to cold in summer, e.g. enjoying the cool in hot summer or taking cooling drinks excessively.

Therapeutic Principle. Relieving the exterior syndrome with drugs pungent in flavor and dispersive in action. For the patient with cold invading zang-fu, warming the middle-energizer.

Yin Syncope

Symptoms. Cold limbs, dark lips, diarrhea, clear and profuse urine.

Pathogenesis. Interior deficiency of yang, exterior deficiency of essence and blood, exhaustion of yang and essence, dysfunction of qi and blood circulation, yin-qi and yang-qi failing to connect smoothly.

Therapeutic Principle. Recuperating depleted yang and rescuing the patient from collapse, nourishing blood to restore normal flow of blood and warming meridians to alleviate cold.

Yin Syndrome

Symptoms. Pale complexion, low voice and breath, cold body and limbs, cold pain in the abdomen, clear and profuse urine, diarrhea, etc.

Therapeutic Principle. Warming middle-energizer to expel coldness, supporting and tonifying yang.

Yintang (Ex-HN 3)

It is one of the extraordinary points.

Location. In the middle between the two eyebrows.

Indication. Headache, vomiting, insomnia, epistaxis, ocular pain, pain of supraorbital bone, facial furuncle, acute or chronic infantile convulsion, postpartum dizziness due to profuse bleeding and eclampsia gravidarum.

Method. Puncture subcutaneously downward 0.5-1 cun or prick to cause little bleeding, and apply moxibustion to the point for 5-10 minutes with warming moxibustion.

Yinwei Meridian

One of the Eight Extra Meridians.

Course. Beginning at the medial side of the shank, it goes upward along the medial side of the thigh to the abdomen, joins the Foot-taiyin Meridian on the chest and the Front Middle Meridian on the neck.

Yinxi (Ex-CA)

An extra acupuncture point.

Location. On the chest, in the 6th intercostal space, 6 cun lateral to the sternal midline.

Indication. The chest and abdominal pain, borborygmus, pain in the chest and hypochondriac region, pneumonia, pleurisy and hepatalgia.

Method. Puncture obliquely 0.3-0.5 cun. Apply moxibustion 5-10 minutes with warming moxibustion.

Yinxi (H 6)

A meridian acupuncture point.

Location. On the palmer side of the forearm and on the radial side of the tendon of the ulnar flexor muscle of the wrist, 0.5 cun above the transverse crease of the wrist.

Indication. Cardiac pain, fright and terror, palpitation, night sweat, hematemesis, epistaxis, and aphasia.

Method. Puncture perpendicularly 0.3-0.5 cun. Apply moxibustion 1-3 moxa cones or 3-5 minutes with warming moxibustion.

Yin-yang Interlocking

Symptoms. High fever which does not reduce fever even after diaphoresis, delirium, anorexia. It belongs to a serious syndrome of the domination of the pathogenic factors over the vital qi.

Pathogenesis. Yang-heat pathogen invading the yin phase, resulting in interlocking of both.

Yin-yang Theory

It refers to one of the basic theories in TCM derived from ancient philosophical concept of dialectics. This theory consist of the concept of yin-yang relative nature, the laws of yin-yang movement and changes, opposition and restriction, interdependence and utilizing each other, waxing and waning, balance and transformation between yin and yang. Since the yin-yang theory permeated the medical field, it has became an important constituent of the theory of TCM and has been widely used in all fields of TCM.

Yin-yang Transmission

Symptoms. Cramping sensation of the lower abdomen, even affecting the pubic region, heaviness in the head and dim eyesight, heavy sensation of body and fatigue.

Pathogenesis. The relapse of febrile disease due to sexual intercourse.

Therapeutic Principle. Warming yang and relieving the symptoms.

Yishe (B 49)

An acupuncture point.

Location. On the back, 3 cun lateral to Jizhong (GV 6), or to the lower border of the spinous process of the 11th thoracic vertebra.

Indication. Abdominal distention, nausea, vomiting, diarrhea, jaundice, backache, etc.

Method. Puncture obliquely 0.5-0.8 cun. Apply moxibustion to the point for 10-15 minutes or 3-7 moxa cones.

Notice. Deep puncture is prohibited.

Yixi (B 45)

An acupuncture point.

Location. On the back 3 cun lateral to Lingtai (GV 10) or to the spinous process of the 6th thoracic vertebra.

Indication. Cough, asthma, fever, lumbago, pain of the shoulder and back, epilepsy, malarial disease, etc.

Method. Puncture obliquely 0.3-0.8 cun. Apply moxibustion to the point for 5-15 minutes or 3-5 moxa cones.

Notice. Deep puncture is prohibited.

Yongquan (K 1)

An acupuncture point.

Location. On the sole of the foot, in the depression on the anterior part of the sole when the foot bent downward.

Indication. Headache, insomnia, swollen sore throat, blurred vision, aphonia, epistaxis, palpitation, jaundice, psychosis, dysuria, dysporia, plantar heat, spasm of lower limbs, infantile convulsion, and hernia.

Method. Puncture perpendicularly 0.5-1 cun and apply moxibustion to the point with 1-3 moxa cones or for 5-10 minutes with warming moxibustion.

Youmen (K 21)

An acupuncture point.

Location. On the upper abdomen, 6 cun above to the umbilicus, and 0.5 cun lateral to the anterior median line.

Indication. Distention and fullness in the chest and abdomen, vomiting, eructation, dyspepsia, abdominalgia, diarrhea, dysentery, etc.

Method. Puncture perpendicularly 0.5-1 cun. Apply moxibustion to the point with 5-7 moxa cones or for 5-15 minutes.

Notice. Deep puncture is prohibited.

Young Bee

It is the young insect of Apis cerana Fabricius (Apidae).

Effect. Eliminating pathogenic wind, detoxication and destroying parasites.

Indication. Erysipelas, nettle rash, abdominal pain due to parasitic malnutrition, and leukorrhea, etc.

Yuanye (G 22)

An acupuncture point.

Location. With the arm lifted, on the midline of the axilla 3 cun below the axilla, in the 4th intercostal space.

Indication. Fullness in chest and costalgia, pain of the shoulder and the upper extremities.

Method. Prick obliquely 0.5-0.8 cun and apply moxibustion to the point for 3-5 minutes with warming moxibustion.

Yuji (L 10)

A meridian acupuncture point.

Location. In the depression proximal to the 1st metacarpophalangeal joint, on the radial side of the midpoint of the 1st metacarpal bone, and at the junction of the red and white skin.

Indication. Cough, hemoptysis, aphonia, sore throat, general fever, breast carbuncle, elbow spasm.

Method. Puncture perpendicularly 0.5-0.8 cun. Moxibustion is applicable.

Yumentou (Ex-CA)

An extra acupuncture point.

Location. On the external genital organs in females, at the head of the clitoris.

Indication. Pundendal sores of women, manic-depressive psychosis.

Method. Puncture 0.3 cun. Apply moxibustion to the point for 3-7 minutes with moxa stick.

Yunmen (L 2)

An acupuncture point.

Location. 6 cun lateral to the anterior midline, in the lower border of the clavicle, or 1 cun above Zhongfu (L 1) on the lateral side of the pectoral triangle.

Indication. Cough, asthma, sudden blindness, deafness, fullness and pain in the chest, pain of the shoulder and arm.

Method. Prick obliquely 0.5-0.8 cun towards the lateral aspect of the chest, and apply moxibustion to the point with 3-5 moxa cones, or for 5-10 minutes with warming moxibustion.

Yunnan Alstonia Twig and Leaf

It is the branch leaf of Alstonia yunnanensis Diels. (Apocynaceae).

Effect. Relieving inflammation, arresting bleeding, rejoining fractured bones and relieving pain.

Indication. Hepatitis.

Yunnan Begonia Herb

It is the whole herb or root and fruit of Begonia Yunnanensis Levl. (Begoniaceae).

Effect. Invigorating the circulation of qi and relieving the pain, promoting blood circulation and dissipating blood stasis.

Indication. Stomachache, irregular menstruation, dysmenorrhea, vomiting and diarrhea in children, traumatic injuries.

Yunnan Glorybower Root

It is the root and rhizome of Clerodendron yunnanense Hu ex Hand.-Mazz. (Verbenaceae).

Effect. Dispelling wind, preventing attack of malaria, promoting flow of qi and inducing diuresis.

Indication. Malaria, wind-dampness syndrome, edema, fullness pain in the abdomen, etc.

Yunnan Larkspur Root

It is the root of Delphinium yunnanense Franch. or Delphinium delavayi Franch. (Ranunculaceae).

Effect. Expelling wind, dissipating dampness, dispersing cold, relieving pain and removing obstruction in the meridians to dissipate blood stasis.

Indication. Arthralgia due to wind-dampness, pain in the stomach due to cold and traumatic injuries.

Yunnan Rhodiola Root

It is the root of Rhodiola yunnanensis Franch. Fu (Crassulaceae).

Effect. Clearing away heat, detoxicating, dissipating blood stasis and arresting pain.

Indication. Laryngitis, cough, diarrhea, dysentery and traumatic injuries.

Yunnan Supplejack Root

It is the root of Berchemia Yunnanensis Franch. (Rhamnaceae).

Effect. Clearing away heat and inducing diuresis.

Indication. Dysentery, jaundice, metrorrhagia, metrostaxis, leukorrhagia, etc.

Yunnanu Wintergreen Stem and Leaf

It is the stem and leaf of Gaultheria yunnanensis (Franch) Rehd. (Ericaceae).

Effect. Dispelling pathogenic wind and eliminating dampness, promoting blood circulation and activating collaterals.

Indication. Rheumatic arthritis, ascites, traumatic injuries, toothache and eczema.

Yuquan (Ex-CA)

An extra acupuncture point.

Location. 6.5 cun below the umbilicus, right in the middle of the penis root.

Indication. Swelling of the scrotum, testitis, etc.

Method. Puncture perpendicularly 0.3-0.5 cun. Apply moxibustion 3-7 moxa cones or 5-15 minutes with warming moxibustion.

Yutang (CV 18)

An acupuncture point.

Location. On the anterior median line of chest, at the level with the 3rd intercostal space.

Indication. Cough, asthma, dyspnea, thoracic pain and vomiting.

Method. Puncture subcutaneously 0.3-0.5 cun and apply moxibustion to the point with 3-5 moxa cones or for 5-10 minutes.

Yutian (Ex-B)

An extra acupuncture point.

Location. On the sacrum, in the depression below the 4th articular sacral crest.

Indication. Difficult labor, pain in the waist and sacrum, etc.

Method. Puncture subcutaneously 0.5-1.0 cun. Apply moxibustion 3-5 moxa cons or 5-10 minutes with warming moxibustion.

Yuwei (Ex-HN)

An extra acupuncture point.

Location. 0.1 cun lateral to the extra canthus.

Indication. Headache, vertigo, dizziness, ocular trouble, facial paralysis.

Method. Puncture 0.2-0.3 cun horizontally.

Yuyao (Ex-HN4)

An extra acupuncture point.

Location. Directly superior to the pupil within the center of eyebrow.

Indication. Migraine, headache, swelling and redness of eyes, nebula and myopia.

Method. Puncture 0.3-0.5 cun subcutaneously. Moxibustion is applicable.

Yuye (Ex-HN13)

Location. On the vein of the right side of the frenulum of tongue.

Indication. Stiff tongue, swelling of the tongue, sore throat, diabetes, vomiting, diarrhea, aphasia.

Method. Prick to cause bleeding.

Yuzhen (B 9)

An acupuncture point.

Location. In the posterior part of the head, 2.5 cun above the posterior hairline and 1.3 cun lateral to Naohu (GV 17).

Indication. Headache, vertigo, vomiting, aversion to wind and cold, ocular pain, stuffy nose, rigid nape and epilepsy.

Method. Puncture subcutaneously 0.3-0.5 cun and apply moxibustion to the point with 1-3 moxa cones or for 3-5 minutes with warming moxibustion.

Yuzhong (K 26)

A meridian acupuncture point.

Location. On the chest, in the 1st intercostal space, 2 cun lateral to Huagai (CV 20).

Indication. Cough, dyspnea, abundant expectoration, fullness in the chest and hypochondrium, profuse sputum, vomiting, breast carbuncle.

Method. Puncture obliquely or subcutaneously 0.5-0.8 cun. Apply moxibustion to the point with 3-5 moxa cones or for 5-10 minutes with warming moxibustion.

Z

Zang-cold
Symptoms. Restlessness, cold limbs and body, feeble pulse, etc., it is a severe syndrome of cold limbs.
Pathogenesis. Due to deficiency of yang-qi and exhaustion of kidney yang.
Therapeutic Principle. Warming up zang organ and emergency treatment.

Zang Organs
Referring to the short form of five zang organs, heart, liver, spleen, lung and kidney, for storing genuine qi and not leaking out and differentiated from six fu organs.

Zangshu (Ex-B)
An extra acupuncture point.
Location. On the back of the body, at the tip of the spinous process of the fifth thoracic vertebra.
Indication. Sudden attack of disease with aversion to wind, inability to raise oneself slightly, numbness, etc.
Method. Performing moxibustion.

Zanzhu (B 2)
An acupuncture point.
Location. On the face, in the depression of the eyebrow, on the superior notch of the orbit.
Indication. Headache, dizziness, pain in the supra-orbital bone, conjunctival congestion, blurred vision, epiphora due to wind, stuffy nose, epistaxis, etc.
Method. Puncture subcutaneously 0.3-0.5 cun, or prick to cause little bleeding. Moxibustion is prohibited.

Zedoary
It is the rhizome of Curcuma zedoaria (Berg) Rosc., C. aromatica Salisb. or C. kwaxgsiensis S. Lee et C.F. Liang (Zingiberaceae).
Effect. Relieving blood stasis, regulating qi and ceasing pain.
Indication. Amenorrhea, abdominal pain, masses in the abdomen resulting from stagnancy of qi and blood stasis and epigastric and abdominal distention and pain.

Zhangmen (Liv 13)
An acupuncture point.
Location. On the lateral side of the abdomen, below the free end of the 11th rib.
Indication. Abdominal distention, diarrhea, costalgia, lump in abdomen, vomiting.
Method. Perpendicularly puncturing 0.5-0.8 cun, and performing moxibustion to the point 3-5 moxa cones, or for 5-10 minutes.

Zhangxiaohengwen
A massage point.
Location. At the start of the ulnar palm print.
Operation. Kneading method.
Function. Clearing the chest, dispersing accumulation of pathogens, decreasing stagnated fever and relieving sputum.
Indication. Dyspnea and cough caused by phlegm-heat, aphthae, whooping cough, slobbering, etc.

Zhaohai (K 6)
An acupuncture point.
Location. Medial to the foot, in the depression of the tip of the medial malleolus.
Indication. Inflammation of the throat, dryness of the throat, pain of the eye, insomnia, epilepsy, chest pain, frequency of

micturition, hernia, irregular menstrua-tion, morbid leukorrhagia, prolapse of uterus, etc.

Method. Puncture perpendicularly 0.5-1.0 cun and perform moxibustion to the point for 5-10 minutes or 3-5 units of moxa cones.

Zhejin (G 23)

A meridian acupuncture point.

Location. On the lateral side of the chest, 1 cun anterior to Yuanye (G 22), parallel to the nipple, and in the 4th intercostal space.

Indication. Pain in the chest and hypochondrium, dyspnea, vomiting, acid regurgitation, pain in the shoulder and back.

Method. Puncture obliquely 0.5-0.8 cun.

Apply moxibustion with 1-3 moxa cones or 3-5 minutes with warming moxibustion.

Notice. Deep puncture is prohibited.

Zhengying (G 17)

An acupuncture point.

Location. On the head, 2.5 cun superior to the anterior hairline and 2.25 cun lateral to the median line of the head, i.e. 1 cun be-hind Muchuang (G 16).

Indication. Headache, dizziness and toothache.

Method. Puncture subcutaneously 0.3-0.5 cun and per form moxibustion to the point with 3-5 units of moxa cones or for 5-10 minutes warming moxibustion.

Zhibian (B 54)

An acupuncture point.

Location. On the buttock, in the fourth posterior sacral foramen, 3 cun lateral to the median sacral crest.

Indication. Lumbosacral pain, dysuria, dysporia, vulvar pain, and hemorrhoid.

Method. Puncturing perpendicularly 1-2 cun and performing moxibustion to the point with 3-7 units of moxa cones or for 5-15 minutes.

Zhigen (Ex-UE)

An extra acupuncture point.

Location. At the midpoint of palmar digi-tal cross striation of the 2nd to the 5th fingers, total 8 points on both sides.

Indication. Hand furuncle, pain in five fingers, abdominal pain, vomiting and fever.

Method. Pricking with a three-edged needle to cause little bleeding.

Zhigou (TE 6)

A meridian acupuncture point.

Location. On the dorsal side of the fore-arm, on the line connecting Yangchi (TE 4) and the tip of the olecranon, 3 cun proximal to the dorsal crease of the wrist and between the radius and ulna.

Indication. Febrile diseases, sudden loss of voice, deafness, tinnitus, soreness and pain in the shoulder and back, vomiting, hypochondriac pain and constipation.

Method. Puncturing perpendicularly 0.5-1 cun. Apply moxibustion with 3-5 moxa cones or 5-10 minutes with warming moxibustion.

Zhigu (Ex-CA)

It is an extra acupuncture point.

Location. On the chest, one finger-width directly below nipples.

Indication. Heat pyrexia in children, cough and dyspnea.

Method. Performing moxibustion with 3-5 moxa cones or 5-10 minutes with warm-ing moxibustion.

Zhili

An acupuncture point and one of the extra acupuncture points.

Location. 4.5 cun directly above and 1.5 cun interior to Weizhong (B 40).

Indication. Sequela of infantile paralysis.

Method. Puncturing 1-2 cun perpen-dicularly.

Zhi Mass (Fetus-like Mass)

Symptoms. Pain in the chest, the abdo-men, the waist and back, to lift distention of the bladder, constant bloody stool and urine, irregular menstruation, sterility, etc.

Pathogenesis. Due to sexual intercourse during menstruation or no more than a month after delivery, damaging the uterine collaterals and leading to an open vaginal orifice and accumulation and stagnation of turbid semen and blood in the uterus.

Therapeutic Principle. Enhancing blood circulation to relieve stasis, soften and resolve the hard mass.

Zhishi (B 52)

An acupuncture point.

Location. In the lumbar region, inferior and 3 cun lateral to the spinous process of the second lumbar vertebra.

Indication. Lumbar rigidity and pain, paralysis of lower limb, seminal emission, impotence, vulvar swelling and pain, dribbling urination, edema, vomiting and diarrhea.

Method. Puncturing obliquely 0.5-0.8 cun. Performing moxibustion to the point with 5-7 units of moxa cones or for 10-20 minutes.

Notice. Deep puncture is prohibited.

Zhiyang (GV 9)

An acupuncture point.

Location. Between the seventh and the eighth spinous process of the thoracic vertebrae.

Indication. Cough, asthma, jaundice, back pain and general fever.

Method. Puncture obliquely upward 0.5-1 cun and apply moxibustion to the point with 3-5 units of moxa cones or for 5 minutes to a quarter.

Zhiyin (B 67)

An acupuncture point.

Location. At the lateral of little toe, 0.1 cun to the toe-nail.

Indication. Headache, stuffy nose, epistaxis, ocular pain, feverish sensation in the sole, etc.

Method. Puncture obliquely 0.1-0.2 cun or prick to cause little bleeding with a triangular needle. Apply moxibustion with 3-5 moxa cones or 5-10 minutes with warming moxibustion.

Zhizheng (SI 7)

A meridiAn acupuncture point.

Location. On the ulnar side of the posterior surface of the forearm, the line connecting Yanggu (SI 5) and Xiaohai (SI 8), and 5 cun above Yanggu.

Indication. Rigidity of the nape, spasm of the elbow, pain in the fingers, chills and fever, headache, dizziness, emotional disorders, diabetes, scabies and wart.

Method. Puncture 0.3-0.5 cun perpendicularly or obliquely. Apply moxibustion with 3-5 moxa cones or 5-10 minutes with warming moxibustion.

Zhongchong (P 9)

An acupuncture point.

Location. In the center of the tip of the superior segment of the middle finger.

Indication. Apoplectic coma, cardialgia, vexation, sunstroke, swelling pain of stiff tongue, infantile night cry, swelling sore throat and palmar heat.

Method. Puncturing perpendicularly 0.1 cun or pricking to cause little bleeding, or performing moxibustion to the point with 1-3 units of moxa ones or for 3-5 minutes.

Zhongdu (Ex-UE)

An extra acupuncture point.

Location. Between the bone junctures of the 3rd and 4th metacarpophalangeal joints.

Indication. Redness and swelling of the hand and arm.

Method. Puncture perpendicularly 0.1 cun. Apply moxibustion if needed.

Zhongdu (G 32)

A meridian acupuncture point.

Location. On the lateral side of the thigh, 2 cun below Fengshi (G 31) or 5 cun above the popliteal crease, between the lateral vastus muscle and biceps muscle of the thigh.

Indication. Flaccidity, numbness and pain of the lower limbs and hemiplegia.

Method. Puncture perpendicularly 1.0-1.5 cun. Apply moxibustion with 3-5 moxa cones or 5-10 minutes with warming moxibustion.

Zhongdu (Liv 6)

A meridian acupuncture point.

Location. On the medial side of the leg, 7 cun above the tip of the medial malleolus, on the midline of the medial surface of the tibia.

Indication. Hypochondriac pain, abdominal distention, diarrhea, hernia, pain in the lower abdomen, metrorrhagia and metrostaxis, and lochiorrhea.

Method. Puncture subcutaneously 0.5-0.8 cun. Apply moxibustion with 1-3 moxa cones or 3-5 minutes with warming moxibustion.

Zhongfeng (Liv 4)

An acupuncture point.

Location. On the dorsum of the foot, 1 cun anterior to the medial malleolus, on the connecting line between Shangqiu (Sp 5) and Jiexi (S 41), in the medial excavation of the anterior cervical tendon.

Indication. Pain in umbilical region, jaundice, seminal emission, dripping urination, hernia, lumbago, knee pain, sore ankle and beriberi.

Method. Puncturing perpendicularly 0.5-0.8 cun, or applying moxibustion with 3-5 moxa cones or 5-10 minutes.

Zhongfengbuyuxue (Ex-B)

An extra acupuncture point.

Location. On the back, at the high point of the spinous processes of the 2nd and 5th thoracic vertebra.

Indication. Aphasia from apoplexy.

Method. Apply moxibustion with 3-5 moxa cones or 5-10 minutes with warming moxibustion.

Zhongfu (L 1)

An acupuncture point.

Location. Exterior and superior to the anterior pectoral region, 1 cun inferior to Yunmen (L 2), parallel to the first intercostal space, and 6 cun lateral to the anterior median line.

Indication. Cough, dyspnea, spitting of pus and blood, pectoralgia, thoracic fullness with dysphagia, laryngitis, sore shoulder and backache.

Method. Puncturing obliquely 0.5-1 cun exterior to the chest wall or performing moxibustion with 3-5 moxa cones or 5-10 minutes with warming moxibustion.

Notice. Do not insert too deeply and it is forbidden to puncture obliquely toward the interior aspect of the chest in order to protect the lung.

Zhongji (CV 3)

An acupuncture point.

Location. In the lower abdomen, 4 cun inferior to the center of the umbilicus.

Indication. Seminal emission, prospermia, impotence, enuresis, retention of urine, frequent micturition, stranguria, hernia, lower abdominalgia, irregular menstruation, amenorrhea, metrorrhagia, metrostaxis, morbid leukorrhea, prolapse of uterus, pruritus vulva and dystocia.

Method. Puncture perpendicularly 1-1.5 cun. Apply moxibustion with 3-7 moxa cones or 10-20 minutes with warming moxibustion.

Zhongju (Ex-HN)

An extra acupuncture point.

Location. In the inner side of the mandible below the mouth cavity, at the intersection of the midline of the mouth base and gingival mucosa.

Indication. Apoplexy, stiff tongue, aphasia and dry tongue, etc.

Method. Puncturing 0.2-0.3 cun perpendicularly. Moxibustion is forbidden.

Zhongkui (Ex-UE4)

Referring to an extra acupuncture point.

Location. On the dorsal side of the middle finger, at the midpoint of the proximal interphalangeal joint.

Indication. Vomiting, obstructive sensation of swallowing, epistaxis, toothache and vitiligo, etc.

Method. Puncture perpendicularly 0.2-0.3 cun, perform moxibustion with 3-7 moxa cones.

Zhongliao (B 33)

An acupuncture point.

Location. In the sacral region, inferior anterior to Ciliao (B 32) at the lower end of the pseudospinal process of the third sacrum..

Indication. Irregular menstruation, leukorrhea with reddish discharge, lumbago, dripping urination, diarrhea and dysporia.

Method. Puncturing perpendicularly 1-1.5 cun and performing moxibustion to the points with 3-7 units of moxa cones or for 5-15 minutes.

Zhonglushu (B 29)

A meridian acupuncture point.

Location. At the sacrum and on the level of the 3rd posterior sacral foramen, 1.5 cun lateral to the midline of sacral region.

Indication. Dysentery, hernia, stiffness and pain in the back and loin, and diabetes.

Method. Puncture perpendicularly 0.8-1.0 cun. Apply moxibustion to the point with 3-7 moxa cones or 5-15 minutes with warming moxibustion.

Zhongping (Ex-UE)

An extra acupuncture point.

Location. At the center of palmar transverse crease of the middle finger.

Indication. Stomatitis.

Method. Puncture perpendicularly 0.2-0.3 cun. Apply moxibustion with 1-3 moxa cones or 3-5 minutes with warming moxibustion.

Zhongquan (Ex-UE 3)

An extra acupuncture point.

Location. At the dorsal crease of the wrist, at the midpoint of the line connecting Yangchi (TE 4) and Yangxi (LI 5).

Indication. Precordial pain, the body inability to lie down, severe distention and fullness of the lung, nebula, feverish sensation in the palms.

Method. Puncturing perpendicularly 0.2-0.3 cun. Applying moxibustion to the point with 3-7 moxa cones or 5-15 minutes with warming moxibustion.

Zhongshu (GV 7)

A meridian acupuncture point.

Location. In the back, on the posterior midline, between the spinal process of the 10th and 11th thoracic vertebra.

Indication. Jaundice, vomiting, fullness of the abdomen, stomachache, poor appetite and pain in the waist and back.

Method. Puncturing obliquely upward 0.5-1.0 cun. Applying moxibustion to the point with 3-5 moxa cones or 5-10 minutes with warming moxibustion.

Zhongting (CV 16)

A meridian acupuncture point.

Location. In the chest, on the thoracic midline, on the level of the 5th intercostal space, 1.3 cun below Danzhong (CV 17).

Indication. Distention and fullness in the chest and abdomen, dysphagia, vomiting, and globus hystericus.

Method. Puncture subcutaneously 0.3-0.5 cun. Apply moxibustion with 3-5 moxa cones or 5-10 minutes with warming moxibustion.

Zhongwan (CV 12)

A meridian acupuncture point.

Location. In the upper abdomen and the anterior midline, 4 cun above the center of the umbilicus.

Indication. Epigastric pain, abdominal distention, vomiting, hiccups, acid regurgitation, anorexia, dyspepsia, infantile malnutrition, tympanites, jaundice, etc.

Method. Puncture perpendicularly 0.5-1.0 cun. Apply moxibustion to the point with 3-7 moxa cones or 10-20 minutes with warming moxibustion.

Zhongwu (Ex-CA)

An extra acupuncture point.

Location. In the lateral side of the chest, about 3 cun lateral to nipples, in the 4th intercostal space.

Indication. Abdominal pain, pain in the chest and hypochondrium and intercostal neuralgia, etc.

Method. Moxibustion with 3-5 moxa cones or 5-10 minutes with warming moxibustion.

Zhongzhijie (Ex-UE)

An extra acupuncture point.

Location. On the dorsal side of the middle finger, in the depression at the anterior border of the distal interphalangeal joint.

Indication. Toothache.

Method. Perform moxibustion.

Zhongzhu (K 15)

A meridian acupuncture point.

Location. In the lower abdomen, 1 cun below the center of the umbilicus and 0.5 cun lateral to Yinjiao (CV 7).

Indication. Irregular menstruation, pain of the waist and abdomen, constipation, diarrhea and dysentery.

Method. Puncture 0.8-1.2 cun. Apply moxibustion with 3-5 moxa cones or 5-15 minutes with warming moxibustion.

Zhongzhu (TE 3)

A meridian acupuncture point.

Location. On the dorsum of the hand, when the fist is clenched, in the depression posterior to the metacarpophalangeal joint between the 4th and 5th metacarpal bones.

Indication. Headache, dizziness, congestive eye, deafness, tinnitus, sore throat, aching pain of the shoulder, back, elbow and arm, inability of fingers to extend, pain of the muscles near the spine.

Method. Puncturing 0.3-0.5 cun. Applying moxibustion to the point with 3-5 moxa cones or 5-10 minutes with warming moxibustion.

Zhoujian (Ex-UE 1)

An extra acupuncture point.

Location. On the posterior side of the elbow, at the tip of the olecranon when the elbow is flexed.

Indication. Scrofula, furuncle and carbuncle, deep-rooted sore.

Method. Apply moxibustion with 3-5 moxa cones or 5-10 minutes.

Zhouliao (LI 12)

A meridian acupuncture point.

Location. With the elbow flexed, on the lateral side of the upper arm, 1 cun above to Quchi (LI 11), on the border of the humerus.

Indication. Pain of the elbow and arm, contracture, numbness and drowsiness.

Method. Puncture perpendicularly 0.5-0.8 cun. Apply moxibustion if needed.

Zhourong (Sp 20)

A meridian acupuncture point.

Location. On the lateral side of the chest and in the 2nd intercostal space, 6 cun lateral to zigong (CV 19) at the midpoint of chest.

Indication. Distention, pain and fullness in the chest and hypochondrium, cough, dyspnea, spitting suppurative blood, poor appetite.

Method. Puncture horizontally or obliquely 0.5-0.8 cun. Apply moxibustion with 3-5 moxa cones or 5-10 minutes with warming moxibustion.

Zhoushu (Ex-UE)

An extra acupuncture point.

Location. On the posterior to the elbow joint, in the depression between the projection of the olecranon and the small head of the radius.

Indication. Diseases of the elbow joint and its surrounding tissues.

Method. Puncture perpendicularly 0.3-0.5 cun. Apply moxibustion with 3-5 moxa cones or 5-10 minutes with warming moxibustion.

Zhouzhui (Ex-B)

An extra acupuncture point.

Location. On the waist, with the patient in prone position, extend the arms. At the junction of the line connecting the two tips of the elbows and the posterior midline, and also 1 cun bilateral to the junction, three points in total.

Indication. Convulsion, vomiting, diarrhea, distending pain of the heart and abdomen.

Method. Apply moxibustion with 3-5 moxa cones or 5-15 minutes with warming moxibustion.

Zhuang

1. It refers to a unit of enumerable times of moxibustion with moxa cones. It is called one zhuang when moxibustion is done with one moxa cone.
2. Referring to moxa cone, e.g. big zhuang moxibustion indicates moxibustion with bigger moxa cones, while small zhuang moxibustion using smaller moxa cones.

Zhuangu (Ex-CA)

An extra acupuncture point.

Location. On the lateral side of the chest, directly below the anterior axillary fold, in the 3rd intercostal space.

Indication. Fullness in the chest and hypochondrium, poor appetite, vomiting and intercostal neuralgia.

Method. Puncture obliquely 0.3-0.5 cun. Apply moxibustion with 3-5 moxa cones or 5-10 minutes with warming moxibustion.

Zhubin (K 9)

A meridian acupuncture point.

Location. At the inner side of the leg, on the line connecting Taixi (K 3) and Yingu (K 10), 5 cun above Taixi, medial and inferior to the gastrocnemius muscle belly.

Indication. Mania, epilepsy, sialemesis, hernia pain, umbilical hernia for children and pain in the inner side of the leg.

Method. Puncture perpendicularly 0.5-0.8 cun. Apply moxibustion with 3-5 moxa cones or 5-10 minutes moxibustion.

Zhushi (Ex-CA)

An extra acupuncture point.

Location. On the lateral position of the chest, at the middle axillary line, in the 7th intercostal space.

Indication. Chronic summer fever, pain of the chest, hypochondrium, and abdominal pain, etc.

Method. Puncture obliquely 0.3-0.5 cun. Apply moxibustion with 3-5 moxa cones or 5-10 minutes with warming moxibustion.

Zhuxia (Ex-UE)

An extra acupuncture point.

Location. At the side of the palm, the midpoint of the radial edge of the 2nd metacarpal bone, opposite to Hegu (LI 4).

Indication. Anorexia in summer, dyspepsia, vomiting and diarrhea.

Method. Puncture perpendicularly 0.3-0.5 cun. Apply moxibustion with 3-7 moxa cones or 5-15 minutes with warming moxibustion.

Zigong (CV 19)

A meridian acupuncture point.

Location. On the chest, at the anterior midline, at the level of the 2nd intercostal space.

Indication. Cough, dyspnea, asthmatic breathing, fullness in the chest and hypochondrium, chest pain, sore throat, hematemesis, vomiting, loss of appetite.

Method. Puncture subcutaneously 0.3-0.5 cun. Apply moxibustion with 3-5 moxa cones or 5-10 minutes with warming moxibustion.

Zigong (Ex-CA1)

An extra acupuncture point.

Location. At the lower abdomen, 4 cun below the center of the umbilicus and 3 cun lateral to Zhongji (CV 3).

Indication. Prolapse of uterus, irregular menstruation, dysmenorrhea, etc.

Method. Puncture perpendicularly 0.5-1.0 cun. Apply moxibustion with 3-7 moxa cones or 5-15 minutes with warming moxibustion.

Zongjin

Referring to a massage point.

Location. In the right middle of the cross-striation of the carpometacarpal joints on the palm side.

Operation. Nipping and kneading manipulations.

Function. Removing pathogenic heat in the heart, reducing fever and adjusting the flow of qi all over the body.

Indication. Infantile convulsion, spasm, night cry, aphthae, hectic fever, toothache, etc.

Zudierzhishang (Ex-LE)

Referring to an extra acupuncture point.

Location. At the instep of the foot, 0.1 cun above the suture between the 2nd and 3rd toes.

Indication. Edema.

Method. Performing moxibustion with the number of moxa cones equal to the patient's age.

Zulinqi (G 41)

A meridian acupuncture point.

Location. At the lateral side of the instep of the foot, anterior to the 4th and 5th metatarsal bones joint, in the depression lateral to the tendon of the extensor muscle of the little toe or 1.5 cun above Xiaxi (G 43), at the end of the toe suture.

Indication. Headache, vertigo, breast abscess, scrofula, pain flaccidity and numbness, swelling and aching of the dorsum of the foot, irregular menstruation.

Method. Puncture perpendicularly 0.5-0.8 cun. Apply moxibustion with 1-3 moxa cones or 5-10 minutes with warming moxibustion.

Zuoguxue (Ex)

An extra acupuncture point.

Location. 1 cun inferior to the middle point of the connecting line between Dazhunzi and the tip of the coccyx.

Indication. Sciatica, paralysis of lower limb, etc.

Method. Puncture perpendicularly 2-3 cun.

Zuqiaoyin (G 44)

A meridian acupuncture point.

Location. At the lateral side of the distal segment of the 4th toe, 0.1 cun lateral to the corner of the toe-nail.

Indication. Headache, dizziness, migraine, vertigo, redness, swelling and pain of the eye, deafness, etc.

Method. Puncture perpendicularly 0.1 cun, or prick to cause a little bleeding. Apply moxibustion with 1-3 moxa cones or 3-5 minutes with warming moxibustion.

Zusanli (S 36)

An acupuncture point.

Location. At the anterior exterior side of the shank, 3 cun directly below to Dubi (S 35), one middle finger-breadth from the anterior border of the tibia.

Indication. Stomachache, nausea, vomiting, borborygmus, diarrhea, constipation, fullness in chest and hypochondrium, dysphagia, arthralgia syndrome, cough with profuse sputum, stranguria, dysuria, enuresis, edema, epilepsy, ophthalmalgia, deafness, laryngitis, fever, headache, palpitation, psychosis, acute mastitis, hemiparalysis, numbness of lower limbs, etc.

Method. Puncturing perpendicularly, with a slight incline to tibia 1-1.5 cun, and performing moxibustion to the point with

5-15 units of moxa cones of for 10-30 minutes.

Zushaoyangxue (Ex-LE)

An extra acupuncture point.

Location. On the midline of the 2nd toe, 1 cun posterior to the 2nd metatarsophalangeal joint, at the instep of the foot.

Indication. Gallbladder stone, abdominal distention and mass.

Method. Puncturing 0.2 cun perpendicularly.

Zutaiyangxue (Ex-LE)

An extra acupuncture point.

Location. In the depression 1 cun posterior to the external malleolus.

Indication. Diabetes, dry throat, stranguria and swelling of the scrotum.

Method. Performing moxibustion.

Zutonggu (B 66)

A meridian acupuncture point.

Location. On the external side of the foot, in the depression in front of the 5th metatarsophalangeal joint, at the junction of the red and white skin.

Indication. Headache, stiff and painful neck, dizziness, fullness in the chest, asthmatic breathing, epistaxis, mania.

Method. Puncture perpendicularly 0.2-0.3 cun. Apply moxibustion with 3-5 moxa cones or 5-10 minutes with warming moxibustion.

Zuwuli (Liv 10)

A meridian acupuncture point.

Location. On the internal side of the thigh, 3 cun directly below Qichong (S 30), below the pubic tubercle and on the external border of the long abductor muscle of the thigh.

Indication. Distention pain in the bilateral lower abdomen, retention of urine, prolapse of the uterus, swelling and pain of the testicle, weakness of the four limbs and scrofula.

Method. Puncture perpendicularly 0.5-0.8 cun. Apply moxibustion to the point with 3-5 moxa cones.

Zuxin (Ex-LE)

An extra acupuncture point.

Location. At the midline of the sole, at the midpoint of the line connecting the tip of the 2nd toe and the posterior border of the heel.

Indication. Metrorrhagia and metrostaxis, headache, dizziness, epilepsy, pain of the sole, and shock, etc.

Method. Puncture perpendicularly 0.3-0.5 cun. Apply moxibustion for 5-15 minutes with warming moxibustion.

Illustrations

Note:
The captions show the titles of the related lexical entries (marked by a blossom symbol and an alphanumeric reference, e.g. ✤ **A-4**) and therefore the pictures do not always match the plant's organ used for medication.

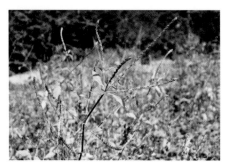

A-1. Achyranthes Root.

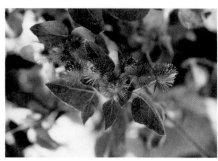

A-4. Arctium Fruit.

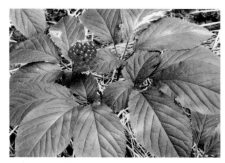

A-2. American Ginseng.

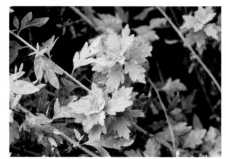

A-5. Argyi Leaf.

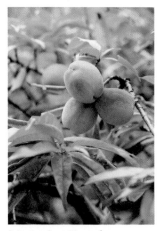

A-3. Apricot Kernel.

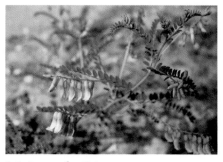

A-6. Astragalus Root.

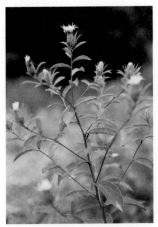

A-7. Atractylodes Rhizome.

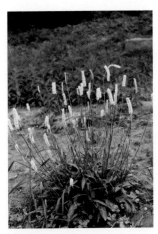

B-3. Bistort Rhizome.

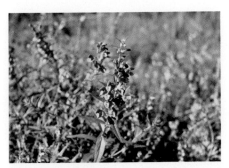

B-1. Baikal Skullcup Root.

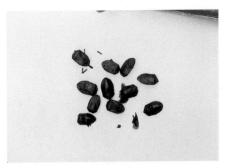

B-4. Boat-fruited Sterculia Seed.

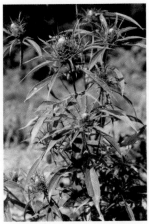

B-2. Bighead Atractylodes Rhizome.

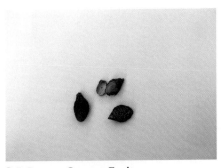

B-5. Broom Cypress Fruit.

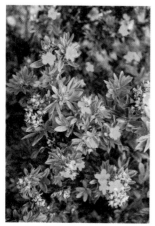

B-6. Bush Cinquefoil Leaf.

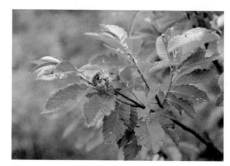

C-3. Chestnut.

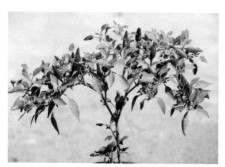

C-1. Cayenne Pepper.

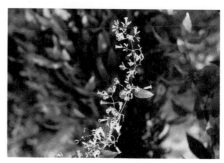

C-4. Chinese Fevervine Herb.

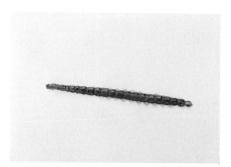

C-2. Centipede.

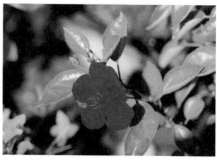

C-5. Chinese Hibiscus Flower.

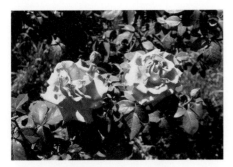

C-6. Chinese Rose.

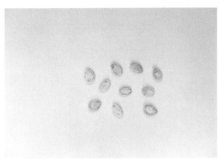

C-9. Chinese Waxgourd Seed.

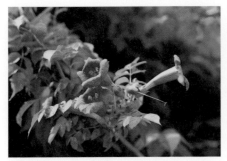

C-7. Chinese Trumpet-creeper Flower.

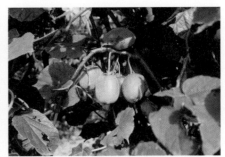

C-10. Chinese Yangtao.

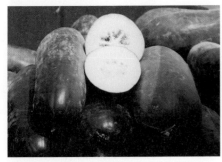

C-8. Chinese Waxgourd.

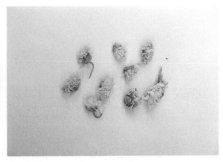

C-11. Chrysanthemum Flower.

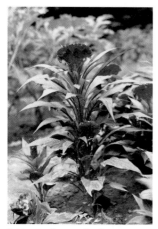

C-12. Cockscomb Flower.

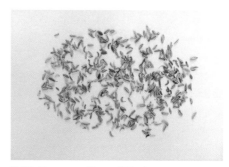

C-15. Common Fennel Fruit.

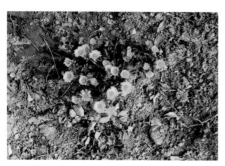

C-13. Coltsfoot Flower.

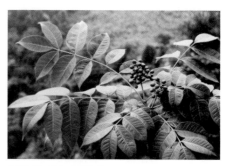

C-16. Corktree Bark.

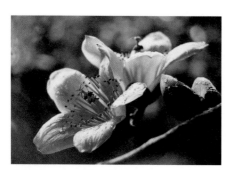

C-14. Common Bombax Bark.

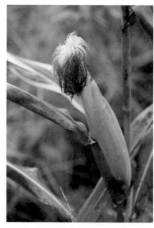

C-17. Corn Stigma.

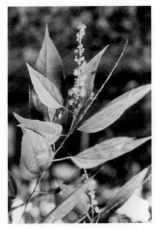

C-18. Croton Seed.

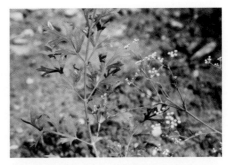

D-3. Divaricate Saposhnikovia Root.

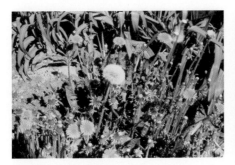

D-1. Dandelion Herb.

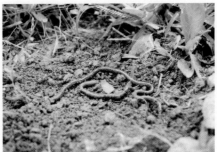

E-1. Earthworm.

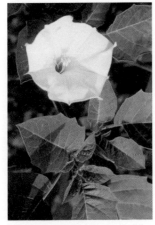

D-2. Datura Flower.

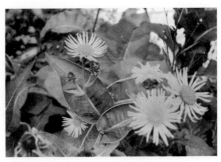

E-2. Elecampane Inula Root.

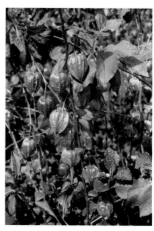

F-3. Franchet Groundcherry Calyx of Fruit.

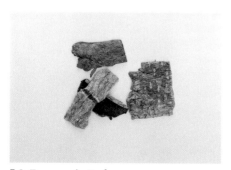

E-3. Eucommia Bark.

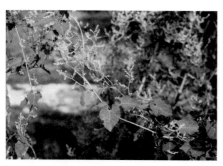

F-1. Fleece-flower Root.

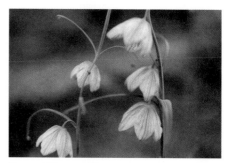

F-4. Fritillary Bulb.

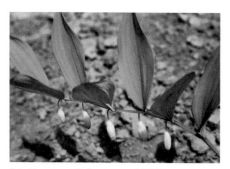

F-2. Fragrant Solomonseal Rhizome.

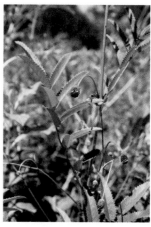

G-1. Garden Burnet Root.

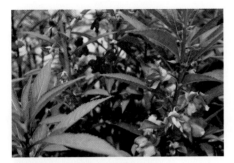

G-2. Garden Balsam Seed.

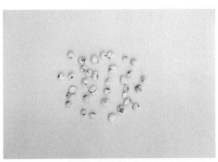

G-5. Gordon Euryale Seed.

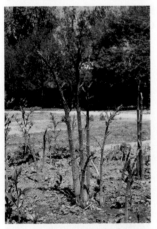

G-3. Giant Knotweed Rhizome.

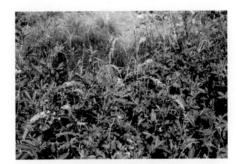

H-1. Hairy-vein Agrimony Seed.

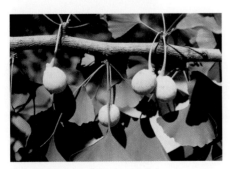

G-4. Ginkgo Leaf.

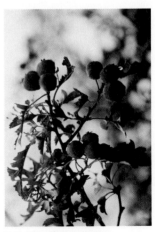

H-2. Hawthorn Fruit.

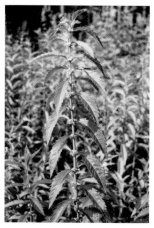

H-3. Hirsute Shiny Bugleweed Herb.

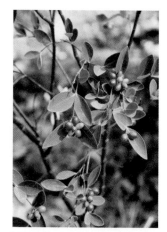

I-2. Indian String-bush Root.

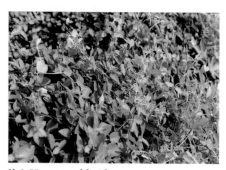

H-4. Honeysuckle Flower.

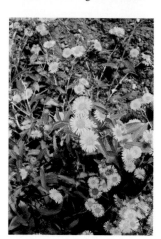

I-3. Inula Flower.

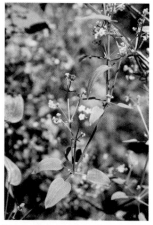

I-1. Indian Madder Stem or Leaf.

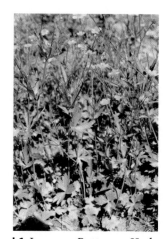

J-1. Japanese Buttercup Herb.

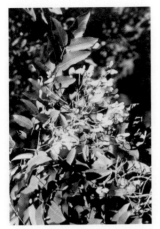

J-2. Japanese Sophora Flower.

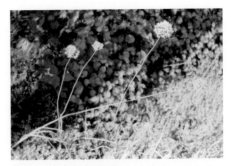

M-1. Macrostem Onion.

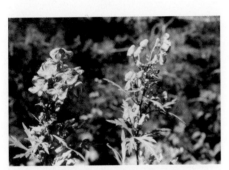

K-1. Kusnezoff Monkshood Root.

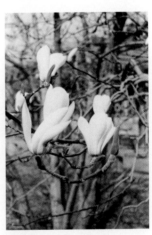

M-2. Magnolia Flower.

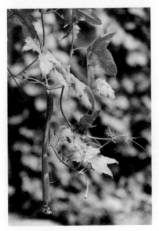

L-1. Luffa.

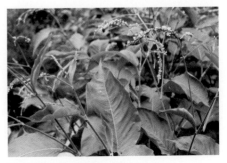

P-1. Prince's-feather Flowert.

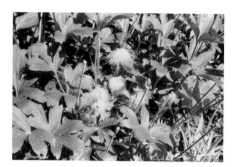

P-2. Pulsatilla Root.

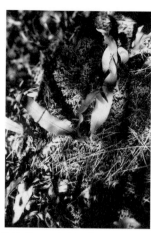

P-5. Pyrrosia Leaf.

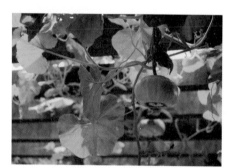

P-3. Pumpkin Fruit.

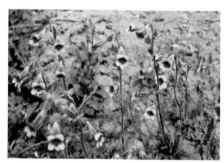

R-1. Rehmannia Dried Root.

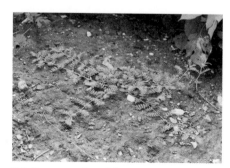

P-4. Puncturevine Caltrop Fruit.

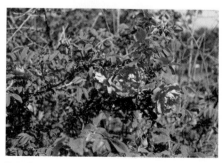

R-2. Rose.

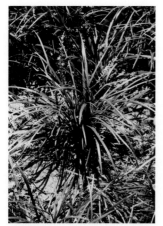

R-3. Rush.

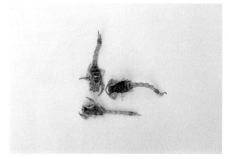

S-3. Scorpion.

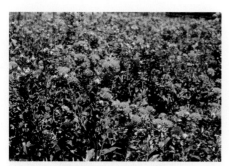

S-1. Safflower.

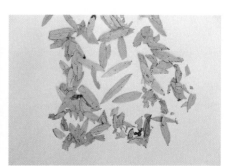

S-4. Senna Leaf.

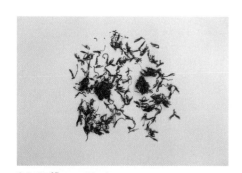

S-2. Safflower Fruit.

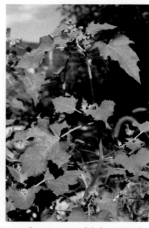

S-5. Siberian Cocklebur Herb.

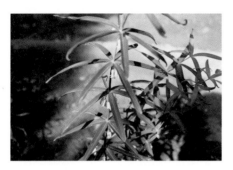

S-6. Siberian Solomonseal Rhizome.

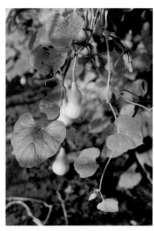

T-2. Toothleaf Goldenray Root.

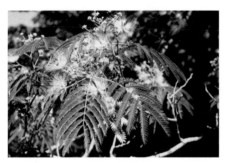

S-7. Silktree Albizzia Bark.

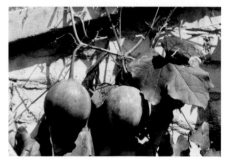

T-3. Trichosanthes Fruit.

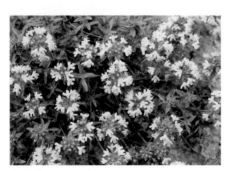

T-1. Thyme Herb.

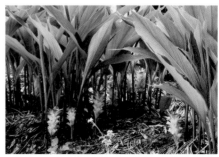

T-4. Turmeric Root.

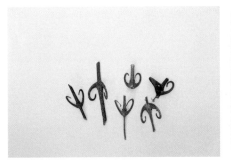

V-1. Villous Amomum Fruit.

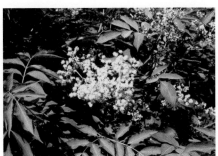

W-3. Williams Elder Twig.

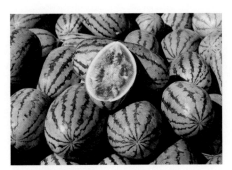

W-1. Water Melon.

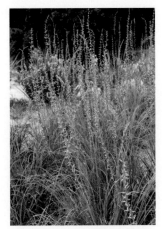

W-4. Wind-weed Rhizome.

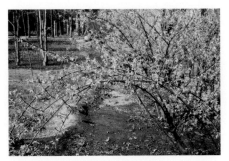

W-2. Weeping Forsythia Fruit.

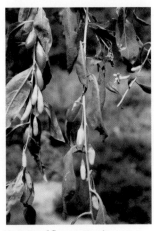

W-5. Wolfberry Fruit.

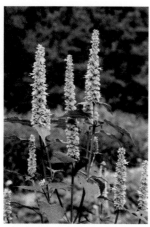

W-6. Wrinkled Giant Hyssop Herb.

Printing: Druckhaus Berlin-Mitte
Binding: Buchbinderei Stein & Lehmann, Berlin